Orthopaedic Decision Making

SECOND EDITION

Orthopaedic Decision Making

SECOND EDITION

Robert W. Bucholz, M.D.

Professor and Chairman
Charles Gregory Distinguished Chair in Orthopaedic Surgery
Department of Orthopaedic Surgery
University of Texas Southwestern Medical School
Dallas, Texas

with 430 illustrations

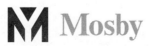 Mosby

St. Louis Baltimore Boston Carlsbad Chicago Naples New York Philadelphia Portland
London Madrid Mexico City Singapore Sydney Tokyo Toronto Wiesbaden

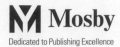

Dedicated to Publishing Excellence

Publisher: Anne S. Patterson
Senior Managing Editor: Lynne Gery
Project Manager: Linda Clarke
Senior Production Editor: Allan S. Kleinberg
Manufacturing Supervisor: Bill Winneberger
Illustrator: Stuart Almond

SECOND EDITION
Copyright © 1996 by Mosby–Year Book, Inc.

Previous edition copyrighted 1984

Composition by The Clarinda Company
Printed in the United States of America by Maple-Vail Press

Mosby–Year Book, Inc.
11830 Westline Industrial Drive
St. Louis, Missouri 63146

Library of Congress Cataloging-in-Publication Data

Orthopaedic decision making/[edited by] Robert W. Bucholz.—2nd
  ed.
       p.   cm.
    Includes bibliographical references and index.
    ISBN 0-8016-7356-9 (HC)
    1. Orthopedics—Handbooks, manuals, etc.   I. Bucholz, Robert W.
    [DNLM: 1. Orthopedics—handbooks.   WE 39 077 1996]
  RD732.5.077   1996
  617.3—dc20
  DNLM/DLC
  for Library of Congress   95-52402
                                                               CIP

96 97 98 99 00/9 8 7 6 5 4 3 2 1

CONTRIBUTORS

B. HUDSON BERREY, JR., M.D.

Associate Professor of Orthopaedic Surgery, University of Texas Southwestern Medical School, Dallas, Texas; Associate Professor of Clinical Surgery, Uniformed Services University of the Health Sciences, Bethesda, Maryland; Consultant, Orthopaedic Surgery, Walter Reed Army Medical Center, Washington, DC

JOHN G. BIRCH, M.D., F.R.C.S.(C)

Associate Professor of Orthopaedic Surgery, University of Texas Southwestern Medical School; Assistant Chief of Staff, Texas Scottish Rite Hospital for Children, Dallas, Texas

H. JAY BOULAS, M.D.

Assistant Professor of Orthopaedic Surgery, University of Texas Southwestern Medical School, Dallas, Texas

MAUREEN A. FINNEGAN, M.D., F.R.C.S.(C)

Associate Professor of Orthopaedic Surgery, University of Texas Southwestern Medical School; Active Attending, Parkland Memorial Hospital, Children's Medical Center, and Zale-Lipshy University Hospital, Dallas, Texas

PAUL L. FLICKER, M.D.

R. Wofford Cain Distinguished Chair in Bone and Joint Research, and Assistant Professor of Orthopaedic Surgery, Internal Medicine, and Radiology, University of Texas Southwestern Medical School, Dallas, Texas

FRANK A. GOTTSCHALK, M.D.

Associate Professor of Orthopaedic Surgery, University of Texas Southwestern Medical School; Distinguished Chair in Orthopaedic Rehabilitation, Dallas Rehabilitation Institute, Dallas, Texas

ROBERT J. HEAPS, M.D.

Chief Resident, Department of Orthopaedic Surgery, National Naval Medical Center, Bethesda, Maryland

ALAN L. JONES, M.D.

Assistant Professor of Orthopaedic Surgery, University of Texas Southwestern Medical School, Dallas, Texas

FREDERICK G. LIPPERT III, M.D.

Professor of Surgery and Head, Division of Orthopaedic Surgery, Uniformed Services University of the Health Sciences; Chairman, Orthopaedic Residency Program, and Head, Foot and Ankle Service, Department of Orthopaedic Surgery, National Naval Medical Center, Bethesda, Maryland

JAMES F. SILLIMAN, M.D.

Clinical Assistant Professor of Orthopaedic Surgery, University of Texas Southwestern Medical School, Dallas, Texas

ROBERT VIERE, M.D.

Assistant Professor of Orthopaedic Surgery, University of Texas Southwestern Medical School; Chief, Spinal Cord Injury Service, Dallas Veterans Administration Medical Center, Dallas, Texas

PREFACE

Since the publication of the first edition of *Orthopaedic Decision Making*, orthopaedic surgery has undergone many changes. Not only have the science and technology of orthopaedic surgery exponentially expanded but there is a new appreciation for systematic, algorithmic approaches to the practice of medicine. This latter phenomenon is attributable to several factors. Firstly, the increasing complexity of medical science has made decision making more difficult and, at times, less intelligible. Secondly, radical changes in health care delivery in the form of managed care have led to a proliferation of practice guidelines, treatment pathways, utilization management programs, and clinical protocols. These decision-making guidelines may be general or specific, depending on the local resources, practice specialization, and managed care environment of an orthopaedic surgery center.

The purpose of this textbook is not to provide strict pathways for the diagnosis and treatment of specific orthopaedic problems. These algorithms primarily reflect the current clinical decision making of the individual authors. Rather, the book is intended to serve as an educational aid for students, orthopaedic residents, and practitioners. The detail of the algorithms is insufficient to act as complete treatment pathways for managed care applications. It may, however, provide a generic starting point or template for the creation of such detailed decision trees based on the treatment preferences and expertise of any given orthopaedic practice. If it does stimulate individual orthopaedists to formulate their own treatment algorithms, then it will be successful in its mission.

I want to thank the orthopaedic surgery academic faculty of the University of Texas Southwestern Medical School for their efforts in contributing algorithms in their respective areas of expertise. Thanks also to Dr. Robert Heaps and Dr. Fred Lippert (a contributor for the first edition) for their units and to Stuart Almond for his help in illustrating the text.

The book would not have been completed in a timely fashion without the organizational and secretarial skills provided by Patrice McWhorter. Lynne Gery, Senior Managing Editor at Mosby–Year Book, has been extremely patient and supportive during the inception, writing, and editing stages of this book.

Robert W. Bucholz, M.D.

CONTENTS

ORTHOPAEDIC TRAUMA

Sternoclavicular Joint Dislocation
Acromioclavicular Joint Subluxation
Acute Traumatic Dislocation of the
   Glenohumeral Joint
Fracture of the Proximal Humerus
Fracture of the Humeral Shaft
Fracture of the Pelvic Ring
Hemorrhage from Pelvic Fracture
Acetabular Fracture
Hip Dislocation
Fracture of the Femoral Neck
Intertrochanteric Fracture
Subtrochanteric Fracture
Fracture of the Femoral Shaft
Closed Intramedullary Nailing of the Femur
Fracture of the Distal Femur
Dislocation of the Knee Joint
Fracture or Dislocation of the Patella
Fracture of the Tibial Plateau
Fracture of the Tibial Shaft
Compartment Syndrome
Fracture Dislocation of the Ankle
Fracture of the Calcaneus
Fracture or Dislocation of the Talus
Tarsometatarsal Fracture-Dislocation

STERNOCLAVICULAR JOINT DISLOCATION

A. Dislocation of the sternoclavicular joint is a relatively rare injury. Motor vehicle accidents are the cause in most cases; the second most common cause is sporting activities. Signs and symptoms include severe pain localized to the sternoclavicular joint which is increased by any movement of the shoulder. The affected shoulder appears shortened and protracted as compared to the unaffected side. In patients with anterior dislocation the medial end of the clavicle appears prominent and can be palpated easily. In contrast, the patient with posterior dislocation is characterized by diminished prominence of the medial clavicle as compared to the normal side. The lateral border of the manubrium can be palpated as well. Because the great vessels, trachea, esophagus and lungs lie directly posterior to the sternoclavicular joint, injury and/or compression of any of these structures can occur with posterior dislocation. Venous congestion in the upper extremity or neck may be present and the patient may complain of a choking sensation. A careful detailed neurologic and vascular examination should be performed prior to any intervention. This is particularly important in cases of posterior dislocation which may have associated injury.

B. X-ray evaluation of the patient with injury to the sternoclavicular joint should consist of an anterior posterior (AP) view and a 40° cephalic tilt view or serendipity view as described by Rockwood. Computed tomography (CT) is the preferred next step in radiographic investigation of sternoclavicular joint injuries when further delineation of the injury is needed.

C. Anterior dislocation of the sternoclavicular joint can be reduced by placing the patient supine on a firm surface with a 3 to 4 inch roll between the shoulder blades and applying gentle pressure over the clavicle, reducing it posteriorly after administration of local anesthesia, intravenous sedation, or general anesthesia. Instability following reduction of anterior sternoclavicular dislocations is common and immediate redislocation may occur, despite application of a figure of eight type splint. If the reduction is stable, the patient should be placed in a figure of eight type splint and maintained for 6 weeks. Treatment of patients with an unsuccessful reduction or unstable reduction is the same. Operative treatment of acute anterior dislocations is not indicated.

D. Evaluation of posterior sternoclavicular dislocations should include a CT scan of both sternoclavicular articulations as well as the thoracic inlet for evidence of associated injury. The need for arteriography or other additional studies should be determined by findings on physical examination and CT scan.

E. Reduction of posterior sternoclavicular joint dislocation is best performed under general anesthesia, although intravenous sedation has been used successfully. Reduction is accomplished by placing the patient supine on a bolster between the shoulders, applying longitudinal traction to the arm and then the medial clavicle is pulled anteriorly, either by directly grasping the bone, or percutaneously using a towel clip or similar instrument (Fig. 1). In contrast to anterior dislocations, most posterior dislocations are stable after reduction. A delay of several days in reduction can increase the difficulty of closed reduction. After successful closed reduction the patient is placed in a figure of eight splint for 4 to 6 weeks.

F. Open reduction of posterior sternoclavicular dislocations is indicated following failed closed reduction. This is performed with the patient on an interscapular bolster with the involved upper extremity draped free. A transverse incision is made along the superior border of the medial clavicle and sternum. The joint is then exposed while preserving as much intact capsule as possible. Entrapped intra-articular disc or in younger patients, the medial clavicular epiphysis may impede reduction and require debridement. Stability is assessed after open reduction. If instability is present, one of several described methods of fixation using fascial reconstruction can be used. If significant articular damage has occurred, excision of the medial clavicle and suture stabilization to the first rib may be performed. Symptomatic chronic or recurrent dislocation is treated with open reduction in a similar fashion. The use of pins or wires for stabilization of the sternoclavicular articulation is contraindicated because of the risk of pin migration.

DISLOCATION OF THE STERNOCLAVICULAR JOINT

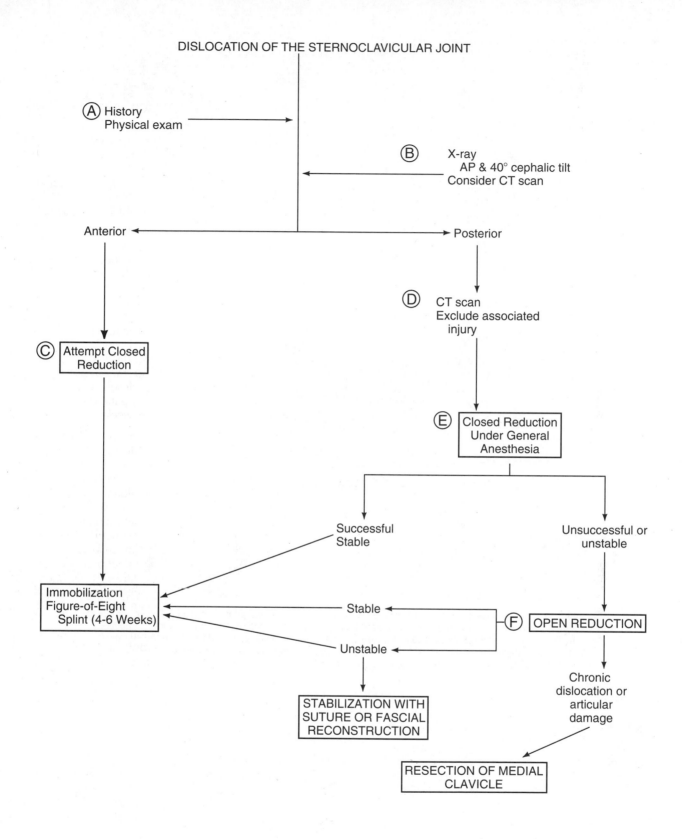

Ⓐ History
Physical exam

Ⓑ X-ray
AP & 40° cephalic tilt
Consider CT scan

Anterior   Posterior

Ⓓ CT scan
Exclude associated
injury

Ⓒ Attempt Closed
Reduction

Ⓔ Closed Reduction
Under General
Anesthesia

Successful   Unsuccessful or
Stable   unstable

Immobilization
Figure-of-Eight
Splint (4-6 Weeks)   Stable   Ⓕ OPEN REDUCTION

Unstable

STABILIZATION WITH   Chronic
SUTURE OR FASCIAL   dislocation or
RECONSTRUCTION   articular
                             damage

RESECTION OF MEDIAL
CLAVICLE

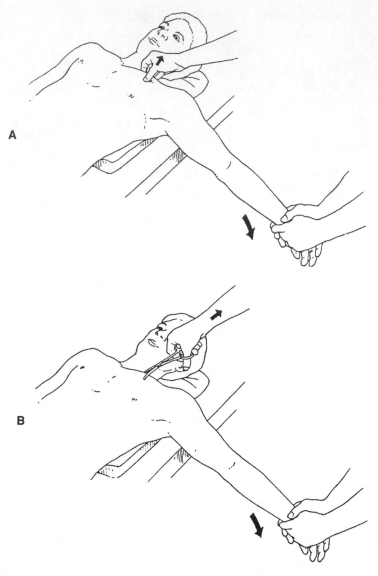

Figure 1 Technique of closed reduction of posterior sternoclavicular joint dislocation. The patient is supine with folded towels under the scapula. The arm is abducted and extended with traction applied. **A**, The proximal end of the clavicle is grasped manually and elevated to dislodge it from the sternum. **B**, A sterile towel clip can be used to dislodge the proximal clavicle if necessary. (From Jobe FW, ed. Operative Techniques in Upper Extremity Sports Injuries. St. Louis: Mosby–Year Book, 1996.)

References

Booth CM and Roper BA. Chronic dislocation of the sterno-clavicular joint: An operative repair. Clin Orthop 1979; 140:17.

Buckerfield CT and Castle ME. Acute traumatic retrosternal dislocation of the clavicle. J Bone Joint Surg 1984; 66-A:379.

Burrows HJ. Tenodesis of subclavius in the treatment of recurrent dislocation of the sterno-clavicular joint. J Bone Joint Surg 1951; 33-B:240.

Clark RL, Milgram JW, and Yawn DH. Fatal aortic perforation and cardiac tamponade due to a Kirschner wire migrating from the right sternoclavicular joint: Case Report. South Med J 1974; 67:316.

Destouet JM, Gilula LA, Murphy WA, and Sagel SS. Computed tomography of the sternoclavicular joint and sternum. Radiology 1981; 138:123.

Eskola A, Vainiopaa S, Vastamaki M, Slatis P, and Bokkanen P. Operation for old sternoclavicular dislocation: Results in 12 cases. J Bone Joint Surg 1989; 71-B:63.

Gunther WA. Posterior dislocation of the sternoclavicular joint: Report of a case. J Bone Joint Surg 1949; 31-A:878.

Lunseth PA, Chapman KW, and Frankel VH. Surgical treatment of chronic dislocation of the sterno-clavicular joint. J Bone Joint Surg 1975; 57-B:193.

Nordback I and Markkula H. Migration of Kirschner pin from clavicle into ascending aorta. Acta Chir Scand 1985; 151:177.

Omer GE. Osteotomy of the clavicle in surgical reconstruction of anterior sternoclavicular dislocation. J Trauma 1967; 7:584.

Pate JW and Wilhite JL. Migration of a foreign body from the sternoclavicular joint to the heart: A case report. Am Surg 1969; 35:448.

Poland J. Traumatic separation of epiphysis of the upper extremity. London, Smith, Elder & Co., 1898, p. 135.

Rockwood CA: Injuries to the sternoclavicular joint. In Rockwood CA, Jr, Green DP, and Bucholz RW, eds. Fractures in Adults. Philadelphia: JB Lippincott, 1991, p. 1253.

Wasylenko MJ and Busse EF. Posterior dislocation of the clavicle causing fatal tracheoesophageal fistula. Can J Surg 1981; 24(6):626.

ACROMIOCLAVICULAR JOINT SUBLUXATION

A. A typical injury history for the acromioclavicular (AC) joint is a fall either on the point of the shoulder or on an outstretched hand. In the older age group, this mechanism can also create a rotator cuff tear and injury. Therefore, the history and physical examination should rule out a rotator cuff tear in the older age group.

B. A radiographic evaluation is essential in classifying the degree of injury to the AC joint. A 15° cephalad AP gives the best view of the AC joint. A trauma series, including an axillary lateral and a transcapular lateral is used to document associated coracoid fractures, AP displacement of the clavicle, and other bony injuries about the shoulder complex. Weighted views are typically not helpful. The most useful classification scheme describes six types of injury: Type I is a sprain of the AC ligaments (Fig. 1), Type II is AC joint disruption (Fig. 2), Type III is disruption of the coracoclavicular ligaments with the coracoclavicular space increased to 25% to 100% greater than in the normal side (Fig. 3), Type IV is posterior displacement of the distal clavicle into or through the trapezius muscle (Fig. 4), Type V is detachment of the deltoid and trapezius muscle from the distal half of the clavicle and marked increase in the coracoclavicular space 100% to 300% greater than in the normal shoulder (Fig. 5), and Type VI is a decrease of the coracoclavicular space with the clavicle inferior to the acromion and coracoid (Fig. 6).

C. Conservative treatment of AC joint injuries includes a sling to relieve distraction on the AC joint with the weight of the arm, a protected range of motion protocol beginning when discomfort will allow, ice, and anti-inflammatory agents. After approximately 3 to 4 weeks, a rehabilitation program including strength training can be initiated. Typically, this will resolve all symptoms in Types I-III patients. Type III patients will have some residual prominence of the distal clavicle. Long-term functional deficits are minimal.

D. In Types IV and VI, closed reduction can be attempted. If reduction is successful, conservative treatment can be followed. Of the three Type VI injuries described in the literature, all were treated surgically. Type V injuries and irreducible Type IV and VI injuries are best treated with open reduction coracoclavicular repair and/or reconstruction. More than 50 surgical procedures have been described for reconstruction of the AC joint and repair or replacement of the coracoclavicular ligaments. Many of these techniques require hardware such as screw fixation of the clavicle to the base of the coracoid, or pin fixation of the acromion to the distal clavicle. Weaver and Dunn described excision of the distal clavicle with coracoacromial ligament transfer to the distal clavicle with or without repair of the coracoclavicular ligaments. This has been modified and augmented with various forms of suture material in a loop fashion around the clavicle and coracoid process.

E. For those patients who have chronic symptoms of pain when returning to activities after AC joint injuries that cannot be resolved by conservative measures, distal clavicle resection is recommended. This is typically recommended in those rare Type II injuries that remain symptomatic. However, in injuries resulting in disruption of the coracoclavicular ligaments, the coracoclavicular reconstruction must be added to the distal clavicle resection for satisfactory results.

ACROMIOCLAVICULAR JOINT SUBLUXATION

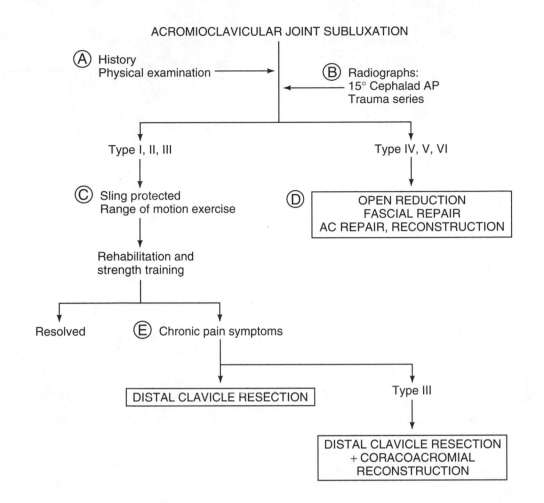

Ⓐ History
Physical examination → Ⓑ Radiographs:
15° Cephalad AP
Trauma series

Type I, II, III

Type IV, V, VI

Ⓒ Sling protected
Range of motion exercise

Ⓓ
OPEN REDUCTION
FASCIAL REPAIR
AC REPAIR, RECONSTRUCTION

Rehabilitation and
strength training

Resolved

Ⓔ Chronic pain symptoms

DISTAL CLAVICLE RESECTION

Type III

DISTAL CLAVICLE RESECTION
+ CORACOACROMIAL
RECONSTRUCTION

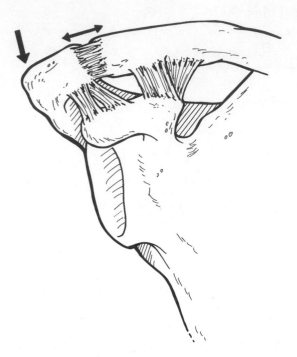

Figure 1   Type I. Sprain of the acromioclavicular ligament.

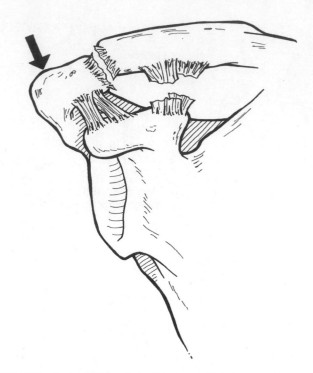

Figure 3   Type III. Disruption of the acromioclavicular and coraco-clavicular ligaments. Coracoclavicular inner-space between 25% and 100% greater than the contralateral shoulder. Deltoid and tra-pezius muscles stripped from the distal end of the clavicle.

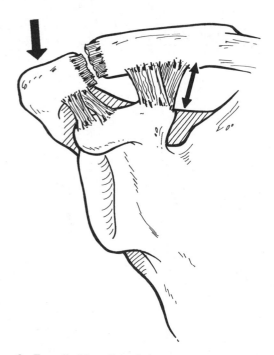

Figure 2   Type II. Disruption of the acromioclavicular ligament, sprain of the coracoclavicular ligaments.

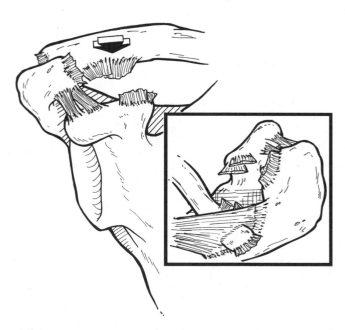

Figure 4   Type IV. Acromioclavicular joint dislocated and clavicle is displaced posteriorly and impaling itself in the trapezius muscle.

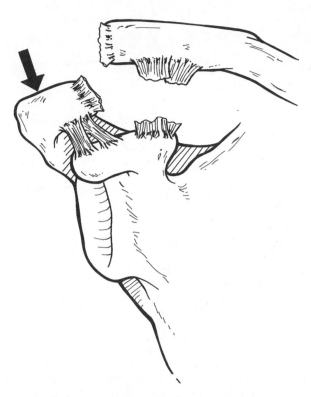

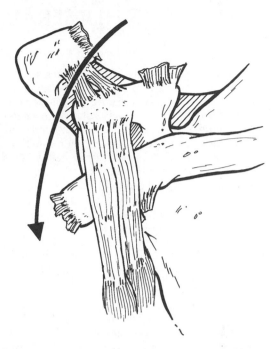

Figure 5 Type V. Coracoclavicular inner-space between 100% and 300% greater than the contralateral shoulder.

Figure 6 Type VI. Acromioclavicular joint dislocated under either the acromion or coracoid process.

References

Bosard PJ, Joyce SM, Manaster BJ, et al. Lack of efficacy of weighted radiographs in diagnosing acute acromioclavicular separation. Ann Emerg Med 1988; 17:47.

Larsen E, Bjerg-Nielsen A, Christensen P. Conservative or surgical treatment of acromioclavicular dislocation: A prospective, controlled, randomized study. J Bone Joint Surg 1986; 68A:552.

Rockwood CA Jr., Williams GR, Young DC. Injuries to the acromioclavicular joint. In Rockwood CA Jr., Green DP, Bucholz RW, eds. Fractures in Adults. 3rd ed. Philadelphia: JB Lippincott, 1991; 1181.

Taft TN, Wilson SC, Oglesby JW. Dislocation of the acromioclavicular joint: an end-result study. J Bone Joint Surg 1987; 69A:1045.

Tibone J, Sellers R, Topine P. Strength testing after third-degree acromioclavicular dislocations. Am J Sports Med 1992; 20:328.

Walsh WM, Peterson DA, Shelton G, et al. Shoulder strength following acromioclavicular injury. Am J Sports Med 1985; 13:153.

Weaver JK, Dunn HK. Treatment of acromioclavicular injuries, especially complete acromioclavicular separation. J Bone Joint Surg 1972; 54A:1187.

ACUTE TRAUMATIC DISLOCATION OF THE GLENOHUMERAL JOINT

The shoulder is the most commonly dislocated joint in the body. The typical mechanism of injury is abduction, extension and external rotation creating an anterior dislocation. Axial loading of the internally rotated and extended arm, violent trauma, electrical shock, or convulsions can produce posterior dislocations. Severe trauma with hyperabduction forces on the upper extremity can produce an inferior dislocation. Due to the bony anatomy of the shallow glenoid and the round humeral head, initial dislocations can become locked by a wedge shaped impression defect in the humeral head. Shoulder dislocations are classified as to the degree of instability (dislocation or subluxation), the chronicity of the instability (acute, chronic or recurrent), the etiology of the instability (traumatic or atraumatic), and the direction of the instability (anterior, posterior or multi-directional).

A. The history, including mechanism of injury, violence of the injury, prior history and treatment of instability, and neurovascular symptoms, is significant. Physical examination can give an understanding of the degree and direction of the instability. Neurovascular examination is critical both before and after reduction, especially in the elderly. The axillary nerve injury is frequently associated with anterior dislocation. Less commonly, axillary artery or venous injuries can present a life or limb threatening situation.

B. Glenohumeral, anteroposterior (AP), axillary lateral, and trans-scapular radiographs are necessary to document the direction and degree of instability (Fig. 1). Hill-Sachs lesion is best demonstrated by an AP view in internal rotation or the Stryker Notch view. An osseous Bankart or glenoid rim fracture is best demonstrated by the axillary West Point view.

C. After a complete neurovascular examination of the upper extremity, a gentle reduction is performed. Suspicion of vascular or neurologic injury is the key to recognition after major trauma. Angiography should be performed when indicated. Most traumatic dislocations are anterior. Some patients need sedation to achieve muscular relaxation. Reduction can be accomplished without sedation by slowly elevating the arm in the seated or supine patient. Relaxation of the deltoid and pectoralis musculature is key. External rotation and slight abduction is added near a reduction. Sometimes, general traction or posterior superior pressure on the humeral head and the axilla is necessary. Posterior dislocations typically reduce spontaneously. Those that present for treatment are typically locked on the glenoid rim and have some degree of impression defect. The physician must rule out a chronic dislocation prior to reduction maneuvers to prevent fracture or even vascular/neurologic injury in the elderly patient. After muscle spasm has been eliminated, gentle traction and anterior force on the head usually accomplishes reduction. If reduction is difficult, slight internal rotation and lateral traction on the proximal humerus may be necessary.

D. In the typical circumstance the shoulder is reduced and placed in a sling. The patient avoids a provocative positioning and begins an early range of motion rehabilitation program. Controversy exists as to whether the natural history can be changed by any specific immobilization or rehabilitation program. Elderly patients with slow return of function should be evaluated for rotator cuff tear. If indicated, an arthrogram is used to document status of the rotator cuff. Ultrasonography and MRI could also be used. If a tear is present, the patient should undergo rotator cuff repair. The recurrence rate of instability varies with the patient's age. Those patients in the youngest age groups have a high likelihood of recurrence.

E. Irreducible or open dislocation becomes an acute surgical indication. Both of these conditions are rare and are usually associated with significant trauma. Open dislocations require irrigation/debridement and repair of the soft tissues as indicated. Irreducible dislocation can present with interposition of soft tissue, i.e., biceps tendon, subscapularis tendon.

F. At the time of glenohumeral dislocation, shear forces can create fractures about the tuberosities or glenoid rim. The tuberosity fractures may actually reduce into an acceptable position at the time of the shoulder reduction. Presence of greater tuberosity fractures lessens the likelihood of recurrent instability. If, at the time of reduction, the tuberosity fractures do not reduce into an acceptable position (i.e. near anatomic in both displacement and rotation), or a large glenoid rim fracture is present, open reduction and internal fixation (ORIF) are indicated.

G. If abnormal vascular examination is present before or after reduction, the patient is taken immediately for arteriography. Vascular injuries are more common in the elderly and after inferior dislocations or dislocations associated with significant trauma. Vascular injury can also occur in the elderly at the time of reduction especially when a chronic dislocation is mistaken for an acute dislocation. The treatment of choice is to restore normal circulation with either a graft or a prosthesis.

ACUTE TRAUMATIC DISLOCATION OF THE GLENOHUMERAL JOINT

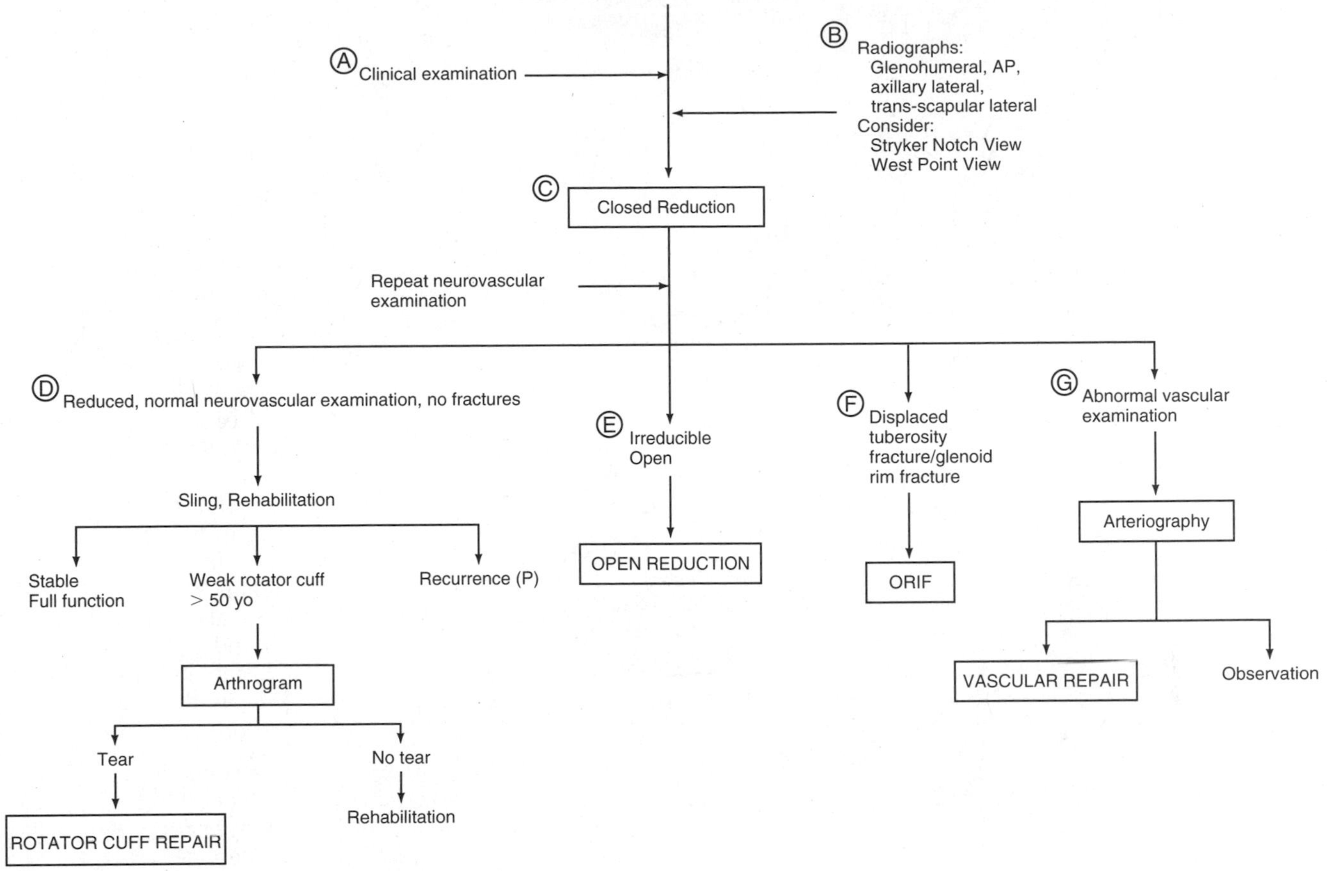

(A) Clinical examination ⟶

(B) Radiographs:
Glenohumeral, AP,
axillary lateral,
trans-scapular lateral
Consider:
Stryker Notch View
West Point View

(C) Closed Reduction

Repeat neurovascular examination ⟶

(D) Reduced, normal neurovascular examination, no fractures

(E) Irreducible
Open

(F) Displaced tuberosity fracture/glenoid rim fracture

(G) Abnormal vascular examination

Sling, Rehabilitation

Stable
Full function

Weak rotator cuff
> 50 yo

Recurrence (P)

OPEN REDUCTION

ORIF

Arteriography

Arthrogram

Tear

No tear

Rehabilitation

ROTATOR CUFF REPAIR

VASCULAR REPAIR

Observation

11

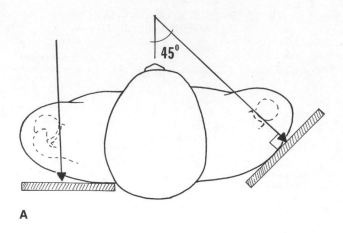

A

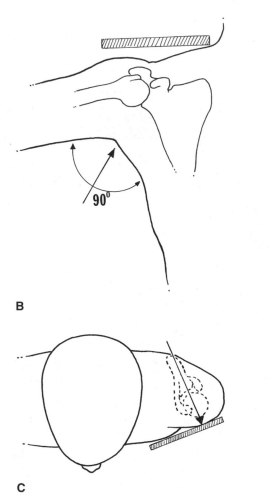

B

C

Figure 1 The trauma series for shoulder evaluation must include **(A)** true glenohumeral AP, **(B)** axillary lateral, and **(C)** trans-scapular lateral views.

References

Aronen JG, Regan K. Decreasing incidence of recurrence of first-time anterior shoulder dislocations with rehabilitation. Am J Sports Med 1984; 12:283-291.

Gibson JMC. Rupture of the axillary artery following anterior dislocation of the shoulder. J Bone Joint Surg 1962; 44B:114-115.

Hawkins RJ. Unrecognized dislocations of the shoulder. Instr Course Lect 1985; 34:258-263.

Hawkins RJ, Neer CS II, Pianta RM, et al. Locked posterior dislocation of the shoulder. J Bone Joint Surg 1987; 69A:9-18.

Hill HA, Sachs MD. The groove defect of the humeral head: The frequently unrecognized complication of dislocation of the shoulder joint. Radiology 1940; 35:690-700.

Hovelius L. Anterior dislocation of the shoulder in teenagers and young adults: A five year prognosis. J Bone Joint Surg 1987; 69A:393-399.

Hovelius L, Ericksson K, Fredlin H, et al. Recurrences after initial dislocations of the shoulder: Results of a prospective study of treatment. J Bone Joint Surg 1983; 65A:343-349.

Lev-El A, Rubinstein Z. Axillary artery injury in erect dislocation of the shoulder. J Trauma 1981; 21:323-325.

Malen WJ, Bassett FH III, Goldner RD. Luxatio erecta: The inferior glenohumeral dislocation. J Orthop Trauma 1990; 4:19-24.

Pavlov H, Warren RF, Weiss CB Jr, Dienes DM. The roentgenographic evaluation of anterior shoulder instability. Clin Orthop 1985; 194:153-158.

Rose CR. Prognosis and dislocation of the shoulder. J Bone Joint Surg 1956; 38A:957-977.

Schulz TJ, Jacobs B, Patterson RL. Unrecognized dislocations of the shoulder. J Trauma 1969; 9:1009-1023.

Silliman JF, Dean MT. Neurovascular injuries to the shoulder complex. JOSPT 1993; 18(2):442-448.

Tietjen R. Occult glenohumeral interposition of a torn rotator cuff. J Bone Joint Surg 64A:458-459, 1982.

Tigmes J, Loyd HM, Tullos HS. Arthrography in acute shoulder dislocations. South Med J 1979; 72:564-567.

FRACTURE OF THE PROXIMAL HUMERUS

A. Most fractures of the proximal humerus result from falling on the outstretched arm, typically in the pronated position. In an elderly person with osteoporosis, this could be from minimal trauma; however, in the younger patient or in the elderly patient with significant displacement of the fragments, significant force is required to produce these injuries. Therefore, a thorough neurovascular examination, due to the close proximity of the brachial plexus, is important.

B. Bi-plane radiography at a minimum is necessary to determine the displacement and the number of fragments involved. It is also very important to note if there is a dislocation associated with the proximal humerus fracture. Glenohumeral, anteroposterior (AP), axillary lateral, and a trans-scapular lateral/shoulder trauma series are necessary to assess the plane and the amount of displacement and rotation of the fragments. If dislocation is noted, reduction becomes a component of the treatment algorithm. Radiographic classification proposed by Neer assists in the practical management of these patients. This classification is based on two factors: (1) the amount of displacement of the fragments, and (2) the amount of angulation of the fragments. Displacement of the fragments >1 cm or angulation ≥45° of a major segment are the criteria for this description. Radiographic classification is very difficult. Accuracy can be improved with computed tomographic scans. Two-part fractures include displaced anatomic neck fractures, displaced surgical neck fractures, greater tuberosity and lesser tuberosity fractures. Three-part fractures include anatomical neck fractures with an associated displaced or rotated tuberosity fracture. Four-part fractures include detachment and displacement of both tuberosities along with displacement of the shaft, head, and neck fragments. High energy injuries with open wounds are treated by external fixation and soft tissue management.

C. Over 80% of proximal humerus fractures are minimally displaced and impacted. These fractures are inherently stable due to the musculotendinous anatomy about the shoulder girdle and the thick fascia that envelops and attaches many of these fragments. Under fluoroscopy, most of these fractures move in unison and, therefore, can be treated with a sling for comfort and protected range of motion (ROM) in order to minimize the adhesions and arthrofibrosis can complicate these injuries. Strengthening exercises are typically begun at approximately six weeks. In most cases, full ROM and return to functional activities is accomplished by twelve weeks.

D. Two-part fractures (Fig. 1, A) are separated into those of the anatomic and surgical necks that should undergo an initial attempt at closed reduction. Displaced fractures typically require general anesthetic and if successful can be treated with a sling for comfort and protected ROM. Greater and lesser tuberosity fractures are analogous to rotator cuff tears and usually require open reduction and internal fixation (ORIF). Fracture fixation depends on the size and quality of the fracture fragments. If the fracture fragments are small and of poor quality, they can be excised and the rotator cuff repaired to a trough and bone as in a rotator cuff tear. Postoperatively, these patients are typically treated as in a rotator cuff reconstruction of a large rotator cuff tear; the arm can be supported in an abduction pillow type splint in a protective ROM protocol with passive assist initiated.

E. Because the three-part fracture (Fig. 1, B) is inherently unstable and because angulation and displacement is not correctable, these fractures require ORIF. This is best accomplished through a deltopectoral splitting incision, using the biceps tendon as a landmark. The head and tuberosity fragments are wired to the humeral shaft. Early motion should be instituted in order to prevent significant arthrofibrosis. Occasionally, some three-part fractures may be amenable to closed treatment. Some elderly patients may be best treated by prosthetic replacement of the head.

F. By definition, a four-part fracture (Fig. 1, C and D) leaves the articular fragment of the humerus completely devoid of soft tissue coverage. These fractures are often associated with dislocation of the head fragments. Therefore, this is a shell fragment and cannot be expected to revascularize and heal. Consequently, the typical treatment is a hemiarthroplasty. Tuberosity segments are identified using the biceps tendon as a landmark and attached both to themselves and to the shaft of the humerus enveloping the prosthetic implant. The implant is cemented in a lengthened position which restores the normal soft tissue tension about the rotator musculature. Postoperatively, these patients should begin passive assisted ROM exercises immediately.

G. Head splitting fractures are amenable to ORIF if the articular segments are intact and comminution is limited. Typically, comminuted fractures require prosthetic replacement.

H. If reduction is not possible or an unstable reduction is present, reduction and fixation is necessary. Unstable reductions can be held with percutaneous pins. Irreducible fractures require open reduction, typically due to interposed soft tissue such as the biceps tendon.

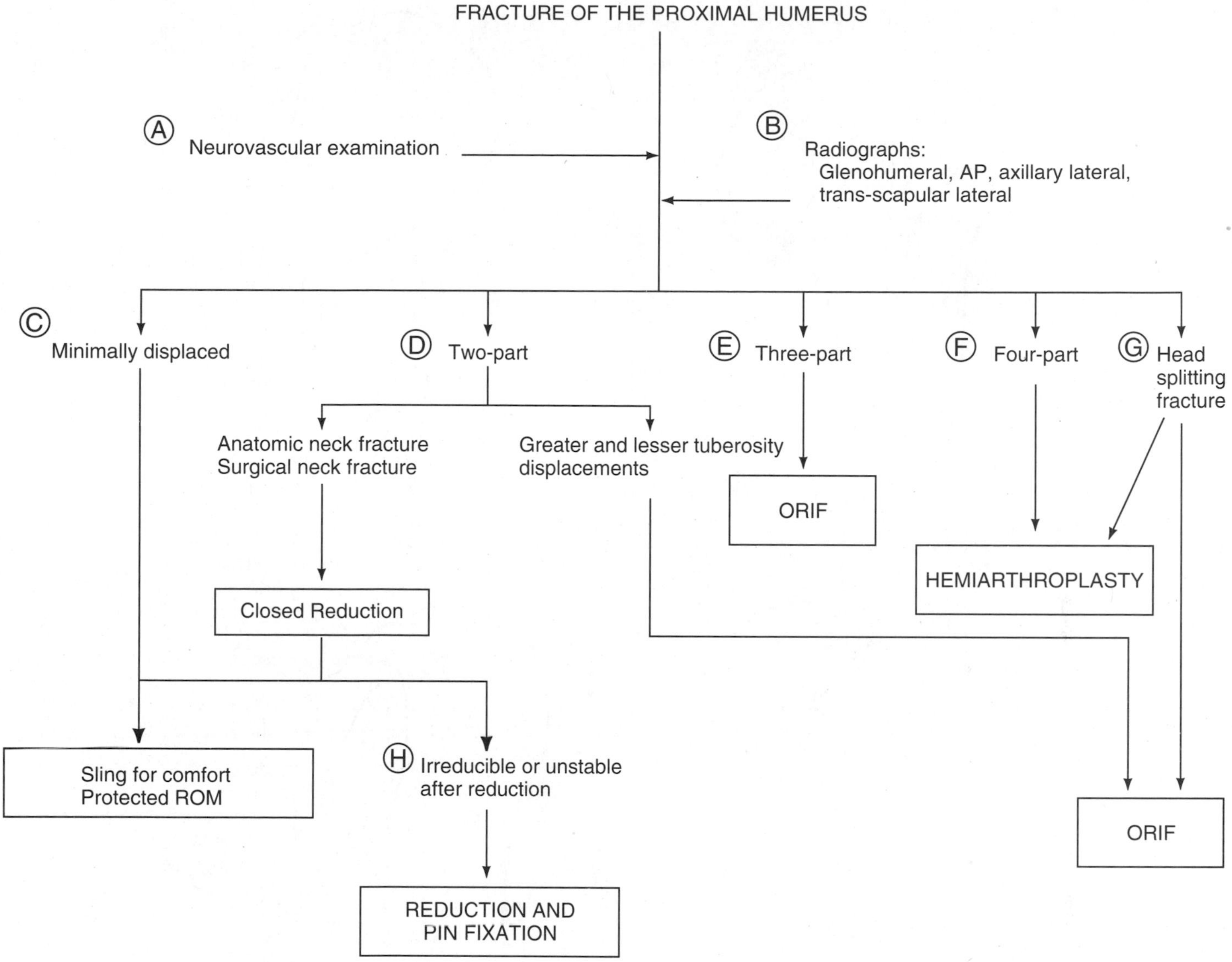

FRACTURE OF THE PROXIMAL HUMERUS

(A) Neurovascular examination ⟶

(B) Radiographs:
Glenohumeral, AP, axillary lateral,
trans-scapular lateral

(C) Minimally displaced

(D) Two-part

Anatomic neck fracture
Surgical neck fracture

Greater and lesser tuberosity
displacements

(E) Three-part

(F) Four-part

(G) Head
splitting
fracture

```
Closed Reduction
```

```
ORIF
```

```
HEMIARTHROPLASTY
```

```
Sling for comfort
Protected ROM
```

(H) Irreducible or unstable
after reduction

```
REDUCTION AND
PIN FIXATION
```

```
ORIF
```

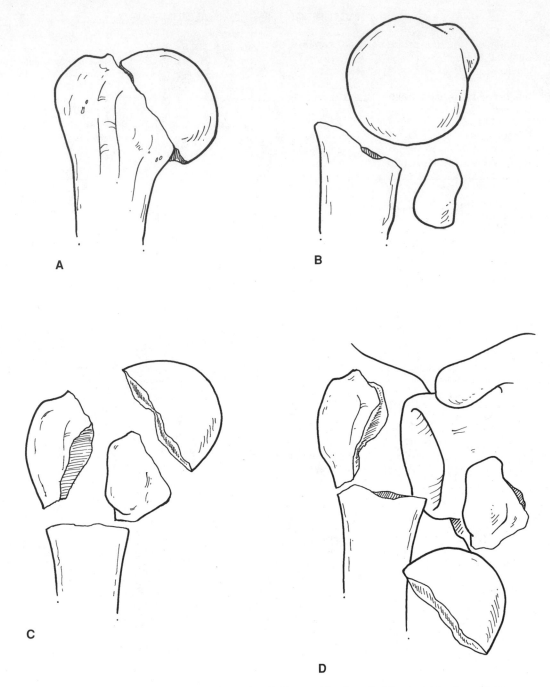

Figure 1 Fractures of the proximal humerus. **A,** Two-part fracture. **B,** Three-part fracture. **C,** Four-part fracture. **D,** Four-part fracture−dislocation.

References

Cofield RH. Comminuted fractures of the proximal humerus. Clin Orthop 1988; 230:49-57.

Hawkins RJ, Angelo RL. Orthop Clin of North America 1987; 18(3).

Hawkins RJ, Bell RH, Gurr K. The three-part fracture of the proximal humerus: Operative treatment. J Bone Joint Surg 1986; 68A:1410-1414.

Jakob RP, Kristiansen T, Mayo K, et al. Classification and aspects of treatment of fractures of the proximal humerus. In Bateman JE, Welsh RP, eds. Surgery of the Shoulder. Philadelphia: BC Decker, 1984.

Kilcoyne RF, Shuman WP, Matzen III FA, et al. The Neer classification of displaced proximal humeral fractures: Spectrum of findings on plain radiographs and CT scans. AJR 1990; 154:1029-1033.

Leyshon RL. Closed treatment of fractures of the proximal humerus. Acta Orthop Scand 1984; 55:48-51.

Neer C. Displaced proximal humeral fractures, part 1: classification and evaluation. J Bone Joint Surg 1970; 52A:1077−1089.

Neer CS II. Displaced proximal humerus fractures, part 2: treatment of three-part and four-part displacement. J Bone Joint Surg 1970; 52A:1090-1103.

Smith DK, Cooney WP. External fixation of high energy extremity injuries. J Orthop Trauma 1990; 4:7-18.

Stableforth PG. Four-part fractures of the neck of the humerus. J Bone Joint Surg 1984; 66B:104-108.

Tanner MW, Cofield RH. Prosthetic arthroplasty for fractures and fracture-dislocations of the proximal humerus. Clin Orthop 1982; 179:116.

Young TB. Conservative treatment of fractures and fracture dislocations of the upper end of the humerus. J Bone Joint Surg 1985; 67B:273-377.

FRACTURE OF THE HUMERAL SHAFT

A. Evaluation and treatment of the patient with suspected fracture of the humerus begin with a history of the injury, and a detailed physical examination. This should include assessment of vascular status, as well as a detailed neurologic examination, with particular attention to radial nerve function. Radial nerve palsy occurs in approximately 11% of humeral shaft fractures. Of patients with radial nerve palsy associated with humeral fracture, laceration of the radial nerve is present in only 10%. Most radial nerve injuries are neuropraxic, and recover with time. Exploration of radial nerve injuries is reserved for those patients that do not demonstrate clinical or electromyographic improvement in three to four months following injury. Other factors such as very proximal or distal fractures, or marked obesity may impair closed treatment of humeral shaft fractures.

B. Treatment of open fractures of the humerus follows the principles applied to other open fractures: extension of the open wound, debridement of devitalized tissue, copious irrigation, and stabilization of the fracture with internal or external fixation (Fig. 1). Internal fixation is preferred for most open fractures of the humeral shaft without gross contamination. Open wounds are not closed primarily, and delayed closure or soft tissue coverage is ideally performed in 5-7 days.

C. Most fractures of the shaft of the humerus are easily treated non-operatively. A commonly used method includes coaptive splinting and sling immobilization initially, followed by a humeral cuff orthosis when acute swelling and discomfort decrease. An adjustable orthosis allows better comfort and stabilization of the fracture as soft tissue swelling subsides. Several series report successful treatment in greater than 90 percent of patients using similar methods. The musculature of the upper extremity allows up to 20° of anterior angulation and up to 30° of varus angulation without compromising function or appearance. Shortening of as much as one inch is also well tolerated. Healing of closed fractures at 6 to 8 weeks after injury is usually sufficient to allow discontinuation of immobilization.

D. Surgical stablization of closed humeral shaft fractures is indicated in selected circumstances, including open fractures, bilateral fractures, fractures in the multiply injured patient, and fractures with associated vascular injury. Multiply injured patients who require a prolonged period of recumbency are more difficult to treat by closed methods because the longitudinal traction afforded by gravity in the upright position is not present. Patients with concomitant lower extremity injuries which require the use of ambulatory aids need a functional upper extremity for ambulation.

E. Types of fixation used for surgical stabilization of humeral shaft fractures include open reduction and internal fixation (ORIF), intramedullary fixation, and external fixation (Fig. 2). The method chosen depends on the geometry of the fracture and the degree of associated soft tissue injury. Most fractures of the humeral shaft are amenable to *ORIF* using plate and screw fixation. Disadvantages include extensive exposure and frequent need for bone grafting to achieve union. *Intamedullary nailing* allows stabilization of humeral shaft fractures using closed techniques, but insertion sites involve violation of the olecranon fossa or rotator cuff. Because of the conical shape of the distal intramedullary canal, fractures in the distal portion of the humeral shaft are best treated with alternative methods of fixation. Intramedullary fixation may provide better fixation for patients who are weight-bearing on their extremity for ambulation. *External fixation* is in general reserved for those fractures with severe associated soft tissue or vascular injury. Bone grafting may be required to acheive union in fractures with severe soft tissue disruption, bone loss, or evidence of delayed union. External fixation is continued until clinical and radiographic union.

FRACTURE OF THE HUMERAL SHAFT

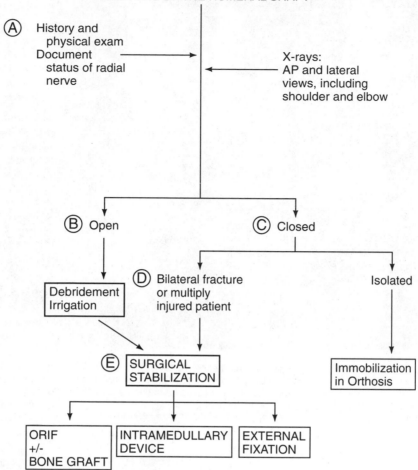

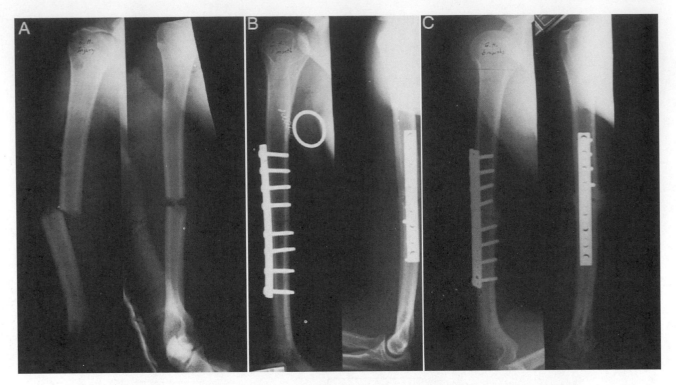

Figure 1 Compression plating of an open humeral shaft fracture. **A,** Displaced, transverse, midshaft humeral fracture. **B,** Compression plating through an anterolateral approach using an eight-hole, 4.5-mm dynamic compression plate. **C,** Abundant callus formation by 6 months after surgery. (From Swanson TV, Gustilo RB. Fractures of the humeral shaft. In: Gustilo RB, Kyle RF, Templeman D, eds. Fractures and Dislocations. St. Louis: Mosby–Year Book, 1993.)

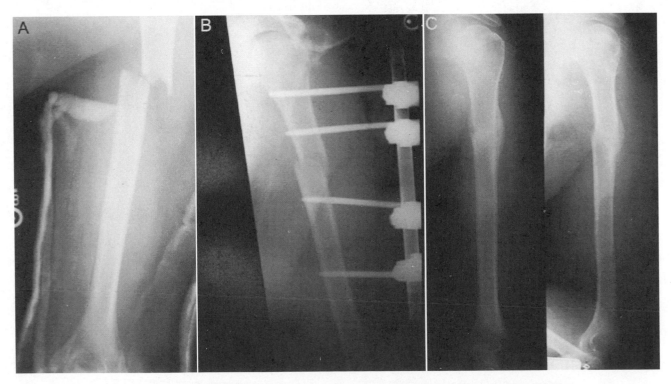

Figure 2 External fixation of a humeral shaft fracture with associated arterial injury. **A,** Displaced, short, oblique fracture of proximal third of humerus. **B,** Stabilization using a four-pin external fixator prior to vascular repair. **C,** Solid union 1 year after injury. (From Swanson TV, Gustilo RB. Fractures of the humeral shaft. In: Gustilo RB, Kyle RF, Templeman D, eds. Fractures and Dislocations. St. Louis: Mosby–Year Book, 1993.)

References

Balfour GW, Mooney V, Ashby ME. Diaphyseal fractures of the humerus treated with a ready-made fracture brace. J Bone Joint Surg 1982; 64-A:11.

Brumback RJ, Bosse MJ, Poka A, Burgess AR. Intramedullary stabilization of humeral shaft fractures in patients with multiple trauma. J Bone Joint Surg 1986; 68A:960.

Fenyo G. On fractures of the shaft of the humerus: A review covering a 12-year period with special consideration of the surgically treated cases. Acta Chir Scand 1971; 137:221.

Garcia A, Jr., Maeck B. Radial nerve injuries in fractures of the shaft of the humerus. Am J Surg 1960; 99:625.

Hall RF, Jr, Pankovich AM. Technique and results of closed intramedullary rodding of diaphyseal fractures of the humerus (abstr). Orthop Trans 1982; 6:359.

Holstein A, Lewis GB. Fractures of the humerus with radial-nerve paralysis. J Bone Joint Surg 1963; 45A:1382.

Kettlekamp DB, Alexander H. Clinical review of radial nerve injury. J Trauma 1967; 7:424.

Klenerman L. Fractures of the shaft of the humerus. J Bone Joint Surg 1966; 48-B:105.

Mast JW, Spiegel PG, Harvey JP, Jr., Harrison C. Fractures of the humeral shaft: A retrospective study of 240 adult fractures. Clin Orthop 1975; 112:254.

Packer JW, Foster RR, Garcia A, Grantham SA. The humeral fracture with radial nerve palsy: Is exploration warranted? Clin Orthop 1972; 88:34.

Pollock FH, Drake D, Bovill EG, et al. Treatment of radial neuropathy associated with fractures of the humerus. J Bone Joint Surg 1981; 63A:239.

Sarmiento A, Kinman PB, Galvin EG, et al. Functional bracing of fractures of the shaft of the humerus. J Bone Joint Surg 1977; 59A:596.

Seddon HJ. Nerve lesions complicating certain closed bone injuries. JAMA 1947; 135:691.

Shaw JL, Sakellarides H. Radial-nerve paralysis associated with fractures of the humerus: A review of forty-five cases. J Bone Joint Surg 1967; 49-A:899.

FRACTURE OF THE PELVIC RING

A. Associated abdominal and thoracic injuries take precedence over the pelvic fracture. Several investigators have outlined excellent emergency management protocols for pelvic fractures and their frequent concomitant visceral injuries. The next algorithm and accompanying comments address the management of severe pelvic hemorrhage following these fractures.

B. High-quality plain radiographs including special inlet and tilt views of the pelvic ring are usually sufficient to diagnose major pelvic ring disruptions. Occult posterior ring fractures and subluxations can be missed if the quality of the film is suboptimal. Computed tomography (CT) aids in the evaluation of the posterior ring injury and the degree of triplane displacement of an unstable pelvic fracture. Routinely obtain CT scans in patients with concomitant acetabular fractures, injuries that necessitate surgical stabilization, and postoperatively in surgically stabilized fractures. Use of three-dimensional reconstructions of CT scans in these injuries is increasing as the quality of the images improve.

C. The Tile classification is useful in determining the preferred treatment for any pelvic disruption. Tile type A injuries are stable including A1 injuries, which are fractures of the pelvis not involving the ring, and A2 injuries, which are minimally displaced fractures of the ring. Tile type B injuries are rotationally unstable but vertically stable (Fig. 1). They include the B1 (open book) injuries, B2 (lateral compression: ipsilateral) injuries, and B3 (lateral compression: contralateral or bucket handle) injuries. Tile type C injuries are both rotationally and vertically unstable (Fig. 2). They may be unilateral (C1), bilateral (C2), or associated with an acetabular fracture (C3).

Minor fracture patterns and stable hemipelvis fractures (Tile type A) retain sufficient posterior stability through the weight-bearing portion of the pelvis that only symptomatic treatment is necessary. Special x-ray studies including stress radiographs of the ring disruption may be useful in distinguishing apparent minor fracture patterns from occult hemipelvis fractures and subluxations. Bed rest followed by protective weight bearing usually suffices for these minor injuries. The uniformly good results arise from the potential for early mobilization of the patient within several days of injury and the low incidence of late disability.

D. The anteroposterior compression or open book injuries (Tile B1) usually involve diastasis of the pubic symphysis and tearing of the anterior sacroiliac ligaments. The stout posterior superior sacroiliac ligament complex remains intact and the hemipelvis hinges open like a book. The pelvis is rendered rotationally unstable but the intact posterior sacroiliac ligaments prevent any significant vertical displacement. If the diastasis of the pubic symphysis is less than 3 cm, there is a tendency for spontaneous closure of the diastasis over time. If the diastasis is greater than 3 cm, however, there is greater likelihood of long-term deformity and pubic pain.

E. Lateral compression injuries are either stable or unstable depending on the degree of impaction of the posterior ring elements. Tile type B2 injuries are rotationally unstable but have little tendency for vertical displacement. If the internal rotational deformity is less than 30°, only symptomatic treatment is indicated. If the deformity is greater than 30°, then the functional and cosmetic result may be unacceptable and closed reduction and anterior ring stabilization is indicated. If the anterior ring disruption with markedly displaced B1 or B2 injuries involves symphyseal disruption, anterior plate fixation is indicated. If, however, the anterior ring injury involves rami fractures, an anterior half pin external fixator is preferred.

F. Vertical shear (Tile type C) injuries may be associated with massive hemorrhage, major visceral injuries, neurologic loss, and late disability including leg length discrepancy, low back pain, sacroiliac arthritis, pelvic obliquity, and lumbosacral plexus palsy.

The preferred treatment depends on the age and functional needs of the patient, the fracture location, the fracture pattern, and the experience of the surgeon. In the young active adult, a rotationally and vertically unstable pelvic ring disruption is best managed by open reduction and internal fixation or closed reduction and percutaneous screw fixation. The best surgical approach and form of stabilization hinges on an accurate assessment of the posterior ring injury. CT scans are especially useful in preoperative planning.

G. Tile C1 injuries frequently involve oblique fractures through the posterior ilium with extension into the anterior portion of the sacroiliac joint. If the posterior soft tissues are not severely contused, a posterior approach with anatomic reduction and plating of the ilium is the preferred treatment.

H. Sacroiliac dislocations may be managed either by closed reduction and screw fixation of the joint or by exposure of the anterior aspect of the joint with plate fixation and fusion. The advantages of an anterior approach include easy exposure of the entire joint surface, unobstructed assessment of the adequacy of the reduction, and the potential for rigid fixation using multiple two- or three-hole plates. The major risk of anterior sacroiliac plating is injury to the L5 nerve root. Percutaneous screw fixation necessitates accurate closed reduction, high quality intraoperative fluoroscopy, and cannulated screws. Supplemental anterior ring fixation is often needed.

FRACTURE OF THE PELVIC RING

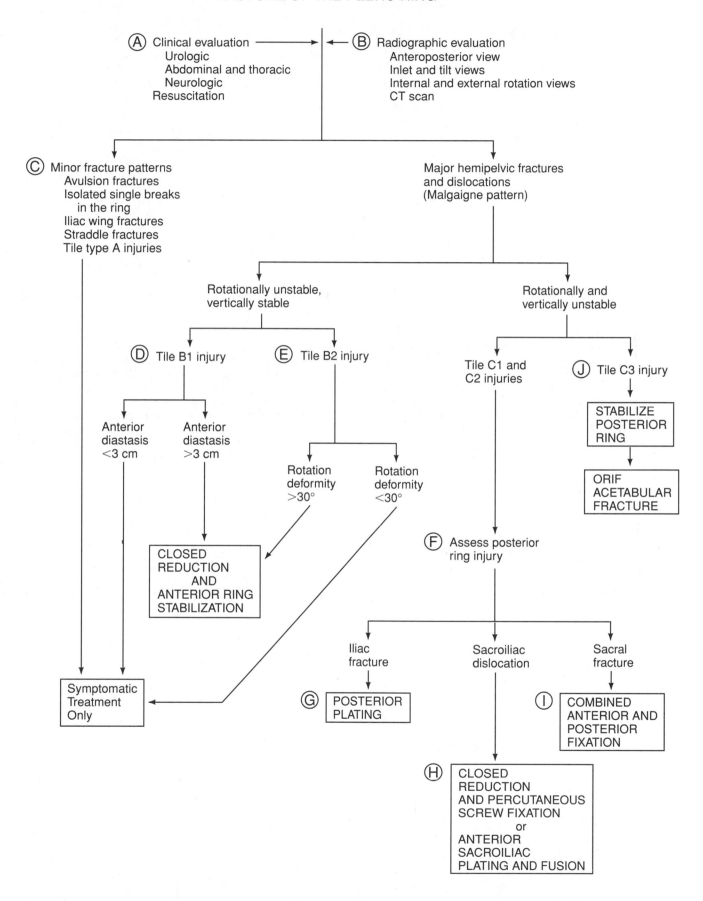

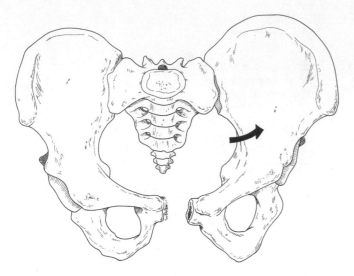

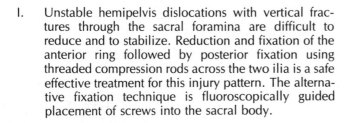

Figure 1 Rotationally unstable but vertically stable injury to the pelvic ring.

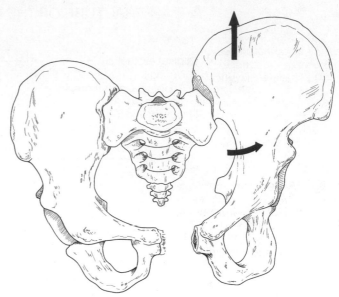

Figure 2 Rotationally and vertically unstable injury to the pelvic ring.

I. Unstable hemipelvis dislocations with vertical fractures through the sacral foramina are difficult to reduce and to stabilize. Reduction and fixation of the anterior ring followed by posterior fixation using threaded compression rods across the two ilia is a safe effective treatment for this injury pattern. The alternative fixation technique is fluoroscopically guided placement of screws into the sacral body.

J. Tile type C3 injuries should be managed first by open reduction and internal fixation (ORIF) of the posterior pelvic ring followed by anatomic reduction and fixation of the acetabular fracture. If only the acetabular fracture is surgically approached, reduction may be very difficult. If both fractures can be stabilized through a single approach (e.g., extended iliofemoral or ilioinguinal approach), improved reductions can be achieved.

References

Bucholz R, Peters P. Assessment of pelvic stability. Instructional course lectures of the AAOS. 1988; 37:119.

Burgess A, Eastridge B, Young J, et al. Pelvic ring disruptions: Effective classification system and treatment protocols. J Trauma 1990; 30:848.

Conolly W, Hedberg E. Observations on fractures of the pelvis. J Trauma 1969; 9:104.

Gill K, Bucholz R. The role of CT scanning in the evaluation of major hemipelvis fractures-dislocations. J Bone Joint Surg 1984; 66A:30.

Harahanju E, Slatis P. External fixation of double vertical pelvic fractures with a trapezoidal compression frame. Injury 1978; 10:142.

Isler B. Lumbosacral lesions associated with pelvic ring injuries. J Orthop Trauma 1990; 4:1.

Lange R, Hansen S. Pelvic ring disruptions with symphysis pubis diastasis: Indications, technique, and limitations of anterior internal fixation. Clin Orthop 1985; 201:130.

Matta J, Sancedo T. Internal fixation of pelvic ring fractures. Clin Orthop 1989; 242:83.

Mears D, Fu F. Modern concepts of external fixation of the pelvis. Clin Orthop 1980; 151:65.

Moed B, Letournel E. Low-dose irradiation and indomethacin prevent heterotopic ossification after acetabular fracture surgery. J Bone Joint Surg 1994; 76B:895.

Pennal G, Tile M, Waddell J, Garside H. Pelvic disruption: Assessment and classification. Clin Orthop 1980; 151:1221.

Poole G, Ward E. Causes of mortality in patients with pelvic fractures. Orthopaedics 1994; 17:691.

Shaw J, Mino D, Werner F, Murray D. Posterior stabilization of pelvis fractures by use of threaded compression rods. Clin Orthop 1985; 192:240.

Simpson L, Waddell J, Leighton R, et al. Anterior approach and stabilization of the disrupted sacroiliac joint. J Trauma 1987; 27:1332.

Slatis P, Huittinen V. Double vertical fractures of the pelvis. Acta Chir Scand 1971; 138:799.

Tile M. Fractures of the pelvis and acetabulum. Baltimore: Williams & Wilkins, 1984.

Tile M. Pelvis ring fractures: Should they be fixed? J Bone Joint Surg 1988; 708:1.

HEMORRHAGE FROM PELVIC FRACTURE

A. The treatment of hemorrhagic shock is the first priority in pelvic fractures (Fig. 1). Bleeding originates from the raw cancellous fracture surfaces as well as ruptured pelvic and lumbar retroperitoneal vessels. Patient movement and manipulation promote further bleeding and therefore should be permitted only when necessary.

B. It is often clinically difficult to localize major sources of bleeding in the polytraumatized patient, especially attempting to differentiate continued pelvic hemorrhage from bleeding at other injury sites. Approximately 10-20% of patients with major pelvic fractures have associated intraabdominal injuries, especially hepatic and splenic lacerations. Bleeding from these intraabdominal sites can be differentiated from pelvic hemorrhage by the use of peritoneal lavage, abdominal computed tomography, or visceral angiography. Although brisk retroperitoneal bleeding is possible without any external manifestation of hemorrhage, an expanding gluteal, scrotal, or perineal hematoma suggests active bleeding at a pelvic fracture.

C. The keystone to treatment is the early institution and continuation of effective blood replacement. The appearance of shock is usually slow to develop, thereby allowing ample time for typing and cross-matching blood. Patients who are hemodynamically unstable on presentation in the emergency room have a very guarded prognosis. Approximately 40% of all patients with major pelvic fractures require transfusions. The average number of transfusions for Malgaigne fracture dislocations is 7.4 units per patient. Fracture patterns which are associated with massive hemorrhage include widely opened Tile type A injuries, type C1 injuries with lateral displacement of the entire hemipelvis, and open pelvic ring injuries.

D. Large vessel injuries occur in only 2% of all pelvic fractures. Physical signs of large vessel injury include diminished or absent distal pulses, a pulsatile hematoma, and an audible pelvic bruit. Massive uncontrollable bleeding may signal a large vessel injury or a concomitant intraabdominal injury. It is advisable to proceed directly with peritoneal lavage or possible arteriography in such situations.

E. Undesirable motion of pelvic fracture fragments may be neutralized by the application of an external fixation device or, alternatively, an external counterpressure suit. The former requires an operative procedure, but has the added advantage of maintaining any fracture reduction and obliterating the potential pelvic dead space created by fracture displacement. Multiple clinical studies demonstrate an approximate 80-90% success rate in controlling hemorrhage by the application of an external fixator and closed reduction of the pelvic fracture.

Pneumatic antishock garments (G-suit, PASG) are easily applied but do not allow for controlled reduction of the fracture. The increased systemic blood pressure recorded after inflation of the trousers is conjectured to be secondary to either an autotransfusion of blood from the legs and pelvis to the upper half of the body, a compression of the bony elements to tamponade small vessel bleeding, or an increase in peripheral vascular resistance. Whatever their mechanism of action, the trousers must be cautiously deflated once their use is no longer indicated. Recent studies have not confirmed a decreased mortality with the aggressive use of PASG in patients with severe blunt trauma. Contraindications to PASG include impaired pulmonary function, cerebral edema, and injuries to the lower extremities which have a high probability of causing a compartment syndrome.

F. There is no absolute point at which either arteriography or surgical exploration is mandatory. Each case much be individualized on the basis of the patient's condition as well as the facilities and expertise at the treatment center. Selective transcatheter arterial embolization is feasible when the bleeding sites are well localized (Fig. 2). Only 10% of bleeds following pelvic fractures are arterial in origin, thereby decreasing the effectiveness of this form of treatment. Prior to selective embolization, an initial abdominal and pelvic flush aortogram is usually performed to survey the pelvic bleeding. A variety of different agents, such as autologous clot, Gelfoam, and detachable silicone balloons have been utilized for vessel occlusion.

Extreme caution must be taken in sending a potentially unstable patient to the radiology suite for arteriography without the benefit of adequate equipment to monitor and resuscitate the patient. If such support is not available in the angiography suite, alternative treatment should be considered.

G. Surgical exploration to attempt direct control of pelvic hemorrhage is rarely indicated. Techniques for halting continued bleeding involve combinations of suture ligation, hypogastric artery ligation, aortic cross-clamping, and compressive packing. Massive intraoperative hemorrhage should be anticipated. Emergency hemipelvectomy has been reported as necessary in several patients as the only method to control hemorrhage. Due to the high operative mortality rate, all alternative methods of controlling hemorrhage should be exhausted before resorting to surgical exploration unless there is a well documented associated intraabdominal or large vessel injury. During laparotomies for intraoperative abdominal trauma, the retroperitoneal hematoma of a pelvic fracture should not be disturbed.

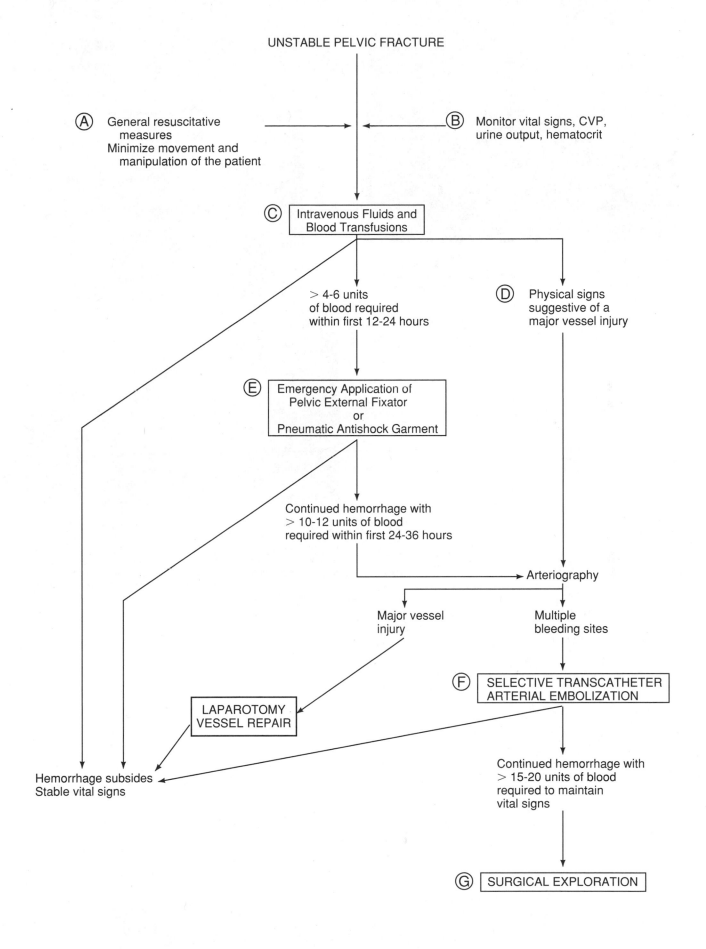

UNSTABLE PELVIC FRACTURE

(A) General resuscitative
measures
Minimize movement and
manipulation of the patient

(B) Monitor vital signs, CVP,
urine output, hematocrit

(C) Intravenous Fluids and
Blood Transfusions

> 4-6 units
of blood required
within first 12-24 hours

(D) Physical signs
suggestive of a
major vessel injury

(E) Emergency Application of
Pelvic External Fixator
or
Pneumatic Antishock Garment

Continued hemorrhage with
> 10-12 units of blood
required within first 24-36 hours

Arteriography

Major vessel
injury

Multiple
bleeding sites

LAPAROTOMY
VESSEL REPAIR

(F) SELECTIVE TRANSCATHETER
ARTERIAL EMBOLIZATION

Hemorrhage subsides
Stable vital signs

Continued hemorrhage with
> 15-20 units of blood
required to maintain
vital signs

(G) SURGICAL EXPLORATION

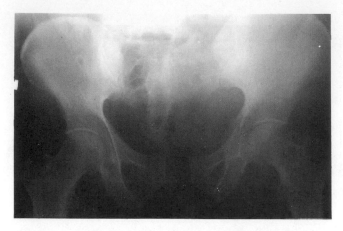

Figure 1 Anterior/posterior radiograph of a severe ipsilateral left hemipelvis disruption and a left acetabular fracture. Despite multiple transfusions, resuscitation was complicated in this patient by continued hypotension and occult bleeding.

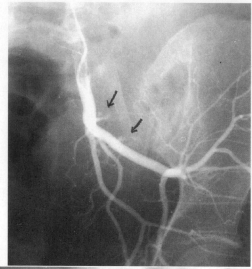

A

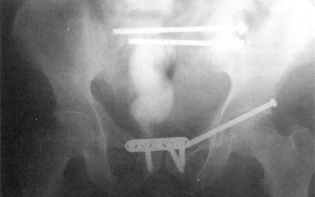

B

Figure 2 **A,** Arteriogram demonstrates multiple sites *(arrows)* of arterial bleeding. Transarterial embolization of these vessels was successfully performed. **B,** Approximately one week later, the patient underwent closed reduction and percutaneous fixation of both his pelvic fracture and his acetabular fracture. The ring fixation was supplemented by an anterior open reduction and internal fixation of the public diastasis.

References

Batalden D, et al. Value of the G-suit in patients with severe pelvic fracture. Arch Surg 1974; 109:326.

Ben-Menachem Y, et al. Therapeutic arterial embolization in trauma. J Trauma 1979; 19:944.

Flint L, et al. Definitive control of bleeding from severe pelvic fractures. Ann Surg 1979; 189:709.

Ganz R, Krushell R, Jakob R. The antishock pelvic clamp. Clin Orthop 1991; 267:71.

Goldstein A, et al. Early open reduction and internal fixation of the disrupted pelvic ring. J Trauma 1986; 26:325.

Hansen C, Perry J. Massive hemorrhage from pelvic fractures. Minn Med 1966; 49:285.

Hawkins L, Pomerantz M, Eiseman B. Laparotomy at the time of pelvic fracture. J Trauma 1970; 10:619.

Moreno C, et al. Hemorrhage associated with major pelvic fracture: A multispecialty challenge. J Trauma 1986; 26:987.

Mucha P, Farrell M. Analysis of pelvic fracture management. J Trauma 1984; 24:379.

Panetta T, et al. Percutaneous transcatheter embolization for massive bleeding from pelvic fractures. J Trauma 1985; 25:1021.

Riska E, et al. Operative control of massive hemorrhages in comminuted pelvic fractures. Acta Orthop Scan 1979; 50:362.

ACETABULAR FRACTURE

A. The proper treatment of acetabular fractures, with or without femoral head subluxation, depends on accurate determination of the fracture pattern. The status of the anterior and posterior acetabular columns as well as the dome of the acetabulum can be defined by careful scrutiny of the anteroposterior (AP) and both oblique (Judet) pelvic radiographs. On the obturator oblique view, the pelvic brim, anterior column, and posterior rim are profiled. The posterior column, iliac crest, and anterior rim are best visualized on the iliac oblique view. Computed tomography (CT) scans should be routinely obtained, especially in operative cases. The CT scan aids in delineating associated pelvic ring fractures, intra-articular osteochondral fragments, fracture lines through the quadrilateral space, and the planes of displacement of the acetabular columns. Three-dimensional reconstructions of the CT sections are helpful but not imperative for preoperative planning.

B. The Letournel classification is useful for defining the indications for surgery and the preferred surgical approaches. This classification includes five simple patterns (posterior wall, posterior column, anterior wall, anterior column, transverse) and five combined patterns (associated posterior wall and posterior column fracture, associated posterior wall and transverse fracture, T-shaped fracture, associated anterior and posterior hemitransverse fractures, and two column fractures) (Fig. 1). The treatment of posterior and anterior wall fractures is discussed in the chapter on hip dislocations.

   In addition to classifying the pattern of acetabular disruption, the amount of fracture displacement and the amount of intact acetabular dome should be measured. Any fracture displacement greater than 2 mm is considered significant. The status of the acetabular dome is assessed by measuring the roof arc angles on the AP and oblique radiographs. The roof arc is measured by drawing a vertical line through the roof of the acetabulum to the geometric center of the femoral head. A second line is drawn through the fracture to the center of the head. The angle subtended by these lines is the roof arc. The roof arc angle can be measured on all three radiographic views.

C. Fractures with displacement of less than 2 mm and satisfactory joint congruity can be managed by variable periods of traction and protected weight bearing. Late displacement of such fractures is infrequent. Certain displaced fracture patterns, such as both column fractures with a congruent joint and low transverse fractures with large roof arc angles, can be similarly treated.

D. The prerequisites for nonsurgical treatment of a displaced acetabular fracture include (1) roof arc angles of greater than 45° on all three radiographic views, (2) congruency of the femoral head with the roof of the acetabulum with longitudinal traction released, and (3) a competent posterior wall of the acetabulum with no tendency for posterior subluxation.

E. The primary cause for poor results with displaced acetabular fractures is residual incongruity of the joint. Articular step-offs of 2 mm or more commonly lead to post-traumatic arthritis. Nearly all patients with major displaced fractures of the acetabulum should be considered for surgical reduction and stabilization. Even elderly patients with displaced acetabular fractures through osteopenic bone should undergo operative reduction to restore acetabular bone stock and anatomy in anticipation of the need for total hip replacement.

F. Open reduction and internal fixation of complex acetabular fractures is ideally performed between 3 and 10 days after the injury, allowing the initial bleeding from the fracture site and the pelvic vessels to subside. The preferred surgical approach is dictated by the fracture pattern. The Kocher-Langenbeck approach allows exposure of the posterior wall, posterior column, and limited access to the acetabular dome. The ilioinguinal incision gives extensile exposure to the anterior column and the iliac crest. The extended iliofemoral approach provides the best access to the entire innominate bone. The tri-radiate incision is an extension of the Kocher-Langenbeck incision and provides more exposure of the acetabular dome and iliac crest.

G. Intraoperative nerve palsies can be minimized by keeping the knee flexed during surgery and avoiding too vigorous intraoperative retraction of the nerves. The incidence of sciatic nerve palsy is highest with the Kocher-Langenbeck incision. Somatosensory evoked potentials can be used intraoperatively to monitor nerve function.

H. Heterotopic ossification complicates any acetabular surgery that involves extensile dissection of the gluteal musculature (such as the extended iliofemoral approach or the Kocher-Langenbeck approach). Brooker Grade III and IV heterotopic ossification can severely limit hip function. This complication is minimized by careful handling of the soft tissues, avoidance of extensive gluteal dissection, and perioperative prophylaxis. Prophylaxis can be accomplished either with indomethacin (25 mg t.i.d. for 8 weeks) or low dose irradiation (500 to 1000 centigrays within 24 hours of surgery).

ACETABULAR FRACTURE

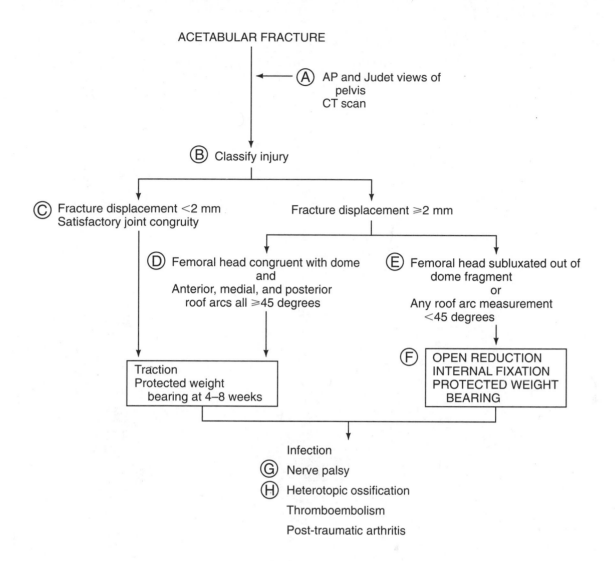

A. AP and Judet views of
pelvis
CT scan

B. Classify injury

C. Fracture displacement <2 mm
Satisfactory joint congruity

Fracture displacement ≥2 mm

D. Femoral head congruent with dome
and
Anterior, medial, and posterior
roof arcs all ≥45 degrees

E. Femoral head subluxated out of
dome fragment
or
Any roof arc measurement
<45 degrees

Traction
Protected weight
bearing at 4–8 weeks

F. OPEN REDUCTION
INTERNAL FIXATION
PROTECTED WEIGHT
BEARING

Infection
G. Nerve palsy
H. Heterotopic ossification
Thromboembolism
Post-traumatic arthritis

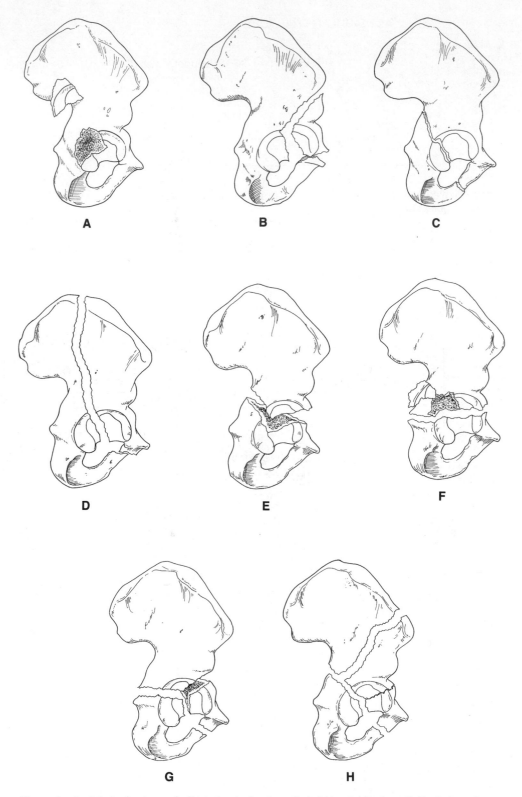

Figure 1 Acetabular fractures. **A,** Posterior rim fracture. **B,** Anterior rim fracture. **C,** Posterior column fracture. **D,** Anterior column fracture. **E,** Transverse fracture. **F,** Transverse fracture with posterior rim fracture. **G,** T-shaped fracture. **H,** Both-column fracture with associated T-shaped fracture.

References

Adam P, Labbe J, Alberge Y, et al. The role of computed tomography in the assessment and treatment of acetabular fractures. Clin Radiol 1985; 36:13.

Bosse M, Poka A, Reinert C, et al. Heterotopic ossification as a complication of acetabular fracture: Prophylaxis with low-dose radiation. J Bone Joint Surg 1988; 70A:1231.

Bray T, Esser M, Fulkerson L. Osteotomy of the trochanter in open reduction and internal fixation of acetabular fractures. J Bone Joint Surg 1987; 69A:711.

Burk D, Mears D, Cooperstein L, et al. Acetabular fractures: Three-dimensional computed tomographic imaging and interactive surgical planning. J Comput Assist Tomogr 1986; 10:1.

Ebraheim N, Coombs R, Jackson W, et al. Percutaneous computed tomography guided stabilization of posterior pelvis fractures. Clin Orthop 1994; 307:222.

Goulet J, Rouleau J, Mason D, et al. Comminuted fractures of the posterior wall of the acetabulum: A biomechanical evaluation of fixation methods. J Bone Joint Surg 1994; 76A:1457.

Heeg M, Oostvogel H, Klasen H. Conservative treatment of acetabular fractures: The role of the weight-bearing dome and anatomic reduction in the ultimate results. J Trauma 1987; 27:555.

Helfet D, Schmeling G. Management of complex acetabular fractures through single nonextensile exposures. Clin Orthop 1994; 305:58.

Judet R, Judet J, Letournel E. Fractures of the acetabulum: Classification and surgical approaches for open reduction. J Bone Joint Surg 1964; 46A:1615.

Letournel E, Judet R. Fractures of the acetabulum. New York: Springer-Verlag, 1981.

Matta J, Anderson L, Epstein H, Hendricks P. Fractures of the acetabulum: A retrospective analysis. Clin Orthop 1986; 205:230.

Matta J, Merritt P. Displaced acetabular fractures. Clin Orthop 1988; 230:83.

Matta J, Mehne D, Roffi R. Fractures of the acetabulum: Early results of a prospective study. Clin Orthop 1986; 205:241.

McLaren A. Prophylaxis with indomethacin for heterotopic bone after open reduction of fractures of the acetabulum. J Bone Joint Surg 1990; 72A:245.

Moed B, Letournel E. Low-dose irradiation and indomethacin prevent heterotopic ossification after acetabular fracture surgery. J Bone Joint Surg 1994; 76B:895.

Reinert C, Bosse M, Poka A, et al. A modified extensile exposure for the treatment of complex or malunited acetabular fractures. J Bone Joint Surg 1988; 70A:329.

Routt C, Swiontkowski M. Operative treatment of complex acetabular fractures: Combined anterior and posterior exposures during the same procedure. J Bone Joint Surg 1990; 72A:897.

Tipton W, D'Ambrosia R, Ryle G. Nonoperative management of central fracture dislocation of the hip. J Bone Joint Surg 1975; 57A:888.

Webb L, Bosse M, Mayo K, et al. Results in patients with craniocerebral trauma and an operatively managed acetabular fracture. J Orthop Trauma 1990; 4:376.

HIP DISLOCATION

A. Motor vehicle accidents cause 70% of hip dislocations. The major forces needed to dislocate an adult hip are also responsible for the frequent concomitant thoracic and abdominal visceral injuries. Sciatic nerve injury occurs in approximately 10% of all posterior fracture dislocations of the hip. Spontaneous neural recovery is expected in a majority of cases if appropriate treatment of the dislocation is instituted.

B. Hip dislocations are often missed in the polytraumatized patient, especially in cases with ipsilateral femoral shaft fracture. A routine anteroposterior (AP) pelvic radiograph should therefore be ordered in all multiply-injured patients. Anterior and Judet (oblique) radiographic views are sufficient to evaluate the dislocation and concomitant posterior and anterior acetabular rim fractures (Fig. 1). The Epstein classification scheme of posterior hip dislocations is useful in treatment planning. The five injury patterns include:

Type I: Pure posterior dislocation without fracture
Type II: Single large posterior acetabular rim fragment
Type III: Acetabular rim comminution
Type IV: Rim comminution and acetabular floor fracture
Type V: Femoral head fracture

The Type V injuries have been further subclassified by Pipkin as follows:

Type I: Fracture caudad to the fovea centralis
Type II: Fracture cephalad to the fovea centralis
Type III: Type I or II with an associated femoral neck fracture
Type IV: Type I or II or III with an associated acetabular fracture

Anterior hip dislocations may be divided into pubic (superior) and obturator (inferior) types.

C. Anterior dislocations result from forced hip abduction whereas posterior dislocations are usually secondary to a force applied to the flexed knee with the hip in flexion. The specific injury pattern dictates the proper manipulative maneuver for reduction. Closed reduction should be performed on an emergency basis. Patient relaxation can be achieved with intravenous medications in the emergency room or, ideally, with general anesthesia in the operating room. A maximum of two or three attempts at closed reduction should be tried prior to resorting to operative reduction.

D. Closed reduction of the femoral head can be blocked by buttonholing of the head through the joint capsule, osteochondral fragments within the joint, infolding of the acetabular labrum, or an interposed pyriformis tendon.

E. After successful closed reduction of a posterior hip dislocation, the hip is flexed to 90° in neutral position relative to adduction/abduction and rotation. The weight of the leg is allowed to rest on the posterior acetabular rim. If redislocation occurs, the hip is deemed unstable (Fig. 2). Anterior dislocations need not be tested for redislocation since post-reduction instability is extremely rare.

F. A stable, reduced dislocation of the hip should then be studied with a computed tomography (CT) scan of the pelvis. If the axial CT slices of 1.5 to 3 mm in thickness demonstrate a nonconcentric reduction with interposition of osteochondral fragments or soft tissue, surgical debridement of the joint is indicated. The CT scan is also useful in assessing the extent of posterior rim fracture (Fig. 3). The percentage of remaining posterior acetabulum can be accurately assessed. Clinical studies demonstrate that if less than 34% of the remaining posterior acetabulum is intact, the hip is unstable. Hips with greater than 55% of intact posterior acetabular rim are stable. Between these values, the hip may be either stable or unstable, depending on the supporting soft tissues of the joint. Clinical testing for stability is critical in this latter patient population. Biomechanical studies on cadaver specimens of pelves have yielded similar results correlating the extent of posterior wall damage and the stability of the joint.

G. A concentric reduction with a small stable acetabular rim fracture can be managed with bed rest, with or without traction. Within 3 to 5 days most patients are sufficiently comfortable to start protected weight bearing. Early weight bearing does not increase the frequency of late complications.

H. Posterior dislocations are approached posteriorly whereas anterior dislocations necessitate an anterior exposure. After careful redislocation of the hip, the joint is debrided of all displaced osseous and soft tissues. Associated femoral head and neck fractures must be reduced and fixed, except for small, comminuted inferior head fragments, which can be discarded. Anterior dislocations often have associated impaction injuries to the superior aspect of the femoral head. If these impaction fractures are at a depth greater than 4 mm, they should be surgically elevated with bone graft inserted under the osteochondral surface. Interfragmental screw fixation is used for acetabular rim fractures. Posterior column buttress plates are occasionally needed for comminuted rim fractures and associated transverse column fractures. Small Pipkin Type I and II fractures can be excised but those Type II fractures involving more than one third of the articular surface are preferably reduced and fixed. Young patients with Pipkin Type III injuries are best managed by fixation of all fractures but the prognosis for these injuries is poor.

HIP DISLOCATION

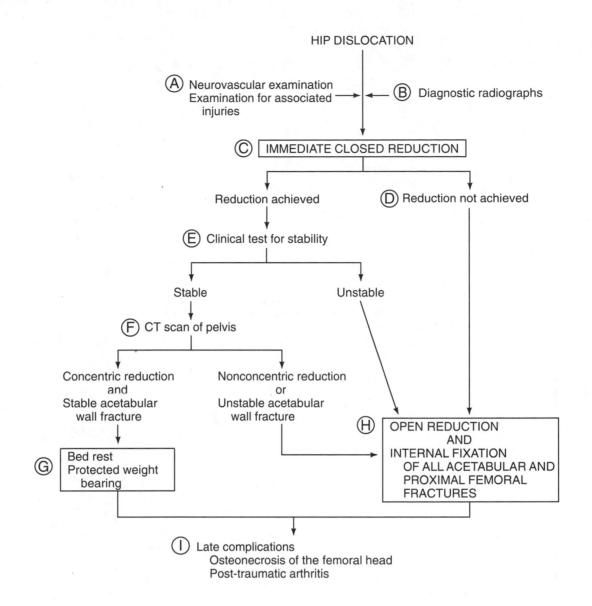

(A) Neurovascular examination
Examination for associated injuries → ← (B) Diagnostic radiographs

(C) | IMMEDIATE CLOSED REDUCTION |

Reduction achieved   (D) Reduction not achieved

(E) Clinical test for stability

Stable   Unstable

(F) CT scan of pelvis

Concentric reduction
and
Stable acetabular
wall fracture

Nonconcentric reduction
or
Unstable acetabular
wall fracture

(H) | OPEN REDUCTION
AND
INTERNAL FIXATION
OF ALL ACETABULAR AND
PROXIMAL FEMORAL
FRACTURES |

(G) | Bed rest
Protected weight
bearing |

(I) Late complications
Osteonecrosis of the femoral head
Post-traumatic arthritis

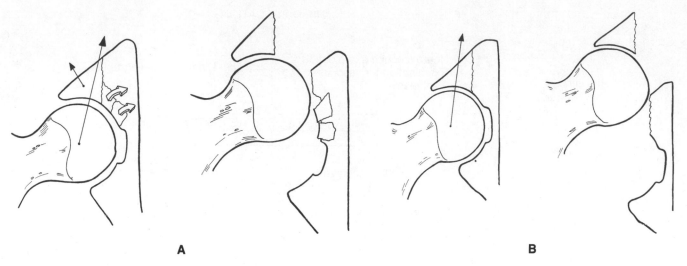

A   B

Figure 1 **A,** Posterior dislocation with the hip in an abducted position at the time of impact may result in marginal impaction fractures to the posterior articular surface. **B,** The size of the posterior rim fracture depends on the position of the hip at the time of impact.

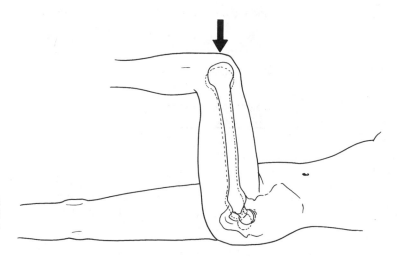

Figure 2 Clinical test for hip instability. The hip and the knee are flexed 90° with the patient lying supine. The hip is deemed unstable if it redislocates with the weight of the leg on the posterior acetabular rim.

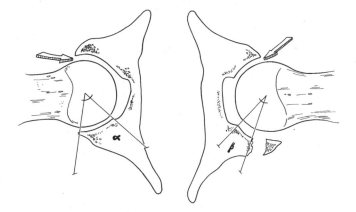

Figure 3 The degree of hip instability following a posterior acetabular rim fracture can be assessed on axial CT views by either widening of the anterior cartilage space *(arrows)* or the size of the posterior rim fragment. The angle subtended by lines drawn from the center of the femoral head to the edge of the posterior rim and the centralmost point of the posterior facet of the acetabular articular surface is compared to that of the contralateral uninjured acetabulum ($\angle\beta$ compared to $\angle\alpha$). If β is less than one third of α, the hip is definitely unstable.

I. Osteonecrosis of the femoral head becomes manifest radiographically at an average of 18 months after injury. The incidence of osteonecrosis varies from 15% for Epstein Type I dislocations to 21% for Epstein Type II to Type V fracture dislocations to 4% to 8% for anterior dislocations. Delays in initial treatment increase the frequency of this complication. The incidence of post-traumatic degenerative arthritis is similar for anterior and posterior dislocations. Recent long-term follow-up studies reveal an incidence from 24% to 60% of osteoarthritis in patients followed for over 15 years.

References

Calkins M, Zych G, Latta L, et al. Computed tomography evaluation of stability in posterior fracture dislocation of the hip. Clin Orthop 1988; 227:152.

DeLee J, Evans J, Thomas J. Anterior dislocation of the hip and associated femoral-head fractures. J Bone Joint Surg 1980; 62A:960.

Epstein H. Traumatic dislocation of the hip. Baltimore: Williams & Wilkins, 1980.

Epstein H, Wiss D, Cozen L. Posterior fracture dislocation of the hip with fractures of the femoral head. Clin Orthop 1985; 201:9.

Goulet J, Rouleau J, Mason D, et al. Comminuted fraction of the posterior wall of the acetabulum: A biomechanical evaluation of fixation methods. J Bone Joint Surg 1994; 76A:1457.

Jacob J, Rao J, Ciccarelli C. Traumatic dislocation and fracture dislocation of the hip: A long-term follow-up study. Clin Orthop 1987; 214:249.

Judet R, Judet J, LeTournel E. Fracture of the acetabulum: Classification and surgical approaches for open reduction. J Bone Joint Surg 1964; 46A:1615.

Keith J, Brewster R, Guilford W. Stability of fracture-dislocation of the hip: Quantitative assessment using computed tomography. J Bone Joint Surg 1988; 70A:711.

Kelly R, Yarborough, S. Posterior fracture-dislocation of the femoral head with retained medial head fragment. J Trauma 1971; 11:97.

Pipkin G. Treatment of grade IV fracture-dislocation of the hip. J Bone Joint Surg 1957; 39:1027.

Upadhyay S, Moulton A, Srikrishnamurthy K. An analysis of the late effects of traumatic posterior dislocation of the hip without fractures. J Bone Joint Surg 1983; 65B:150.

FRACTURE OF THE FEMORAL NECK

A. Simple anteroposterior (AP) and true lateral radiographs of the hip are usually sufficient to distinguish displaced from nondisplaced femoral neck fractures (Fig. 1). The Garden stage I and II fractures do not require preoperative manipulation prior to in situ pinning. Attempts to disimpact Stage I fractures and improve their reduction should not be made. The incidence of complications in undisturbed Stage I and II fractures that have been adequately stabilized is low. Approximately 10% to 15% of impacted femoral neck fractures displace with nonoperative treatment. Nonoperative treatment for Stage I and II fractures should be reserved for fractures that are 3 to 4 weeks old and have not yet displaced and for fractures in patients who are extremely poor operative risks. In the latter category of patients, percutaneous pinning can often be performed under local anesthesia.

B. The principles in the management of displaced femoral neck fractures include early anatomic reduction, fracture impaction, and rigid fixation. Treatment is aimed at restoring the osseous anatomy and stability of the proximal femur. In a selected population of patients, however, primary replacement of the femoral head with a hemiarthroplasty or a total hip replacement is indicated.

C. Primary femoral head replacement should be reserved mainly for elderly patients who have a limited life expectancy. Physiologic age is a better criterion than chronologic age in deciding to resort to hemiarthroplasty. Many patients over 70 years of age who have no significant medical problems should be treated by closed reduction and pinning. On the other hand, patients under 70 years of age who have an ipsilateral hemiplegia, other neurologic disease with ipsilateral spasticity, Parkinson's disease, or pathologic fracture are good candidates for primary femoral head replacement. Uncemented hemiarthroplasties should be cautiously utilized in this patient population since better results are reported with cemented hemiarthroplasty and cemented total hip replacement.

D. Any patient over the age of 50 years with pre-existing rheumatoid arthritis or osteoarthritis of the hip, metastatic disease to the acetabulum, or severe osteopenia involving both sides of the hip joint should be treated with a primary total hip replacement if the femoral neck fracture is markedly displaced. The presence of these pre-existing hip pathologies precludes a successful result with hemiarthroplasty alone.

E. The ideal time for reduction and stabilization of displaced femoral neck fractures varies with the age of the patient and the number of associated medical problems. Many retrospective studies suggest that if the patient is medically stable at the time of presentation, the morbidity and mortality associated with the femoral neck fracture is decreased if emergent reduction and stabilization is performed. If the patient has multiple unstable medical problems, however, surgery should be delayed until these problems have been adequately managed. Young patients with high-energy injuries to the femoral neck should always undergo emergency reduction and stabilization. Various techniques of closed reduction on a fracture table have been described. Impaction of the fracture fragments is essential since there is no periosteum along the femoral neck that can produce callus across the fracture site. Only an anatomic or slight valgus reduction should be accepted before proceeding with internal fixation.

F. Open reduction of a displaced femoral neck fracture can be performed through either anterior or posterior approaches. If a posterior approach is utilized, some authors recommend supplementing the fixation with a quadratus femoris muscle pedicle graft. Such a graft theoretically reduces the incidence of avascular necrosis with late segmental collapse. The results of various clinical studies do not consistently show improved results with this grafting technique. Its use is occasionally indicated in young adults with displaced subcapital or transcervical fractures and in the occasional older adult with fractures necessitating open reduction. More extensive surgery may increase the incidence of operative infection.

G. Either multiple pins (Knowles, Deyerle, Hagie, Steinmann, cancellous screws, cannulated screws) or a sliding nail or screw device can be used for internal fixation. Although some recent studies suggest improved results with multiple pin fixation, the selected implant is of less importance than the adequacy of the reduction and proper placement of the device across the fracture (Fig. 2). Risk factors for a failed fixation include advanced age, inaccurate reduction, poor mental status of the patient, inadequate number of pins, and low level of preinjury function. Several clinical studies note a higher incidence of osteonecrosis with the use of the compression hip screw as compared with the multiple cancellous screw technique. Important operative principles of internal fixation of these fractures include (1) the use of two to four pins for adequate stabilization of the fracture in all planes, (2) parallel placement of the pins, (3) placement of the threads of these pins up to the subchondral bone of the femoral head, (4) central or bull's-eye positioning of the screws within the femoral head, (5) avoiding the use of long screw threads that may span the fracture site, and (6) intraoperative impaction of the fracture.

FRACTURE OF THE FEMORAL NECK

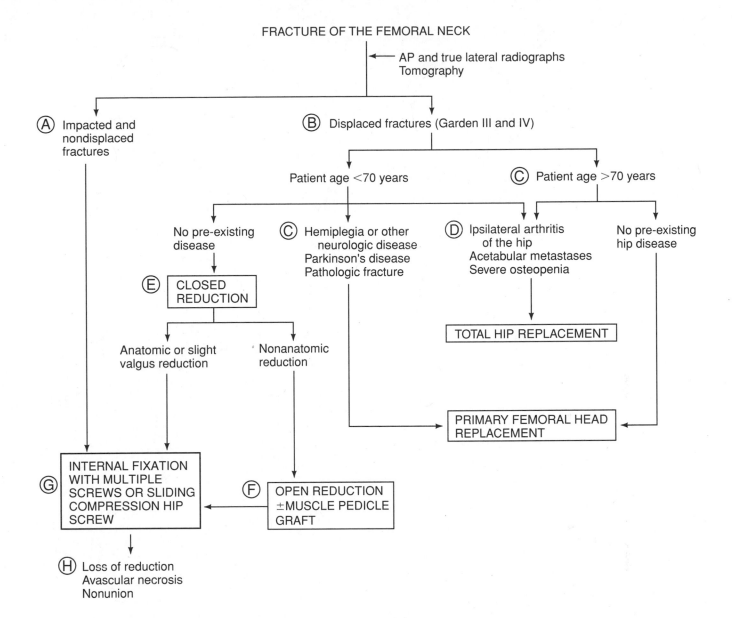

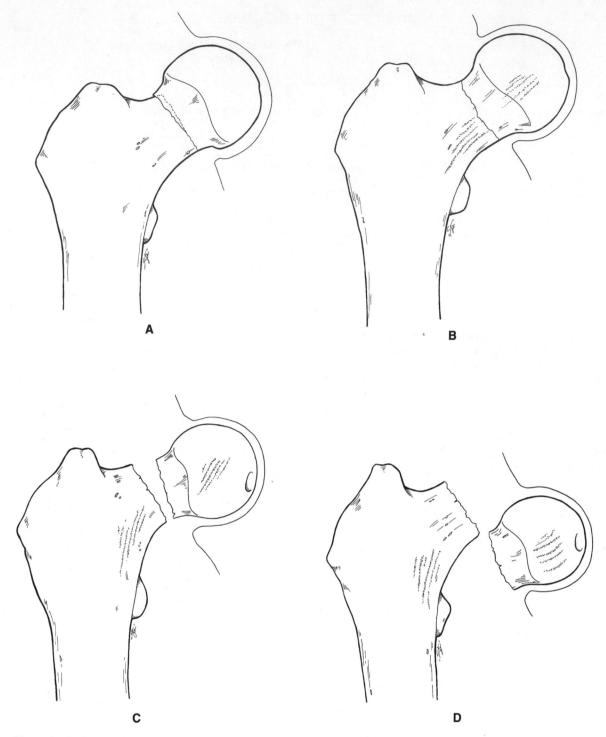

Figure 1 **A,** Garden I incomplete fracture with valgus impaction. **B,** Garden II complete, nondisplaced fracture. **C,** Garden III displaced fracture with substantial contact remaining between major fracture fragments. **D,** Garden IV completely displaced fracture.

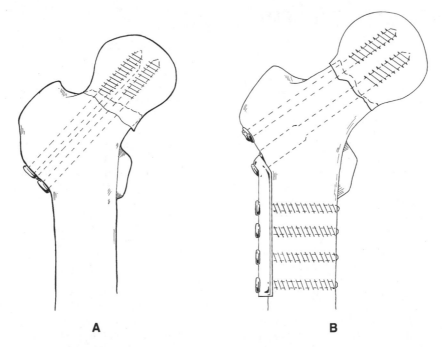

Figure 2 **A,** Ideal placement of multiple cancellous screws for the fixation of a femoral neck fracture. The screw threads completely cross the fracture site, and the shanks of the screws are parallel. **B,** Fixation of a transcervical femoral neck fracture with a compression hip screw supplemented with an interfragmental cancellous screw.

H. Avascular necrosis with segmental collapse and fracture nonunion occur most frequently in Stage III and IV displaced fractures that are incompletely reduced and inadequately stabilized. Specific variables associated with various late complications of femoral neck fractures have been well defined. The incidence of nonunions reported in the literature ranges from 10% to 30% while that of osteonecrosis ranges from 15% to 33%.

References

Barnes R, Brown J, Garden R, Nicoll E. Subcapital fractures of the femur—a prospective review. J Bone Joint Surg 1976; 58B:2.

Bentley G. The case for internal fixation of impacted femoral neck fractures. Orthop Clin North Am 1974; 5:729.

Boriani S, Bettelli G, Zimerly H, et al. Results of the multicentric Italian experience on the Gamma nail: A report on 648 cases. Orthopaedics 1991; 14:1307.

Dorr L. Treatment of femoral neck fractures with total hip replacement versus cemented and noncemented hemiarthroplasty. J Arthroplasty 1986; 1:21.

Eiskjaer S, Ostgard S. Risk factors influencing mortality after bipolar hemiarthroplasty in the treatment of fracture of the femoral neck. Clin Orthop 1991; 270:295.

Evarts M. The use of quadratus femoris muscle pedicle bone graft for the treatment of displaced femoral neck fractures. Orthopedics 1985; 8:972.

Garden RS. Reduction and fixation of subcapital fractures of the femur. Orthop Clin North Am 1974; 5:683.

Leung K, So W, Lam T, et al. Treatment of ipsilateral femoral shaft fractures and hip fractures. Injury 1993; 24:41.

Linde F. Avascular femoral head necrosis following fracture fixation. Injury 1986; 17:159.

Madsen F. Fixation of displaced femoral neck fractures: A comparison between sliding screw plate and four cancellous bone screws. Acta Orthop Scand 1987; 58:212.

Meyers M, Moore T, Harvey J. Displaced fracture of the femoral neck treated with a muscle pedicle graft with emphasis on the treatment of those fractures in young adults. J Bone Joint Surg 1975; 51A:718.

Mullen J, Mullen N. Hip fracture mortality: A prospective multifactorial study to predict and minimize death risk. Clin Orthop 1992; 280:214.

Sexson S, Lehner J. Factors affecting hip fracture mortality. J Orthop Trauma 1988; 1:290.

Swiontkowski M, Winquist R, Hansen S. Fractures of the femoral neck in patients between the ages of twelve and forty-nine years. J Bone Joint Surg 1984; 66A:837.

Welch R. The rationale for primary hemiarthroplasty in the treatment of fractures of the femoral neck in elderly patients. Hip 1983; 11:42.

INTERTROCHANTERIC FRACTURE

A. Intertrochanteric fracture, predominantly an injury of the elderly, has a high mortality rate. Rapid patient mobilization following surgical stabilization of the fracture lessens the frequency of life-threatening complications such as cardiopulmonary failure and thromboembolic disease. It also minimizes the incidence of decubitus ulcers and limb contractures. Most intertrochanteric fractures are four-part injuries with a secondary comminution of the greater and lesser trochanters. Proper classification of these injuries necessitates a good quality anteroposterior (AP) radiograph with the hip in internal rotation.

B. Surgical reduction and internal fixation should be performed as soon as the patient is medically stable. Although the incidence of osteonecrosis and other healing problems are not influenced by the timing of surgery, the potential for medical complications is significantly lessened by early surgical intervention. Closed reduction should be performed with the patient under anesthesia on a fracture table. With the hip in slight abduction and external rotation, direct traction is applied to the leg and the reduction is confirmed by fluoroscopy. The goal of the closed reduction should be to restore the normal neck shaft angle.

C. Successful reduction restores the osseous stability by achieving medial cortical abutment or impaction of the major fracture fragments in a normal or slight valgus alignment. A sliding nail or screw plate device is preferred since it permits controlled intraoperative compression of the fracture and telescopes postoperatively. This allows the fracture to settle in a stable position and prevents nail protrusion through the femoral head. The sliding characteristics of a screw plate device, such as the dynamic hip screw, depends on the angle of the device used (the 150° device has improved sliding characteristics) and the proper selection of the screw length so that the shank of the screw deeply engages the barrel on the plate (Fig. 1). The device should act effectively as an internal splint. Recent retrospective studies show that the adequacy of the reduction is as important a variable as the above mechanical considerations in determining the sliding characteristics of a compression hip screw. All sliding occurs during the first 30 days after fixation.

The stability afforded by a screw plate device is largely dependent on (1) the bone quality, (2) the fragment geometry, (3) the adequacy of the reduction, (4) the implant placement, and (5) the implant design. Complications arise when the surgical construct is inadequate to withstand the major forces to which the proximal femur is subjected. Complications include varus settling of the fracture, cutting out or protrusion of the nail or screw, and fatigue failure of the implant. Relative contraindications to surgery are a contaminated wound at the operative site, septicemia, and a delay in treatment of more than 3 weeks.

D. The preferred treatment for unstable intertrochanteric fractures depends more on the physiologic age of the patient and the degree of osteopenia of the proximal femur than on the strict chronologic age of the patient. Many healthy patients over 70 years of age who have good bone stock should be treated with anatomical reduction of all major fracture fragments so as to avoid the complications of shortening and external rotation at the fracture site.

E. Reconstitution of the medial buttress of unstable fractures by interfragmental compression screws decreases the likelihood of limb shortening and abductor insufficiency. Most patients under 70 years of age, and active patients over 70 years of age, benefit from this additional surgery. Severe medial comminution or advanced osteoporosis may preclude successful interfragmental fixation. Consider routine cancellous bone grafting of the medial cortical defect, especially in young patients with unstable fractures.

F. Elderly nonambulatory patients who have minimal symptoms related to their fracture can be treated with early mobilization out of bed. Shortening, varus angulation of the fracture site, and external rotation of the leg are expected with this treatment.

INTERTROCHANTERIC FRACTURE

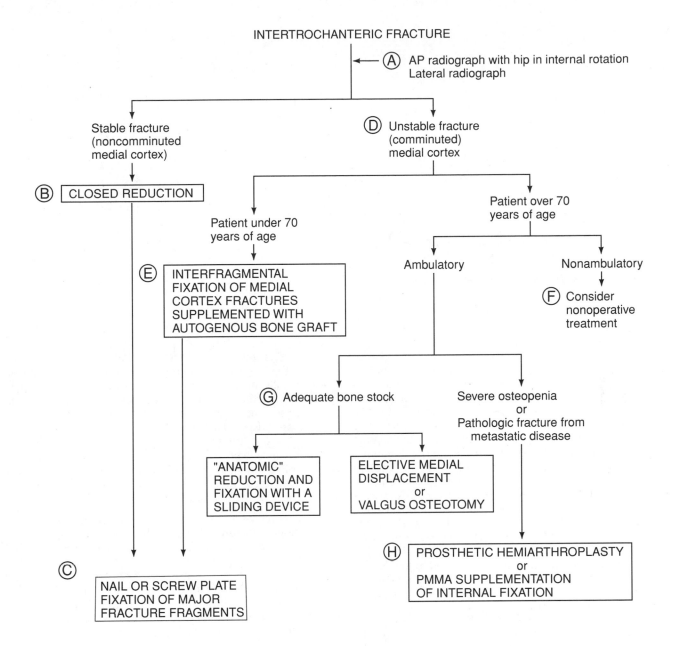

A AP radiograph with hip in internal rotation
   Lateral radiograph

Stable fracture
(noncomminuted
medial cortex)

D Unstable fracture
   (comminuted)
   medial cortex

B CLOSED REDUCTION

Patient under 70
years of age

Patient over 70
years of age

E INTERFRAGMENTAL
   FIXATION OF MEDIAL
   CORTEX FRACTURES
   SUPPLEMENTED WITH
   AUTOGENOUS BONE GRAFT

Ambulatory

Nonambulatory

F Consider
   nonoperative
   treatment

G Adequate bone stock

Severe osteopenia
or
Pathologic fracture from
metastatic disease

"ANATOMIC"
REDUCTION AND
FIXATION WITH A
SLIDING DEVICE

ELECTIVE MEDIAL
DISPLACEMENT
or
VALGUS OSTEOTOMY

H PROSTHETIC HEMIARTHROPLASTY
   or
   PMMA SUPPLEMENTATION
   OF INTERNAL FIXATION

C

NAIL OR SCREW PLATE
FIXATION OF MAJOR
FRACTURE FRAGMENTS

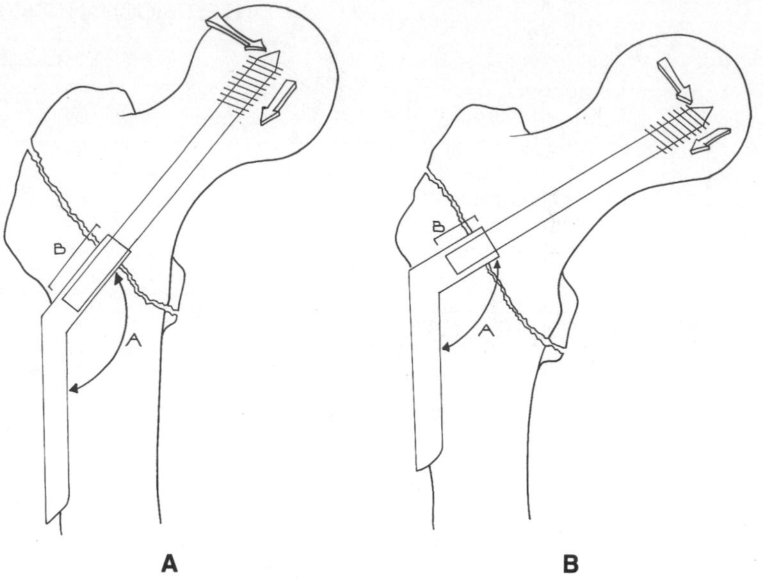

Figure 1 The sliding properties of a compression hip screw depend on the angle of the barrel/plate **(A)** and the engagement of the shank of the lag screw in the barrel **(B)**. A 135° barrel/plate implant has poorer sliding properties than one with a 150° angle. Minimal engagement of the lag screw in the barrel **(B)** lessens its sliding properties.

A **B**

G. Unstable fractures in elderly ambulatory patients with adequate bone stock may be managed by one of two techniques. First, the major head/neck and shaft fragments are aligned on the fracture table so that the femoral length is restored without concern for the trochanteric fractures. A sliding nail or screw plate implant allows postoperative settling and stabilization of the fracture as necessary. This technique is referred to as an "anatomic" reduction. Alternatively, intraoperative medial bony contact and stability are achieved by medial displacement of the shaft fragment or valgus osteotomy. Although these procedures obviate the need for "anatomically" nailed fractures to migrate into a stable position, they do shorten the limb and the abductor mechanism. Limb shortening, limp, and often external rotation can be expected following this type of surgery. The versatile compression hip screw is the most popular device for unstable fractures managed by any of these techniques.

Condylocephalic nails (Enders, Harris) have been advocated for the fixation of intertrochanteric fractures. Theoretically, these implants involve less blood loss, a lower rate of infection, and less surgical time than the use of compression hip screw. Clinical results, however, have been disappointing with a high rate of complications, including knee pain at the distal tips of the nails, external rotation deformities, and varus settling of the fracture.

New intramedullary rod/screw implants (e.g., the Gamma nail) have been recommended for unstable intertrochanteric fractures but data from clinical trials with these nails show few advantages, if any, over those of the compression hip screw.

H. Patients with markedly advanced osteopenia or pathologic fracture of the intertrochanteric area from metastatic disease may not be adequately stabilized by any of the above methods. Prosthetic hemiarthroplasty using a Leinbach, Rosenfield, or other calcar replacement prostheses can be used in such patients. Alternatively, a nail or screw plate implant supplemented with polymethylmethacrylate (PMMA) can be employed for stabilization of such injuries.

References

Cobilli N, Sadler A. Ender rod versus compression screw fixation of hip fractures. Clin Orthop 1985; 201:123.

Dimon J, Hughston J. Unstable intertrochanteric fractures of the hip. J Bone Joint Surg 1967; 49A:440.

Goldhagen P, O'Connor D, Schwarze D, et al. A prospective comparative study of the compression hip screw and the Gamma nail. J Orthop Trauma 1994; 8:367.

Gurtler R, Jacobs R, Jacobs C. Biomechanical evaluation of the Ender's pins, the Harris nail, and the dynamic hip screw for the unstable intertrochanteric fracture. Clin Orthop 1986; 206:109.

Harrington K. The use of methylmethacrylate as an adjunct in internal fixation of unstable comminuted intertrochanteric fracture in osteoporotic patients. J Bone Joint Surg 1975; 57A:744.

Kaufer H, Mathews L, Sonstegard D. Stable fixation of intertrochanteric fractures. J Bone Joint Surg 1974; 56A:899.

Kyle R. Fixation of intertrochanteric hip fractures with sliding devices. AAOS Instructional Course Lectures 1984; 33:197.

Kyle R, Wright T, Burstein A. Biomechanical analysis of the sliding characteristics of compression hip screws. J Bone Joint Surg 1980; 62A:1308.

Lindsey K, Teal P, Probe R, et al. Early experience with the Gamma interlocking nail for pertrochanteric fractures of the proximal femur. J Trauma 1991; 31:1649.

Mahaisavariya B, Laupattarakasem W. Cracking of the femoral shaft by the Gamma nail. Injury 1992; 23:493.

Mahomed N, Harrington I, Kellam J, et al. Biomechanical analysis of the Gamma nail and sliding hip screw. Clin Orthop 1994; 304:280.

Radford P, Needoff M, Webb J. A prospective randomised comparison of the dynamic hip screw and the Gamma locking nail. J Bone Joint Surg 1993; 75B:789.

Sarmiento A, Williams E. The unstable intertrochanteric fracture; treatment with a valgus osteotomy and I-beam nail plate. J Bone Joint Surg 1970; 52A:1309.

Steinberg G, Desai S, Kornwitz N, et al. The intertrochanteric hip fracture: A retrospective analysis. Orthopedics 1988; 11:265.

Stern M, Angerman A. Comminuted intertrochanteric fractures treated with a Leinbach prosthesis. Clin Orthop 1987; 218:75.

Stern M, Goldstein T. The use of the Leinbach prosthesis in intertrochanteric fractures of the hip. Clin Orthop 1977; 128:325.

Williams W, Parker B. Complications associated with the use of the Gamma nail. Injury 1992; 23:291.

SUBTROCHANTERIC FRACTURE

A. Subtrochanteric fractures of the femur may be either high-energy injuries from motor vehicle accidents or, in elderly patients, low-energy injuries from falls. The preferred treatment and expected outcomes are different for these two types of injuries. The major problems with subtrochanteric fractures are malunion and nonunion. These frequent complications can be attributed to the slow healing of the cortical bone in the subtrochanteric area, the strong muscle forces acting on the bone, and the major biomechanical stresses at this level with normal ambulation. Nonoperative management has traditionally yielded unsatisfactory results because of the persistence of deformity and shortening at the fracture site. The successful surgical management of these injuries hinges on an accurate assessment of the fracture geometry and proper selection of fixation implants.

B. The Seinsheimer classification of subtrochanteric fractures is based on the number of parts to the fracture (Fig. 1):
   I. Nondisplaced or minimally displaced (less than 2 mm in any plane)
   II. Two-part fractures
      A. Transverse fracture
      B. Oblique or spiral fracture with the lesser trochanter attached to the proximal fragment
      C. Oblique or spiral fracture with the lesser trochanter attached to the distal fragment
   III. Three-part fractures
      A. Spiral fracture with the lesser trochanter as a third fragment
      B. Spiral fracture with a lateral butterfly fragment
   IV. Comminuted fractures with four or more major fragments
   V. Subtrochanteric—intertrochanteric fractures

The stability of subtrochanteric fractures depends on the integrity of the medial cortex. If the medial cortex is intact, a lateral plate can act as a tension band fixation. If, however, the medial cortex is absent, bending (and therefore tensile) stresses are placed on the lateral plate. Therefore, an accurate assessment of the degree of comminution of both the greater trochanter and the medial cortical buttress of the proximal femur is imperative in the proper selection of a fixation implant.

C. The goal of surgery is to create a stable osteosynthesis of the subtrochanteric fracture. No single implant or method of fixation is effective for all fracture patterns. Because of the high incidence of implant failure, it is critical that the proper implant be chosen. This decision is based mainly on the fracture geometry and the anticipated problems with fracture healing.

D. True subtrochanteric fractures with intact greater trochanters and lesser trochanters are ideally treated with closed reduction and stabilization with a locked intramedullary nail. Closed reduction decreases the likelihood of postoperative infection and minimizes any additional soft tissue injury that may impede fracture union. Locked intramedullary nails have a mechanical advantage over any form of blade or screw plate device. It is important that the fracture be distal enough to allow for the proximal locking screw to engage both the greater trochanter and the medial cortex of the proximal fragment. Recent reports note a 98% union rate and a very low implant failure rate with the use of commercially available interlocking nails.

E. Subtrochanteric fractures with comminution of the medial cortex (Seinsheimer Types IIIA and IV) are not amenable to first-generation locked intramedullary nailing. The choice of implants depends on the degree of comminution and the experience of the surgeon. Preferred implants include the condylar blade or screw plate fixation with bone grafting (Fig. 2), the Zickel nail, or the Russell-Taylor femoral reconstruction nail. The Seinsheimer Type IIIA fractures, especially those with long spiral components greater than 8 cm in length, account for many of the implant failures with more traditional forms of fixation. Seinsheimer Type IIC fractures are also difficult to manage despite the lack of medial comminution because of the major shear forces acting at the fracture site. These particular fractures are ideally treated with a femoral reconstruction nail. Many variants of second-generation interlocking nails are now available.

   Problems during extraction of Zickel nails have recently been described. Due to the rigid, curved design of the Zickel nail, refracture of the proximal femur at a level different from the original fracture can occur during its removal in young patients. The device is therefore not recommended in young patients with subtrochanteric fractures.

F. The technical difficulties with each of these forms of fixation vary. If a blade or screw plate device is used, it is important to supplement the proximal fragment fixation with two screws from the plate into that fragment. The purchase of the blade or screw alone is usually not sufficient to provide stable osteosynthesis. The dynamic condylar screw, designed for use in the distal femur, has been applied to these difficult fracture patterns and has been found to provide improved purchase of the proximal fragment. Supplementary bone graft in all of these patients is recommended as is delayed weight bearing until complete fracture healing has occurred.

   Enders nails have been largely abandoned as a form of fixation because of their high rate of complications and reoperations. Gamma nails (intramedullary nail/sliding screw device) have recently been introduced for high subtrochanteric fractures.

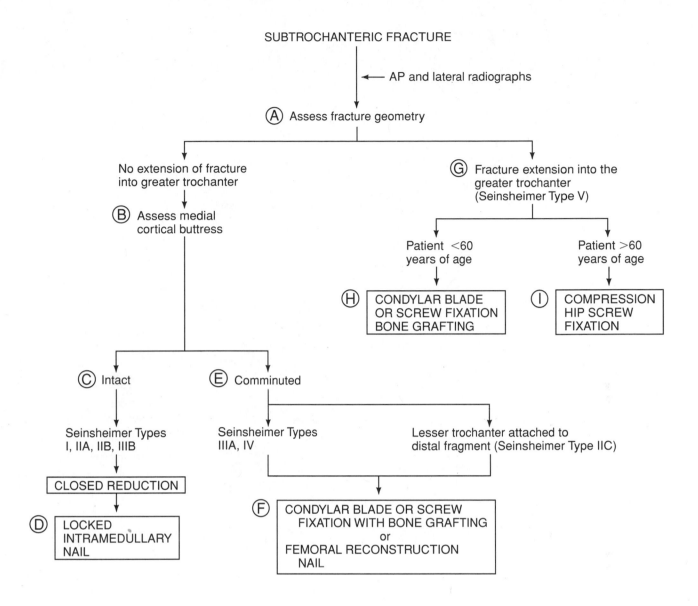

SUBTROCHANTERIC FRACTURE

← AP and lateral radiographs

Ⓐ Assess fracture geometry

No extension of fracture into greater trochanter

Ⓑ Assess medial cortical buttress

Ⓖ Fracture extension into the greater trochanter (Seinsheimer Type V)

Patient <60 years of age

Patient >60 years of age

Ⓗ CONDYLAR BLADE OR SCREW FIXATION BONE GRAFTING

Ⓘ COMPRESSION HIP SCREW FIXATION

Ⓒ Intact

Ⓔ Comminuted

Seinsheimer Types I, IIA, IIB, IIIB

Seinsheimer Types IIIA, IV

Lesser trochanter attached to distal fragment (Seinsheimer Type IIC)

CLOSED REDUCTION

Ⓓ LOCKED INTRAMEDULLARY NAIL

Ⓕ CONDYLAR BLADE OR SCREW FIXATION WITH BONE GRAFTING or FEMORAL RECONSTRUCTION NAIL

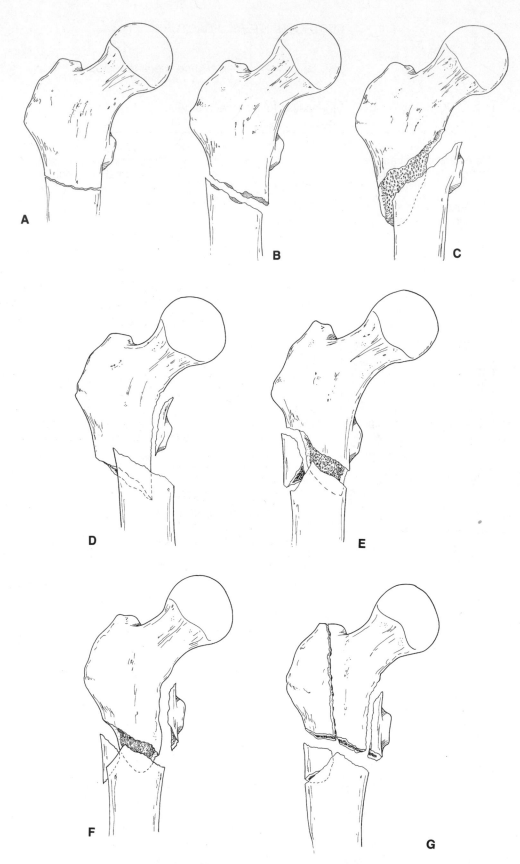

Figure 1 Seinsheimer classification of subtrochanteric fractures. **A,** Nondisplaced (Type I). **B,** Two-part fracture (Type IIB). **C,** Two-part fracture with lesser trochanter attached to the distal fragment (Type IIC). **D,** Type IIIA fracture. **E,** Type IIIB fracture. **F,** Comminuted subtrochanteric fracture (Type IV). **G,** Subtrochanteric—intertrochanteric fracture (Type V).

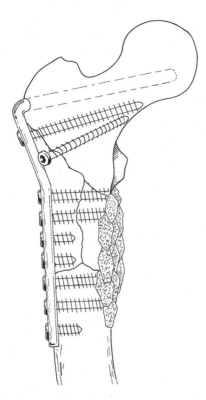

Figure 2 Fixation of a Type IV subtrochanteric fracture with a 95° condylar blade plate and autogenous bone grafting.

G. Subtrochanteric fractures with comminution extending up to the greater trochanter (Seinsheimer Type V) are not amenable to intramedullary fixation. The preferred implant in such comminuted fractures is dependent on the physiologic age of the patient, the degree of comminution of the fracture, the fracture geometry, and the quality of the bone stock.

H. Patients under 60 years of age who have adequate bone stock can be managed with a condylar blade or screw plate fixation. Consider supplemental stabilization of the greater trochanter with interfragmental screws and routine bone grafting of the medial cortical defects.

I. While the compression hip screw can be used for nearly any pattern of subtrochanteric fracture, it is ideally suited for the comminuted Seinsheimer Type V injuries in elderly patients with osteopenia. The compression hip screw permits controlled shortening at the fracture site with maintenance of the normal neck-shaft angle.

References

Alho A, Ekeland A, Stromsoe K. Subtrochanteric femoral fracture treated with locked intramedullary nails. Acta Orthop Scand 1991; 62:573.

Blatter G, Janssen M. Treatment of subtrochanteric fractures of the femur: Reduction on the traction table and fixation with dynamic condylar screw. Arch Orthop Trauma Surg 1994; 113:138.

Brien W, Wiss D, Becker V, et al. Subtrochanteric femur fractures: A comparison of the Zickel nail, 95 degree blade plate, and interlocking nail. J Orthop Trauma 1991; 5:458.

Brumback R, Garbarino J, Poka A, Burgess A. Closed interlocking intramedullary nailing of subtrochanteric fractures. Presentation to the 54th Annual Meeting of the AAOS, 1987.

Dobozi W, Larson B, Zindrick M, et al. Flexible intramedullary nailing of subtrochanteric fractures of the femur: A multicenter analysis. Clin Orthop 1986; 212:68.

Fielding W, Cochran G, Zickel R. Biomechanical characteristics and surgical management of subtrochanteric fractures. Orthop Clin North Am 1974; 5:629–650.

Mullaji A, Thomas T. Low-energy subtrochanteric fractures in elderly patients: Results of fixation with the sliding screw plate. J Trauma 1993; 34:56.

Ovadia D, Chess J. Intraoperative and postoperative subtrochanteric fracture of the femur associated with removal of the Zickel nail. J Bone Joint Surg 1988; 70A:239.

Ruff M, Zubbers L. Treatment of subtrochanteric fractures with a sliding screw-plate device. J Trauma 1986; 26:75.

Schatzker J, Waddell J. Subtrochanteric fractures of the femur. Orthop Clin North Am 1980; 11:539.

Seinsheimer F. Subtrochanteric fractures of the femur. J Bone Joint Surg 1978; 60A:300.

Thomas W, Villar R. Subtrochanteric fractures: Zickel nail or nail-plate? J Bone Joint Surg 1986; 68B:255.

Trafton P. Subtrochanteric-intertrochanteric femoral fractures. Orthop Clin North Am 1987; 18:49.

Waddell J. Subtrochanteric fractures of the femur: A review of 130 patients. J Trauma 1979; 19:582.

Wiss D, Brien W, Peter K, Merritt P. Subtrochanteric fractures of the femur. Presentation to the 54th Annual Meeting of the AAOS, 1987.

Zickel R. Subtrochanteric femoral fractures. Orthop Clin North Am 1980; 11:555.

FRACTURE OF THE FEMORAL SHAFT

Femoral shaft fractures in adults are ideally treated by a rigid intramedullary nail, preferably inserted by the closed technique. Available implants, including the Kuntscher, ASIF, and a variety of interlocking nails, allow early mobilization and functional use of the injured extremity with maintenance of satisfactory length and alignment of the fracture. Therapeutic decision making centers on the timing of closed nailing, the potential for intraoperative and postoperative complications, and the need for adjunctive locking screws.

A. Evaluate preoperative femur radiographs for fracture location, anatomy, and comminution. Seek radiographic evidence for nondisplaced longitudinal cortical splits in otherwise simple transverse or short oblique fractures. The Winquist classification for comminution includes: Type I fracture, which has a very small butterfly fragment involving 25% or less of the width of the bone; Type II fracture, in which a larger butterfly fragment involves up to 50% or less of the width of the bone; Type III fracture, which consists of a very large butterfly fragment representing more than 50% of the width of the bone with only a very small spike of bone remaining intact; and Type IV fracture, which has comminution over an entire segment of bone (Fig. 1). A routine pelvis radiograph detects concomitant hip fractures or dislocations. The presence of an ipsilateral intertrochanteric or femoral neck injury may necessitate the selection of an alternative form of fixation, such as a femoral reconstructive nail, for the femoral shaft fracture.

B. Most femoral shaft fractures are high energy injuries and thus are often associated with major abdominal, pelvic, or thoracic visceral injuries and significant bleeding into the thigh. Immobilize the shaft fractures with skeletal traction during the emergency evaluation of blood loss and possible life-threatening injuries. If nailing is delayed for more than several days, it is imperative to radiographically document distraction of the fracture. Longitudinal traction with 25 to 40 lbs of weight usually ensures adequate distraction.

　　The thigh contains three distinct fascial compartments. The anterior compartment encases the quadriceps femoris, sartorius, iliacus, psoas, and pectineus muscles, as well as the femoral artery and vein, femoral nerve, and lateral femoral cutaneous nerve. The medial compartment contains the gracilis, adductor longus, adductor brevis, adductor magnus, and obturator externus muscles along with the profundus femoris artery, obturator artery and vein, and the obturator nerve. The contents of the posterior compartment include the biceps femoris, semitendinosus, semimembranosus, and a portion of the abductor magnus muscles as well as branches of the profundus femoris artery, sciatic nerve, and posterior femoral cutaneous nerve. The thick lateral intermuscular septum divides the anterior and posterior compartments. The medial and posterior intermuscular septa are

much thinner. Due to the high volume of these three compartments, compartmental syndrome of the thigh is much less common than that of the leg. Significant bleeding into one or more compartments is necessary to elevate the compartment pressure above the critical level. The distinction between the normal swelling and hemorrhage after a shaft fracture and the findings of an early thigh compartmental syndrome often requires the measurement of intracompartmental pressures.

C. The preferred treatment for open femoral shaft fractures has changed significantly in the last 10 years. Traditionally these injuries have been managed by thorough wound debridement, delayed wound closure, and either delayed nailing or traction/cast brace treatment. Recent series indicate a low infection and nonunion rate with primary nailing of open femoral shaft fractures immediately following thorough debridement of the wound. Individualize the treatment of Grade III open fractures based on the soft tissue loss and the degree of contamination of the soft tissues. Never perform an immediate nailing of an open femoral shaft fracture with gross medullary contamination. Utilize external fixation if there is inadequate muscular coverage of the fracture or gross contamination of the wound.

D. The ideal timing for closed nailing of femoral shaft fractures depends largely on the presence or absence of multiple injuries. The incidence of pulmonary complications including adult respiratory distress syndrome is increased in polytrauma patients if nailing is delayed. The benefits of immediate nailing of isolated femur fractures are less evident and elective nailing is not associated with an unacceptably high rate of pulmonary complications.

E. Classify fracture comminution preoperatively and intraoperatively to determine the degree of locking of fracture fragments necessary to achieve a stable surgical construct. Midshaft fractures with no comminution or Type I comminution can be safely managed by an unlocked nail or a dynamically locked nail. Most Type II, III, and IV fractures, especially when they are far proximal or distal to the medullary isthmus, should undergo static nailing with both proximal and distal locking screws. At many trauma centers, all shaft fractures, regardless of their degree of comminution, are treated with static locking. Routine dynamization of statically locked fractures by removal of the proximal and/or distal bolts is not necessary for the stimulation of fracture healing and remodeling. The clinical results of large series of femoral shaft fractures managed by interlocking nails has demonstrated far superior results to those reported with other forms of treatment. The improved results are even greater if only severely comminuted (Winquist Type III or IV) injuries are considered.

FEMORAL SHAFT FRACTURE

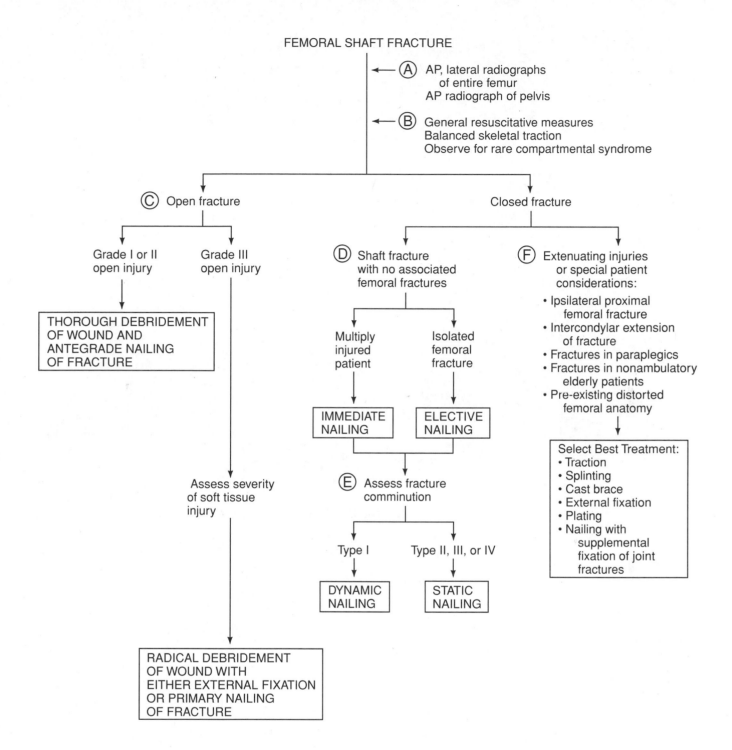

Ⓐ AP, lateral radiographs
of entire femur
AP radiograph of pelvis

Ⓑ General resuscitative measures
Balanced skeletal traction
Observe for rare compartmental syndrome

Ⓒ Open fracture

Closed fracture

Grade I or II
open injury

Grade III
open injury

Ⓓ Shaft fracture
with no associated
femoral fractures

Ⓕ Extenuating injuries
or special patient
considerations:

- Ipsilateral proximal
  femoral fracture
- Intercondylar extension
  of fracture
- Fractures in paraplegics
- Fractures in nonambulatory
  elderly patients
- Pre-existing distorted
  femoral anatomy

THOROUGH DEBRIDEMENT
OF WOUND AND
ANTEGRADE NAILING
OF FRACTURE

Multiply
injured
patient

Isolated
femoral
fracture

IMMEDIATE
NAILING

ELECTIVE
NAILING

Select Best Treatment:
- Traction
- Splinting
- Cast brace
- External fixation
- Plating
- Nailing with
  supplemental
  fixation of joint
  fractures

Assess severity
of soft tissue
injury

Ⓔ Assess fracture
comminution

Type I

Type II, III, or IV

DYNAMIC
NAILING

STATIC
NAILING

RADICAL DEBRIDEMENT
OF WOUND WITH
EITHER EXTERNAL FIXATION
OR PRIMARY NAILING
OF FRACTURE

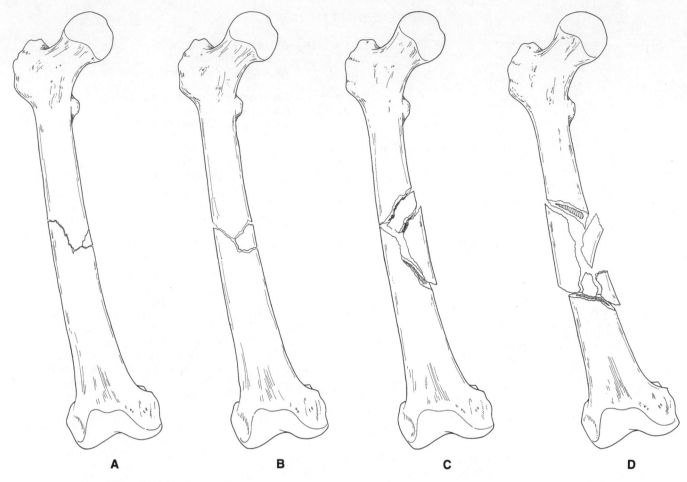

Figure 1 Winquist classification of femoral shaft fractures. **A,** Type I. **B,** Type II. **C,** Type III. **D,** Type IV.

F. Treatment other than interlocking nailing is indicated in certain complex injury patterns and in special patient populations. Ipsilateral proximal femoral fractures or intercondylar extension of distal third fractures may preclude the successful use of standard interlocking nails. Fractures in paraplegic patients and in nonambulatory elderly patients can often be treated with simple splinting and/or careful casting. Patients with pre-existing distorted anatomy of the femoral canal from previous injury or systemic bone disease are often best treated using other forms of internal or external support.

References

Berhman M, Tornetta P, Kerira M, et al. Femur fractures caused by gunshots: Treatment by immediate reamed intramedullary nailing. J Trauma 1993; 34:783.

Bone L, et al. Early versus delayed stabilization of femoral fractures. A prospective randomized study. J Bone Joint Surg 1989; 71A:336.

Bosse M, Coras A, Anderson L. A preliminary experience with the Russell-Taylor reconstruction nail for complex femoral fractures. J Trauma 1992; 32:71.

Browner B. Pitfalls, errors and complications in the use of locking Kuntscher nails. Clin Orthop 1986; 212:192.

Brumback R. Fracture healing with static interlocking femoral fixation: Is dynamization necessary? J Bone Joint Surg 1988; 70A:1453.

Brumback R, et al. Intramedullary nailing of open fractures of the femoral shaft. J Bone Joint Surg 1989; 71A:1324.

Brumback R, Ellison T, Poka A, et al. Intramedullary nailing of femoral shaft fractures: Part III—Long-term effects of static interlocking fixation. J Bone Joint Surg 1992; 74:106.

Brumback R, Reilly T, Poka A, et al. Decision errors with interlocking intramedullary femoral fixation: To lock or not to lock? J Bone Joint Surg 1988; 70A:1441.

Bucholz R, Jones A. Current concepts review: Fracture of the shaft of the femur. J Bone Joint Surg 1991; 73A:1561.

Dabezies E, D'Ambrosia R, Shoji H, et al. Fractures of the femoral shaft treated by external fixation with the Wagner device. J Bone Joint Surg 1984; 66A:360.

Grosse A, Christie J, Taglang G, et al. Open adult femoral shaft fracture treated by early intramedullary nailing. J Bone Joint Surg 1993; 75B:562.

Kempf I, Grosse A, Beck G. Closed locked intramedullary nailing: Its application to comminuted fractures of the femur. J Bone Joint Surg 1985; 67A:709.

Kuntscher G. Practice of intramedullary nailing. Springfield, IL: Charles C Thomas, 1967.

Llowe D, Hansen S. Immediate nailing of open fractures of the femoral shaft. J Bone Joint Surg 1988; 70A:812.

Meggitt B, Juett D, Smith J. Cast-bracing for fractures of the femoral shaft. J Bone Joint Surg 1981; 63B:12.

Montgomery S, Mooney V. Femur fractures: Treatment with roller traction and early ambulation. Clin Orthop 1981; 165:196.

Pape H, Aufimokolk M, Paffrath T, et al. Primary intramedullary femur fixations in multiple trauma patients with associated lung contusion: A cause of posttraumatic ARDS? J Trauma 1993; 34:540.

Riemer B, Butterfield S, Burke C, et al. Immediate plate fixation of highly comminuted femoral diaphyseal fractures in blunt polytrauma patients. Orthopaedics 1992; 15:907.

Tarlow S, Achterman C, Hayhurst J, et al. Acute compartmental syndrome in the thigh complicating fractures of the femur. A report of three cases. J Bone Joint Surg 1986; 68A:1439.

Thoresen B, Alho A, Ekeland A, et al. Interlocking intramedullary nailing in femoral shaft fractures: A report of 48 cases. J Bone Joint Surg 1985; 67A:1313.

Winquist R, Hansen S, Clawson K. Closed intramedullary nailing of femoral fractures. A report of 520 cases. J Bone Joint Surg 1984; 66A:529.

Wu C, Shih C, Veng W, et al. Treatment of segmental femoral shaft fractures. Clin Orthop 1993; 287:224.

CLOSED INTRAMEDULLARY NAILING OF THE FEMUR

A. Most femoral shaft fractures are ideally treated by intramedullary nailing within 24 hours of the time of injury. If the surgical procedure is delayed, preoperative traction of the fracture, using skeletal traction of 25 to 40 lbs, facilitates fracture reduction on the operative table. If the nailing is delayed for more than 2 to 3 days, obtain a lateral radiograph of the femur demonstrating satisfactory distraction of the fracture fragments. If a complete stock of nails of variable length and width is not available, preoperative measurement of femoral length is necessary to anticipate nail length and width. Preoperative measurement can be accomplished by clinical measurement of the contralateral femur from the trochanter to the knee joint, radiographic determination of femoral length by taping a nail of known length to the thigh of the opposite leg, or the use of the Kuntscher ossimeter. The probable width of the nail to be used is 1 to 2 mm greater than the isthmal medullary width measured on the anteroposterior (AP) radiograph. Smaller diameter nonslotted nails can also be used without increased risk of implant failure.

B. Supine positioning of the patient on the fracture table is preferred in cases of multiple injuries, bilateral femur fractures, unstable spinal fractures, and major pelvic ring disruptions. Lateral positioning is indicated in obese patients and patients with fractures in the proximal third of the shaft (Fig. 1). Nail most femoral shaft fractures using the most familiar position. If the full lateral position on a McKay or comparable fracture table is used, place the patient's hip at slight adduction and moderate flexion. Apply traction through the proximal tibial or distal femoral Steinmann pin, thus permitting flexion of the knee. For most femoral shaft fractures inserting a distal femoral pin as far anterior and distal in the femoral condyles as possible is preferred. Insert such a pin under fluoroscopic control prior to turning the patient on the fracture table. Flex the knee 60° or more to avoid sciatic nerve stretch injury. Internal rotation of the leg of 10° to 15° in relation to the floor usually guarantees correct rotatory alignment of fracture fragments. Achieve satisfactory reduction of the fracture in both the AP and lateral planes before the preparation and draping of the leg. The proximal fragment is usually flexed and adducted in relation to the distal fragment. Correct adduction by lowering the leg or supporting the proximal fragment with a crutch under the thigh. Easily overcome flexion by gentle external pressure over the anterior proximal aspect of the thigh. The entire femur from the femoral neck to the femoral condyles must be easily visible in both planes on the image intensifier.

C. If near anatomic reduction in both planes is not accomplished, manipulation of the leg out of traction may be necessary. Correct minor degrees of fracture translation intraoperatively by the techniques described below.

D. The ideal location for the trochanteric entrance hole is the trochanteric fossa, located just medial to the tip of the trochanter and slightly posterior to the midline of the trochanter. This point is in the center of the longitudinal axes of the medullary canal in both the AP and mediolateral planes (Fig. 2). Eccentric reaming and medial comminution of the proximal fragment are complications that occur frequently when an entrance hole is made too far laterally. Such intraoperative comminution is especially common in proximal third fractures in which supine positioning of the patient is utilized.

E. Use any standard medullary instrumentation with flexible reamers. Pass a straight bulb-tipped guide rod across the fracture into the distal fragment down to the distal femoral subchondral bone. If minor residual translatory displacement of the fracture makes passage of the guide rod difficult, use the following maneuvers: bend the end of the guide rod; place external pressure on the thigh with crutches, lead-gloved hands, or retractors; or insert a narrow 9 or 10 mm nail into the proximal fragment to serve as a lever for fracture reduction.

F. Commence reaming with a 9-mm end cutting flexible reamer and then proceed at 0.5-mm increments. In proximal and midshaft fractures, cortical contact of the nail of at least 2 to 3 cm on either side of the fracture is desirable in simple Kuntscher nailings. Overreaming of the proximal fragment of 0.5-mm greater than the nail to be used is recommended to avoid incarceration and operative comminution of the fracture. Use overreaming of 1.0 to 1.5 mm for interlocking nails, especially those with an unslotted design, such as the Russell-Taylor nail. The variable degree of anterior bow of the proximal fragment makes routine overreaming of 1 full mm advisable in all distal shaft fractures whether a simple Kuntscher nail or an interlocking nail is being used.

G. Intraoperative measurement of the guide rod in the femur yields a precise optimal length for the nail. For fractures with Winquist IV comminution it is important to consider not only the length of the guide rod but also its location in the distal fragment and the preoperative measurements of the ideal femoral length. The selected pre-bent nail is then driven over a nail guide rod. When the tip of the nail reaches the fracture site, achieve anatomic reduction again by external pressure on the thigh. If the fracture is located at the femoral isthmus, release longitudinal traction once the nail is several centimeters across the fracture site to avoid distraction of the fracture. Also check rotation of the distal fragment prior to fully driving the nail down into the distal fragment. The proximal tip of the nail should be level with the tip of the greater trochanter.

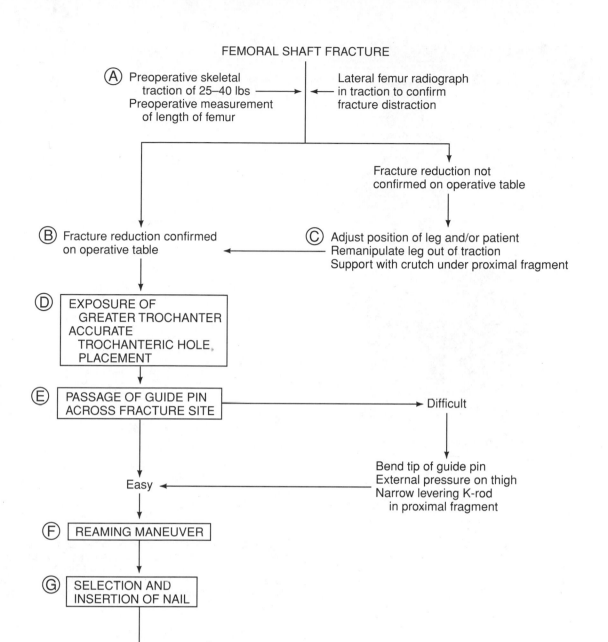

FEMORAL SHAFT FRACTURE

Ⓐ Preoperative skeletal
traction of 25–40 lbs ⟶ ← Lateral femur radiograph
in traction to confirm
Preoperative measurement fracture distraction
of length of femur

Fracture reduction not
confirmed on operative table

Ⓑ Fracture reduction confirmed   Ⓒ Adjust position of leg and/or patient
on operative table   Remanipulate leg out of traction
                                           Support with crutch under proximal fragment

Ⓓ | EXPOSURE OF
    GREATER TROCHANTER
    ACCURATE
    TROCHANTERIC HOLE,
    PLACEMENT |

Ⓔ | PASSAGE OF GUIDE PIN
    ACROSS FRACTURE SITE | ⟶ Difficult

Bend tip of guide pin
External pressure on thigh
Easy ← Narrow levering K-rod
        in proximal fragment

Ⓕ | REAMING MANEUVER |

Ⓖ | SELECTION AND
     INSERTION OF NAIL |

Ⓗ | PROXIMAL AND/OR
     DISTAL SCREW ⟶ Ⓘ Rehabilitation
     INSERTION |

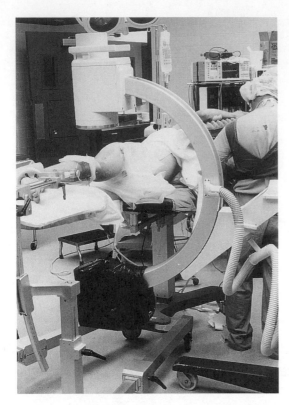

Figure 1 Proper lateral positioning of the patient for closed intramedullary nailing.

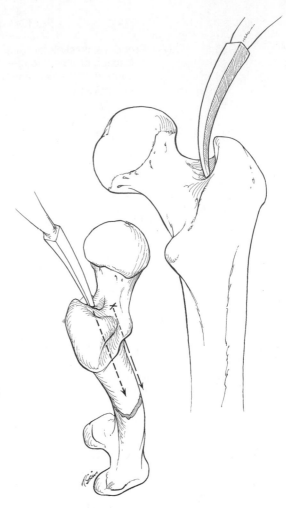

Figure 2 The preferred entrance portal for the insertion of an intramedullary nail is in the pyriformis fossa. This point should be centered in the longitudinal axis of the shaft in both the anteroposterior and mediolateral planes. Excessive anterior placement of the hole can result in inadvertent penetration of the anterior femoral cortex.

H. Once the nail has been fully seated, visualize the entire length of the femur on the fluoroscope to detect any unrecognized preoperative comminution or longitudinal splits that might compromise the stability of the surgical construct. Then lock the nail with the major proximal and distal fracture fragments as indicated. Most proximal targeting devices attach firmly to internal threads on the proximal tip of the nail. It is critical that the proximal locking screw obtains purchase on at least two intact cortices of the proximal fragment. Accomplish distal targeting by the use of a nail mounted targeting jig, a C-arm mounted targeting jig, or a variety of free hand techniques. Insert at least one screw into the distal fragment to adequately control the length of the femur. Two screws are necessary for all infraisthmal and supracondylar fractures to ensure fracture stability in the sagittal plane. Confirm the proper positioning of the screws by fluoroscopy prior to closure.

I. The postoperative management depends on the reliability of the patient and the stability of the fixation. If a stable surgical construct is achieved, begin progressive weight bearing as tolerated. If a distal third fracture within 5 cm of the proximal most of the two distal screws of the nail is fixed, then delay weight bearing until there is clear evidence of fracture union. Early weight bearing may result in fatigue failure of the nail at this level. Begin quadriceps strengthening exercises within several weeks and encourage active range of motion exercises.

References

Baumgaertal F, Dahlen C, Stiletto R, et al. Technique of using the AO-femoral distractor for femoral intramedullary nailing. J Orthop Trauma 1994; 8:315.

Braten M, Terjessen T, Rossvoll I. Torsional deformity after intramedullary nailing of femoral shaft fractures: Measurement of anteversion angles in 110 patients. J Bone Joint Surg 1993; 75:799.

Browner B. Pitfalls, errors, and complications in the use of locking Kuntscher nails. Clin Orthop 1986; 212:192.

Bucholz R, Browner B. Fracture of the femoral shaft. In: Evarts M, ed. Surgery of the musculoskeletal system. New York: Churchill Livingstone, 1988.

Bucholz R, Ross S, Lawrence K. Fatigue fracture of the interlocking nail in the treatment of fractures of the distal part of the femoral shaft. J Bone Joint Surg 1987; 69A:1391.

Coetzee J, van der Merwe E. Exposure of surgeons-in-training to radiation during intramedullary fixation of femoral shaft fractures. S Afr Med J 1992; 81:312.

Dugas R, D'Ambrosia R. The Grosse-Kempf interlocking nail: Technique of femoral and tibial fractures. Orthopaedics. 1985; 8:1363.

Hajek P, Bicknell H, Bronson W, et al. The use of one compared with two distal screws in the treatment of femoral shaft fractures with interlocking intramedullary nailing: A clinical and biomechanical analysis. J Bone Joint Surg 1993; 75A:519.

Hansen S, Winquist R. Closed intramedullary nailing of fracture of the femoral shaft—Technical considerations. In: Instructional Course Lectures of the AAOS, 1978.

Kuntscher G. Practice of intramedullary nailing. Springfield, Charles C Thomas, 1967.

MacMillan M, Gross R. A simplified technique of distal femoral screw insertion for the Grosse-Kempf interlocking nail. Clin Orthop 1988; 226:252.

McFerran M, Johnson K. Intramedullary nailing of acute femoral shaft fractures without a fracture table: Technique of using a femoral distractor. J Orthop Trauma 1992; 6:271.

Tencer A, Sherman M, Johnson K. Biomechanical factors affecting fracture stability of femoral bursting in closed intramedullary rod fixation of femur fractures. J Biomech Eng 1985; 107:104.

FRACTURE OF THE DISTAL FEMUR

A. Supracondylar and intercondylar fractures of the femur are usually secondary to either high-velocity injuries in young patients or low-velocity injuries in elderly patients. The ASIF classification scheme for distal femur fractures is based on the distinction between supracondylar injuries, isolated condylar fractures, and supracondylar fractures with intercondylar extension in one or more planes (Fig. 1). Accurate radiographic assessment is essential in the selection of the ideal treatment, the preoperative planning of any surgical procedures, and the prediction of long-term complications. The tunnel view of the intercondylar notch is helpful in judging the extent of displacement of vertical fractures into the joint.

B. Improved techniques of internal fixation introduced over the last 15 years have yielded results superior to those achieved with traditional nonoperative management. There are currently, however, a number of good indications for nonoperative treatment of fractures of the distal femur. The rare nondisplaced and impacted supracondylar fractures usually occur in elderly patients and can be treated with casting. Long spiral fractures through the length of the distal femoral metaphysis are also easily aligned and stabilized by nonoperative means. Paraplegic and nonambulatory patients with low-energy supracondylar fractures can be treated by simple splinting of the extremity. Higher-energy injuries and displaced intra-articular fractures in ambulatory elderly patients are better treated with surgery. Nonoperative treatment of these latter injuries often results in varus and internal rotation malalignment, knee contractures, and increased hospitalization.

C. Early attempts at internal fixation of distal femur fractures yielded unacceptably high rates of malunion, nonunion, and infection. A wide variety of currently available implants provide the surgeon with much improved techniques for rigid fixation of these fractures. The preferred implant for any given fracture depends on a careful assessment of the fracture pattern.

D. Extra-articular supracondylar fractures (ASIF Type A) can be subdivided into infraisthmal fractures 8 cm or more above the knee joint and low supracondylar fractures less than 8 cm above the joint. The former fractures can be best treated as distal shaft fractures with the use of a statically locked intramedullary nail. The nail must be driven down to the intercondylar notch area, with care taken to avoid excessive varus or valgus deformity at the fracture. Two distal locking screws should be used to ensure fracture stability in the sagittal plane. Because of the proximity of the fracture to the proximalmost of the two distal holes of the interlocking nail, fatigue failure of the nail is a recognized complication. Delayed weight bearing on the extremity is indicated until there is evidence of advanced healing (usually at 2 to 3 months).

E. Displaced type A fractures within 8 cm of the knee joint in patients with normal bone stock are preferably managed with either a dynamic condylar blade plate or dynamic condylar screw. The condylar screw is easier to use than the blade plate since rotation of the device in the sagittal plane can be adjusted. All fractures with comminution (Type A2 and A3) must undergo autogenous bone grafting.

F. Type A fractures in elderly patients with severe osteopenia are difficult to stabilize rigidly with a condylar blade plate or screw. The GSH (Green, Seligson, Henry) supracondylar nail supplemented with a cast brace offers an excellent alternative in these patients. While healing of the fracture can predictably be expected, some degree of motion at the fracture site can be expected. Early knee motion is feasible when the supracondylar nail is used for fixation.

G. Isolated condylar fractures may occur in either the sagittal or the frontal plane. These intra-articular fractures require anatomic reduction and rigid internal fixation, especially in young, active patients. Grossly unstable shear injuries of either the medial or lateral condyles may necessitate buttressing with a plate.

H. Supracondylar/intercondylar fractures (ASIF Type C) are frequently due to very high energy injuries. In Type C1 and C2 fractures, the sagittal plane fracture into the intracondylar notch should be anatomically reduced prior to stabilization of the supracondylar component of the fracture. Because of the simple nature of the intercondylar extension of the fracture, a dynamic condylar screw is an excellent implant for fixation.

Five to ten percent of supracondylar/intercondylar fractures are open. After thorough debridement of these injuries, employ the same principles utilized for the management of all open intra-articular fractures, including immediate rigid stabilization of the fracture with plates and screws and open treatment of the wound. Grade III injuries that are grossly contaminated are preferably managed with debridement and external fixation of the supracondylar fracture following anatomic reduction and limited internal fixation of any intra-articular extension.

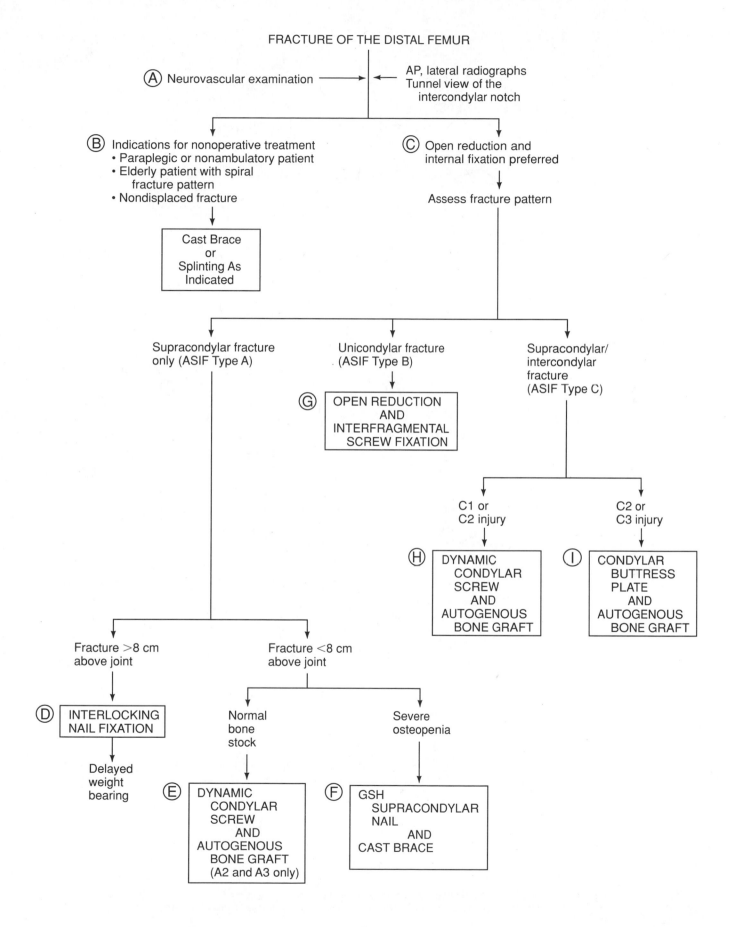

FRACTURE OF THE DISTAL FEMUR

Ⓐ Neurovascular examination ← → AP, lateral radiographs
Tunnel view of the
intercondylar notch

Ⓑ Indications for nonoperative treatment
• Paraplegic or nonambulatory patient
• Elderly patient with spiral
  fracture pattern
• Nondisplaced fracture

Ⓒ Open reduction and
internal fixation preferred

Assess fracture pattern

Cast Brace
or
Splinting As
Indicated

Supracondylar fracture
only (ASIF Type A)

Unicondylar fracture
(ASIF Type B)

Supracondylar/
intercondylar
fracture
(ASIF Type C)

Ⓖ OPEN REDUCTION
AND
INTERFRAGMENTAL
SCREW FIXATION

C1 or
C2 injury

C2 or
C3 injury

Ⓗ DYNAMIC
CONDYLAR
SCREW
AND
AUTOGENOUS
BONE GRAFT

Ⓘ CONDYLAR
BUTTRESS
PLATE
AND
AUTOGENOUS
BONE GRAFT

Fracture >8 cm
above joint

Fracture <8 cm
above joint

Ⓓ INTERLOCKING
NAIL FIXATION

Normal
bone
stock

Severe
osteopenia

Delayed
weight
bearing

Ⓔ DYNAMIC
CONDYLAR
SCREW
AND
AUTOGENOUS
BONE GRAFT
(A2 and A3 only)

Ⓕ GSH
SUPRACONDYLAR
NAIL
AND
CAST BRACE

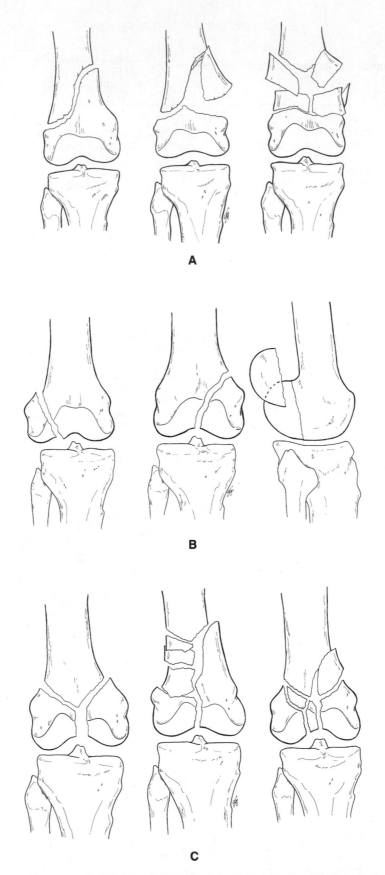

Figure 1 **A,** ASIF Type A fractures involving only the supracondylar area of the femur. **B,** ASIF Type B condylar fractures of the distal femur. **C,** ASIF Type C supracondylar/intercondylar fractures of the femur.

I. Low C2 fractures and most C3 fractures are difficult to stabilize with a condylar screw device. The condylar buttress plate is more versatile for these fractures and allows for individualized placement of multiple cancellous screws for purchase of the distal fragment. Although the ease of application of the buttress plate is useful in these complex injuries, the plate is relatively weak compared with the condylar screw device. Postoperative settling of the fracture into varus is common in fractures with medial comminution. A second buttress plate placed medially across the fracture is necessary in such cases.

Severely comminuted supracondylar/intercondylar fractures with fracture lines in multiple planes occasionally require an extensile surgical approach. The Mercedes incision has been used in these complex injuries but carries a high incidence of soft-tissue slough and infection. Combined medial and lateral incisions are less risky and are preferred by most orthopedists.

References

Bankston A, Keating M, Saha S. The biomechanical evaluation of intramedullary nails in distal femoral shaft fractures. Clin Orthop 1992; 276:277.

Bucholz R, Ross S, Lawrence K. Fatigue fracture of interlocking nails in distal femoral shaft fractures. J Bone Joint Surg 1987; 69A:1391.

Butler M, Brumback R, Ellison T, et al. Interlocking intramedullary nailing for ipsilateral fractures of the femoral shaft and distal part of the femur. J Bone Joint Surg 1991; 73A:1492.

Chapman M. The use of immediate internal fixation in open fractures. Orthop Clin North Am 1980; 11:579.

Charnley J. The closed treatment of common fractures. 3rd Ed. Edinburgh: Churchill-Livingstone, 1972.

Giles J, DeLee J. Supracondylar-intercondylar fractures of the femur treated with a supracondylar plate and lag screw. J Bone Joint Surg 1982; 64A:864.

Healy W, Brooker A. Distal femoral fractures: Comparison of open and closed methods of treatment. Clin Orthop 1983; 174:166.

Iannocone W, Bennett F, DeLong W, et al. Initial experience with treatment of supracondylar femoral fractures using the supracondylar intramedullary nail. J Orthop Trauma 1994; 8:322.

Lucas S. Seligson D, Henry S. Intramedullary supracondylar nailing of femoral fractures: A preliminary report of the GSH supracondylar nail. Clin Orthop 1993; 196:200.

Mize R, Bucholz R, Grogan D. Surgical treatment of displaced, comminuted fractures of the distal end of the femur. J Bone Joint Surg 1982; 64A:871.

Mooney V, Nickel V, Harvey J, et al. Cast-brace treatment for fractures of the distal part of the femur. J Bone Joint Surg 1970; 52A:1563.

Neer C, Grantham S, Shelton M. Supracondylar fracture of the adult femur: A study of one hundred and ten cases. J Bone Joint Surg 1967; 49A:591.

Pritchett J. Supracondylar fractures of the femur. Clin Orthop 1984; 184:173.

Sanders R, Swiontkowski M, Raven J, et al. Double-plating of comminuted unstable fractures of the distal part of the femur. J Bone Joint Surg 1991; 73A:341.

Schatzker J, Lambert D. Supracondylar fracture of the femur. Clin Orthop 1979; 138:77.

Zickel R, Fietti V, Lansing J. A new intramedullary fixation device for the distal third of the femur. Clin Orthop 1977; 125:185.

DISLOCATION OF THE KNEE JOINT

Knee dislocation is a true emergency. Many patients present with severe soft tissue disruption and often neurologic and vascular compromise. Knee dislocation can present after spontaneous reduction. Whenever severe ligamentous disruptions occur in multiple planes, the examiner should suspect a complete dislocation. The most accepted definition of knee dislocation is complete disruption of both cruciate and one collateral complex. However, some reports include cases where only one cruciate is disrupted. These injuries occur in association with multiple trauma and high velocity events as opposed to an isolated injury and low velocity trauma, such as a sporting event. Knee dislocations are classified in terms of the tibial displacement with respect to the femur (Figs. 1 to 4).

A. The vascular status of the limb takes precedence. A thorough, brief neurovascular examination is performed prior to reduction.

B. After documentation of the neurovascular status of the limb, a closed reduction is attempted. This is typically easily accomplished by gentle longitudinal traction, lifting the femur or tibia to avoid further injury to the popliteal vascular structures.

C. After reduction, a thorough examination to assess neurovascular, bony and ligamentous stability is performed. Palpable pulses do not guarantee the absence of vascular injury. Careful assessment of both peroneal and tibial nerve injury is necessary. Posterolateral dislocations are associated with a high prevalence of peroneal nerve injury. Recovery after nerve injury is poor and treatment is controversial.

D. These injuries are often associated with fractures. AP, lateral, and both obliques detail the bony anatomy. MRI can be helpful in preoperative planning for elective ligamentous repair. All knee dislocations should undergo arteriography. Even knees that present with palpable pulses and a reduced knee but have multiplanar instability have a high prevalence of vascular injury.

E. Irreducible or open dislocations are taken urgently for reduction, irrigation, debridement, and vascular repair if necessary. Intraoperative arteriography is performed.

F. Open dislocations are treated by thorough irrigation, debridement, and closure over drains. Capsular, collateral ligament, and meniscal injuries can also be addressed at the initial operation. Rarely, external fixation is required for stability and soft tissue healing in severe open wounds. Rotatory or posterolateral dislocations are associated with irreducibility due to "button-holing" of the medial femoral condyle through the medial capsule. Open reduction is required. If ideal conditions exist, capsular and ligamentous repair may be performed at that time.

G. Dislocations in the anterior posterior plane are associated with popliteal artery disruptions in up to 40% of cases. If disruption is identified, immediate repair (within six to eight hours) is indicated. Grafting is most successful with interpositional collateral saphenous veins. If successful, a four-compartment fasciotomy is performed. If vascular integrity is not reestablished, amputation is indicated.

H. Operative repair or reconstruction of the ligamentous injuries and open reduction and internal fixation of the periarticular fractures yields the best long-term results. Limited extra-articular repair is performed on an acute basis if the dislocation is irreducible or if the vascular repair is necessary. Delaying for two to three weeks allows resolution of swelling and appropriate planning. Limited arthroscopy or preoperative MRI is helpful in planning incisions. Primary repair is performed for avulsive cruciate injuries. Reconstruction may be necessary for mid-substance tears. Some conditions warrant closed treatment. A stable knee with 90° of painless motion can be achieved with cast immobilization.

SUSPECTED KNEE DISLOCATION

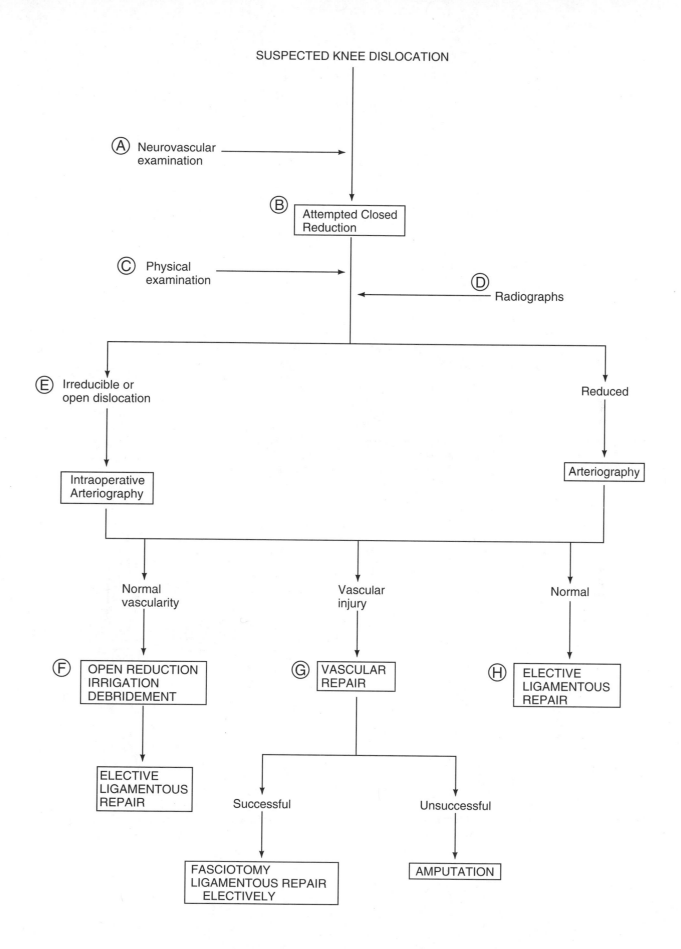

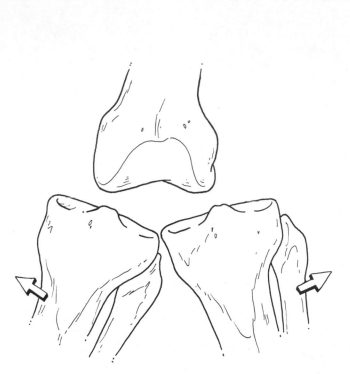

Figure 1   The dislocation is described by the relative position of the tibia to the femur. Medial and lateral dislocations often have a rotatory component.

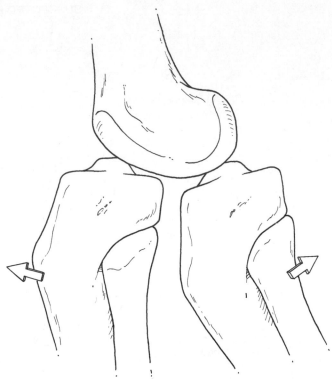

Figure 3   Anterior and posterior dislocation.

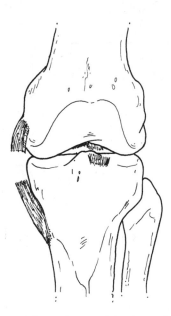

Figure 2   Both cruciates and one collateral complex are disrupted.

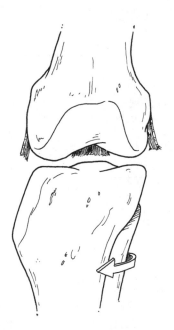

Figure 4   Rotation may create irreducibility by interposition of skin and soft tissue.

References

Ertl TJ, Marder RA. Traumatic knee dislocations. In Chapman MW, Madison M, eds: Operative Orthopaedics. Philadelphia, Lippincott, 1993; pp 2131-2149.

Green NE, Alan BL. Vascular injuries associated with dislocations of the knee joints. J Bone Joint Surg 1977; 59A:236.

Kennedy JC. Complete dislocation of the knee joint. J Bone Joint Surg 45A:889-904, July 1963.

Kremcheck TE, Welling RE, Kremcheck EJ. Traumatic dislocation of the knee. Orthop Rev 1989; 18:1051.

McCutchon JD, Gillham NR. Injury to the popliteal artery associated with dislocation of the knee: Palpable pulses do not negate the requirement for arteriography. Injury 1989; 20:307.

Meyers MH, Moore TM, Harvey PJ Jr. Traumatic dislocations of the knee joints. J Bone Joint Surg 1975; 57A:430-433.

Shields L, Mitel M, Cave EF. Complete dislocation of the knee: Experience at the Massachusetts General Hospital. J Trauma 1969; 9:192.

Taylor A, Arden P, Riney HA. Traumatic dislocation of the knee: A report of 40 cases, 3 cases with special reference to conservative treatment. J Bone Joint Surg 1972; 54B:96.

Varnell RN, Coldwell DM, Sangezoran BJ, Johansen KH. Arterial injury complicating knee disruption. Am Surg 1989; 55:699.

Wand JS. Physical findings in noting irreducibility of the dislocated knee. J Bone Joint Surg 1989; 71B:862.

FRACTURE OR DISLOCATION OF THE PATELLA

A. Fracture displacement and intra-articular incongruity are evaluated best on the lateral radiograph while anteroposterior (AP) and sunrise (tangential) views aid in visualizing vertical fractures and osteochondral fragments. Bipartite patellas with the characteristic superolateral ossicles should not be mistakenly diagnosed as fractured. Lateral dislocations of the patella often reduce spontaneously. Tenderness over the medial aspect of the patella and a positive apprehension test should alert the physician to a probable reduced lateral dislocation.

B. The patella increases the mechanical advantage of the knee extensor mechanism (quadriceps tendon). The medial and lateral extensions of the vastus muscles around the patella constitute the extensor retinacula. Sparing of the retinacula during a complete fracture of the patella may permit some active knee extension. Retinacular disruption and total loss of active extension usually occur in fractures with greater than 3 to 4 mm of displacement. If the amount of displacement is borderline, test the patient for active knee extension. Prevent a false positive test by aspirating the hemarthrosis and injecting a local anesthetic into the joint prior to the test. If a transverse patellar fracture is allowed to heal in a displaced position, permanent extension lag may be expected.

C. The prerequisites for cast treatment (a long leg or cylinder cast for 4 to 6 weeks) include an intact articular surface with less than 3 mm of translation or distraction of the major fracture fragments and active knee extension. Chronic patellofemoral symptoms may result from direct cartilage trauma or from failure to reconstitute the articular congruity.

D. As with quadriceps and patellar tendon ruptures, the goal of surgery is to restore the extensor mechanism. Tension band wiring offers dynamic fixation of simple fractures (Fig. 1). Anchorage of the wire directly to the patella, using two vertical Steinmann pins, is probably necessary if early knee motion is anticipated. Following visual confirmation of patellar articular reconstitution, repair the extensor retinacula. Transverse fractures with good interdigitation of the major fracture fragments and proper positioning of a tension band wire can be mobilized early. In cases with less than optimal fixation, or extensive comminution of the fracture, 3 to 6 weeks of postoperative immobilization is indicated.

E. Partial patellectomy may be required in cases with severe comminution of either the proximal or distal poles. Save as much of the patella as possible to preserve its mechanical benefit. Suture the remaining tendon adjacent to the articular surface of the intact patellar fragment, thereby preventing tilting of the patellar fragment into the femoral condyles (Fig. 2). Postoperative mobilization is necessary for a minimum of 4 to 6 weeks to achieve solid tendon-to-bone healing. Full return of motion and function of the knee often requires 6 to 12 months of rehabilitation.

Extensive comminution necessitates total patellectomy. Approximately one third the strength of the quadriceps is lost following patellectomy. The degree of functional loss following patellectomy is controversial and may be contingent on the specific indication for patellectomy. Open fractures commonly are displaced and comminuted, thus requiring partial or total patellectomy during surgical debridement.

Severely comminuted fractures have also been treated by cerclage of the major fragments with no attempt to restore anatomically the articular surface of the patella. Satisfactory results following early motion of the knee can be achieved with this technique.

F. Patellar dislocations are usually secondary to twisting injuries in which the femur rotates internally on a fixed foot. Young patients should routinely have their uninjured leg checked for possible predisposing factors to patellar dislocations. These include an increased Q-angle, a dysplastic vastus medialis obliquus muscle, external rotation deformity of the tibia, patella alta, a shallow femoral sulcus, and generalized ligamentous laxity. The presence of one or more of these predisposing factors worsens the prognosis for recurrent patellar dislocations. Approximately two thirds of patients will have a predisposition for dislocation. Recurrence is less frequent in patients who have their first dislocation when they are older than 14 years of age.

G. Following closed reduction by gentle extension of the knee, patellar dislocations must be evaluated radiographically to detect concomitant medial patellar facet fractures and lateral femoral condyle fractures. If these osteochondral fractures are displaced, arthroscopic debridement or fixation of the fragments is necessary. Splint all patellar dislocations for 2 to 3 weeks, during which time early quadriceps exercises can be performed. Continue the splint or knee immobilizer for up to 6 weeks or until the knee is nontender to palpation. Most patients with a first time dislocation and no predisposing factors for dislocation will have an excellent clinical result with this treatment regimen.

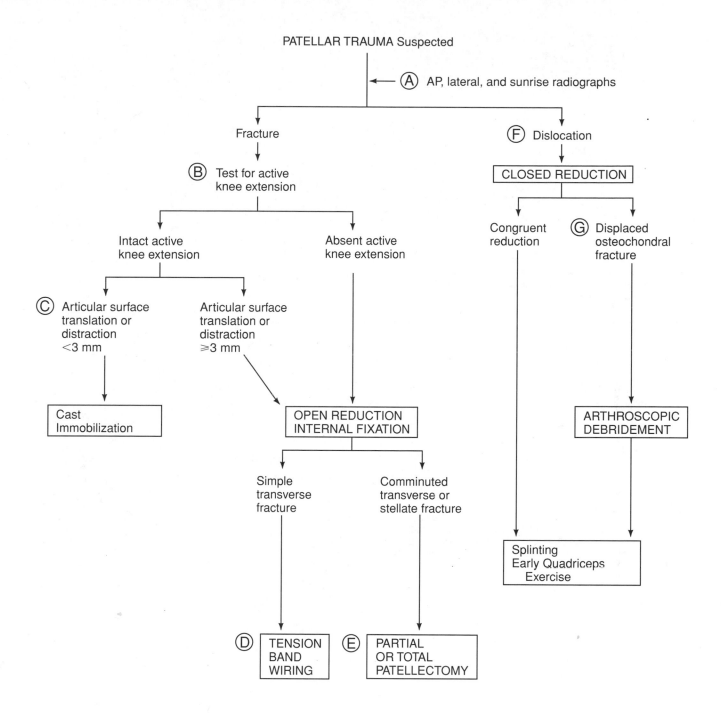

PATELLAR TRAUMA Suspected

(A) AP, lateral, and sunrise radiographs

Fracture

(F) Dislocation

(B) Test for active
knee extension

CLOSED REDUCTION

Intact active
knee extension

Absent active
knee extension

Congruent
reduction

(G) Displaced
osteochondral
fracture

(C) Articular surface
translation or
distraction
<3 mm

Articular surface
translation or
distraction
≥3 mm

Cast
Immobilization

OPEN REDUCTION
INTERNAL FIXATION

ARTHROSCOPIC
DEBRIDEMENT

Simple
transverse
fracture

Comminuted
transverse or
stellate fracture

Splinting
Early Quadriceps
Exercise

(D) TENSION
BAND
WIRING

(E) PARTIAL
OR TOTAL
PATELLECTOMY

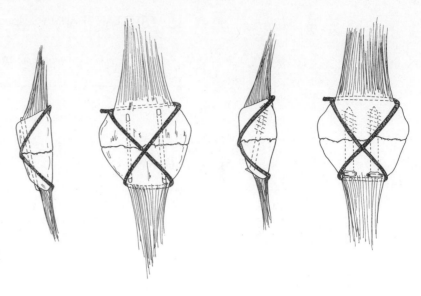

Figure 1 Standard fixation of simple, transverse fractures of the patella using a tension band wire and either parallel Steinmann pins or cancellous screws.

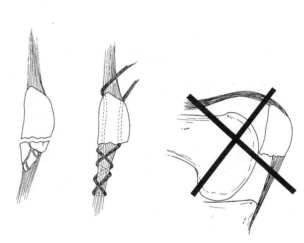

Figure 2 Following partial patellectomy, the patellar tendon should be reattached to the articular side of the remaining patella. Reattachment to the superficial side *(right diagram)* causes tilting of the patella and possible patellofemoral symptoms.

References

Burrant J, Thomas K, Alexander R, et al. Evaluation of methods of internal fixation of transverse patella fractures: A biomechanical study. J Orthop Trauma 1994; 8:147.

Cash J, Hughston J. Treatment of acute patellar dislocation. Am J Sports Med 1988; 16:144.

Haajanen J, Karaharju E. Fractures of the patella: One hundred consecutive cases. Ann Chir Gynaecol 1981; 70:32.

Hawkins R, Bell R, Anisette G. Acute patellar dislocations. Am J Sports Med 1986; 14:117.

Hung L, Lee S, Leong K, et al. Patial patellectomy for patellar fracture: Tension band wiring and early mobilization. J Orthop Trauma 1993; 7:252.

Jakobsen J, Christensen K, Rasmussen O. Patellectomy—A 20-year follow-up. Acta Orthop Scand 1985; 56:430.

Johnson E. Fractures of the patella. In Rockwood and Green's Fractures, 3rd ed. Philadelphia: Lippincott, 1991.

Kaufer H. Mechanical function of the patella. J Bone Joint Surg 1971; 53A:1551.

Muller M, Allgower M, Schneider R, Willenegger H. Manual of internal fixation. 2nd ed. New York: Springer-Verlag, 1979.

Pritsch M, Velkes S, Levy O, et al. Suture fixation of osteochondrial fractures of the patella. J Bone Joint Surg 1995; 77B:154.

Saltzman C. Results of treatment of displaced patellar fractures by partial patellectomy. J Bone Joint Surg 1990; 72A:1279.

Watkins M, et al. Effect of patellectomy on the function of the quadriceps and hamstrings. J Bone Joint Surg 1983; 65A:390.

Weber M, et al. Efficacy of various forms of fixation of transverse fractures of the patella. J Bone Joint Surg 1980; 62A:215.

FRACTURE OF THE TIBIAL PLATEAU

A. The tibial condylar surface slopes posteroinferiorly 10° to 15°. Accurate assessment of the amount of depression of articular fragments therefore necessitates an anteroposterior (AP) radiograph with the beam directed 10° to 15° inferiorly. Tomograms may be required in questionable cases. Although coronal reconstructions of computed tomography (CT) scans avoid the problem of radiographic magnification, tomography is still preferred by most investigators.

Since the depression of the weight-bearing portion of the plateau may lead to varus or valgus instability, routinely obtain stress radiographs in the evaluation of plateau fractures. The presence of 5° to 10° or more of valgus or varus angulation greater than the uninjured knee is a good indication for anatomical reduction and rigid fixation of the fracture. Perform stress testing with the knee in full extension.

B. Diagnostic radiographs may reveal avulsion fractures signaling associated ligamentous injuries. The most common bony avulsion involves the intercondylar eminence, signifying a disruption of the anterior cruciate ligament. The incidence of concomitant ligamentous injury is approximately 10% for all plateau fractures, except for central depression fractures where ligamentous injury is rare. Following rigid internal fixation of the plateau fracture, always test the knees in full extension to detect occult ligamentous disruptions.

C. The goal of any treatment is to restore knee motion, alignment, and stability. Dense intra-articular adhesions with resultant mechanical blockage of knee motion are a predictable consequence of prolonged immobilization. Nondisplaced fractures and stable central depression fractures should therefore be managed with early cast bracing. Commence full weight bearing once early union is apparent, usually at 6 to 8 weeks.

D. The criteria for displaced fractures include condylar widening of greater than 5 mm, condylar depression of greater than 5 mm, central articular depression of greater than 10 mm, and valgus or varus instability of 5° to 10° greater than the opposite knee with stress testing. Thoroughly assess and classify fractures with one or more of these findings prior to operation.

The best classification scheme for plateau fractures is a modification of that proposed by Hohl, Schatzker, and the ASIF group. The six major fracture patterns are split or wedge fractures, central depression fracture, split depression fracture, total condylar fracture, bicondylar fracture, and condylar fracture associated with extensive metaphyseal comminution (Fig. 1).

E. Isolated central depression fractures, usually in the anterior aspect of the lateral condyle, that are less than 10 mm depressed and do not cause valgus instability can be treated by early motion and a cast brace. Minor degrees of central depression of the articular surface do not predispose the joint to post-traumatic degenerative arthritis.

F. Central depression fractures depressed greater than 10 mm are commonly associated with major varus/valgus instability and should be elevated and stabilized. Autogenous cortical cancellous bone graft (or alternatively, allograft or synthetic bone graft substitutes) is used to fill the subarticular cavity under the raised osteocartilagenous fragment, thereby preventing postoperative settling of the condylar surface.

Arthroscopy may occasionally be useful for the assessment of intra-articular pathology, including meniscal injuries, cruciate ruptures, and intra-articular loose bodies. Its primary use for reduction of plateau fractures is technically demanding and should be limited to very simple fracture patterns.

G. Displaced split, split compression, and total condylar fractures are best treated by anatomic reduction, elevation of all major fracture fragments, autogenous bone grafting of metaphyseal defects, and plate buttressing of all major condylar fragments. The long-term results are mainly dependent on the restoration of stability of the knee and the accuracy of reduction achieved at surgery. Total condylar fractures of the medial aspect of the plateau have an especially guarded prognosis. Accept no residual depression of the medial condyle, which results in a varus malalignment of the mechanical axis of the leg. Following anatomic reduction and rigid fixation of these fractures, examine the knee under anesthesia for any ligamentous instability.

H. Bicondylar fractures and severely comminuted tibial plateau fractures are best treated by anatomic reduction and rigid fixation. Late complications of degenerative joint disease, knee contractures, and knee instability are minimized by accurate anatomic reduction and early active motion. Open reduction and internal fixation of complex plateau fractures, however, may present formidable challenges to the surgeon. Temper surgical enthusiasm by consideration of such variables as patient age, functional demands, soft tissue status, associated injuries, and operative experience.

I. Specific indications for primary skeletal traction and/or cast brace treatment include major skin loss and elderly patients with minimal functional demands. Selected bicondylar fractures with extensive comminution of the metaphysis can be successfully managed by closed reduction and percutaneous pinning of the articular fragments followed by external fixation across the area of metaphyseal comminution (Fig. 2). The alternative treatment of a dynamic compression plate spanning the metaphyseal defect is associated with a high incidence of soft tissue complications.

TIBIAL PLATEAU FRACTURE

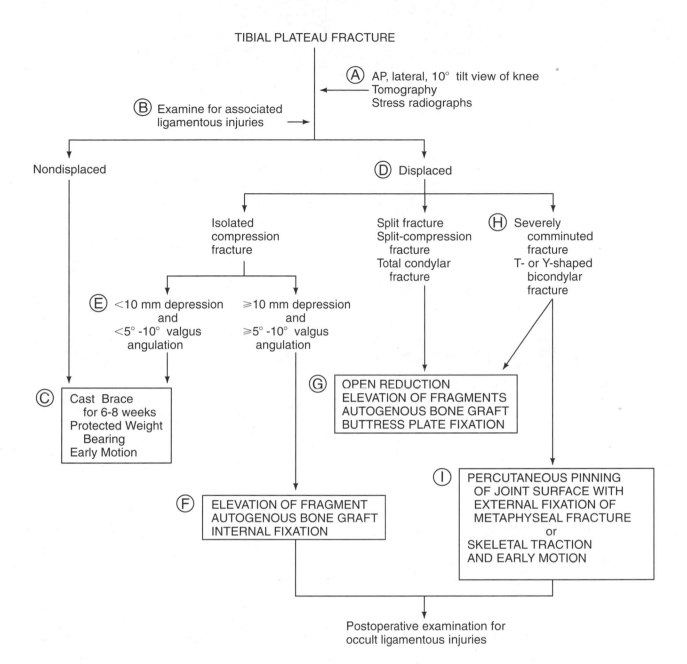

(A) AP, lateral, 10° tilt view of knee
Tomography
Stress radiographs

(B) Examine for associated ligamentous injuries

Nondisplaced

(D) Displaced

Isolated compression fracture

Split fracture
Split-compression fracture
Total condylar fracture

(H) Severely comminuted fracture
T- or Y-shaped bicondylar fracture

(E) <10 mm depression and <5°-10° valgus angulation

≥10 mm depression and ≥5°-10° valgus angulation

(C) Cast Brace for 6-8 weeks
Protected Weight Bearing
Early Motion

(G) OPEN REDUCTION
ELEVATION OF FRAGMENTS
AUTOGENOUS BONE GRAFT
BUTTRESS PLATE FIXATION

(F) ELEVATION OF FRAGMENT
AUTOGENOUS BONE GRAFT
INTERNAL FIXATION

(I) PERCUTANEOUS PINNING OF JOINT SURFACE WITH EXTERNAL FIXATION OF METAPHYSEAL FRACTURE
or
SKELETAL TRACTION AND EARLY MOTION

Postoperative examination for occult ligamentous injuries

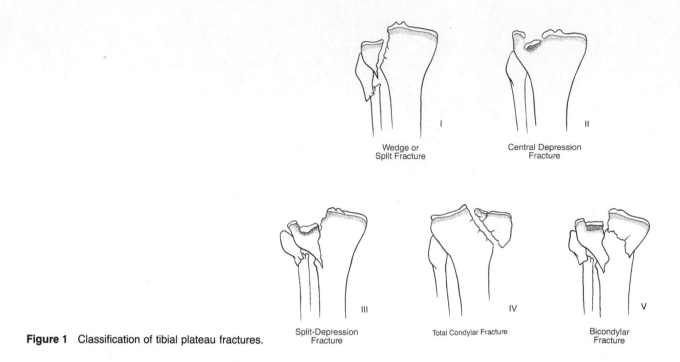

Wedge or
Split Fracture

I

Central Depression
Fracture

II

Split-Depression
Fracture

III

Total Condylar Fracture

IV

Bicondylar
Fracture

V

Figure 1 Classification of tibial plateau fractures.

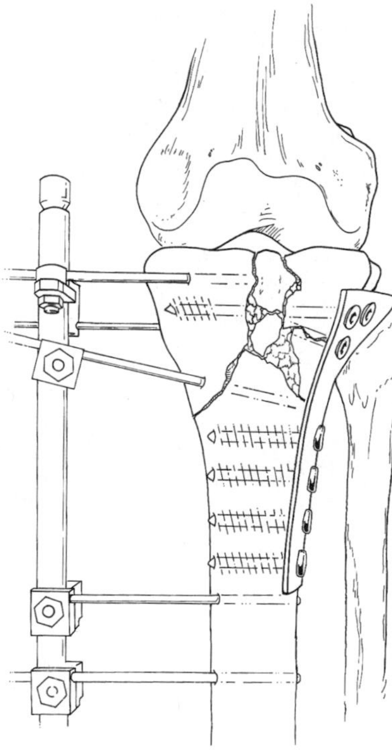

Figure 2 Fixation of a Schatzker Type V tibial plateau fracture using limited internal fixation and a half-pin medial external fixator.

References

Benirschke S. Immediate internal fixation of open, complex tibial plateau fractures: Treatment by a standard protocol. J Orthop Trauma 1992; 6:78.

Blokker C, Rorabeck C, Bourne R. Tibial plateau fractures—An analysis of the results of treatment in 60 patients. Clin Orthop 1984; 182:193.

Bucholz R, Carlton A, Holmes R. Interporous hydroxyapatite as a bone graft substitute in tibial plateau fractures. Clin Orthop 1989; 240:53.

Caspari R, Hutton P, Whipple T, et al. The role of arthroscopy in the management of tibial plateau fractures. Arthroscopy 1985; 1:76.

Delamarter R, Hohl M, Hopp E. Ligament injuries associated with tibial plateau fractures. Clin Orthop 1990; 250:226.

Dias J, et al. Computerized axial tomography for tibial plateau fractures. J Bone Joint Surg 1987; 69B:84.

Hohl M. Tibial condylar fractures. J Bone Joint Surg 1967; 49A:1455.

Jensen D. Tibial plateau fractures: A comparison of conservative and surgical treatment. J Bone Joint Surg 1990; 72B:49.

Koval K. Indirect reduction and percutaneous screw fixation of displaced tibial plateau fractures. J Orthop Trauma 1991; 5:237.

Lansinger O, Bergman B, Korner L, et al. Tibial condylar fractures—A twenty-year follow-up. J Bone Joint Surg 1986; 68A:13.

Moore T, Patzakis M, Harvey J. Tibial plateau fractures: Definition, demographics, treatment rationale, and long-term results of closed traction management or operative reduction. J Orthop Trauma 1987; 1:97.

Muller M, Allgower M, Schneider R, Willenegger H. Manual of internal fixation. Berlin: Springer-Verlag, 1979.

Schatzker J, McBroom R, Bruce D. The tibial plateau fracture—The Toronto experience 1968–1975. Clin Orthop 1979; 138.

Scotland T, Wardlaw D. The use of cast-bracing as treatment for fractures of the tibial plateau. J Bone Joint Surg 1981; 63B:575.

Waddell J, Johnston D, Neidre A. Fracture of the tibial plateau: A review of ninety-five patients and comparison of treatment methods. J Trauma 1981; 21:376.

FRACTURE OF THE TIBIAL SHAFT

A. The variables that most affect the outcome of tibial shaft fractures are the degree of initial displacement, the extent of fracture comminution, the severity of the soft tissue wounds, and the adequacy of reduction. Most closed tibial shaft fractures are ideally treated with either closed reduction with cast/brace immobilization or intramedullary nailing. The latter treatment is strongly indicated in patients with ipsilateral femoral fracture (floating knee), ipsilateral knee ligament injuries, vascular injuries necessitating repair, bilateral tibial fractures, pathologic fractures, and segmental diaphyseal fractures.

B. The introduction of interlocking nails has significantly expanded the indications for intramedullary fixation of tibial shaft fractures. Limit the use of nonlocked nails to simple transverse and short oblique fractures in the midshaft area. Use interlocking nails for any shaft fracture from 4 cm distal to the tibial tuberosity to 5 cm from the ankle joint. Static locking of the nails prevents postoperative shortening and/or malrotation. Using a closed technique, complications including delayed union, nonunion, and infection occur in less than 5% of patients (Figs. 1 to 3).

C. Acceptable reductions for tibial shaft fractures generally fall within 10° of varus or valgus, 10° of anterior or posterior angulation, and 5° of rotation compared to the normal contralateral tibia. Recent long-term follow-up studies suggest that even greater degrees of malalignment are not inconsistent with excellent long-term knee and ankle function. While any fracture distraction must be avoided, shortening of up to 5 to 10 mm may be accepted, especially in comminuted, oblique fracture patterns. Translatory displacement of the major fragments is of less functional significance.

Severely displaced comminuted fractures of the tibia and fibula may be very difficult to maintain in satisfactory alignment in a cast. Such unstable patterns are preferably treated with interlocking nailing in selected patients. If closed treatment is elected, it is imperative to carefully monitor the fracture and correct any reangulation or shortening. Temporary nonweight-bearing casts, cast wedgings, remanipulations, or occasionally, reverting to external or internal fixation may be necessary to ensure healing in a satisfactory position. Large cassette radiographs that permit visualization of the entire tibia and the adjacent joints are necessary to provide the essential information for subsequent therapeutic decisions.

D. Early weight bearing appears to have a propitious effect on the healing process. Besides improving muscle and joint function, the cyclical loading of the fracture with weight bearing accelerates the formation of callus. The frequent problems of shortening and reangulation demand close radiographic follow-up.

By 4 to 8 weeks, conversion to a total contact below-knee cast is feasible for most fractures. The average time to union for closed tibial shaft fractures is 3 to 5 months. The absence of progressive healing on radiographs over a 2- to 3-month period is diagnostic of a delayed union. Additional treatment in the form of autogenous bone grafting or closed intramedullary nailing may be indicated in such patients.

E. Following thorough debridement and irrigation, open wounds are re-examined and debrided under sterile conditions at 3 to 5 days. The presence of an open fracture does not preclude the development of a compartment syndrome. Autopedestrian victims with severe Grade III open injuries are especially prone to compartment syndromes, which should be managed by emergency fasciotomy. Treat all open fractures with a short course of antibiotic therapy. Small Grade I or II wounds may be closed in a delayed fashion but often, especially in Grade III injuries, a large anterior or anteromedial wound remains. Ideally, cover proximal third tibial wounds with a medial gastrocnemius flap, middle third wounds by a soleus flap, and distal third wounds by a free latissimus flap. Once soft tissue coverage is achieved, direct attention towards achieving fracture union with minimal functional loss of the extremity.

F. After wound debridement and subsequent closure, Grade I and II fractures can be definitively managed in one of several ways. Stable fracture patterns can be treated as closed injuries in a long leg cast with early weight bearing. Unstable patterns are preferably treated with nonreamed intramedullary nailing. The nailing may be performed immediately after the emergency debridement of the wound if there is minimal contamination of the bone and soft tissues. Either small diameter (8 to 10 mm) interlocking nails or flexible medullary pins (e.g., Enders pins) may be used. If statically locked nails are used, subsequent surgery aimed at achieving union may be necessary. Preferred secondary procedures include dynamization of the nail, exchange nailing, and autogenous bone grafting. Avoid nails that require reaming. If a delayed intramedullary nailing is chosen, it should not be performed after an external fixation device has been in place for longer than 2 to 3 weeks. The incidence of postoperative infection is prohibitive in such cases due to the colonization of the pin sites of the fixator.

Selected Grade I and II injuries, especially those with persistent anteromedial wounds necessitating local myoplasties or distant flaps, are often treated with external fixation. If the fracture pattern is unstable, then use the fixator as the definitive mode of immobilization.

TIBIAL SHAFT FRACTURE

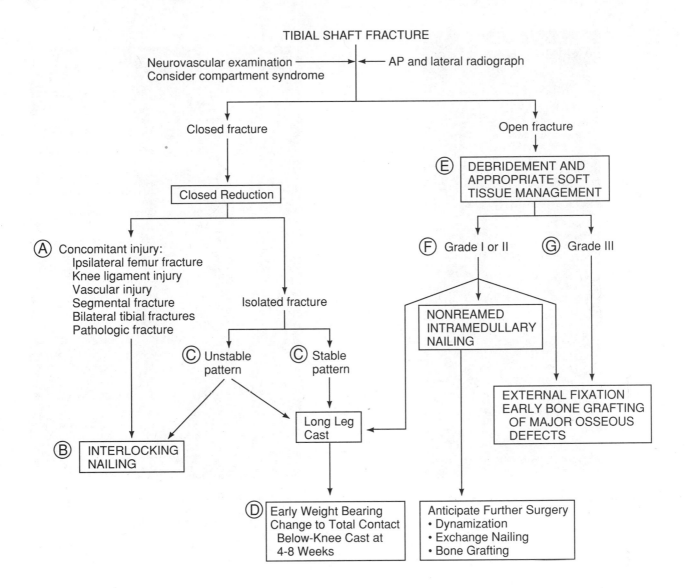

Neurovascular examination ⟶ ⟵ AP and lateral radiograph
Consider compartment syndrome

Closed fracture

Open fracture

Closed Reduction

Ⓔ DEBRIDEMENT AND APPROPRIATE SOFT TISSUE MANAGEMENT

Ⓐ Concomitant injury:
　　Ipsilateral femur fracture
　　Knee ligament injury
　　Vascular injury
　　Segmental fracture
　　Bilateral tibial fractures
　　Pathologic fracture

Ⓕ Grade I or II

Ⓖ Grade III

Isolated fracture

NONREAMED INTRAMEDULLARY NAILING

Ⓒ Unstable pattern

Ⓒ Stable pattern

Long Leg Cast

EXTERNAL FIXATION EARLY BONE GRAFTING OF MAJOR OSSEOUS DEFECTS

Ⓑ INTERLOCKING NAILING

Ⓓ Early Weight Bearing Change to Total Contact Below-Knee Cast at 4-8 Weeks

Anticipate Further Surgery
• Dynamization
• Exchange Nailing
• Bone Grafting

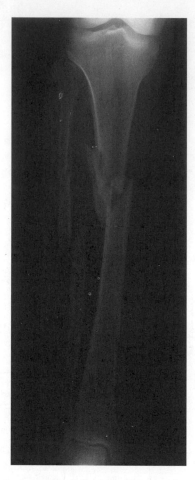

Figure 1 Anteroposterior radiograph of a comminuted fracture of the tibia.

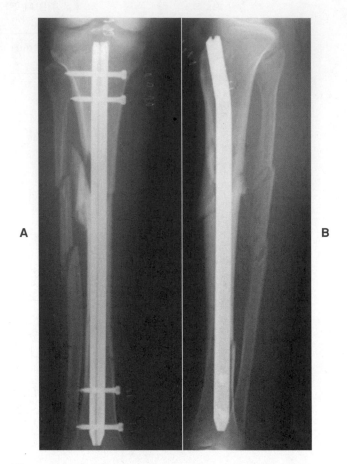

Figure 2 **A** and **B,** Anteroposterior and lateral radiographs postoperatively following closed statically locked interlocking nailing of the fracture. The length and alignment of the tibia have been restored.

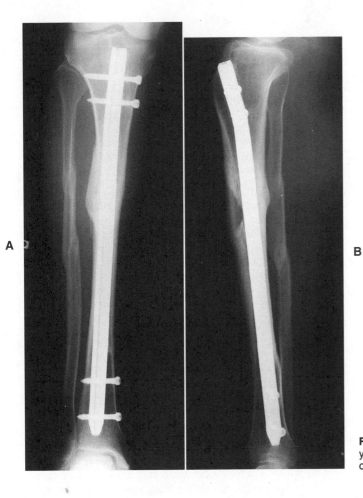

Figure 3 **A** and **B,** Anteroposterior and lateral radiographs at 1 year demonstrate complete consolidation of the fracture with no loss of position.

G. The first priority for Grade III open tibial shaft fractures is debridement of the wound followed by prompt wound coverage. Remove all devascularized bone fragments along with necrotic muscle. Grade III A and III B wounds can both be successfully managed by local myoplasties or free flap coverage. Due to the extensive comminution of these injuries, triangulated (delta) external fixation frames are necessary. Following soft tissue coverage, early bone grafting, preferably through a posterolateral approach, of all major osseous defects is indicated.

The treatment of Grade III C open fractures must be individualized. Temper attempts to salvage these limbs with severe vascular injuries with an understanding of the prolonged hospitalization and multiple operations that might be required. Amputation may be the preferred primary treatment. Guidelines for the selection of treatment in these severely damaged extremities have been proposed.

References

Blick S, et al. Compartment syndrome in open tibial fractures. J Bone Joint Surg 1986; 68:1348.

Bone L, Johnson K. Treatment of tibial fractures by reaming and intramedullary nailing. J Bone Joint Surg 1986; 68A:877.

Brown P, Urban J. Early weight-bearing treatment of open fractures of the tibia. J Bone Joint Surg 1969; 51A:59.

Dehne E, Metz C, Deffer P. Nonoperative treatment of the fractured tibia by immediate weight bearing. J Trauma 1961; 1:514.

Dietz F, Merchant P. Long-term follow-up of shaft fractures of the tibia and fibula. J Bone Joint Surg 1989; 71A.

Gustilo R, Anderson J. Prevention of infection in the treatment of one thousand and twenty-five open fractures of long bones. J Bone Joint Surg 1976; 58A:453.

Hansen S. Editorial—The Type III C tibial fracture. J Bone Joint Surg 1987; 69A:799.

Klemm K, Borner M. Interlocking nailing of complex fractures of the femur and tibia. Clin Orthop 1986; 212:89.

McAndrew M, Pontarell W. The long-term follow-up of ipsilateral tibial and femoral diaphyseal fractures. Clin Orthop 1988; 232:190.

McGraw J, Lim E. Treatment of open tibial-shaft fractures. External fixation and secondary intramedullary nailing. J Bone Joint Surg 1988; 70:900.

Nesbakken A, et al. Open tibial fractures treated with Hoffmann external fixation. Arch Orthop Trauma Surg 1988; 107:248.

Puno R, et al. Critical analysis of results of treatment of 201 tibial shaft fractures. Clin Orthop 1986; 212:113.

Sarmiento A. A functional below-the-knee cast for tibial fractures. J Bone Joint Surg 1967; 49A:855.

Wiss D. Flexible medullary nailing of acute tibial shaft fractures. Clin Orthop 1986; 212:122.

COMPARTMENT SYNDROME

A. Injuries predisposing to compartment syndrome include all events that increase the contents of the compartment or restrict compartment expansion. These may involve bleeding diatheses (hemophilia, AV malformation), inadvertent administration of intravenous fluids or drugs, snake or insect bites, burns, crush syndrome, or high-energy trauma. Any muscle that has a restrictive fascial envelope may develop compartment syndrome including the foot, thigh, and gluteal muscles as well as the more common forearm and leg compartments.

B. Any limb that is predisposed to compartment syndrome should have a specific and frequent physical examination. Gentle palpation of the compartment can give a feel for the amount of intracompartmental swelling. Pain on passive stretch of the involved compartments—usually by dorsiflexion or volarflexion of the fingers or toes—is the most sensitive test of compartment tightness.

C. Patients with mild discomfort to passive stretch of the involved compartment can be observed if re-examined frequently. The affected limb must be elevated *only* to heart level and no higher. No circumferential dressing should be placed; therefore, casts, if needed for reduction, must be split, as must the cast padding. Ice in plastic bags or surgical gloves placed over the involved compartment may decrease swelling. Pain medication should be kept to a minimum. Most potential compartment syndromes have declared themselves within 48 hours of the most recent traumatic event. If the clinical examination demonstrates decreased swelling and pain, then treatment and mobilization may proceed. If in doubt, continue monitoring.

D. The key to clinical monitoring of compartment pressures is level of pain; therefore, patients who cannot determine pain (head injury, spinal cord injury) or who cannot communicate pain require direct compartment measurement.

E. Increasing pain or increasing demand for pain medication in a patient whose limb is splinted and nondependent equals impending compartment syndrome until ruled out by compartment measurements.

F. Palpation of very firm or rock hard compartments or severe pain with passive stretch of the involved compartment should raise a high suspicion of compartment syndrome. Loss of pulse, not restorable by realignment of displaced fracture/dislocated joint and not associated with an arterial injury, is *end stage compartment syndrome.*

G. Each individual compartment should be measured. There are numerous commercially available measuring devices. One can also set up a fairly simple system as demonstrated in Figure 1. A catheter with a larger measuring surface such as a wick catheter is more accurate than a needle. Accurate calibration of the device is imperative. One needs to be aware that the pressures measured at the fracture site will be higher than in the remainder of the compartment.

H. Patients with normal blood pressure can be expected to have pressures within specific ranges. Correlate pressure measurements with clinical examination, and perform fasciotomies earlier rather than later. In the face of equivocal pressure measurements and a suspicious physical exam, fasciotomies should be performed.

I. Hypotensive patients will have lower diastolic pressures and therefore the intracompartment pressure precipitating a compartment syndrome will be lower. Thus the difference between the diastolic and compartment pressures, rather than absolute numbers, is used.

J. Undertake complete fasciotomies including skin incisions that are the same length as the fasciotomy. Adjacent tunnels such as the carpal tunnel may also need surgical release. Accomplish closure by either delayed primary closure or delayed skin graft.

K. Accomplish continual monitoring in one of two ways. Use commercially available indwelling catheters to provide continuous pressure measurements. Most clinical situations do not warrant this expense or potential morbidity. In these cases, two or three serial measurements provide the necessary information to make the appropriate decision.

INJURY PREDISPOSING TO COMPARTMENT SYNDROME

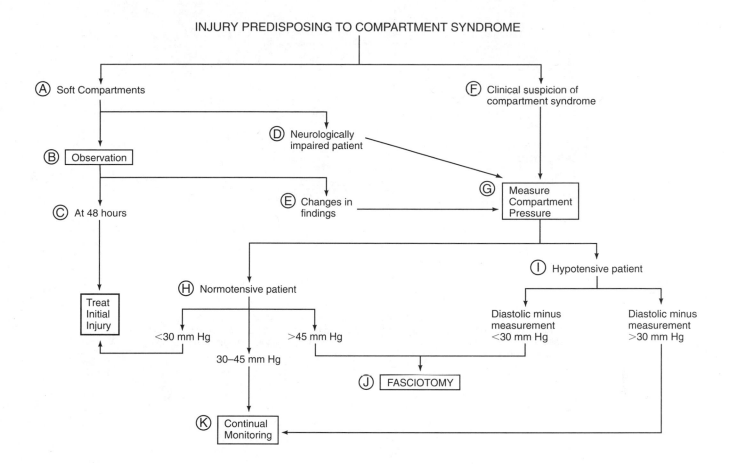

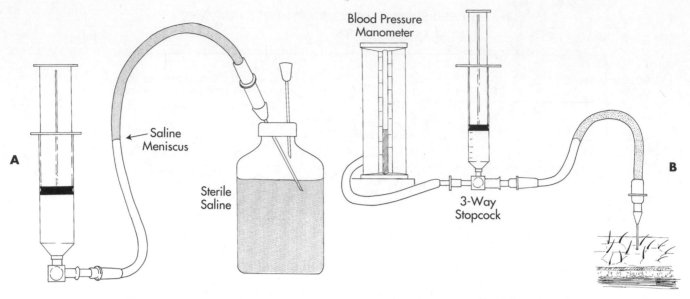

Figure 1 **A,** A syringe, hooked up to a 3-way stop cock, is used to aspirate sterile saline into an IV extension tube. **B,** A blood pressure manometer is then connected to the 3-way stop cock. Compartment pressure is measured as that pressure needed to move the saline meniscus in the tubing towards the compartment.

References

Bourne RB, Rorabeck CH. Compartment syndromes of the lower leg. Clin Orthop 1989; 240:97.

Buck SS, Brumback RJ, Poka A, et al. Compartment syndrome in open tibial fractures. J Bone Joint Surg 1986; 68(A):1348.

Gurvender SV, Smith RC, Sherk HH, Mooar P. Accurate compartment pressure measurement using the intravenous alarm control pump—Report of a technique. J Orthop Trauma 1992; 6(1):87.

Lagerstrom CF, Reed II RL, Rowlands BJ, Fischer RP. Early fasciotomy for acute clinically evident posttraumatic compartment syndrome. Am J Surg 1989; 158:36.

Matsen FA. Compartment syndrome—A unified concept. Clin Orthop 1975; 113:8.

McDougall CG, Johnston GH. A new technique of catheter placement for measurement of forearm compartment pressure. J Trauma 1991; 31(10):1404.

Moed BR, Fakhouri AJ. Compartment syndrome after low velocity gunshot wounds to the forearm. J Orthop Trauma 1991; 5(2):134.

Mubarek SJ, Hargens AR, Owen CA, et al. The Wick catheter technique for measurement of intramuscular pressure. J Bone Joint Surg 1976; 58(A):1016.

Mubarek SJ, Owen CA. Double-incision fasciotomy of the leg for decompression in compartment syndromes. J Bone Joint Surg 1977; 59(A):184.

Whitesides TE, Haney TC, Harada H, et al. A simple method for tissue pressure determination. Arch Surg 1975; 110:1311.

Willis RB, Rorabeck CH. Treatment of compartment syndrome in children. Orthop Clin North Am 1990; 21(2):401.

FRACTURE DISLOCATION OF THE ANKLE

A. The stability of the ankle joint depends on the structural integrity of the bones (medial and lateral malleoli, tibial plafond, and talus), the ligaments (lateral collateral, deltoid, and syndesmotic), and, to a lesser degree, the capsular and muscular tissues. A minimum of two breaks, either osseous or ligamentous, in the ankle mortise is necessary for significant talar shift to occur. A weight-bearing line drawn down the center of the tibial shaft should pass through the center of the talus on the anteroposterior (AP) radiograph. On the lateral radiograph, such a line should intersect the most proximal point of the talar dome. Talar shift of more than 1 or 2 mm in any plane, with or without asymmetry in the articular clear space or evident widening of the distal tibiofibular syndesmosis, is diagnostic of an unstable injury. Stress radiographs and comparable views of the opposite normal ankle may assist in evaluating equivocal fractures.

B. Single breaks in the mortise, commonly isolated fractures of the lateral malleolus, are stable and merely require external immobilization. Closely monitor the injury with serial radiographs during the first 4 weeks of treatment to ensure maintenance of the fracture reduction.

C. The goal of surgery is anatomic positioning and stabilization of the talus in the ankle mortise. Radiographs following closed reduction and the use of either the Lauge-Hansen or ASIF (Fig. 1) classification schemes aid in the preoperative planning for unstable injuries. The Lauge-Hansen scheme is especially useful in fractures amenable to closed treatment, while the ASIF (Association for the Study of Internal Fixation) classification is preferable for injuries requiring operative reduction. Closed treatment with casting only is unsatisfactory because of difficulties in achieving acceptable reductions, loss of reductions in plaster necessitating remanipulations, and stiffness and disuse atrophy from prolonged immobilization.

D. Because of the stout lateral collateral ligament complex and the buttressing role of the lateral malleolus, talar shift correlates directly with the plane and extent of lateral malleolar displacement. Restoration of the length and stability of the lateral malleolus is therefore the first priority of surgery. If the lateral malleolus is severely comminuted, precise restoration of the mortise is best achieved by first reducing and stabilizing the medial malleolar fragment. Anatomic reduction is ensured only when intraoperative radiographs show the subchondral bone plate of the distal tibia to be continuous with that of the lateral malleolar articular surface. An alternative measure of the restoration of the anatomy of the ankle mortise is the talocrural angle. Restoration of the talocrural angle is important to achieve a satisfactory functional result. Cadaveric studies have shown that 1 mm of displacement of the talus results in a 42% reduction in the tibiotalar contact, predisposing the joint to post-traumatic arthritis. Interposition of medial malleolar fragments or portions of the deltoid ligament in the joint occasionally blocks the lateral reduction and requires a medial incision for extraction prior to fixation of the lateral malleolus.

E. The joint space must be equal width throughout the mortise after lateral malleolar stabilization. In the presence of a deltoid ligament rupture, persistent medial widening implies probable infolding of the ligament. Fraying of the ligament makes rigid repair impractical, but reapproximation and apposition of the ligament ends should be attempted.

F. Most posterior malleolar fragments are firmly attached to the lateral malleolus and will reduce with accurate realignment of the lateral malleolar fracture. Potentially unstable fractures involving more than one third of the articular surface of the distal tibia warrant interfragmental screw fixation. Recent studies have shown that separate reduction and stabilization of the posterior malleolar fragment is not required in the majority of trimalleolar fractures.

G. The syndesmosis consists of the anterior and posterior distal tibiofibular ligaments and the extension of the interosseous membrane. Injury to these ligaments can be deduced from the level of the fibular fracture. The syndesmosis remains intact with transverse fibular fractures below the joint line. Spiral fibular fractures beginning at the joint line are associated with partial syndesmotic disruption. When the entire fibular fracture is located above the joint, complete rupture can be anticipated. A widened or unstable syndesmosis permits slight lateral displacement of the talus, thereby significantly increasing talotibial joint force and predisposing to degenerative arthritis. Following fixation of all high fractures, evaluate the syndesmosis radiographically and manually, using a bone hook or bone clamp to check for excessive laxity. A transfixion or position screw is commonly needed to hold the distal tibiofibular joint in a reduced position during the healing of the supporting ligaments. The ASIF group recommends repair of the syndesmotic ligaments in place of position screws, reserving the latter for the more severe disruptions, e.g., those seen with very proximal (Maisonneuve) fibular fractures. Randomized studies comparing various postoperative regimens for bimalleolar and trimalleolar fractures have shown no significant difference in various treatment methods. The long-term radiographic and functional results are the same whether casting and/or protected weight bearing are used or not, assuming that a stable osteosynthesis has been achieved.

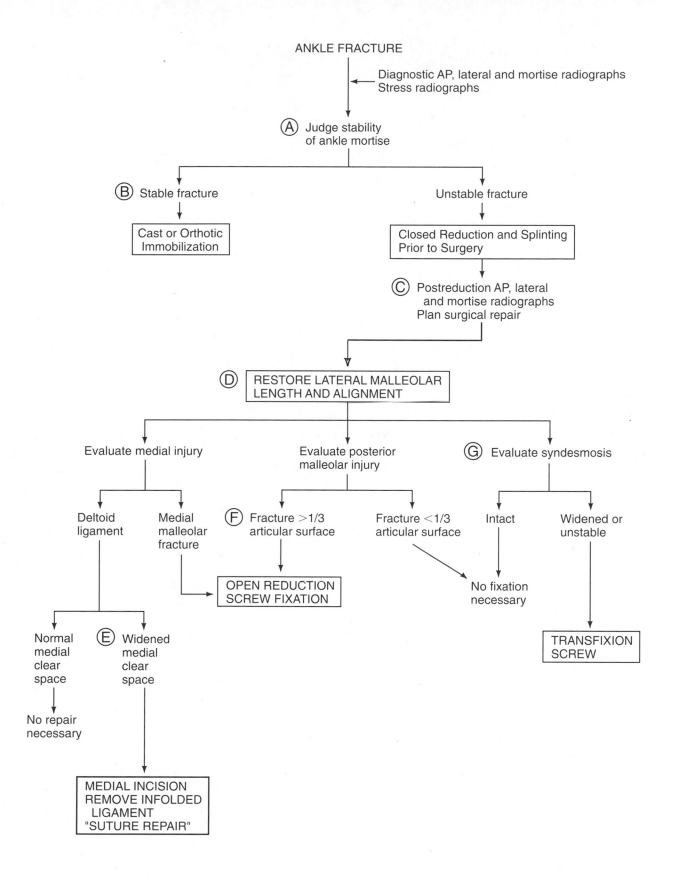

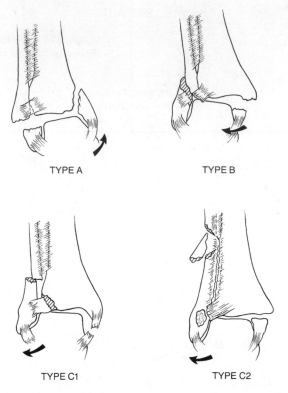

Figure 1   ASIF (Weber) classification of ankle fractures.

Open ankle fractures are ideally managed by thorough debridement, immediate open reduction and internal fixation, and delayed primary closure of any open wounds. A high union rate can be expected from such treatment, but often open fractures are associated with significant cartilage damage resulting in early post-traumatic arthritis.

References

Baird R, Jackson S. Fractures of the distal part of the fibula with associated disruption of the deltoid ligament. J Bone Joint Surg 1987; 69A:1346.

Bucholz R, Henry S, Henley M. Fixation with bioabsorbable screws for the treatment of fractures of the ankle. J Bone Joint Surg 1994; 76A:319.

Finsen V, et al. Early postoperative weight-bearing and muscle activity in patients who have a fracture of the ankle. J Bone Joint Surg 1989; 71A:23.

Franklin J, Johnson K, Hansen S. Immediate internal fixation of open ankle fractures. J Bone Joint Surg 1984; 66A:1245.

Harper M. The deltoid ligament—An elevation of need for surgical repair. Clin Orthop 1988; 226:156.

Harper M. Posterior malleolar fractures of the ankle associated with external rotation-abduction injuries: Results with and without internal fixation. J Bone Joint Surg 1988.

Joy G, Patzakis M, Harvey J. Precise evaluation of the reduction of severe ankle fractures. J Bone Joint Surg 1974; 56A:979.

Lauge-Hansen N. Fractures of the ankle: II. Combined experimental-surgical and experimental-roentgenologic investigations. Arch Surg 1950; 60:957.

Limbird R, Aaron R. Laterally comminuted fracture-dislocation of the ankle. J Bone Joint Surg 1987; 69A:881.

Lindsjo V. Classification of ankle fractures: The Lauge-Hansen or AO system? Clin Orthop 1985; 199:12.

Muller M, Allgower M, Schneider R, Willenegger H. Manual of internal fixation. Berlin: Springer-Verlag, 1991.

Phillips W, et al. A prospective, randomized study of the management of severe ankle fractures. J Bone Joint Surg 1985; 67A:67.

Ramsey P, Hamilton W. Changes in tibiotalar area of contact caused by lateral talar shift. J Bone Joint Surg 1976; 58A:356.

Yablon I, Heller F, Shouse L. The key role of the lateral malleolus in displaced fractures of the ankle. J Bone Joint Surg 1977; 59A:169.

FRACTURE OF THE CALCANEUS

A. Accurate delineation of all fracture lines necessitates multiple radiologic views. By demonstrating the extension of fractures into the subtalar joint, the loss of the tuberosity-joint (Bohler's) angle, and the degree of posterior facet depression the lateral radiograph serves as the basis for most traditional classification schemes (Fig. 1). The anteroposterior (AP) radiograph demonstrates the calcaneocuboid joint, while the sustentaculum tali, cortical margins of the tuberosity, and the varus/valgus alignment are best seen on the axial view. Oblique radiographs (especially Broden's views) aid in defining the extent of depression and comminution of the posterior facet.

Computed tomography (CT) scanning has replaced plain radiography in the assessment of complex intra-articular fractures of the calcaneus (Fig. 2). Both coronal (perpendicular to the posterior facet) and plantar CT sections are routinely obtained. A CT scan of the opposite hindfoot is used for reference. Recent classification schemes are based on the pathoanatomy of the fracture revealed by the CT scan. The traditional measurement of the Bohler's angle has been found to be less important than an accurate assessment of the amount of posterior facet disruption. CT scanning is imperative if surgical reduction of the calcaneus is planned.

B. Since most calcaneal fractures are the result of falls from heights, the 10% incidence of associated compression fractures of the lumbar spine is understandable. A mandatory part of the work-up of all calcaneal fractures is a thorough lumbosacral spine examination, usually including radiographs.

C. Isolated extra-articular chip or avulsion fractures of the tuberosity, sustentaculum tali, or anterior process of the calcaneus and minimally displaced body and tuberosity fractures have an excellent prognosis for full return of function. Direct treatment at the soft tissues. After 2 to 3 days of elevation, compressive bulky dressings, and ice, begin early motion. Delay weight bearing for 6 to 8 weeks on any comminuted fracture with subtalar extension prone to displacement. Avoid cast immobilization because it leads to muscle atrophy, joint contractures, and slow functional recovery.

D. Avulsion fractures of the calcaneal tendon insertion comprise less than 5% of all calcaneal fractures. While avulsion fractures displaced less than 5 mm may be treated in plaster casts, those with complete separation from the tuberosity require operative reduction and interfragmental screw fixation.

E. The multitude of recommended approaches in the orthopaedic literature to displaced intra-articular calcaneal fractures attests to the fact that no single treatment regimen is indisputably superior. The loss of Bohler's angle (normally 30° to 40°) implies fracture and impaction of the posterior calcaneal facet. Although specific fracture variants have been classified, there is no universally accepted classification scheme for intra-articular fractures. Most recent classifications have been based on the degree of comminution of the posterior facet as demonstrated on the coronal CT sections. Minimally displaced (CT type I) fractures result in little functional impairment with standard conservative treatment.

F. Intra-articular fractures associated with shortening and widening of the hindfoot, lateral subluxation of the tuberosity with impingement on the lateral malleolus and/or soft tissue structures, or significant varus deformity of the heel are ideally treated by reduction and fixation of the fracture. Closed manipulative and percutaneous techniques yield unpredictable results. Operative techniques are often difficult and may be fraught with significant soft tissue complications. The best indications for operative treatment are displacement of the posterior facet or the tuberosity fragment with loss of Bohler's angle and/or incongruity of the joint surface of the posterior facet. There may be extenuating conditions, such as edematous or contused soft tissues, severe osteopenia or comminution, or systemic problems such as diabetes mellitus, that might increase the risk of open surgery. It is preferable to manage such cases by traditional conservative means.

G. Any aggressive surgical approach demands a complete understanding of the pathologic anatomy of a given fracture. The goals of surgery include (1) anatomic reduction of the joint surfaces of the hindfoot, (2) restoration of the normal width and height of the calcaneus, and (3) relief of any lateral impingement of displaced fracture fragments on the surrounding soft tissues (Fig. 3). Intra-articular fractures may be approached through a medial, lateral, or combined lateral/medial surgical exposure. Medially comminuted tongue fractures are especially amenable to medial approaches while comminuted posterior facet fractures are best visualized through a lateral approach. Careful soft tissue handling is critical to avoid postoperative wound sloughs. The precise indications for bone grafting of calcaneal body defects have not been defined.

The role of primary subtalar or triple arthrodesis in the management of calcaneal fractures is unknown. This technique, however, should be reserved for severely comminuted, irreducible fractures.

FRACTURE OF THE CALCANEUS

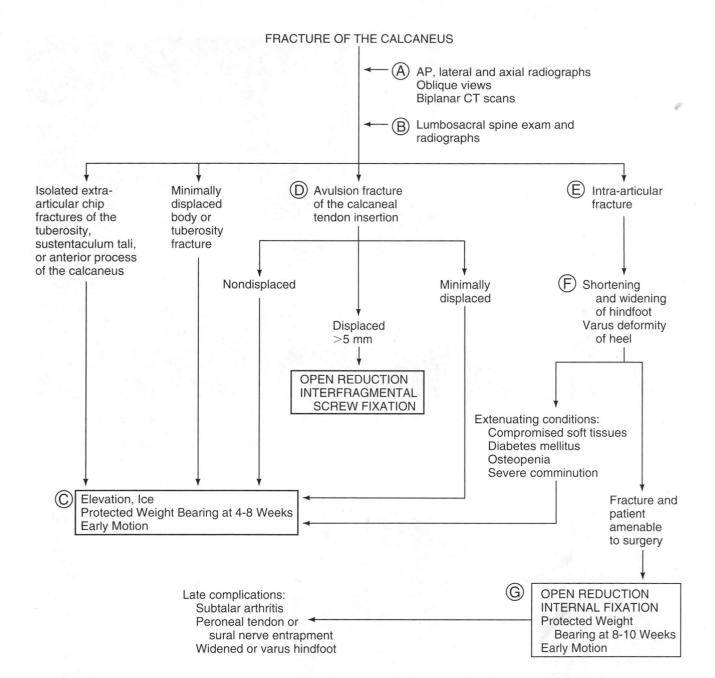

Ⓐ AP, lateral and axial radiographs
Oblique views
Biplanar CT scans

Ⓑ Lumbosacral spine exam and
radiographs

Isolated extra-articular chip fractures of the tuberosity, sustentaculum tali, or anterior process of the calcaneus

Minimally displaced body or tuberosity fracture

Ⓓ Avulsion fracture of the calcaneal tendon insertion

Ⓔ Intra-articular fracture

Nondisplaced

Minimally displaced

Displaced
>5 mm

Ⓕ Shortening and widening of hindfoot
Varus deformity of heel

OPEN REDUCTION
INTERFRAGMENTAL
SCREW FIXATION

Extenuating conditions:
Compromised soft tissues
Diabetes mellitus
Osteopenia
Severe comminution

Ⓒ Elevation, Ice
Protected Weight Bearing at 4-8 Weeks
Early Motion

Fracture and patient amenable to surgery

Late complications:
Subtalar arthritis
Peroneal tendon or
sural nerve entrapment
Widened or varus hindfoot

Ⓖ OPEN REDUCTION
INTERNAL FIXATION
Protected Weight
Bearing at 8-10 Weeks
Early Motion

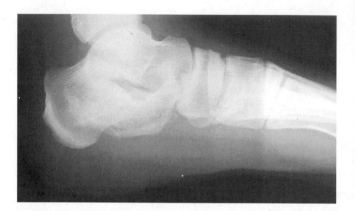

Figure 1 Lateral radiograph of an intra-articular fracture of the calcaneus.

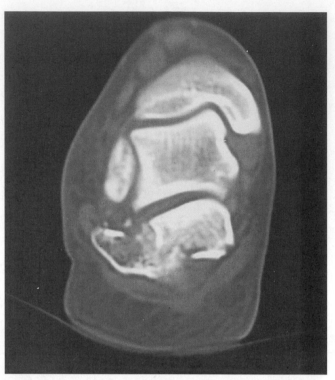

Figure 2 Preoperative CT scan demonstrates intra-articular fracture of the posterior facet of the calcaneus with extrusion of the lateral wall of the calcaneus. Multiple fragments of the lateral wall are impinging against the lateral malleolus.

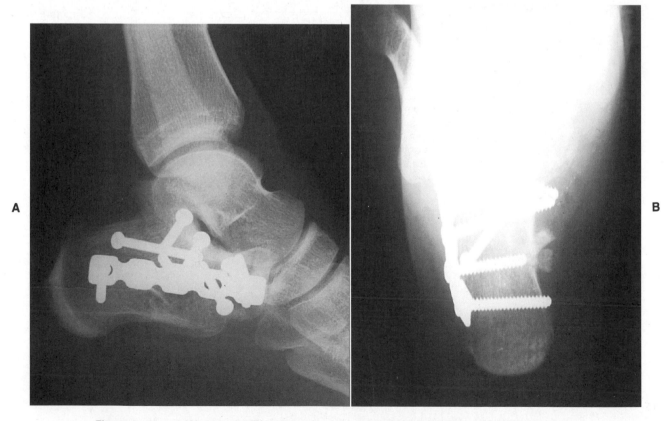

A

B

Figure 3 Lateral **(A)** and axial **(B)** radiographs postoperatively demonstrate restoration of the position of the posterior facet of the calcaneus and reduction of the displaced lateral wall.

References

Bowe C, Sakellarides H, Freeman P, Sorbie C. Fractures of the os calcis: A long-term follow-up study of 146 patients. JAMA 1963; 184:920.

Burdeaux B. Reduction of calcaneal fractures by the McReynolds medial approach technique and its experimental basis. Clin Orthop 1983; 177:87.

Carr J. Surgical treatment of the intra-articular calcaneus fracture. Orthop Clin North Am 1994; 25:665.

Crosby L, Fitzgibbons T. Computerized tomography scanning of acute intra-articular fractures of the calcaneus: A new classification system. J Bone Joint Surg 1990; 72A:852.

Essex-Lopresti P. The mechanism, reduction, technique, and results in fracture of the os calcis. Bone J Surg 1951; 39:395.

Giachino A, Uhthoff H. Intra-articular fractures of the calcaneus. J Bone Joint Surg 1989; 71A:784.

Kerr P, James A, Cole A, et al. The use of the axial CT scan in intra-articular fractures of the calcaneum. Injury 1994; 25:359.

Kitaoka H, Schaap E, Chao E, et al. Displaced intra-articular fractures of the calcaneus treated non-operatively: Clinical results and analysis of motion and ground-reaction and temporal forces. J Bone Joint Surg 1994; 76A:1531.

Lance E, Carey E, Wade P. Fractures of the os calcis: Treatment by early mobilization. Clin Orthop 1963; 30:76.

McReynolds I. Trauma to the os calcis and heel cord. In: Jahss MH, ed. Disorders of the foot. Vol. 2. Philadelphia: W.B. Saunders, 1982: 1497.

O'Farrell D, O'Byrne J, McCabe J, et al. Fractures of the os calcis: Improved results with internal fixation. Injury 1993; 24:263.

Parmar H, Triffitt T, Gregg P. Intra-articular fracture of the calcaneus treated operatively or conservatively: A prospective study. J Bone Joint Surg 1994; 76B:851.

Stephenson J. Treatment of displaced intra-articular fractures of the calcaneus using medial and lateral approaches, internal fixation, and early motion. J Bone Joint Surg 1987; 69A:115.

Thompson K. Treatment of comminuted fractures of the calcaneus by triple arthrodesis. Orthop Clin North Am 1973; 4:189.

Warrick C, Bremner A. Fractures of the calcaneum with an atlas illustrating the various types of fractures. J Bone Joint Surg 1953; 35B:33.

FRACTURE OR DISLOCATION OF THE TALUS

A. Talar neck fractures are usually secondary to hyperextension forces, whereas body fractures are due to severe axial loads. Cast nondisplaced neck fractures with the ankle in neutral or slight equinus. It is imperative that the fracture be truly nondisplaced since minor degrees of displacement of the talar neck can alter the biomechanics of the hindfoot. Do not allow weight bearing on the leg until there is radiographic evidence of union.

The Hawkins classification is widely used for the categorization of talar neck fractures (Fig. 1). Hawkins Type I injuries are nondisplaced while Hawkins Type II injuries include displaced talar neck fractures with or without obvious subluxation of the subtalar joint. Hawkins Type III fractures are associated with subluxation or complete dislocation of both the subtalar and tibiotalar joints. Type IV injuries are Type III injuries with additional disruption of the talonavicular joint.

B. Minimally displaced neck and body fractures occasionally can be manipulated and casted. Maintenance of reductions in casts is difficult, however, and redisplacement frequently occurs. Anatomic reduction and internal fixation yield better functional results in most cases. Most displaced talar neck fractures are associated with some degree of subtalar subluxation.

Many different surgical approaches and techniques of fixation have been advocated. Screw fixation is generally preferable to the use of K-wires or Steinmann pins. Anteromedial and/or anterolateral incisions are most commonly used, though occasionally a medial malleolar osteotomy is required for adequate exposure of a displaced body fracture. Interfragmental screws placed anteroposteriorly or posteroanteriorly are usually sufficient for rigid internal fixation. Be careful not to further disrupt the tenuous blood supply to the talus.

C. Treat a talar neck or body fracture associated with a complete subtalar dislocation the same as an isolated neck or body fracture after the dislocation has been reduced.

D. A simple subtalar dislocation without associated fracture can often be reduced under general anesthesia by closed manipulation alone. Carefully inspect the postreduction radiographs to ensure an accurate reduction. The incidence of late subtalar post-traumatic arthritis is low. Evaluate associated fractures on the postreduction film and treat appropriately. Infrequently the closed reduction of a pure subtalar dislocation may be blocked by interposed soft tissues, either tendinous or capsular. Lateral subtalar dislocations are commonly associated with injuries to the posterior tibial artery, vein, and nerve.

E. Closed reduction of complete talar dislocations (Hawkins Type III) is usually impossible because of massive soft tissue swelling, triplane displacement and rotation of the talus, and interposed osteochondral fragments. At open reduction, a transcalcaneal pin may be helpful, providing additional distraction of the ankle and thus facilitating talar reduction. Following rigid internal fixation of any associated talar fractures, test the stability of the ankle. If there is a tendency for residual subluxation of the talus, then maintain anatomic reduction of the talus by an external fixator spanning the ankle joint.

F. In an open complete talar dislocation, leave the soft tissue open after surgical reduction of the talus. A delayed primary closure or skin grafting can be performed at 5 to 7 days.

G. Osteochondral dome fractures are also called flake fractures or osteochondritis dissecans. Lateral dome osteochondral fractures are the most common pattern and can be diagnosed on either the mortise view or tomography of the ankle. Arthroscopy or arthrography occasionally is needed to diagnose pure cartilaginous lesions.

H. Displaced transchondral fractures may mechanically block full joint motion and cause persistent ankle pain. Operative treatment with extraction of all loose fragments, curettage of the defect, and drilling of all exposed subchondral bone has been reported as offering the best long-term results. In the rare case where there is a minimally comminuted, large osteochondral fragment, open reduction and internal fixation with countersunk screws or Herbert screws may be possible. Early postoperative ankle motion stimulates fibrocartilaginous resurfacing of any defect in cases where the fragment has been excised. Lateral dome lesions are usually anterior and easily amenable to arthroscopic debridement. Medial lesions are usually posterior and may require either a posterior portal for arthroscopic debridement or a transmalleolar osteotomy for open debridement.

I. A radiographic zone of bone resorption under the subchondral plate of the dome of the talus at 1 to 2 months postinjury signifies adequate preservation of the vascular supply to the bone (Hawkins sign). Owing to the tenuous blood supply of the talus, avascular necrosis is a frequent sequela of talar injuries. The incidence of this complication varies from 13% in isolated neck fractures to 50% in subtalar fracture-dislocations to 84% in complete talar fracture-dislocations. Due to the high incidence of osteonecrosis with complete talar dislocations, primary tibiotalar arthrodesis has been advocated for these injuries. Most complete talar dislocations, however, are preferably managed by open reduction and internal fixation. Pantalar arthrodesis can then be performed at a later date if segmental collapse of the talar dome occurs.

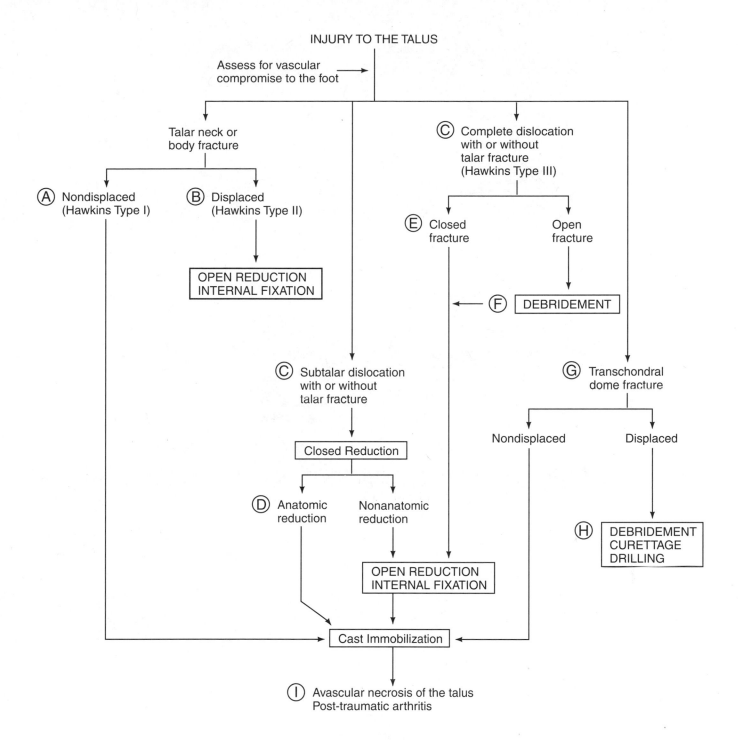

INJURY TO THE TALUS

Assess for vascular compromise to the foot

Ⓐ Nondisplaced (Hawkins Type I)

Ⓑ Displaced (Hawkins Type II)

Talar neck or body fracture

OPEN REDUCTION INTERNAL FIXATION

Ⓒ Complete dislocation with or without talar fracture (Hawkins Type III)

Ⓔ Closed fracture

Open fracture

Ⓕ DEBRIDEMENT

Ⓒ Subtalar dislocation with or without talar fracture

Closed Reduction

Ⓓ Anatomic reduction

Nonanatomic reduction

OPEN REDUCTION INTERNAL FIXATION

Ⓖ Transchondral dome fracture

Nondisplaced

Displaced

Ⓗ DEBRIDEMENT CURETTAGE DRILLING

Cast Immobilization

Ⓘ Avascular necrosis of the talus
Post-traumatic arthritis

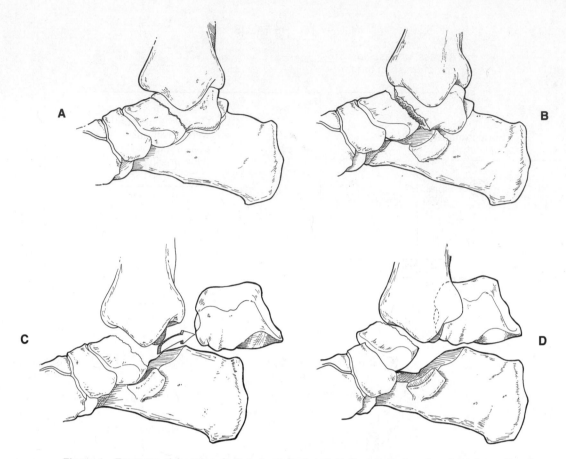

Figure 1 Fractures of the talus. **A,** Type I nondisplaced. **B,** Type II displaced neck fracture with subtalar subluxation. **C,** Type III fracture with complete talar dislocation. **D,** Type IV injury with complete talar dislocation and disruption of the talonavicular joint.

References

Alexander H, Lichtman D. Surgical treatment of transchondral talar dome fractures (osteochondritis dissecans). J Bone Joint Surg 1980; 62A:646.

Baker C, Andrews J, Ryan J. Arthroscopic treatment of transchondral talar dome fractures. Arthroscopy 1986; 2:82.

Berndt A, Harty M. Transchondral fractures of the talus. J Bone Joint Surg 1959: 41A:988.

Canale T, Kelly F. Fractures of the neck of the talus. J Bone Joint Surg 1978; 60A:143.

Daniels T, Smith J. Talar neck fractures. Foot Ankle 1993; 14:225.

Grob D, Simpson L, Weber B, Bray T. Operative treatment of displaced talus fractures. Clin Orthop 1985; 199:88.

Kelly P, Sullivan C. Blood supply of the talus. Clin Orthop 1963; 30:37.

Ly P, Fallat L. Trans-chondral fractures of the talus: A review of 64 surgical cases. J Foot Ankle Surg 1993; 32:352.

Monson S, Ryan J. Subtalar dislocation. J Bone Joint Surg 1981; 63A:1156.

Pennal G. Fractures of the talus. Clin Orthop 1963; 30:53.

Pritsch M, Horoshovski H, Farine I. Arthroscopic treatment of osteochondral lesions of the talus. J Bone Joint Surg 1986; 68A:862.

Saltzmann C, Marsh J, Tearse D. Treatment of displaced talar fractures: An arthroscopically assisted approach. Foot Ankle 1994; 15:630.

Shea M, Mandi A. Osteochondral lesions of the talar bone. Foot Ankle 1993; 14:48.

Swanson T, Bray T. Talar neck fractures. A mechanical and histomorphometric study of fixation. Presented at the 1988 OTA Meeting.

Szyszkowitz R, Reschaver R, Seggl W. Eighty-five talus fractures treated by ORIF with five to eight years of follow-up study of 69 patients. Clin Orthop 1985; 199:97.

TARSOMETATARSAL FRACTURE-DISLOCATION

A. The stability of the tarsometatarsal (Lisfranc) joint is attributable to a thick plantar ligamentous complex and the locking of the second metatarsal base in the cuneiform recess. Disruption of these supporting structures may result from direct or indirect forces applied to the forefoot. Direct injuries secondary to crushing of the forefoot result in plantar or dorsal dislocations with significant fracture comminution and open wounds. Indirect injuries may occur from severe abduction or plantar flexion loads, most commonly axial loading of a plantar flexed and fixed foot.

The joint injury may be total, partial, or divergent. The three most common patterns are lateral dislocation of the entire forefoot, lateral dislocation of the second through the fifth metatarsals, and medial displacement of the first metatarsal (Fig. 1). Divergent injuries with medial dislocation of the first ray and lateral dislocation of the lateral four rays are rare. Nearly 20% of tarsometatarsal fracture-dislocations are missed at the time of initial patient evaluation. Most patients, however, will have severe forefoot pain and will report a clunking or snapping sensation in the foot. Radiographic abnormalities may be subtle. A fracture of the base of the second metatarsal or an anterior compression fracture of the cuboid is often the only evidence for significant joint disruption. In such cases, stress radiographs with the patient under regional or general anesthesia are helpful in detecting spontaneously reduced unstable tarsometatarsal injuries.

B. Complete forefoot dislocations, especially those secondary to direct trauma, can result in injury to the dorsalis pedis artery. Persistent forefoot ischemia after manipulative realignment of the joint is an absolute indication for vessel exploration and internal fixation of the joint.

C. Longitudinal traction through a Chinese finger trap applied to the forefoot aids in obtaining a closed reduction. Closed reduction may fail because of marked instability of the joint or interposition of soft tissues or osteochondral fragments. The most common tissues interposed in these dislocations are the anterior tibial tendon between the first and second metatarsals and comminuted fragments of the base of the second metatarsal blocking its reduction.

D. Prior to percutaneous Steinmann pin fixation, confirm anatomic reduction in all planes with anteroposterior (AP), lateral, and oblique radiographs. Most total fracture-dislocations require two pins, one through the first metatarsal into the medial cuneiform and one through the fifth metatarsal into the cuboid. The middle three metatarsals generally do not need to be pinned since they are tethered to the fifth metatarsal by the intermetatarsal ligaments. Individualize modifications in pin placement for partial and divergent injuries. Postoperatively, place the patient in a well molded, nonweight-bearing, short leg cast. Elevation of the foot for several days with monitoring of the neurovascular status is imperative. Remove the percutaneous Steinmann pins at 6 to 8 weeks after insertion. Rehabilitation of the foot may be slow.

E. Residual forefoot displacement or joint widening of greater than 1 mm in active patients and gross instability of a satisfactorily reduced dislocation are indications for open reduction and internal fixation. Longitudinal skin incisions, usually one medially and one laterally, suffice in exposing the entire disrupted joint. The location of the incisions is dependent on the fracture pattern. The medial incision is usually made just lateral to the extensor hallucis longus tendon with care to avoid injury to the dorsalis pedis artery and the multiple dorsal veins. This incision is critical for proper visualization of the base of the second metatarsal. A lateral longitudinal incision, parallel to the medial incision may be required for visualization of the lateral column of the foot. Wide transverse incisions lead to marginal skin necrosis, dorsal sensory loss, and unsightly scarring, and therefore should be avoided.

Secure fixation with multiple Steinmann pins or screws. Use either 4 mm cancellous screws or malleolar screws. Avoid interfragmental compression of the joint and remove the screws 16 to 20 weeks after insertion. The postoperative management is identical to that for percutaneous pinning.

F. Late complications, frequently encountered in improperly managed injuries, include joint incongruity with degenerative arthritis, forefoot deformity, and plantar callosities secondary to prominent metatarsal heads. The variables associated with poor results include crush injuries, delayed diagnosis, and residual displacement of greater than 2 mm or residual angulation of greater than 15°. If anatomic reduction is achieved and maintained, excellent functional results can be anticipated, but are not guaranteed. There is no indication for primary arthrodesis of a Lisfranc joint in the management of a tarsometatarsal fracture-dislocation.

INJURY TO LISFRANC JOINT

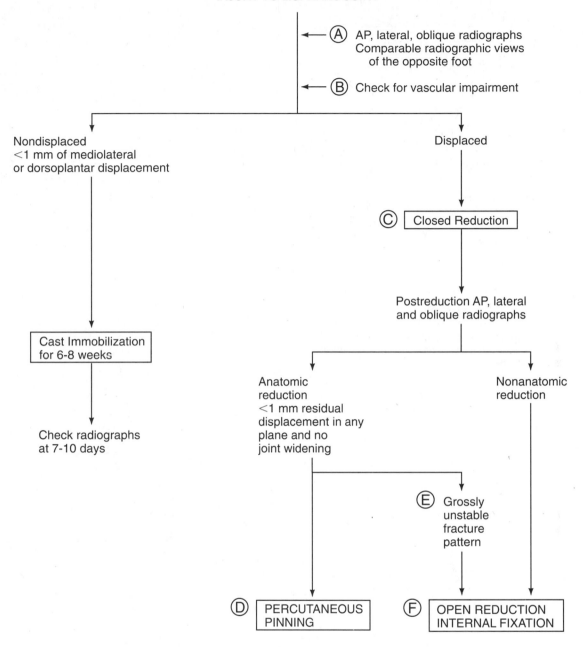

A AP, lateral, oblique radiographs
Comparable radiographic views
of the opposite foot

B Check for vascular impairment

Nondisplaced
<1 mm of mediolateral
or dorsoplantar displacement

Displaced

C Closed Reduction

Postreduction AP, lateral
and oblique radiographs

Cast Immobilization
for 6-8 weeks

Anatomic
reduction
<1 mm residual
displacement in any
plane and no
joint widening

Nonanatomic
reduction

Check radiographs
at 7-10 days

E Grossly
unstable
fracture
pattern

D PERCUTANEOUS
PINNING

F OPEN REDUCTION
INTERNAL FIXATION

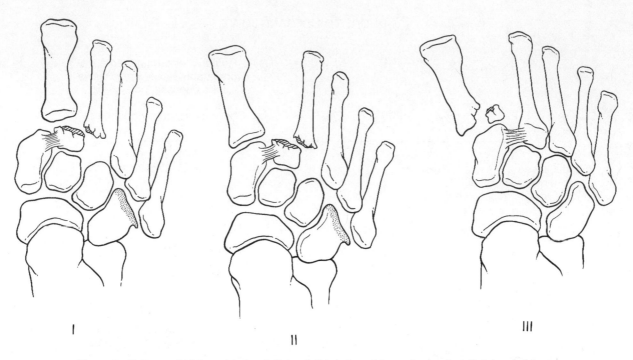

Figure 1 Patterns of Lisfranc injuries. **I,** Lateral dislocation of the entire forefoot. **II,** Lateral dislocation of the second through fifth metatarsals with an intact first ray. **III,** Medial displacement of the first metatarsal.

References

Aitken A, Poulson D. Dislocation of the tarsometatarsal joint. J Bone Joint Surg 1963; 45A:246.

Arntz C, Veith R, Hansen S. Fractures and fracture-dislocations of the tarsometatarsal joint. J Bone Joint Surg 1988; 70A:173.

Curtis M, Meyerson M, Szura D. Tarsometatarsal joint injuries in the athlete. Am J Sports Med 1993; 21:497.

Faciszewski T, Burks R, Manaster B. Subtle injuries of the Lisfranc joint. J Bone Joint Surg 1990; 72A:1519.

Gissane W. A dangerous type of fracture of the foot. J Bone Joint Surg 1951; 33B:535.

Goossens M, DeStoop N. Lisfranc fracture-dislocations— Etiology, radiology, and results. Clin Orthop 1983; 176:154.

Hardcastle P, Reschaver R, Kutacha-Lissberg E, Schoffman W. Injuries to the tarsometatarsal joint: Incidence, classification and treatment. J Bone Joint Surg 1982; 64B:349.

Leenen L, Werken C. Fracture dislocation of the tarsometatarsal joint: A combined anatomical and computed tomographic study. Injury 1992; 21:51.

Myerson M, et al. Fracture dislocations of the tarsometatarsal joints: End results correlated with pathology and treatment. Foot Ankle. 1986; 6:225.

Vuori J, Aro H. Lisfranc joint injuries: Trauma mechanisms and assorted injuries. J Trauma 1993; 35:40.

Wiley J. The mechanism of tarsometatarsal joint injuries. J Bone Joint Surgery 1971; 53B:474.

Wilpula E. Tarsometatarsal fracture-dislocation—Late results in 26 patients. Acta Orthop Scand 1973; 44:335.

Yamamoto H, Furuy A, Munetz T, et al. Neglected Lisfranc's joint dislocation. J Orthop Trauma 1992; 6:129.

RECONSTRUCTIVE SURGERY

Arthritis of the Shoulder
Osteonecrosis of the Shoulder
Impingement Syndrome
Rotator Cuff Tear
Elbow Pain
Surgery for Elbow Arthritis
Hip Pain
Osteonecrosis of the Femoral Head
Arthritis of the Hip
Hip Pain Following Total Hip Replacement
Dislocation Following Total Hip Replacement
Infected Total Hip Replacement
Rheumatoid Arthritis of the Knee
Degenerative Arthrosis of the Knee
Hemophilic Arthropathy of the Knee
Painful Total Knee Replacement
Chronic Ankle Pain
Medial Arch Pain
Heel Pain
Achilles Tendinitis
Metatarsalgia
Diabetic Foot
Hallux Valgus
Focal Bone Lesion
Soft Tissue Mass
Metastatic Lesions of Bone

ARTHRITIS OF THE SHOULDER

Relative to the weight bearing joints, the glenohumeral joint is rarely involved in arthritic conditions or systemic disease. Rheumatoid arthritis (RA), however, can involve the glenohumeral joint both from changes in the rotator cuff musculature and destruction of the joint itself. Patients with arthritic conditions about the shoulder typically present with pain, loss of function, and occasionally swelling. Activities of daily living become difficult due to loss of range of motion (ROM) and weakness. Treatment plans are designed to focus on pain relief. By gaining a pain-free arc of motion, activities of daily living are improved and therefore, function is also benefitted.

A. The most common complaint of patients with arthritis of the shoulder is pain. Typically, the pattern of pain is worsened with activities and somewhat relieved by rest. Often patients complain of night pain during recumbency. It is important to note a medication history with particular attention to oral steroids which may cause osteonecrosis. Patients with RA are affected by mechanical changes from rotator cuff dysfunction as well as joint destruction in the glenohumeral joint. A general history combined with a physical examination should allow the physician to limit the number of ancillary diagnostic tests to determine the etiology of the arthritic condition. It is important to examine patients in a relaxed atmosphere with full visualization of the entire upper trunk. Observation of ROM with notation of scapulothoracic rhythm is helpful in determining what portion of the range is coming from the glenohumeral joint. Muscle examination includes strength measurement and examination for wasting or atrophy. Assessment of rotator cuff integrity, stability, and the patient's ability to perform activities such as combing hair, reaching the buttock and donning clothing is assessed. Particular attention should be paid to loss of rotation; that can be addressed at the time of therapeutic maneuvers, i.e. Z-plasty or lengthening of the subscapularis tendon.

B. Aspiration of joint effusion or biopsy of periarticular inflammatory tissue can be used in differentiating inflammatory disease of the shoulder. Aspirated fluid is analyzed for its microscopic characteristics, glucose content, protein content, and crystals. Sedimentation rate, uric acid, rheumatoid factor, and anti-nuclear antibody studies are sometimes necessary to determine the etiology of an inflammatory arthritis. If sepsis is part of the differential, culture and sensitivities on the aspiration and a CBC with differential along with the sedimentation rate are an essential part of the diagnostic plan. X-rays in three views are helpful to assess joint destruction. An AP of the glenohumeral joint, axillary lateral and trans-scapular lateral views are a minimum requirement. Identification of a high-riding humeral head suggests rotator cuff insuffi-

ciency. Post-traumatic changes from old fractures about the proximal humerus are also readily apparent on x-ray. Integrity of the rotator cuff may be documented by arthrography or magnetic resonance imaging (MRI). Preoperative templating with two-plane radiography of the humeral shaft is also a necessity if arthroplasty is considered. Some attention should be paid to the acromioclavicular joint; degeneration of this joint can add to the pain component and if untreated can adversely affect the outcome of shoulder arthroplasty.

C. Patients with RA have varying degrees of shoulder symptoms. The great majority of these patients with systemic involvement have shoulder symptoms. Patients have been identified with a mild form of RA which affects only the shoulder joint and is exclusively found in women between 35 and 55 years of age. Patients with RA present with special problems in that the quality of their skin and bone is affected by the systemic disease. Subchondral cysts appear in the humeral head and, at times, in the glenoid. Often times, the contractures around the shoulder joint limit rotation significantly. More of the patients present with rotator cuff tears. Of those patients requiring total shoulder arthroplasty, up to 30-40% have rotator cuff tears. Patients are first placed in a medical treatment program involving a rheumatologist and a physical therapist. Occasional subacromial and intra-articular injections of lidocaine and corticosteroids may be beneficial. Physical therapy focuses on maintaining ROM for activities of daily living and strengthening those muscles around the shoulder girdle. Particular attention is paid to scapulothoracic mobilization and a strong and stable scapular platform. A patient who improves with this program should be placed in a maintenance program and observed for development of changes about the shoulder girdle. If unimproved, early intervention can prevent aggressive soft tissue and bony destruction. Although somewhat controversial, patients in the early stages of disease with minimal radiographic changes often benefit from synovectomy and rotator cuff repair. If significant radiographic changes are present, the most beneficial procedure is total shoulder arthroplasty with rotator cuff repair if necessary (Fig. 1). Other options include arthrodesis, osteotomy and resection arthroplasty, but these have been fraught with significant difficulties and do not provide the functional result seen with total shoulder arthroplasty. Preoperative assessment with CT scanning is appropriate if erosions or subluxation is of concern. Acromioclavicular arthroplasty or anterior acromioplasty can be performed simultaneous to the total shoulder arthroplasty if necessary.

ARTHRITIS OF THE SHOULDER

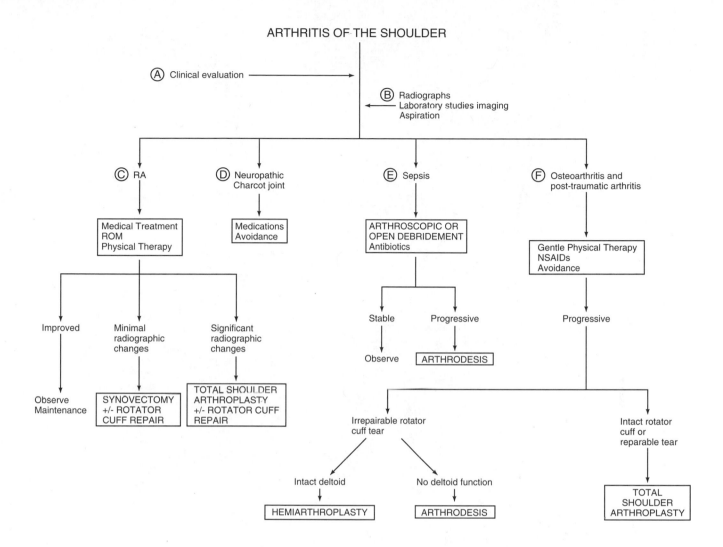

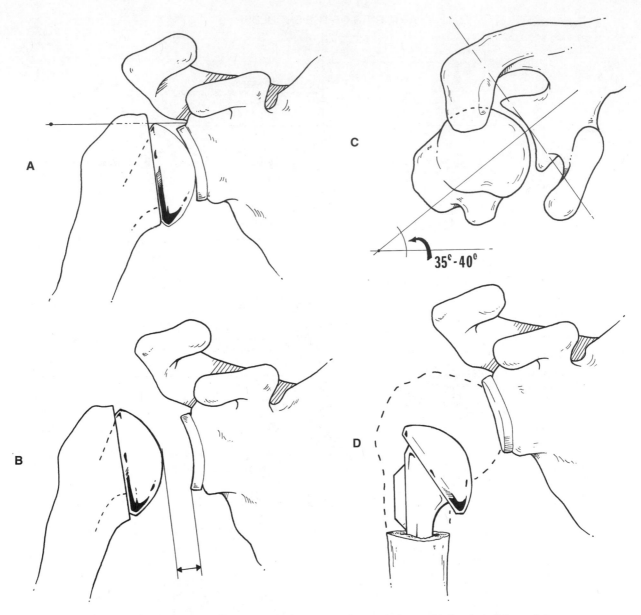

Figure 1 Total shoulder replacement requires anatomic resurfacing and balancing of the soft tissues. **A,** The prosthesis must sit cephalad to the greater tuberosity to prevent impingement on the acromion. **B,** The prosthesis must fill the glenoid or instability will result. Overfill will reduce rotation. **C,** Humeral version should match the glenoid. If no deformity or erosion is present, 35°-40° of retroversion of the humeral component is necessary. **D,** Appropriate humeral length is necessary to restore capsular and muscular tension. Instability and deltoid dysfunction result when humeral length is not preserved.

D. The most common cause of Charcot joint in the shoulder is cervical syringomyelia. The etiology may be cervical spine trauma or idiopathic syringomyelia. Radiographically, the shoulder shows bony destruction with fragmentation and osseous debris in the joint. MRI is the study of choice to diagnose the cervical syrinx. Most commonly, these patients present with a painless joint; however, at times, there is some limitation of function and pain in the shoulder girdle due to soft tissue distention. These patients are typically treated with medications and avoidance of exacerbating activities.

E. Most patients with septic arthritis have significant associated disease that compromises their immune mechanism or had recent joint aspiration or intra-articular injection. It is also not uncommon for patients who are IV drug abusers to present with septic arthritis of the shoulder. Patients are treated with arthroscopic or open debridement and antibiotic therapy which yields better results than repeated aspirations. If the disease is stabilized, these patients can be observed and involved in a functional rehabilitation program. If it progresses and leads to painful arthritis, arthrodesis is the treatment of choice.

F. Osteoarthritis, both primary and secondary, can be treated initially with gentle activities, nonsteroidal anti-inflammatory drugs (NSAIDs), and avoidance. If the pain is progressive and unabated by conservative measures, surgery is indicated. Patients with intact or reparable rotator cuff tear benefit from total shoulder arthroplasty. Those with massive rotator cuff tears with an intact deltoid and coracoacromial arch can successfully undergo hemiarthroplasty. If no functioning deltoid is present arthrodesis should be considered.

References

Arntz CT, Jackins S, Matsen FA III. Prosthetic replacement of the shoulder for the treatment of defects in rotator cuff and the surface of the glenohumeral joint. J Bone Joint Surg 1993; 75-A:485–491.

Curran JF, Ellman MH, Brown NL. Rheumatologic aspects of painful conditions about the shoulder. Clin Orthop 1983; 173:27.

Friedman RJ, Thornhill TS, Thomas WH, Sledge CB. Non-constrained total shoulder replacement in patients who have rheumatoid arthritis in Class IV function. J Bone Joint Surg 1989; 71:494-498.

Leslie DM, Harris JM III, Driscoll D. Septic arthritis of the shoulder in adults. J Bone Joint Surg 1989; 71A:1516-1522.

Neer CS II. Reconstructive surgery and rehabilitation of the shoulder. In Kelley WN, Harris ED Jr, Ruddy S, and Sledge CB (eds): Textbook of Rheumatology. Philadelphia: WB Saunders, 1981; Vol. 11: p 1944.

Neer CS II. Shoulder Reconstruction. Philadelphia: WB Saunders, 1990; p 166.

Pahle JA. The shoulder joint in rheumatoid arthritis: Synovectomy. Reconstr Surg Traumatol 1981; 18:33-47.

Peterson CJ. Painful shoulders in patients with rheumatoid arthritis. Scand J Rheum 1986; 15:275-279.

Rhoades CE, Neff JR, Rengachary SS, et al. Diagnosis of post-traumatic syringohydromyelia presenting as neuropathic joints. Clin Orthop 1983; 180:182-187.

Rowe CR. Arthrodesis of the shoulder used in treating painful conditions. Clin Orthop 1983; 173:92.

OSTEONECROSIS OF THE SHOULDER

Osteonecrosis of the humeral head is associated with trauma, use of systemic steroids, or is idiopathic. Proximal humeral fractures, in particular those with four-part displacement or anatomic neck fractures, often result in interruption of the proximal blood supply to the humeral head. Systemic diseases such as alcoholism, sickle cell disease, decompression sickness, hyperlipidemia, lupus, and others have been implicated in osteonecrosis of the humeral head. Increases in serum lipids from steroid use may precipitate fat embolism into the humeral head blood supply. The radiographic staging system introduced by Ficat is helpful in determining treatment protocols. Stage I disease has no radiographic changes, but may have changes on MRI or bone scanning; Stage II shows segmental bony sclerosis or cyst formation in the humeral head; Stage III shows subchondral bone fracture; Stage IV shows distortions in the humeral head with collapse; and Stage V shows humeral head and glenoid changes (Fig. 1).

A. A thorough history determines if the osteonecrosis is caused by trauma or by systemic diseases or agents. A history of previous fractures of the upper end of the humerus, including dislocations of the upper end of the humerus, history of alcoholism, radiation, scuba diving, sickle cell anemia, Gaucher's disease, or hyperlipidemia can all contribute to the understanding of the etiology of these changes. Obviously, the previous use of steroid medication for any systemic disease is important to note.

B. The standard shoulder series in plain x-ray is the most helpful study in staging the disease. Patients with shoulder pain and history suggestive of osteonecrosis, but with normal radiographs could undergo MRI or bone scanning to determine that changes in the marrow have already occurred. Radiographic examination of the hips and knees should also be done to rule out multifocal osteonecrosis. Laboratory studies are indicated to rule out those systemic diseases which often cause osteonecrosis. Preoperative computed tomography (CT) is used for evaluation of significant changes in the glenohumeral anatomy and is preferred to differentiate Stage II and Stage III disease.

C. Many studies have shown benefits from nonsteroidal anti-inflammatories and, at times, continuing steroid therapy along with gentle physical therapy and range of motion (ROM) preservation. This appears to benefit not only patients in Stage I, II, or III disease, but also patients in Stage IV disease who have a relatively sedentary lifestyle.

D. Patients who fail conservative measures and have Stage I, II or III disease should be recommended for core decompression. In Urquhart's series, all patients with Stage I and II disease had good to excellent results with core decompression and 70% of those patients with Stage III disease had significant pain relief. Not all shoulders with Stage II or III disease progress. Many of these patients can be effectively treated with continued maintenance of ROM and occasional use of medication for pain control. Occasionally, arthroscopic removal of large debris and loose bodies improves function and alleviates mechanical impingement.

E. Patients with recalcitrant Stage IV or V disease can be recommended to undergo hemiarthroplasty or total shoulder replacement depending on the status of the articular cartilage and glenoid surfaces. In a review of the literature, approximately 5% of patients who require prosthetic shoulder arthroplasty have osteonecrosis. Pain relief can be expected in approximately 90% of these patients, most having functional ROM. The rotator cuff is typically intact in these patients. The decision to perform hemiarthroplasty versus total shoulder replacement in the face of an intact glenoid is somewhat controversial. With glenoid articular erosion, total shoulder replacement is indicated.

OSTEONECROSIS OF THE SHOULDER

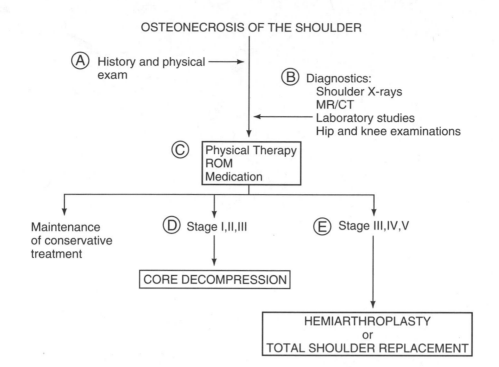

A History and physical ——→
   exam

B Diagnostics:
   Shoulder X-rays
   MR/CT
   Laboratory studies
   Hip and knee examinations

C Physical Therapy
   ROM
   Medication

Maintenance
of conservative
treatment

D Stage I,II,III

   CORE DECOMPRESSION

E Stage III,IV,V

   HEMIARTHROPLASTY
   or
   TOTAL SHOULDER REPLACEMENT

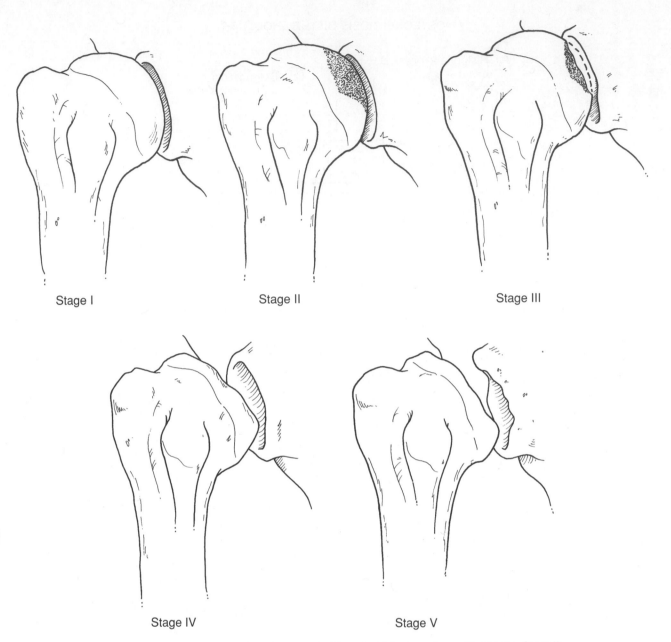

Stage I

Stage II

Stage III

Stage IV

Stage V

Figure 1 Ficat staging system for osteonecrosis. Stage I—Pain; no radiographic change. Stage II—Segmental bony sclerosis or cyst formation in humeral head. Stage III—Localized changes in humeral head. Stage IV—Generalized changes in humeral head. Stage V—Glenoid changes.

References

Cofield RH. Osteonecrosis. In Friedman RJ, ed: Arthroplasty of the Shoulder. New York: Thieme Publishers, 1994; pp 170-182.

Cruess RL. Steroid induced avascular necrosis of the head of the humerus: Natural history and management. J Bone Joint Surg (Br) 1976; 58:313-317.

Ficat P, Arlet J. Necrosis of the femoral head. In Ischaemia and Bone Necrosis. Baltimore: Williams and Wilkins, 1980; pp 53-75.

Fisher DE, Bickel WH, Holley KE, Ellefson, RD. Corticosteroid-induced aseptic necrosis: Experimental study. Clin Orthop 1972; 84:200-206.

Rutherford CS, Cofield RH. Osteonecrosis of the shoulder. Orthop Trans 1987; 11:239.

Urquhart MW, Mont MA, Maar DC, et al. Results of core decompression for avascular necrosis of the humeral head. Orthop Trans 1992; 16:780.

IMPINGEMENT SYNDROME

Any condition that decreases the functional space between the rotator cuff tendons and the rigid subacromial arch can cause impingement. Cadaver studies have been used to determine the morphologic changes in the acromion. Three types have been described (Fig. 1): Type 1, flat; Type 2, curved; and Type 3, hooked. Most rotator cuff tears are associated with Type 3 acromions. Unfused acromion (os acrominale), degeneration and spurring of the acromion and acromioclavicular (AC) joint, bursal thickening and inflammation, tendinopathies and thickening, and fracture malunions can structurally diminish the normal 1–1.5 cm subacromial space. Weak or restricted scapular motion, loss of normal humeral head depression (weak cuff musculature), capsular laxity (instability), and tight posterior capsular structures can functionally diminish the space. Neer described three stages of impingement: Stage I, reversible edema and hemorrhage, usually in the twenty-five year old and under age group; Stage II, fibrosis and tendinosis, in the twenty-five to forty year old age group; and Stage III, bony changes and tendon tears, in the over forty age group. Jobe described the overlap between impingement and instability in the athletic population with anterior shoulder pain.

A. The most consistent complaint is pain, which is exacerbated by daily activities, throwing, or sleeping on the affected side. Most commonly, it is located in the lateral upper arm, deltoid insertion, or the periacromial area. Inspection may reveal deltoid or infraspinatus atrophy, scapular winging and scapular dyskinesia. The anterolateral acromion, biceps groove and AC joint may be tender. Internal rotation may be limited due to posterior capsular tightness. Crossed arm adduction is usually painful. Maximal passive forward elevation can recreate the pain. Abduction and external rotation weakness may be apparent. A complete cervical examination is necessary to rule out cervical radiculopathy.

B. Plain radiographs consisting of glenohumeral, AP, trans-scapular lateral with the beam angled between 10° and 40° caudad, and axillary lateral are necessary. Subacromial sclerosis, spurring or hooking of the anterior lateral acromion, AC joint arthritis, calcific tendinitis, os acrominale, and tuberosity malunion can all be detected. More specific imaging techniques such as single or double contrast arthrography, ultrasonography or MRI are reserved for those patients who fail conservative treatment and have confusing presentations.

C. Injection of 1% lidocaine into the subacromial space is useful in determining the location of the patient's pain. AC, glenohumeral, and, occasionally, bicipital groove injections can assist in differentiating the various contributions of pathologic conditions in these areas to the overall pain pattern. If patients have no relief following subacromial injections, continued diagnostic work-up is necessary.

D. Patients with impingement often respond well to stretching (to eliminate posterior capsular tightness), scapular strengthening (to improve scapular stability), and rotator cuff strengthening (to improve depressor function). Over 90% of patients with Stage I and Stage II impingement will respond to conservative treatment. Due to the damaging effects of steroids on tendon tissue, subacromial steroid injections should be used judiciously. Modification of the patient's activity level in overhead or provocative positioning may prevent symptoms. Use of non-steroidal anti-inflammatory drugs (NSAIDs) in the acute phases can allow early rehabilitation to alleviate symptoms.

E. Patients who improve with rehabilitation are rarely asymptomatic. A maintenance program of rotator cuff strengthening, posterior capsular stretching and scapular stabilization can prevent recurrence. Patients are trained to avoid working or playing in provocative positions such as overhead activities. Weight lifting programs are modified to prevent anterior stresses.

F. If no improvement is achieved with an adequate trial of proper rehabilitation, open or arthroscopic acromioplasty is recommended. Both procedures should give good to excellent long-term results in the 85–95% range. Patients on workers' compensation do less well in most series. If the AC joint is involved in the process distal clavicle resection is indicated. Creating a flat acromion is essential to the success of the procedure. Also, infraclavicular spurs and AC joint hypertrophy should be addressed. In experienced hands, arthroscopic procedures and open procedures are technically similar.

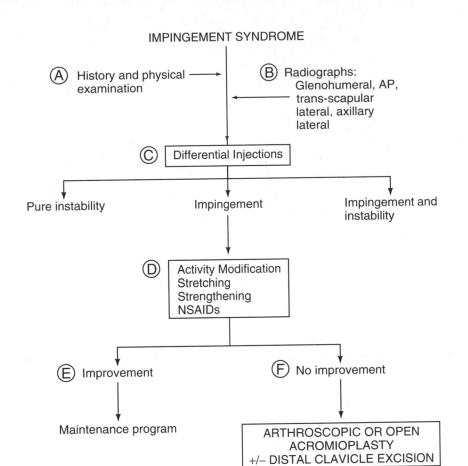

IMPINGEMENT SYNDROME

(A) History and physical examination → (B) Radiographs: Glenohumeral, AP, trans-scapular lateral, axillary lateral

(C) Differential Injections

Pure instability   Impingement   Impingement and instability

(D) Activity Modification
Stretching
Strengthening
NSAIDs

(E) Improvement   (F) No improvement

Maintenance program   ARTHROSCOPIC OR OPEN
ACROMIOPLASTY
+/– DISTAL CLAVICLE EXCISION

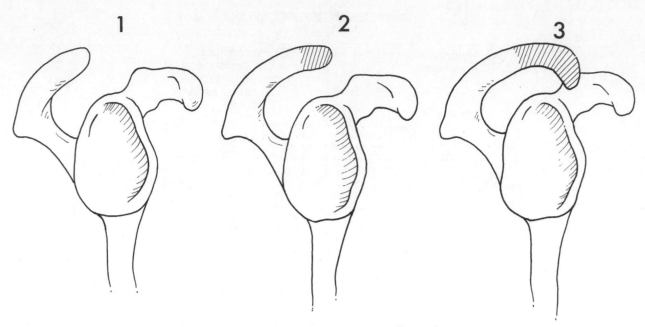

Figure 1 Types of acromion changes found in impingement syndrome. Type 1—Flat acromion. Type 2—Curved acromion. Type 3—Hooked acromion.

References

Altchek DW, Warren RF, Wikiewicz TL, et al. Arthroscopic acromioplasty: Technique and results. J Bone Joint Surg 1990; 72A:1198-1207.

Bigliani LU, Morrison DS, April EW. The morphology of the acromion and its relationship to rotator cuff tears. Orthop Trans 1986; 10:228.

Gartsman GM. Arthroscopic acromioplasty for lesions of the rotator cuff. J Bone Joint Surg 1990; 72A:169-180.

Harryman DT II, Sidles JA, Clark JM, et al. Translation of the humeral head on the glenoid with passive glenohumeral motion. J Bone Joint Surg, 1990 72A:1334-1343.

Hawkins RJ, Brock RM, Abrams JS, et al. Acromioplasty for impingement with an intact rotator cuff. J Bone Joint Surg 1988; 70B:795-797.

Jobe FW, Tibone JE, Jobe CW, et al. The shoulder in sports. In Rockwood CA Jr, Matsen FA III, eds: The Shoulder. Philadelphia, WB Saunders Co., 1990; 961-989.

Litchfield R, Hawkins RJ, Dillman CJ, Atkins JA, Hagerman G. Rehabilitation of the overhead athlete. JOSPT, 1993; 18:433-441.

Neer CS II. Anterior acromioplasty for chronic impingement syndrome in the shoulder: A preliminary report. J Bone Joint Surg 1972; 54A:41-50.

Neer CS II. Impingement lesions. Clin Orthop 1983; 173:70-77.

ROTATOR CUFF TEAR

The pathophysiology of rotator cuff failure is multifactorial. It has been postulated that rotator cuff failure results from fatigue failure of cuff tissue such as in overhead athletes, mechanical failure which is associated with subacromial impingement, and intrinsic etiology such as hypovascularity and intrinsic tendinopathy. Rotator cuff pathology is prevalent in a wide range of patients from overhead athletes to sedentary elderly. Treatment is based on the patient's pain, dysfunction, and anatomy of the tear. The demands of the patient's lifestyle and expectations are also considered.

A. Most tears occur in patients >40 years old. About one-half of the patients can relate a traumatic event which initiated their symptoms. The most common complaint is pain. Usually, the pain is associated with a mild to moderate dysfunction and some limitation of range of motion. Night pain is very consistent as is an inability to sleep on the involved side. As the tear progresses, weakness in elevation and "cracking and popping" become evident. Physical examination may reveal findings of ruptured proximal biceps tendon, infraspinatus wasting, significant subacromial crepitance, and limitation of range of motion (ROM). The supraspinatus strength is tested by downward pressure on the abducted (90°), flexed (90°), and maximally internally rotated arm. Strength of the infraspinatus and teres minor is tested with the arm at the side and the elbow flexed 90°. Demonstrable weakness of external rotation is related to the size of the rotator cuff tear. Large tears can be palpated in thin individuals. The acromioclavicular (AC) joint is also examined for tenderness and hypertrophy.

B. True AP views of the glenohumeral joint may reveal superior migration of the humeral head with narrowing of the acromial humeral interval to 5 mm or less. Greater tuberosity sclerosis, spurring and cyst formation along with subacromial spurring are associated with chronic rotator cuff disease. Glenohumeral or AC degenerative joint disease (DJD) may be apparent. Scapular outlet views demonstrate the morphology of the acromion. Axillary views, 30° caudal tilt views and AC views are also helpful. Stress views with active deltoid firing in the 90° abducted arm may accentuate the humeral head migration. History and physical examination and plain film x-rays are often not specific or sensitive for full-thickness rotator cuff tears. Single or double contrast arthrography is cost effective and highly accurate in detecting full-thickness rotator cuff tears. Ultrasonography is a non-invasive test which is operator dependent. At some centers, this is the imaging method of choice. MRI is also a non-invasive technique which can be very sensitive and specific in some centers.

C. Nonoperative management of full-thickness rotator cuff tears consists of rehabilitation, non-steroidal anti-inflammatory drugs (NSAIDs), ROM preservation, and activity modification. In elderly patients who are poor operative candidates or patients with minimal residual symptoms, a maintenance program can be continued.

D. Arthroscopy or open evaluation of all acute tears and chronic symptomatic tears in active patients is indicated. The best long-term relief and return to function is seen with rotator cuff repair.

E. Many patients with partial thickness tears can be managed with conservative measures. Those that remain symptomatic can benefit from arthroscopic debridement, bursectomy and acromioplasty with or without distal clavicle resection. Most athletes with partial thickness tears are able to return to their previous activities after arthroscopic debridement, acromioplasty, and postoperative rehabilitation.

F. Small, medium and large tears are debrided to normal cuff tissue, mobilized to reduce tension on the repair, and repaired to a trough and bone with nonabsorbable sutures (Fig. 1). Combined subtotal bursectomy, anterior inferior acromioplasty, coracoacromial ligament excision, and distal clavicle resection may be indicated. These patients can expect pain relief. Many will also note improvement and strength in ROM. Patients whose repairs remain intact function better than those who have a "re-tear". However, patients who "re-tear" continue to be satisfied with their pain relief. In younger patients with large-to-massive tears, consideration can be given to transfers (i.e., latissimus dorsi) or rotation coverage (i.e., subscapularis transfer). The results of these procedures are inconsistent.

G. Irreparable tears occur when the quality or quantity of cuff tissue is not sufficient to close a defect. This is seen in cases with significant superior migration, significant loss of external rotation strength, multiple steroid injections, older patients, and atraumatic etiology. Muscle transfers, fascial grafts, and synthetic implants have not performed well. Treatment of patients with massive cuff deficiency and DJD should be individualized based on their demands and status of the deltoid musculature. Those with low demand should undergo bursectomy and cuff debridement if conservative measures have failed. Patients with normal deltoid function may benefit from hemiarthroplasty; those without deltoid function are offered arthrodesis. Irreparable tears in patients with little or no destruction of the glenohumeral articulation benefit from arthroscopic or open debridement of the remaining cuff tissue. These patients may progress to rotator cuff arthropathy.

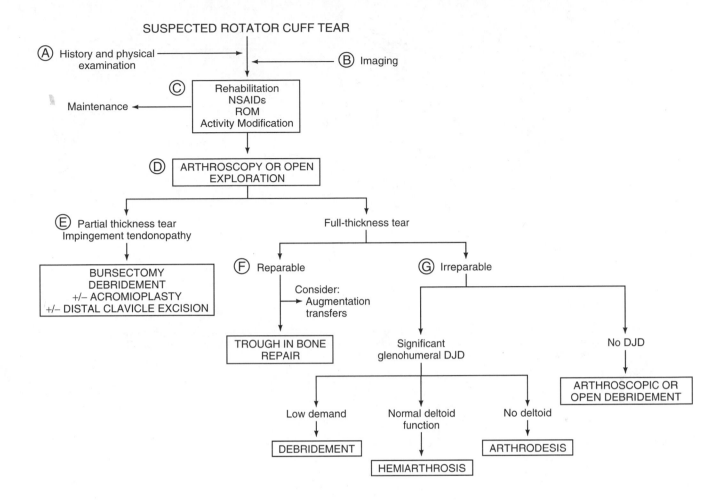

SUSPECTED ROTATOR CUFF TEAR

(A) History and physical examination ⟶

(B) Imaging

(C) Rehabilitation
NSAIDs
ROM
Activity Modification

Maintenance ⟵

(D) ARTHROSCOPY OR OPEN EXPLORATION

(E) Partial thickness tear
Impingement tendonopathy

Full-thickness tear

BURSECTOMY
DEBRIDEMENT
+/− ACROMIOPLASTY
+/− DISTAL CLAVICLE EXCISION

(F) Reparable

(G) Irreparable

Consider:
Augmentation
transfers

TROUGH IN BONE
REPAIR

Significant
glenohumeral DJD

No DJD

ARTHROSCOPIC OR
OPEN DEBRIDEMENT

Low demand

Normal deltoid
function

No deltoid

DEBRIDEMENT

HEMIARTHROSIS

ARTHRODESIS

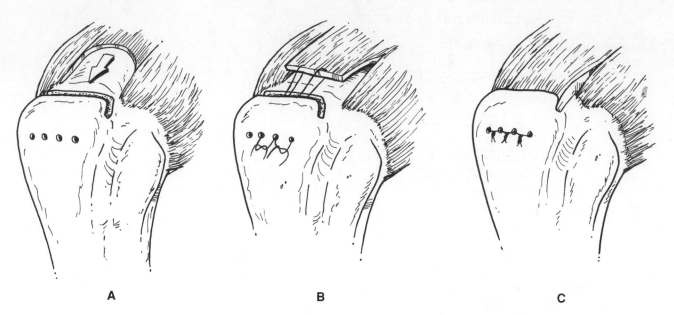

Figure 1   Open or arthroscopic reconstruction of the torn rotator cuff involves reapproximation of viable cuff tendon to a bony trough. **A,** Creation of bony trough and debridement of necrotic cuff. **B,** Reapproximation of the cuff tendon, **C,** Final closure.

References

Andrews JR, Broussard TS, Carson WG. Arthroscopy of the shoulder and the management of partial tears of the rotator cuff: A preliminary report. Arthroscopy 1985; 1:117.

Bigliani LU, Morrison DS, April EW. The morphology of the acromion and its relationship to rotator cuff tears. Orthop Trans 1986; 10:228.

Bloom RA. The active abduction view: A new maneuver in the diagnosis of rotator cuff tears. Skeletal Radiol 1991; 20:255-258.

Brems JJ. Digital muscle strength measurement in rotator cuff tears. Paper presented at the ASES 3rd Open Meeting, San Francisco, January, 1987.

Burkhart SS. Arthroscopic treatment of massive rotator cuff tears. Clin Orthop 1991; 26:45-56.

Harryman DT II, Mack LA, Wang KY, Jackins SE, Richardson ML, Matsen FA III. Repairs of the rotator cuff. J Bone Joint Surg 1991; 73A:982.

Hawkins RJ, Misamore GW, Hobeika PE. Surgery for full-thickness rotator cuff tears. J Bone Joint Surg 1985; 67A:1349-1355.

Iannotti JP, Zlatkin MB, Esterhai JL, et al. Magnetic resonance imaging of the shoulder: Sensitivity specificity and predictive value. J Bone Joint Surg 1991; 73A:17-29.

Matsen FA III, Arntz CT. Rotator cuff tendon failure in the shoulder. In Matsen FA III, Rockwood CA Jr (eds): The Shoulder. Philadelphia, WB Saunders, 1990; pp 647-675.

Misamore GW, Woodward C. Evaluation of degenerative lesions of the rotator cuff: A comparison of arthrography and ultrasonography. J Bone Joint Surg 1991; 73A:704-706.

Neer CS II, Flatow EL, Lech O. Tears of the rotator cuff: Long-term results of anterior acromioplasty and repair. Orthop Trans 1988; 12:673-674.

Resnick D. Shoulder arthrography. Radiol Clin North Am 1981; 19:243-252.

Samilson RL, Binder WF. Symptomatic full-thickness tears of the rotator cuff: An analysis of 292 shoulders in 276 patients. Orthop Clin North Am 1975; 6:449-466.

Silliman JF, Hawkins RJ. Current concepts and recent advances in the athlete's shoulder. Clin Sports Med 1991; 10:693.

Snyder SJ, Pachelli AF, et al. Partial thickness rotator cuff tears: Results of arthroscopic treatment. Arthroscopy 1991; 7(1):1-7.

ELBOW PAIN

A. Medial epicondylitis results from valgus-tension stress injury, such as occurs when serving in tennis or during the acceleration phase of throwing. Radiographs may show medial calcification or spur formation. Treatment is generally conservative; medial release must avoid injury to the medial collateral ligament (MCL). Rehabilitation involves careful stretching and strengthening of the flexor-pronator group.

B. Attenuation of the MCL results from chronic valgus stress injury (Figs. 1 and 2), such as occurs in pitching and racquet sports. The flexor-pronator muscle mass, normally the first line of defense, is overcome, and the resultant instability leads to osteophyte and loose body formation from medial olecranon tip impingement in its fossa and lateral radio-capitellar compression.

   Diagnosis is confirmed by a gravity stress radiograph of the elbow. With the patient supine, the shoulder is abducted and externally rotated such that a cross-table anteroposterior (AP) view of the joint may be taken with the extremity supported only by a bump under the humerus. Opening of the medial joint space indicates MCL insufficiency.

   Ulnar nerve symptoms may also occur due to impingement from local structures, i.e., MCL, capsule, and spurs, as well as an increased carrying angle.

C. Lateral epicondylitis commonly results from improper stroke mechanics in racquet sports. While excessive stress on the extensor origin, particularly the extensor carpi radialis brevis (ECRB), has been implicated with associated microscopic tears and inflammation, its true pathophysiology, as well as the role of radial nerve compression in the radial tunnel, remains unclear (Fig. 3).

   Early treatment is key, with conservative measures stressing activity reduction and relaxation of the extensor origin, accomplished progressively by counterforce bracing, wrist dorsiflexion splinting, or ultimately long arm splinting. Owing to its degenerative effects on the tendon, steroid injection is reserved for refractory cases and severe pain.

   Options for operative intervention vary but usually involve release and excision of the ECRB origin and should be reserved for failure of prolonged conservative management, as success rates are often suboptimal. Rehabilitation following conservative or operative management involves careful stretching and strengthening of the extensor origin and is crucial to preventing recurrence.

D. The use of steroid injection in the treatment of olecranon bursitis is not recommended due to an increased incidence of secondary infection.

E. Triceps tendinitis results from valgus-extension overload, as seen in throwing, racquet sports, gymnastics, boxing, and weight lifting. Microscopic tendon tears with inflammation are seen in association with loose bodies from olecranon tip impingement in its fossa. Steroid injection should be avoided due to risk of tendon degeneration and subsequent rupture.

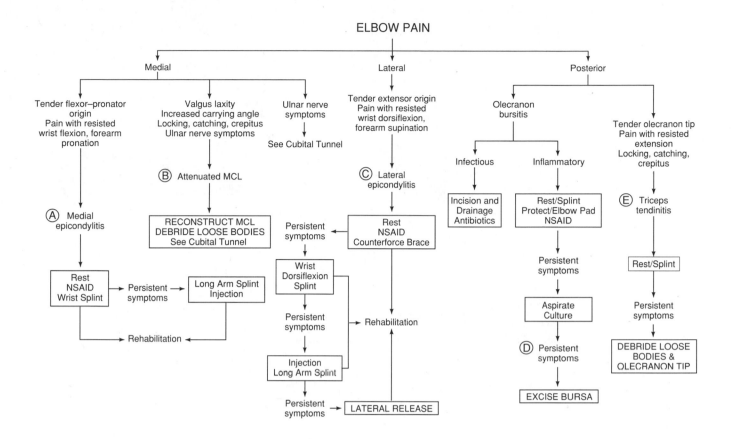

ELBOW PAIN

Medial

Tender flexor–pronator origin
Pain with resisted wrist flexion, forearm pronation

(A) Medial epicondylitis

→ Rest
NSAID
Wrist Splint

→ Persistent symptoms → Long Arm Splint
Injection

→ Rehabilitation

Valgus laxity
Increased carrying angle
Locking, catching, crepitus
Ulnar nerve symptoms

(B) Attenuated MCL

RECONSTRUCT MCL
DEBRIDE LOOSE BODIES
See Cubital Tunnel

Ulnar nerve symptoms

See Cubital Tunnel

Lateral

Tender extensor origin
Pain with resisted wrist dorsiflexion, forearm supination

(C) Lateral epicondylitis

Rest
NSAID
Counterforce Brace

Persistent symptoms ←

Wrist Dorsiflexion Splint

Persistent symptoms

Injection
Long Arm Splint

Persistent symptoms → LATERAL RELEASE

→ Rehabilitation

Posterior

Olecranon bursitis

Infectious

Incision and Drainage
Antibiotics

Inflammatory

Rest/Splint
Protect/Elbow Pad
NSAID

Persistent symptoms

Aspirate
Culture

(D) Persistent symptoms

EXCISE BURSA

Tender olecranon tip
Pain with resisted extension
Locking, catching, crepitus

(E) Triceps tendinitis

Rest/Splint

Persistent symptoms

DEBRIDE LOOSE BODIES &
OLECRANON TIP

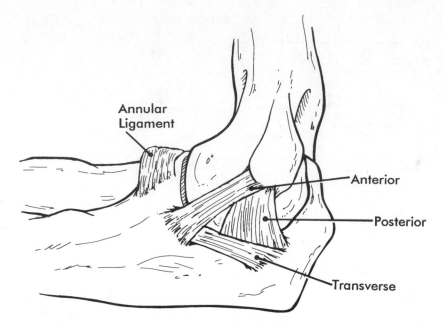

Figure 1 Medial ligaments.

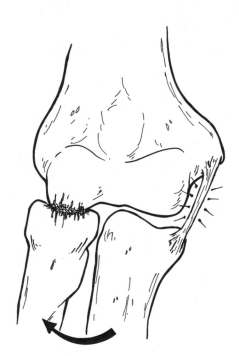

Figure 2 Valgus injury.

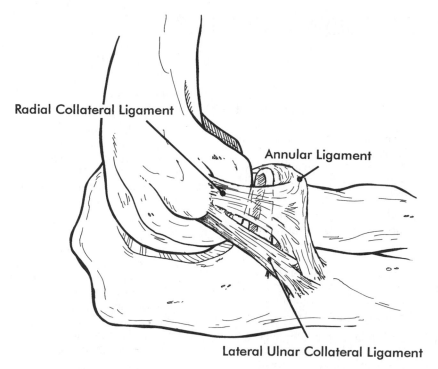

Figure 3 Lateral ligaments.

References

Bennett J, Tullos H. Ligamentous and articular injuries in the athlete. In Morrey BF, ed. The Elbow and Its Disorders. Philadelphia: W.B. Saunders, 1985; 502.

Bennett JB, Tullos HS. Acute injuries to the elbow. In: Nicholas JA, Hershman EB, eds. The Upper Extremity in Sports Medicine. St. Louis: C.V. Mosby, 1990; 319.

Broberg MA, Morrey BF. Results of delayed excision of the radial head after fracture. J Bone Joint Surg 1986; 68A:669.

Conway JE, Jobe FW, Glousman RE, Pink M. Medial instability of the elbow in throwing athletes: Treatment by repair or reconstruction of the ulnar collateral ligament. J Bone Joint Surg 1992; 74A:67.

Froimson AI. Tenosynovitis and tennis elbow. In: Green DP, ed. Operative Hand Surgery. 2nd ed. New York: Churchill Livingstone, 1988; 2127.

Goldberg I, Peylan J, Yosipovitch Z. Late results of excision of the radial head for an isolated closed fracture. J Bone Joint Surg 1986; 68A:675.

Morrey BF. Loose bodies. In: Morrey BF, ed. The Elbow and Its Disorders. Philadelphia: W.B. Saunders, 1985; 736.

Morrey BF. Bursitis. In: Morrey BF, ed. The Elbow and Its Disorders. Philadelphia: W.B. Saunders, 1985; 745-751.

Nirschl RP. Muscle & tendon trauma: Tennis elbow. In: Morrey BF, ed. The Elbow and Its Disorders. Philadelphia: W.B. Saunders, 1985; 481.

Nirschl RP, Pettrone FA. Tennis elbow. J Bone Joint Surg 1979; 61A:832.

Parkes JC. Overuse injuries of the elbow. In: Nicholas JA, Hershman EB, eds. The Upper Extremity in Sports Medicine. St. Louis: C.V. Mosby, 1990; 335.

Regan W, Korinek S, Morrey B, An K-N. Biomechanical study of ligaments around the elbow joint. Clinical Orthop 1991; 271:170.

SURGERY FOR ELBOW ARTHRITIS

A. In stage I disease, there is mild-to-moderate synovitis without radiographic changes. Stage II disease consists of persistent synovitis despite medical management with mild associated radiographic changes. With stage III disease, more extensive joint destruction exists with concurrent ligamentous instability. Synovectomy is indicated for stage II disease before significant joint destruction or instability has occurred, provided a satisfactory range of motion (ROM) still exists.

B. Synovectomy is directed at reducing inflammation, pain, and joint destruction in rheumatoid arthritis and diminishing the potential for recurring joint hemorrhages in hemophilia, when conservative measures have failed. Radial head excision through a lateral approach facilitates synovectomy and is also indicated in cases of radio-capitellar arthritis. Common flexor/extensor origin releases may improve ROM.

C. In cases of chronic hemophilic arthropathy with unremitting pain, arthroplasty may be indicated, though long-term results of such treatment are unknown.

D. Isolated radio-capitellar arthritis may result from the late sequelae of osteochondritis dissecans or previous fracture and/or dislocation of the radio-capitellar joint. Results of late radial head excision following fracture approximate those of early excision. Silastic replacement is not recommended due to potential for silastic synovitis and is usually performed only as a temporizing measure in cases of instability.

E. Limited joint debridement may be effective in cases with marginal impinging osteophytes where adequate joint space is preserved as well as for removal of loose bodies. Otherwise, most cases of elbow arthritis can often be managed nonoperatively.

F. Elbow arthrodesis provides stability but is rarely indicated due to its attendant restriction of function. The contralateral elbow should demonstrate good motion in such instances. Lack of motion proximal and distal to the elbow also is a relative contraindication to elbow arthrodesis. Optimal positioning varies according to patient demands but is generally around 90° of flexion.

G. Ulno-humeral arthroplasty (Fig. 1) is indicated in those instances of primary degenerative arthritis of the elbow in which the ulno-humeral joint is principally involved. In cases of more extensive arthritic involvement or ankylosis, distraction/soft tissue interposition arthroplasty (Fig. 2) provides improved ROM but is technically difficult to perform and associated with high complication rates.

H. Total elbow prosthetic arthroplasty is most indicated in older, low-demand individuals. Resurfacing replacement has been associated with a high failure rate mostly due to dislocation, loosening, and infection. Results appear to be somewhat better with semi-constrained implants. Relative contraindications to arthroplasty include previous infection, severe soft tissue contracture, lack of sufficient elbow motors, and a young or uncooperative patient who might place unreasonable demands on the implant.

ELBOW ARTHRITIS

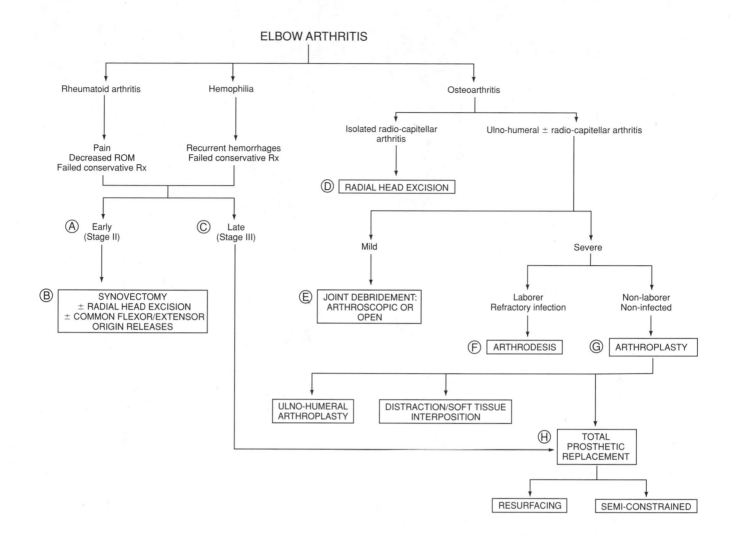

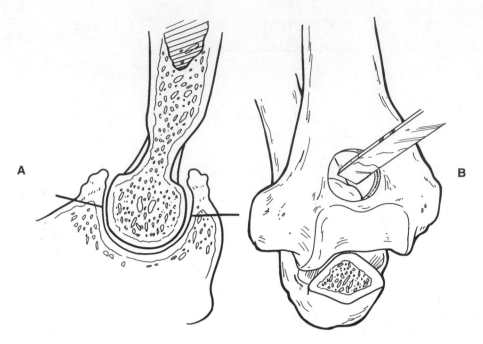

A   B

Figure 1   Ulno-humeral arthroplasty.

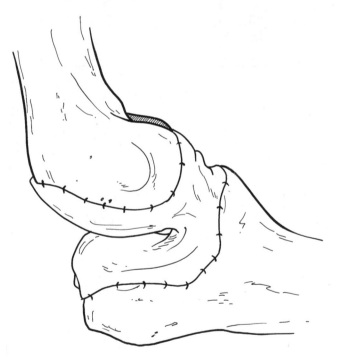

Figure 2   Soft tissue interposition arthroplasty.

References

Beckenbaugh RD. Arthrodesis. In: Morrey BF, ed. The Elbow and Its Disorders. 2nd ed. Philadelphia: W.B. Saunders, 1993; 696.

Bell S, Gschwend N, Steiger U. Arthroplasty of the elbow: Experience with the Mark III GSB prosthesis. Aust N Z J Surg 1986; 56:823.

Figgie HE, Inglis AE, Ranawat CS, et al. Results of total elbow arthroplasty as a salvage procedure for failed elbow reconstructive operations. Clin Orthop 1987; 219:185.

Frassica F, Coventry MB, Morrey B. Ectopic ossification about the elbow. In: Morrey BF, ed. The Elbow and Its Disorders. 2nd ed. Philadelphia: W.B. Saunders, 1993; 505.

Friedman RJ, Ewald FC. Arthroplasty of the ipsilateral shoulder and elbow in patients who have rheumatoid arthritis. J Bone Joint Surg 1987; 69A:661.

Inglis AE, Figgie M. Rheumatoid arthritis. In: Morrey BF, ed. The Elbow and Its Disorders. 2nd ed. Philadelphia: W.B. Saunders, 1993; 751.

Le Balch T, Ebelin M, Laurian Y, et al. Synovectomy of the elbow in young hemophiliac patients. J Bone Joint Surg 1987; 69A:264.

London J. Custom arthroplasty and hemiarthroplasty of the elbow. In: Morrey BF, ed. The Elbow and Its Disorders. 2nd ed. Philadelphia: W.B. Saunders, 1993; 623.

Morrey B. Primary degenerative arthritis of the elbow: Treatment by ulnohumeral arthroplasty. J Bone Joint Surg 1992; 74B:409.

Morrey BF. Revision of failed total elbow arthroplasty. In: Morrey BF, ed. The Elbow and Its Disorders. 2nd ed. Philadelphia: W.B. Saunders, 1993; 676.

Morrey B, Adams R. Semiconstrained arthroplasty for the treatment of rheumatoid arthritis of the elbow. J Bone Joint Surg 1992; 74A:479-490.

Morrey B, Adams R. Semiconstrained elbow replacement arthroplasty: Rationale, technique, and results. In: Morrey BF, ed. The Elbow and Its Disorders. 2nd ed. Philadelphia: W.B. Saunders, 1993; 638.

Morrey B, Adams R, Bryan R. Total replacement for posttraumatic arthritis of the elbow. J Bone Joint Surg 1991; 73B:607.

Morrey BF, Askew LJ, An K-N. Strength function after elbow arthroplasty. Clinical Orthop 1988; 234:43.

Morrey BF, Bryan RS. Revision total elbow arthroplasty. J Bone Joint Surg 1987; 69A:523.

Morrey B, Bryan R, Dobyns J, Linscheid R. Total elbow arthroplasty: a five-year experience at the Mayo Clinic. J Bone Joint Surg 1981; 63A:1050.

Roper BA, Tuke M, O'Riordan SM, et al. A new unconstrained elbow: A prospective review of 60 replacements. J Bone Joint Surg 1986; 68B:566.

Ross AC, Sneath RS, Scales JT. Endoprosthetic replacement of the humerus and elbow joint. J Bone Joint Surg 1987; 69B:652.

Sourmelis SG, Burke FD, Varian JP. A review of total elbow arthroplasty and an early assessment of the Liverpool elbow prosthesis. J Hand Surg 1986; 11B:407.

Trancik T, Wilde AH, Borden LS. Capitellocondylar total elbow arthroplasty: Two- to eight-year experience. Clinical Orthop 1987; 223:175.

Tsuge K, Murakami T, Yasunaga Y, et al. Arthroplasty of the elbow: Twenty years' experience with a new operation. J Bone Joint Surg 1987; 69B:116.

Wevers HW, Siu DW, Broekhoven LH, et al. Resurfacing elbow prosthesis: Shape and sizing of the humeral component. J Biomed Eng 1985; 7:241.

Wright PE, Froimson A, Steward M. Interposition arthroplasty of the elbow. In: Morrey BF, ed. The Elbow and Its Disorders. 2nd ed. Philadelphia: W.B. Saunders, 1993; 611.

HIP PAIN

True hip pain most often presents in the groin. Occasionally it may present as referred pain to the knee or may radiate laterally and infrequently posteriorly. Trochanteric pain presents as lateral buttock or proximal lateral thigh pain. Other complaints include limp and stiffness. Pain may be acute or chronic, continuous or intermittent. Relationship of pain to activity and position are important.

A. Determine the onset of pain, relieving and aggravating factors, and any relationship to activities. Solicit history of trauma, recent or remote; any change in activity level, whether increased or decreased; and any history of inflammatory disease or risk factors for osteonecrosis. Previous surgery to hip is significant.

B. An accurate diagnosis hinges on a complete examination. Have patient undress and watch walking. Check Trendelenburg sign. Any limp or antalgic gait may indicate a hip problem. Examine low back and ipsilateral knee. Document range of motion of both hips. Leg length discrepancy must be measured. Note evidence of muscle atrophy in buttock and/or thigh. Localize pain to buttock area, lateral thigh, or groin or anterior hip area. Buttock pain or iliolumbar area pain is usually indicative of a lumbar spine problem or sacroiliac pathology. Specific radiographs and examination will help elucidate these spinal problems. Groin pain is more specific for the hip joint. Lateral pain localized to the trochanter suggests a problem of muscle or tendon in this area. Hip flexion contracture is assessed using Thomas' test whereby the contralateral thigh is held flexed against the chest and the affected thigh does not rest against the table.

C. If clinical examination and history suggest a hip problem, appropriate radiographs of the pelvis and hips are recommended (Fig. 1). Standing radiographs help show deformity and pelvic obliquity. The cross table lateral view shows the femoral neck area and hip joint in another profile.

D. If groin pain is present, and there is a normal range of hip motion, with no discomfort, extra-articular pathology may be present (Fig. 2). Inguinal or femoral hernia may present with pain. Referred pain from abdominal viscera or lumbar spine may cause anterior hip pain. Palpation of the femoral pulse may reveal a vascular abnormality. Additional investigations such as bone scan or magnetic resonance imaging may be necessary. Evaluation of a total hip replacement may require additional special investigations or arthrogram. (See p.136.)

E. Abnormal hip movement usually implies primary joint pathology. Internal rotation is usually reduced first. Abduction gradually decreases and a fixed external rotation and adduction deformity may be noted. Occasionally abnormal movement may be more than is usual, as in developmental dysplasia of the hip or a fractured neck of femur.

F. Trochanteric pain may result from a fracture of the greater trochanter (Fig. 3). Inflammatory conditions are not commonly associated with radiographic changes of the trochanter. Snapping of the fasciae latae over the greater trochanter may produce pain in the hip area.

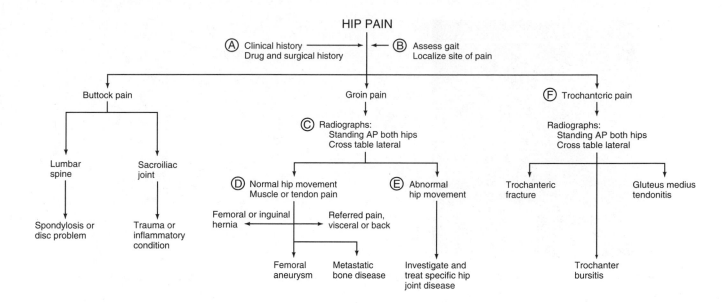

HIP PAIN

A Clinical history ──→ ◄── **B** Assess gait
Drug and surgical history   Localize site of pain

Buttock pain

Lumbar spine

Sacroiliac joint

Spondylosis or disc problem

Trauma or inflammatory condition

Groin pain

C Radiographs:
Standing AP both hips
Cross table lateral

D Normal hip movement
Muscle or tendon pain

E Abnormal hip movement

Femoral or inguinal hernia ◄──   ──► Referred pain, visceral or back

Femoral aneurysm

Metastatic bone disease

Investigate and treat specific hip joint disease

F Trochanteric pain

Radiographs:
Standing AP both hips
Cross table lateral

Trochanteric fracture

Gluteus medius tendonitis

Trochanter bursitis

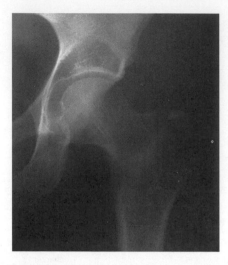

Figure 1 Radiograph of basal fracture of the femoral head.

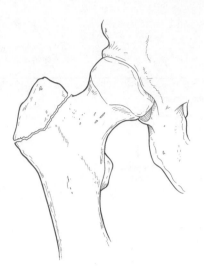

Figure 3 Diagram of fractured trochanter of the hip.

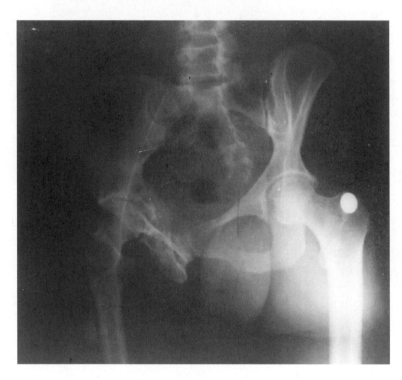

Figure 2 Radiograph of metastatic disease to bone.

References

Brignall CG, et al. The snapping hip. J Bone Joint Surg 1991; 73B:253.

Hoppenfeld S. Physical Examination of the Spine and Extremities. Englewood Cliffs: Prentice-Hall, 1976.

Maquet PC. Biomechanics of the Hip. Berlin: Springer-Verlag, 1985.

McGann WA. History and physical examination. In: Steinberg ME, ed. The Hip and Its Disorders. Philadelphia: W.B. Saunders, 1991.

OSTEONECROSIS OF THE FEMORAL HEAD

Osteonecrosis is a common cause of hip pain in young and middle-aged patients and ultimately results in severe degeneration of the hip joint. The exact pathogenesis of osteonecrosis is unknown, but interference of the blood supply to the femoral head is the common pathway. Factors thought to be important in the pathogenesis of osteonecrosis are extraosseous or intraosseous interruptions of the venous or arterial blood flow. Increased intraosseous pressure, due to disruption of venous outflow or increased fat cell size may ultimately lead to ischemia by preventing arterial inflow. Traumatic injuries to the arterial system such as secondary to femoral neck fracture or hip dislocation can cause osteonecrosis.

A. The most common causes of osteonecrosis are steroid use, alcohol use, trauma, gout, metabolic problems and genetic problems. Idiopathic osteonecrosis is a diagnosis of exclusion. High-dose corticosteroids for only 2 to 3 weeks or low-dose steroid use for long duration produce osteonecrosis. There is a direct correlation between the dose and duration of corticosteroid use in development of osteonecrosis. Joints other than the hip may also be involved and include shoulders, knees, ankle (talus) and occasionally elbow. Osteonecrosis of the hips is a bilateral disease, but each side may present at different stages. Most patients present with pain in the hip during activity. Pain may be either acute or insidious in onset. Examination of the hip may reveal normal or near normal range of motion in the early stages of the disease. With progression of the disease process, motion and function of the hip decrease. Pain with internal rotation of the hip is a frequent early finding on physical examination.

B. In the early stages, radiographs may show *no* bony abnormality. Most classification systems rely on the radiographic changes. The most significant factors on the radiographs are extent of involvement, subchondral fracture, and preservation of the shape of the femoral head. Magnetic resonance imaging (MRI) should be done, especially if the radiographs are normal and the diagnosis of osteonecrosis is suspected. Changes in the bone marrow can be detected by MRI and are fairly specific for osteonecrosis. Changes noted on MRI include an altered signal intensity of the marrow of the femoral head. A localized or circumscribed area in the femoral head, usually in the anterosuperior segment, is noted. The marrow cavity in normal femoral heads emits a strong magnetic resonance signal from the hydrogen rich fat. The early changes occur before any change in trabecular architecture.

C. Other causes of hip pain that may present with symptoms similar to those of osteonecrosis include: gout, femoral or inguinal hernia, pigmented villonodular synovitis, stress fracture of femoral neck, and rheumatoid arthritis.

D. Osteonecrosis is classified into several radiographic stages that aid with prognosis and treatment. The radiographic staging systems developed by Ficat and Enneking for osteonecrosis are the most frequently used and differ very slightly. Ficat described five stages and Enneking six stages. The staging system outlined here is that by Ficat. Stage 0 shows no changes on plain radiographs but a positive MRI; Stage I—mottled densities or osteopenia; Stage II—an area of increased density in the femoral head (Fig. 1); Stage IIA—crescent sign with subchondral fracture or very early flattening of part of femoral head (Fig. 2); Stage III—depression of femoral head (Fig. 3); Stage IV—flattening and collapse of femoral head (Fig. 4); Stage V—degenerative arthrosis. Initially the osteonecrotic segment is localized to the anterosuperior portion of the femoral head. The size of the lesion increases with ongoing ischemia to the femoral head until whole head involvement occurs. In the earlier stages, the size of head involvement helps to determine appropriate treatment.

E. Core decompression seems to offer the best chance of healing of the necrotic segment in Stages I and II (Fig. 5). However, results of this treatment are controversial and mixed according to various reports. In femoral heads with up to Stage II lesions, a 5 to 7 mm core and multiple smaller drill holes may reverse the radiographic changes. Bone grafting by reversing the core or fibular grafting of the core do not appear to provide any additional benefits. Complications and fractures following core decompression vary from 10% to 60%. Electrical stimulation has no beneficial effect. The critical differences occur between Stages IIA and III, since more failures are seen in Stages III and above. Cross table lateral radiographs or tomograms help differentiate Stage IIA (crescent sign) from Stage III.

F. If the area of necrosis is localized and the originating cause is not ongoing, a rotational osteotomy may sometimes benefit the patient. The joint space should be intact and the disease process localized to a small segment of the femoral head. Patients should still have a good range of motion of the hip, and the posterior femoral head contour should be normal. No acetabular changes should be noted on the radiograph. A combined segmental angle measured on the anteroposterior (AP), and lateral radiographs of less than 200° is one of the prerequisites for a rotational osteotomy. Different types of osteotomies include valgus/flexion osteotomy to rotate the posterior femoral head into the weight-bearing area. This osteotomy cut is at the intertrochanteric level. The Sugioka rotational osteotomy is done at the base of the femoral neck and rotates the femoral head almost 180° to move the affected area out of the weight-bearing zone. Nonoperative treatment includes anti-inflammatory medications and crutches.

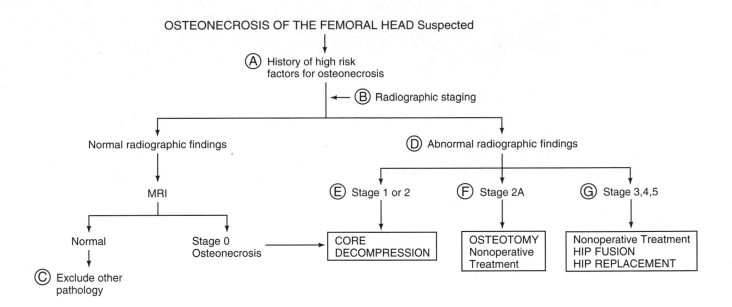

OSTEONECROSIS OF THE FEMORAL HEAD Suspected

Ⓐ History of high risk factors for osteonecrosis

Ⓑ Radiographic staging

Normal radiographic findings

Ⓓ Abnormal radiographic findings

MRI

Ⓔ Stage 1 or 2

Ⓕ Stage 2A

Ⓖ Stage 3,4,5

Normal

Stage 0 Osteonecrosis

Ⓒ Exclude other pathology

CORE DECOMPRESSION

OSTEOTOMY Nonoperative Treatment

Nonoperative Treatment HIP FUSION HIP REPLACEMENT

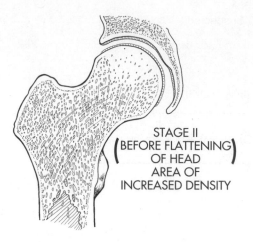

Figure 1 Osteonecrosis Stage II—increased density in the area of maximum loading of the femoral head.

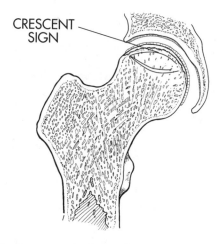

Figure 2 Osteonecrosis Stage IIA—the "crescent sign" with subchondral fracture.

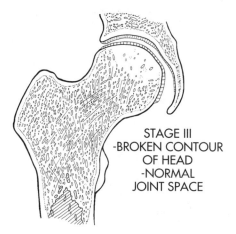

Figure 3 Osteonecrosis Stage III—flattening of the femoral head.

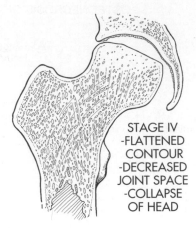

Figure 4 Osteonecrosis Stage IV—collapse of the femoral head and loss of normal contour.

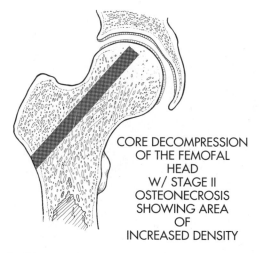

Figure 5 Diagram of core decompression of femoral head for Stage II osteonecrosis.

G. Disease that has progressed to degenerative arthrosis and is symptomatic ultimately requires a joint replacement. Hip fusion is only offered in rare instances. The results of total hip replacement for osteonecrosis are not as good as for other hip problems. This most likely is due to the young age (50 years) of patients with osteonecrosis as compared to patients with osteoarthrosis. The failure rate of hip replacement in these patients is approximately 40% at 7 years. Hip fusion is offered in patients under 30 years of age who have no other problems and who are expected to have high activity levels that would predispose to early loosening of a hip replacement. Nonoperative treatment is offered before any surgery to treat patients symptomatically for as long as possible.

References

Callaghan JJ, Brand R, Pedersen D. Hip arthrodesis. J Bone Joint Surg 1985; 67A:1328.

Camp JF, Colwell CW. Core decompression of the femoral head for osteonecrosis. J Bone Joint Surg 1986; 68A:1313.

Canadell J, Aguilella L, Azcarate JR, Valenti JR. The place of intertrochanteric osteotomy in the treatment of idiopathic necrosis of the head of the femur. Intern Orthop 1986; 10:41.

Ficat RP. Idiopathic bone necrosis of the femoral head. Early diagnosis and treatment. J Bone Joint Surg 1985; 67B:3.

Gottschalk F. Indications and results of intertrochanteric osteotomy in osteonecrosis of the femoral head. Clin Orthop 1989; 249:219.

Hopson CN, Siverhus SW. Ischemic necrosis of the femoral head. Treatment by core decompression. J Bone Joint Surg 1988; 70A:1048.

Hungerford DS, Zizic TM. Pathogenesis of ischemic necrosis of the femoral head. The Hip 1983; 249.

Maistrelli G, Fusco U, Avai A, Bombelli R. Osteonecrosis of the hip treated by intertrochanteric osteotomy. J Bone Joint Surg 1988; 70B:761.

Marcus ND, Enneking WF, Massam RA. The silent hip in idiopathic aseptic necrosis. Treatment by bone-grafting. J Bone Joint Surg 1973; 55A:1351.

Warner J, Philip J, Brodsky G, et al. Studies of nontraumatic osteonecrosis: The role of core decompression in the treatment of non traumatic osteonecrosis of the femoral head. Clin Orthop 1987; 225:104.

ARTHRITIS OF THE HIP

A. Any of the rheumatic disorders may involve the hip. Diagnosis of a specific condition requires a good history and physical examination. The duration of involvement of the disease, and other joint involvement may help in the diagnosis. Precipitating factors such as trauma, childhood hip problems, medications, and general medical problems are important in helping to establish the cause of arthritis as well as planning investigations and treatment. Hip examination should determine range of motion, degree of discomfort, presence or absence of deformity, and gait pattern. Evaluate the back and knee joint for evidence of involvement.

B. Radiographs of both hips should be done with the patient standing whenever possible. Obtain cross table lateral views. When appropriate, also obtain radiographs of the lumbar spine and the knees. The presence of joint space narrowing and the amount of involvement as well as the presence or absence of osteophytes, lytic and sclerotic areas will help in the differentiation of the type of arthritis. Obtain laboratory investigations if an inflammatory process is noted and a previous diagnosis has not been made. Test for rheumatoid factor, uric acid levels, erythrocyte sedimentation rate, and antinuclear antibodies. Computed tomography (CT) or magnetic resonance imaging (MRI) may be indicated if radiographs and laboratory tests are equivocal.

C. Degenerative or post-traumatic arthrosis is noted by the presence of osteophytes, asymmetrical joint involvement, areas of sclerosis and/or lucency in the femoral head and acetabulum (Fig. 1). The hip may be the only joint affected and the patient's function compromised by the hip problem.

D. If degenerative or post-traumatic arthrosis is present, depending on the severity of symptoms and degree of joint deterioration noted on the radiographs, the initial treatment is nonoperative. This includes anti-inflammatory medication, physical therapy, and modification of activities. The use of a cane or crutches for a short time may help reduce symptoms.

E. When treatment is not effective, or there is combined deterioration of symptoms and radiographic findings, and the patient is under 40 years old, the surgical options should be tailored to the patient's life style, type of hip problem, and severity of radiographic changes. In very young patients with a very active life style and a very limited range of motion, a hip fusion may be the best option. If a good range of motion with some preservation of joint space is present, especially in a dysplastic hip (Fig. 2), consider a rotational osteotomy. An uncemented total hip replacement may be performed if neither of the previous two options are indicated. Inform patients about the longevity of the implants and the need for future surgery.

F. Patients older than 40 years, who have not responded to nonoperative treatment and have significant functional impairment may be candidates for total hip replacement. Those under 60 years should have an uncemented hip replacement and those over 60 years should have a hybrid total hip replacement.

G. Inflammatory arthritis is noted radiographically by diffuse joint involvement with symmetrical narrowing of the joint space. Osteophytes are often absent and the bone shows evidence of osteopenia. Small erosions are noted in the femoral head and acetabulum. Although there are several types of inflammatory arthritis, the treatment is similar for all. The seronegative spondyloarthropathies include ankylosing spondylitis (Fig. 3), Reiter's syndrome, psoriatic arthropathy, and reactive arthropathies associated with inflammatory bowel disease. Many of these patients have the HLA-B27 antigen on peripheral blood lymphocytes. Initial treatment should be nonoperative with anti-inflammatory medication, physical therapy, and walking aids. Deterioration of the hip joint is best treated by total hip replacement, hybrid or uncemented depending on bone quality and patient age.

H. Arthritis of the hip resulting from infection often has severe joint destruction noted on the radiographs. The changes that are noted occur some time after the initial infection and lead to widespread joint destruction. Hip infections appear to be more prevalent in patients with chronic disease, immunosuppression, or extra-articular infection. Infection may go undiagnosed for weeks to months. When hip infection is suspected, perform aspiration under aseptic conditions and examine joint fluid for bacteria and white cells.

I. Once the causative organism has been identified, treatment goal is to eradicate the infection and preserve or restore joint integrity and function. Gram-negative organisms are more difficult to eradicate because of their resistance to many antibiotics. Several debridements may be necessary and these may result in a resection arthroplasty or a fusion. Total hip replacement may not be possible if the organisms cannot be eradicated.

J. The presence of gram-positive organisms that are sensitive to a host of antibiotics usually results in eradication of the infection. Staged surgery to debride the hip followed by replacement allows restoration of hip function. In a younger active patient, a hip fusion may be the procedure of choice.

ARTHRITIS OF THE HIP

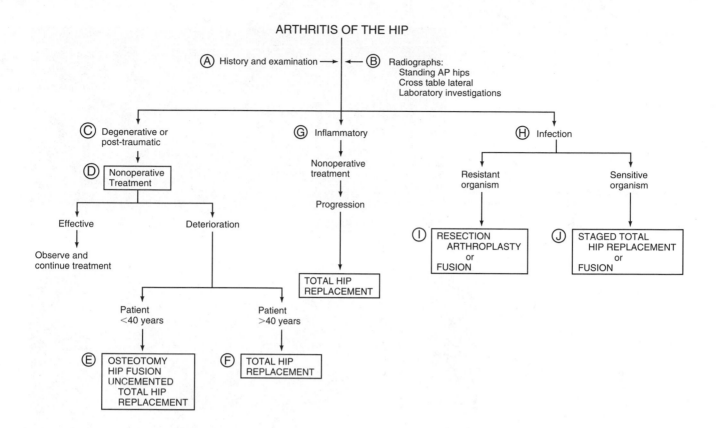

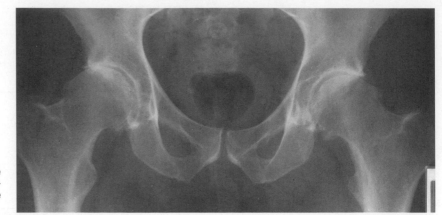

Figure 1 Radiograph of bilateral degenerative arthrosis of the hips. Joint space narrowing, osteophyte formation, and increased areas of bone density are noted around the hips.

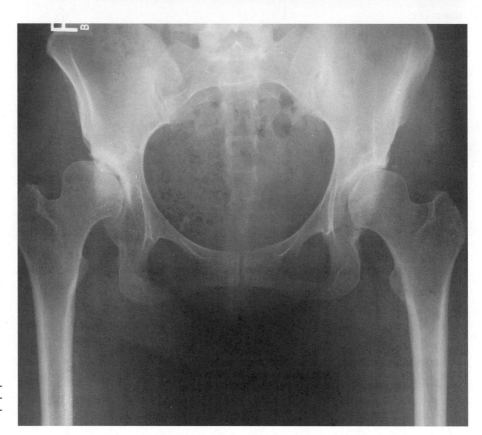

Figure 2 Radiograph of bilateral hip dysplasia with subluxation of the right hip. Increased bone density is noted in the superolateral portion of the right hip.

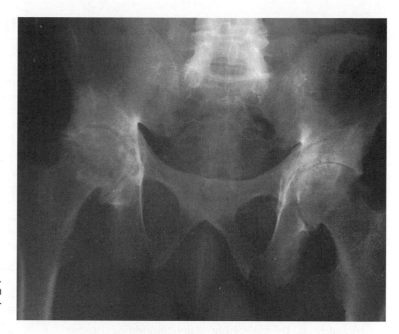

Figure 3 Radiograph of hips with ankylosing spondylitis. More joint destruction is noted than would be seen in degenerative arthrosis and the sacroiliac joints are ankylosed.

References

Bonalaski JS, Schumacher HR. Arthritis and allied conditions. In: Steinberg M, ed. The hip and its disorders. Philadelphia: WB Saunders, 1991.

Collins DN, Nelson CL. Infections of the hip. In: Steinberg M, ed. The hip and its disorders. Philadelphia: WB Saunders, 1991.

Esterhai JL, et al. Adult septic arthritis. Orthop Clin North Am 1991; 22:503.

Milgram JW, et al. Resection arthroplasty for septic arthritis of the hip in ambulatory and nonambulatory adult patients. Clin Orthop 1991; 272:181.

Persselin JE. Diagnosis of rheumatoid arthritis. Medical and laboratory aspects. Clin Orthop 1991; 265:73.

HIP PAIN FOLLOWING TOTAL HIP REPLACEMENT

Pain following total hip reconstruction may occur early or late in the postoperative period. Failure or impending loosening of a component is often heralded by pain. Groin pain may be associated with loosening or failure of the acetabular component, whereas thigh pain and lateral hip pain are indicative of a problem with the femoral component. Most often pain is not present at rest, but as start up pain on initiation of activity such as arising from a chair or walking. Initially the pain may be intermittent, but with progressive loosening or failure of an implant, the pain becomes continuous with the activity. Pain resulting from an acute infection is intense and continuous and not related to activity. Chronic pain may start several years after an initial successful procedure.

A. Examination of the affected hip may reveal an altered range of motion in all directions, associated with discomfort. Patient will have an antalgic gait and possibly a Trendelenburg gait. Shortening of the affected extremity may also be present. Skin changes around the previous incision may indicate chronic infection. Radiographs of the hip should be done with patient standing for the anteroposterior (AP) view and a cross table lateral to show the hip and proximal femur. Loosening of the components is noted from the lucent lines around the stem or acetabulum, subsidence of the femoral component, or migration of the acetabular component. Osteolysis is indicative of particle debris and may be associated with loosening. Cracks in bone cement and lucent lines around the cement are radiographic signs of loosening (Fig. 1).

B. Acute pain after total hip reconstruction may be caused by a variety of conditions. Pain occurring in the early postoperative situation may be caused by hematoma, heterotopic bone formation, infection, trochanter fracture, or dislocation. Acute pain in the late postoperative phase (several years) is most often caused by sudden displacement of a component, whether loosening or dissociation of a modular component (Fig. 2). Acute infection as a result of hematogenous seeding produces severe pain and fever. Femoral fracture at or below the implant, may occur from acute trauma or at an area of weakened bone.

C. Hematomata occur after surgery and cause some pain. If a large hematoma is present it should be evacuated to reduce pain and the risk of hematogenous infection. In many circumstances an active source of the bleeding cannot be found. Patients on anticoagulants for the prevention of deep vein thrombosis are at risk for hematoma formation.

D. Heterotopic bone formation (Fig. 3) occurs in patients who have some predisposing cause such as ankylosing spondylitis, disseminated idiopathic hyperostosis, previous hip surgery with bone formation, and osteoar-

throsis with large osteophyte formation. In high-risk patients, the formation of heterotopic ossification can be prevented by low-dose irradiation using one exposure of 6Gy or 6 weeks of indomethacin. The treatment should be started within 48 hours of surgery.

E. Trochanter fracture or displacement may occur during surgery or postoperatively. This may be a cause of hip pain. An undisplaced fracture may be observed and the patient restricted from specific activities. A displaced trochanteric fragment, by more than 2 mm, should be reattached to improve muscle function and reduce the chance of nonunion.

F. Surgery is necessary in the late postoperative situation, when acute pain develops as a result of a femur fracture, component displacement, or infection. If the femur fracture occurs around the prosthesis (Fig. 4), a long stem femoral component should be inserted. Fractures distal to the stem may be internally fixed or a long stem used depending on the fracture pattern (Fig. 5). Component displacement—dislocation, dissociation, or migration—requires revision surgery. If acute hematogenous infection is suspected, aspirate the hip prior to surgery to try and identify the organism.

G. Chronic hip pain most often is associated with loosening of one or both components of a total hip replacement. It is important to exclude chronic infection as the prime source of loosening. The preoperative investigations should include blood tests, isotope scans, and, when indicated, hip aspiration. If the erythrocyte sedimentation is normal and the quantitative C-reactive protein is normal, then infection is unlikely. A technetium scan and gallium or indium scan may provide sufficient information to help prove or exclude infection around a component. Radiographic evidence of infection, much as periosteal reaction and endosteal irregularities, may obviate the need for isotope scans. Aspirate the hip to try and identify an organism.

H. Loose implants require surgical revision. Often there is bone loss that requires grafting, either autograft or allograft. Special revision components may also be used.

I. If infection is present, perform a two-stage revision. At the first operation remove components and all infected tissue. Use antibiotic impregnated methylmethacrylate as a spacer or in bead form. Place revision implants at the second operation, 4 to 6 weeks later. Certain patients, such as those with gram-negative infections, failure to respond to multiple surgical debridements, or those with severe bone loss, may not be candidates for reimplantation and should be treated definitively with a resection arthroplasty.

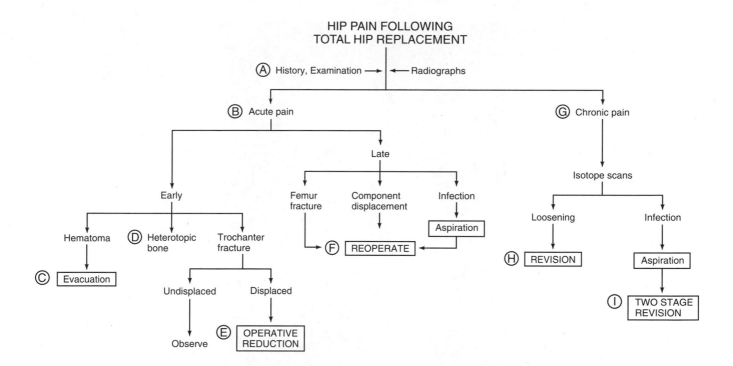

HIP PAIN FOLLOWING TOTAL HIP REPLACEMENT

(A) History, Examination ⟶ ⟵ Radiographs

(B) Acute pain

(G) Chronic pain

Late

Isotope scans

Early

Femur fracture

Component displacement

Infection

Loosening

Infection

Hematoma

(D) Heterotopic bone

Trochanter fracture

Aspiration

(H) REVISION

Aspiration

(C) Evacuation

(F) REOPERATE

(I) TWO STAGE REVISION

Undisplaced

Displaced

Observe

(E) OPERATIVE REDUCTION

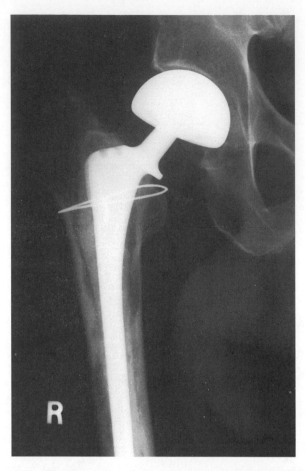

Figure 1   Radiograph of loose right total hip replacement. Lucency and erosions are seen at the bone-cement interface.

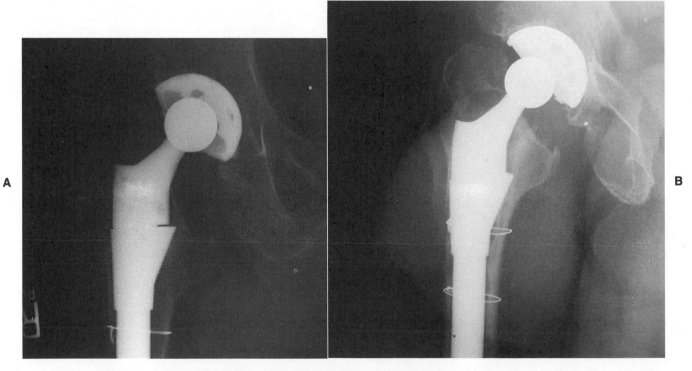

Figure 2   **A,** Immediate postoperative radiograph of total hip replacement. **B,** Radiograph 1 year later with subsidence of femoral component and subluxation of femoral head.

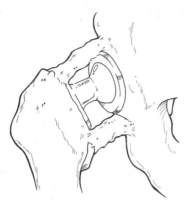

Figure 3 Diagram of heterotopic bone formation around the hip following total hip replacement.

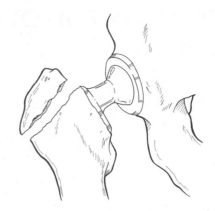

Figure 5 Diagram of hip replacement showing fracture of the greater trochanter.

References

Ayers DC, Evarts CM, Parkinson JR. The prevention of heterotopic ossification in high-risk patients by low dose radiation therapy after total hip arthroplasty. J Bone Joint Surg 1986; 68A:1423.

Barrack RL, Harris WL. The value of aspiration of the hip joint before revision total hip arthroplasty. J Bone Joint Surg 1993; 75A:66.

Gruen TA, McNeice GM, Amstutz HC. "Modes of failure" of cemented stem-type femoral components: A radiographic analysis of loosening. Clin Orthop 1979; 141:17.

Heekin RD, Callaghan JJ, Hopkinson WJ, et al. The porous-coated anatomic total hip prosthesis, inserted without cement. J Bone Joint Surg 1993; 75A:77.

Horne G, Rutherford A, Schemitsch E. Evaluation of hip pain following cemented total hip arthroplasty. Orthopedics 1990; 13:415.

Levitsky KA, Hozack WJ, Balderston, et al. Evaluation of the painful prosthetic joint: Relative value of bone scan, sedimentation rate, and joint aspiration. J Arthrop 1991; 6:237.

Lieberman JR, Huo MH, Schneider R, et al. Evaluation of painful hip arthroplasties: Are technetium bone scans necessary? J Bone Joint Surg 1993; 75B:475.

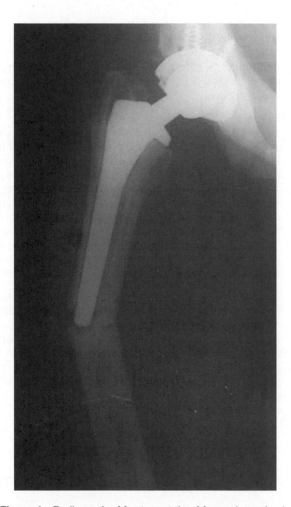

Figure 4 Radiograph of fracture at tip of femoral prosthesis.

DISLOCATION FOLLOWING TOTAL HIP REPLACEMENT

Total hip arthroplasty is one of the most frequently performed orthopedic procedures with over 150,000 replacements annually performed in the United States. Despite significant advances in component design, postoperative dislocation is the second most common complication in total hip arthroplasty. The incidence of dislocation is between 3% and 5%. An important risk factor for dislocation is prior hip surgery. Dislocation after revision total hip replacement appears to occur more frequently than after primary surgery.

A. Early dislocation occurs within 30 days of the operation. Numerous factors have been implicated in contributing to dislocation. Surgical approach and component orientation have been identified as the most important factors leading to early dislocation. The posterior surgical approach has a two- to three-fold prevalence of dislocation compared to the antero-lateral (AP) exposure of the hip. Component head size has not been shown to correlate with the incidence of dislocation of the hip. There is no correlation between limb length and the incidence of dislocation. Myofascial tension related to lengthening or shortening of the extremity does not appear to be a significant factor for joint stability.

B. Radiographic evaluation of joint stability and component orientation is important (Fig. 1). If implant alignment is satisfactory and the hip stable in full range of motion, no surgery is indicated. The acetabulum should be positioned in 15° of anteversion and 45° of abduction. The femoral component should be in 10° of anteversion since retroversion results in a higher incidence of dislocation. If a trochanteric osteotomy was done, continued maintenance of the trochanter in its reattached position as close to a normal anatomic situation as possible is important.

C. If the implants are noted to be in a malposition, it is important to evaluate under fluoroscopy the range of motion and the stability of the hip. If a good range of motion is present and there is no tendency to dislocate, the patient can be treated nonoperatively. Evidence of instability requires revision surgery.

D. Patients who have had an early postoperative dislocation and are compliant should be placed in a hip orthosis for 6 to 12 weeks. The prevalence of redislocation is low after this treatment and patients can then function at the usual level. If the patient is not compliant, apply a hip spica until the soft tissues have healed at 3 months.

E. A persistent unstable situation requires revision surgery. Malposition of the components must be corrected. If the trochanter is avulsed, reattachment is important to contribute to stability. The hip may need to be protected by a hip spica for up to 3 months postoperatively.

F. Late dislocation occurs after the first 4 to 5 weeks. In most reported series dislocation occurred after 1 year and was attributed to a greater range of motion of the hip than in those patients that had not dislocated. However, the incidence of late dislocation is less than 1% of all total hip replacement. With the advent of modular hip systems, dissociation of one of the components may present as a dislocation. Although not common, dissociation of the polyethylene from the metal acetabular shell or the femoral head from the neck of the implant have been noted. In both situations surgery is indicated.

G. Trochanter fracture or migration may contribute to a late dislocation. In some patients with a greater range of motion, an expanded pseudocapsule developed, which was associated with a tendency to late dislocation. Recurrence of dislocation is more common in patients who have had late dislocation, but the prevalence is less than 1%. The most successful procedures to prevent redislocation are reorientation of a component and trochanter advancement.

DISLOCATION FOLLOWING TOTAL HIP REPLACEMENT

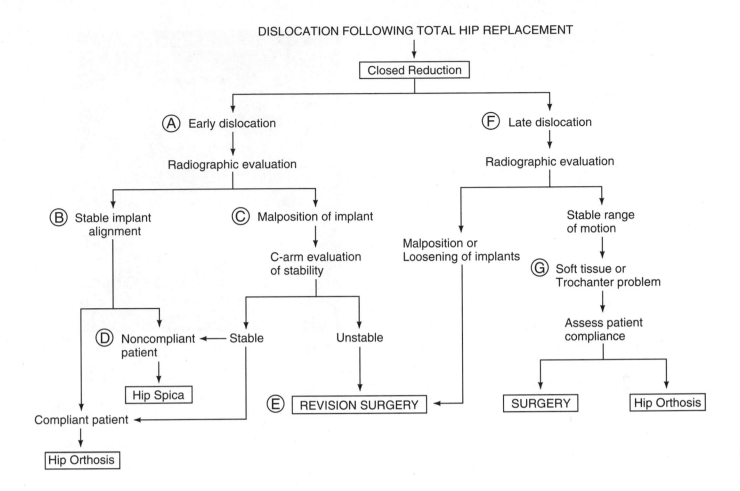

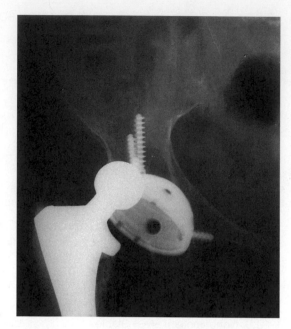

Figure 1 Radiograph of dislocated right total hip replacement.

References

Ackland MK, Bourne WB, Uhthoff HR. Anteversion of the acetabular cup. J Bone Joint Surg 1986; 68B:407.

Beaver RJ, Schemitsch ER, Gross AE. Disassembly of a one-piece metal-backed acetabular component. J Bone Joint Surg 1991; 73B:908.

Kaplan SJ, Thomas WM, Poss R. Trochanteric advancement for recurrent dislocation after total hip arthroplasty. J Arthroplasty 1987; 2:119.

Kitziger KJ, DeLee JC, Evans JA. Disassembly of a modular acetabular component of a total hip replacement arthroplasty. J Bone Joint Surg 1990; 72A:621.

McCollum DE, Gray WJ. Dislocation after total hip arthroplasty. Causes and prevention. Clin Orthop 1990; 261:159.

Morrey BF. Instability after total hip arthroplasty. Orthop Clin North Am 1992; 23:237.

Olerud K. Recurrent dislocation status post total hip replacement. J Bone Joint Surg 1985; 67B:402.

Pellici PM, Haas SB. Disassembly of a modular femoral component during closed reduction of the dislocated femoral component. J Bone Joint Surg 1990; 72A:619.

Rao JP, Bronstein R. Dislocations following arthroplasties of the hip: Incidence, prevention, and treatment. Orthop Rev 1991; 20:261.

Woo R, Morrey B. Dislocations after total hip arthroplasty. J Bone Joint Surg 1982; 64A:1295.

INFECTED TOTAL HIP REPLACEMENT

Infection after total hip replacement occurs in less than 1% of patients. Patients at risk for infection are those who have had previous hip surgery, a prior hip infection, a compromised immune system, obesity, or a bacteremia or septicemia from another source in the body. The risk of infection increases about 5% with each previous operation. Persistent pain in the first 3 months after surgery may indicate infection. Drainage from the wound, erythema, and fever are virtually diagnostic for infection of the joint. In the early postoperative phase, plain radiographs of the hip are not usually helpful for excluding infection. Blood investigations may help to confirm the diagnosis but a normal result does not exclude infection. The white blood cell count has no correlation with the presence of an infected total hip joint. The sedimentation rate has a sensitivity of 56% and an accuracy of 73% when infection is present, whereas the C-reactive protein is elevated when infection is active. Patients who develop radiographic changes of loosening (Fig. 1) should have isotope studies to help exclude infection, when infection is suspected as a cause of the loosening or pain. Technetium[99] scanning is positive in 38% of infected cases and is associated with increased blood flow and an increase in alkaline phosphatase activity. Gallium scans depend on monocyte accumulation and with the technetium scan provides approximately a 60% sensitivity. The Indium[111] labeled white cell scan is taken up at sites of acute inflammation and is about 70% accurate.

The host immune system is important in combating infection. Type A hosts have a normal ability to counter infection both locally and systemically. Type B hosts have a locally compromised situation because of poor blood supply or increased scar tissue. Type C hosts do not have the ability to counter the infection either locally or systemically.

A. Acute infection may occur within the first 3 weeks after surgery or may present several years later as a result of hematogenous spread from another site. Deep infections are insidious and may be accompanied by surface signs. Patients will have pain with movement of the joint and usually are pyrexial. The white cell count is usually elevated. The erythrocyte sedimentation rate is not useful in the early postoperative phase for assessing the presence or absence of infection. A deep hematoma may present with acute pain, and must be distinguished from acute infection. Infection may be accompanied by a drop in the hemoglobin or hematocrit level. Heterotopic bone formation may produce pain similar to acute infection and should be considered in the differential diagnosis.

B. When infection of the total joint is suspected and blood tests and isotope studies have been obtained, aspirate the joint to identify the organism. Aspiration should be done under radiographic imaging and 1 to 2 cc of contrast injected to confirm the position of the needle in the joint. If a dry aspiration is obtained, inject 30 cc of saline and then reaspirate. Preoperative aspiration in the presence of infection is 80% accurate. However, intraoperative cultures and frozen section are the most accurate. In the early weeks of an acute infection, there are no diagnostic radiographic changes. Radiographs do help exclude other causes of acute hip pain such as component dissociation, fracture, or component displacement.

C. Perform surgery as soon as possible to debride the hip joint. Leave components that are not loose in place and after pulsatile lavage, place antibiotic impregnated methylmethacrylate beads. Leave these in the joint area for 2 to 4 weeks and then remove. Place the patient on appropriate intravenous antibiotics for 6 weeks, followed by 6 to 12 weeks of oral antibiotics.

D. If the infection persists or is chronic, removal of the implants is mandatory. Perform an adequate debridement and insert antibiotic impregnated methylmethacrylate beads into the cavity (Fig. 2). These allow antibiotic elution into the surrounding tissue for up to 6 weeks. At the time of bead removal, between 2 and 6 weeks, undertake a revision implant if no evidence of infection is detected (Fig. 3). Do an intraoperative frozen section looking for white cells as well as a gram stain if necessary. More than five polymorphonucleocytes per high power field suggests an ongoing infection, as does the presence of bacteria on the gram stain. The revision components may be cemented or uncemented, depending on bone quality and age of patient.

E. Chronic infection occurs in long-standing total joint replacement and presents with long-standing pain. A chronic draining sinus may be present. Many present 1 or more years after the index operation. Complications with the first operation include wound infection, drainage, and prolonged postoperative pain.

F. Blood investigations should include a white cell count, erythrocyte sedimentation rate, and a quantitative C-reactive protein. These are usually elevated when chronic infection is present. Radiographs often show evidence of loosening of the implant. Bone resorption and periosteal reaction may be evident. Isotope studies help to confirm the diagnosis. Hip aspiration should be done to identify the organism present. Less virulent organisms such as *Staphylococcus aureus* and *epidermidis,* which are susceptible to routine intravenous antibiotics, should be managed by a two-stage revision operation. More resistant or virulent organisms such as *Pseudomonas* or *Klebsiella* require more radical surgery.

INFECTED TOTAL HIP REPLACEMENT

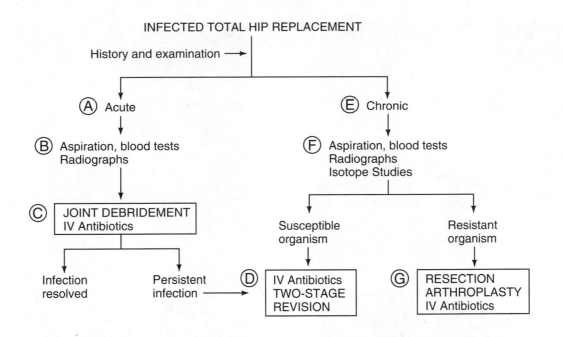

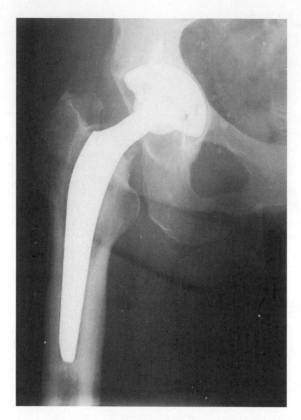

Figure 1 Radiograph of a loose total hip replacement. Aspiration revealed growth of gram-positive cocci.

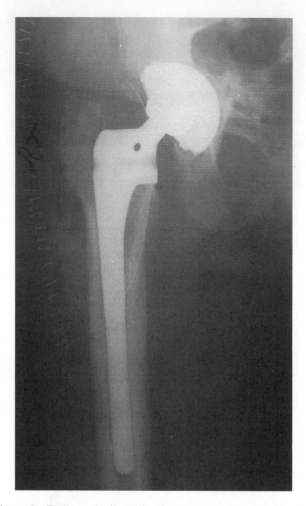

Figure 3 Radiograph of revision hip replacement several weeks after initial placement of antibiotic beads.

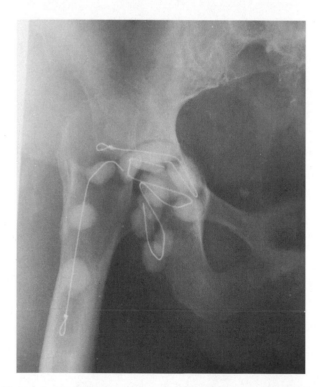

Figure 2 Radiograph showing removal of the components and placement of antibiotic impregnated methylmethacrylate beads.

G. Resection arthroplasty or removal of all foreign material and dead bone may be the best solution for infection by resistant and virulent organisms. Reimplantation of prosthetic devices is not recommended. Place patient on intravenous antibiotics for 4 to 6 weeks to help eradicate the infection. The antibiotics necessary are usually more toxic and may have more severe side effects. The host's ability to counter infection may be important in deciding on a resection arthroplasty.

References

Antti-Poika I, Josefsson G, Konttineu Y, et al. Hip arthroplasty infection: Current concepts. Acta Orthop Scand 1990; 61:163.

Cierny G, Mader JT. Approach to adult osteomyelitis. Orthop Rev 1987; 16:259.

Cierny G, Mader JT, Penninck JJ. A clinical staging system for adult osteomyelitis. Cont Orthop 1985; 10:17.

Collins DN, McKenzie JM. Infections at the site of a hip implant: Successful and unsuccessful management. Clin Orthop 1991; 269:9.

Eftekhar N. Infection in joint replacement surgery. St. Louis: Mosby, 1984.

Horne G, Rutherford A, Schemitsch E. Evaluation of hip pain following cemented total hip arthroplasty. Orthopedics 1990; 13:415.

McDonald DJ, Fitzgerald RH, Ilstrup DM. Two-stage reconstruction of a total hip arthroplasty because of infection. J Bone Joint Surg 1989; 71A:828.

Perry CR, Pearson RL. Local antibiotic delivery in the treatment of bone and joint infections. Clin Orthop 1991; 263:215.

Shutzer SF, Harris WH. Deep wound infection after total hip replacement under contemporary aseptic conditions. J Bone Joint Surg 1988; 70A:724.

Struhl S, Harwin S, Stern R, Kulick R. Infected uncemented hip arthroplasty: Preserving the femoral stem with a two-stage revision procedure. Orthop Rev 1989; 18:707.

Trippel SB. Antibiotic-impregnated cement in total joint arthroplasty. J Bone Joint Surg 1986; 68A:1297.

RHEUMATOID ARTHRITIS OF THE KNEE

Rheumatoid arthritis of the knee should be evaluated and treated in the context of a systemic disease involving multiple organs and joints. Rarely are the knee symptoms the initial presentation and patients most often are taking medication for rheumatoid arthritis.

A. Assessment of acute swelling of the knee requires a good history and physical examination. If the patient does not have a history of being treated for rheumatoid arthritis, blood studies to confirm the diagnosis are required. Blood tests should include cell counts, erythrocyte sedimentation rate, quantitative C reactive protein, rheumatoid factor, and antinuclear antibodies. A random serum uric acid level on three different occasions will help to exclude hyperuricemia. Other causes of acute inflammation should be excluded. These include crystal arthropathy, hemophilia, and infection. Acute infection is not uncommon in the knee joint in patients on immunosuppressive medication for rheumatoid arthritis and knee aspiration with culture of the joint fluid may be indicated.

B. Acute synovitis is managed medically and includes nonsteroidal anti-inflammatory drugs (NSAIDs) and specific drugs for rheumatoid arthritis, (e.g., gold, methotrexate). Patients with severe boggy synovitis frequently respond to an intra-articular steroid injection. These should not be repeated more than a few times a year. Septic arthritis must be excluded prior to injecting any steroid. Steroid preparations that have reduced solubility are injected so as to provide a longer duration of effectiveness without being rapidly absorbed and resulting in any systemic effect. The dose of medication varies from 20 mg to 50 mg depending on the type of steroid used. Bracing of the joint with an acute exacerbation helps in preventing deformity and relieving pain. Intra-articular injections of cytotoxic agents or osmic acid have been used to try and control the synovitis but may cause local irritation. Injections of radioactive isotopes are also noted to provide control of the synovitis. Gold 198, yttrium 90, and dysprosium 165 are experimental in the United States and studies are still in progress to assess the long-term effectiveness of these compounds. Physical therapy should include range of motion exercise of the knee as well as muscle strengthening of the lower extremity. A knee orthosis or brace should be used to help rest the joint and allow for some motion, but reduce the possibility of joint contracture.

C. Chronic synovitis with no articular damage that is unresponsive to medical management is a good indication for an arthroscopic synovectomy followed by intensive physical therapy. Most patients should have had at least 6 months of treatment with medication and physical therapy prior to recommending surgery. Arthroscopic synovectomy can usually be done as a day surgery procedure. Additional portals around the patella and posterior knee joint are often necessary to obtain a complete synovectomy. In most patients, the synovectomy is sufficient to allow symptoms to be controlled by pharmacologic agents, and long-term, patients do not require additional procedures. Patients who have a chronic synovitis with significant articular damage and joint deformity are more appropriately treated by total knee arthroplasty, rather than synovectomy alone.

D. The presence of articular damage usually results in severe functional impairment. These patients benefit from a total knee replacement. The presence of a deformity, usually valgus, with minimal joint damage may be an indication for an osteotomy in the younger patient. The survival rate of total knee replacement in patients with rheumatoid arthritis appears to be lower than that for degenerative arthrosis. However, patient function is greatly enhanced following knee replacement surgery. Knee replacement surgery in a patient with rheumatoid arthritis often requires modification of the standard technique. The soft tissues are more friable, especially if the patient is on corticosteroids, and healing may be delayed. Contractures of the joint require additional release and in most patients the bone is severely osteopenic, requiring that all components be cemented in place. A complete synovectomy should be done at the time of the knee arthroplasty.

RHEUMATOID ARTHRITIS OF THE KNEE

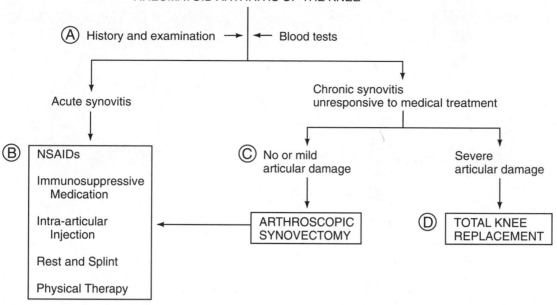

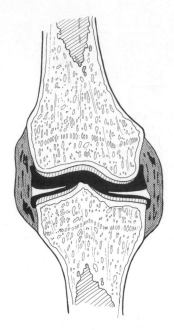

Figure 1 Diagram of the knee showing thickening of the synovium and fluid in the joint in the early stages of the disease.

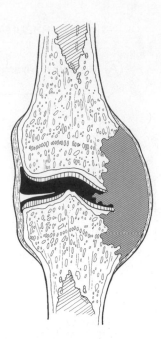

Figure 3 Diagram of the knee showing hypertrophy of the synovium and bony erosion and osteopenia.

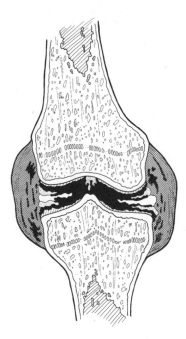

Figure 2 Diagram of the knee showing progression of the synovitis. The synovial tissue is thickened and a pannus involves the articular cartilage, contributing to erosion.

References

Arthritis and Rheumatism Council Multicentre Radiosynovior-thesis Trial Group. Intra-articular radioactive yttrium and triamcinolone hexacetonide. Ann Rheum Dis 1984; 43:620.

Laskin RS. Total condylar knee replacement in patients who have rheumatoid arthritis. J Bone Joint Surg 1990; 72A:529.

Meijers KA, Valkenburg HA, Cats A. A synovectomy trial and the history of early knee synovitis in rheumatoid arthritis: A multicentre study. Rheumatol Int 1983; 3:161.

Menkes CJ. Is there a place for chemical and radiation synovectomy in rheumatic diseases? Rheumatol Rehabil 1979; 18:65.

Multicenter evaluation of synovectomy in the treatment of rheumatoid arthritis: Report of results at the end of three years. Arthritis Rheum 1977; 20:765.

Neustadt DH. Intra-articular therapy in rheumatoid synovitis of the knee: Effects of post injection rest regimen. Clin Rheumatol Practice 1985; 3:65.

Ogilvie-Harris DJ, Basinski A. Arthroscopic synovectomy of the knee for rheumatoid arthritis. Arthroscopy 1991; 7:91.

Sledge CB, Atcher RW, et al. Intra-articular radiation synovectomy. Clin Orthop 1984; 182:37.

Sledge CB, Zuckerman JD, Shortkroff S, et al. Synovectomy of the rheumatoid knee using intra-articular injection of dysprosium-165-ferric hydroxide macroaggregates. J Bone Joint Surg 1987; 69A:970.

DEGENERATIVE ARTHROSIS OF THE KNEE

A. Nonoperative treatment is the first choice for degenerative arthrosis of the knee. Nonsteroidal anti-inflammatory drugs (NSAIDs), weight loss, physical therapy, and orthoses often provide significant symptomatic relief. In some situations intra-articular injections of steroids provides symptomatic relief for some time. Occasionally urethane shoe inserts to cushion impact loading may help reduce knee discomfort. Some patients should modify their activities and avoid impact loading stresses to the knees. These treatment modalities are most likely to help in the earlier stages of the disease. The mechanical alignment of the leg may influence the rate of deterioration as well as the effectiveness of the nonoperative treatment.

B. Total knee replacement is the preferred treatment in older patients with tricompartmental disease. Patients who are 60 years or older generally derive great benefit from knee replacement surgery, which has a better than 90% success rate at 10 years. Younger, more active patients are at greater risk for failure of the implants due to loosening and wear of the components. Unless there is severe deformity, osteotomy does not provide satisfactory results.

C. Medial compartment degenerative disease (Fig. 1) frequently follows a previous medial meniscectomy or trauma. The increasing varus deformity perpetuates the degenerative process. This results in a change in the mechanical alignment of the leg and decreased functional activity.

D. Many patients benefit from a high tibial osteotomy (Fig. 2), which shifts the mechanical axis towards the lateral compartment and unloads the medial compartment (Fig. 3). Indications for a high tibial osteotomy include age less than 60 years, predominantly medial compartment arthrosis, vigorous occupation, and satisfactory knee motion. Flexion should be to 80° to 90° and a flexion contracture of less than 15°. The varus deformity should be less than 15°. If there is doubt about the isolated nature of the arthrosis, a technetium bone scan may be helpful. Contraindications to osteotomy include severe flexion contractures (greater than 15°), ligament instability, and reduced range of motion. The results of high tibial osteotomy depend on adequate correction and are expected to last about 10 years.

E. Unicompartmental knee replacement appears to be less effective in the degenerative knee, but is reported to be satisfactory for post-traumatic arthrosis involving only one compartment. Unicompartmental knee replacement is indicated in the nonobese patient older than 60 years who is sedentary and has no major deformities of the knee. The articular cartilage of the other two compartments should be normal. The results of unicompartmental knee replacement in selected patients are generally 90% good at 10 years.

F. In older patients with equivocal radiographs for isolated medial compartment disease, arthroscopic inspection of the joint may be helpful to stage the disease. If severe cartilage loss and eburnated bone is evident in the lateral and/or patellofemoral compartments, total knee replacement is indicated.

G. Lateral compartment arthrosis with a valgus deformity is less frequent. In the younger patient (less than 60 years), a distal femoral osteotomy is beneficial to correct the mechanical axis. Unicompartmental knee replacement, although less frequent for lateral compartment arthrosis, has the same indications and contraindications as for the medial compartment.

H. Patellofemoral arthrosis is most often associated with arthrosis of the other compartments. Pseudogout (chondrocalcinosis) may present as isolated patellofemoral pain. Nonoperative treatment includes physical therapy and appropriate anti-inflammatory medication.

I. Arthroscopy does not appear to have uniformly successful results but may be the best approach in the elderly patient with isolated patellofemoral disease. If symptoms persist, consider patellectomy or total knee arthroplasty.

J. Patients less than 60 years of age with isolated patellofemoral symptoms, who are unresponsive to nonoperative care, may benefit from elevation of the tibial tubercle (Maquet) to decrease the patellofemoral contact stress area. Patellectomy, which has the disadvantage of reducing the mechanical efficiency of the quadriceps mechanism, should be reserved for the most recalcitrant cases. The Maquet procedure is indicated when symptoms are predominantly patellofemoral, with discomfort and pain during extension from 60° to 20°. Patients should have aggressive physical therapy to strengthen the quadriceps mechanisms and, where indicated, arthroscopic surgery to confirm cartilage damage at the patellofemoral interface. Complications following a Maquet procedure include skin necrosis, wound infection, and nonunion of the bony shingle.

DEGENERATIVE ARTHROSIS OF THE KNEE

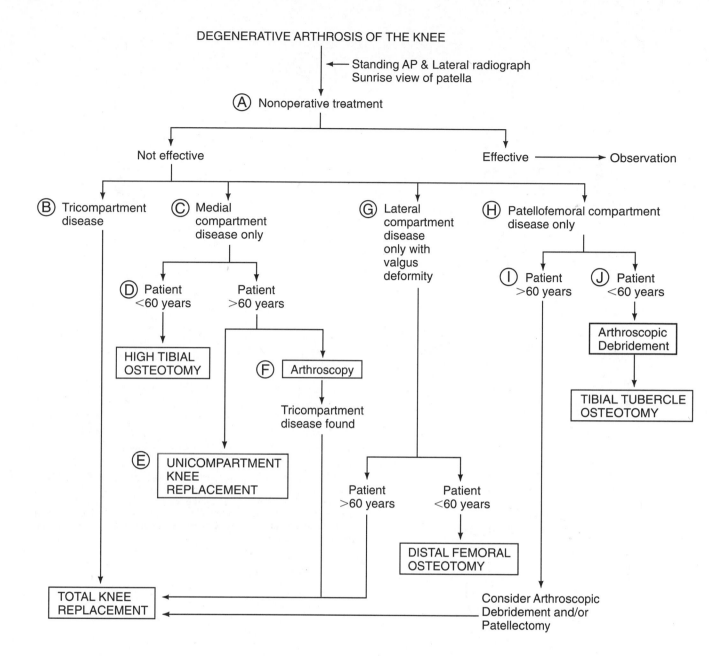

Standing AP & Lateral radiograph
Sunrise view of patella

Ⓐ Nonoperative treatment

Not effective   Effective ──→ Observation

Ⓑ Tricompartment disease

Ⓒ Medial compartment disease only

Ⓖ Lateral compartment disease only with valgus deformity

Ⓗ Patellofemoral compartment disease only

Ⓓ Patient <60 years   Patient >60 years

Ⓘ Patient >60 years   Ⓙ Patient <60 years

HIGH TIBIAL OSTEOTOMY

Ⓕ Arthroscopy

Arthroscopic Debridement

Tricompartment disease found

Ⓔ UNICOMPARTMENT KNEE REPLACEMENT

TIBIAL TUBERCLE OSTEOTOMY

Patient >60 years   Patient <60 years

DISTAL FEMORAL OSTEOTOMY

TOTAL KNEE REPLACEMENT

Consider Arthroscopic Debridement and/or Patellectomy

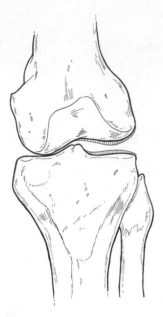

Figure 1 Preoperative medial compartment joint space loss with bone-on-bone contact.

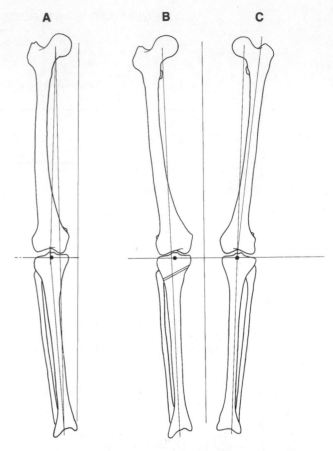

Figure 3 **A,** Mechanical alignment of the leg with medial compartment joint space narrowing. The mechanical axis of the limb passes through the medial side of the knee. **B,** Mechanical alignment of the leg after osteotomy with the mechanical axis shifted to just lateral of the mid portion of the knee. **C,** Normal mechanical alignment of the leg.

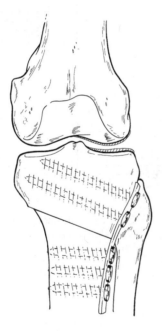

Figure 2 Diagram of a proximal tibial osteotomy to realign tibia and reduce load on the medial compartment.

References

Coventry MB, Ilstrup DM, Wallrichs SL. Proximal tibial osteotomy. J Bone Joint Surg 1993; 75A:196.

Ferguson AB. Elevation of the insertion of the patellar ligament for patellofemoral pain. J Bone Joint Surg 1982; 64A:766.

Insall JN, Joseph DM, Msika C. High tibial osteotomy for varus gonarthrosis. J Bone Joint Surg 1984; 66A:1040.

Kozinn SC, Scott R. Unicondylar knee arthroplasty. J Bone Joint Surg 1989; 71A:145.

McDermott AG, Finkelstein JA, Farine I, et al. Distal femoral varus osteotomy for valgus deformity of the knee. J Bone Joint Surg 1988; 70A:110.

Moran CG, Pinder IM, Lees TA. Survivorship analysis of uncemented porous-coated anatomic knee replacement. J Bone Joint Surg 1991; 73A:848.

Radin EL. The Maquet procedure—anterior displacement of the tibial tubercle. Clin Orthop 1986; 213:241.

Rand JA. Total knee arthoplasty. New York: Raven, 1993.

Rudan JF, Simurda MA. High tibial osteotomy: A prospective clinical and roentgenographic review. Clin Orthop 1990; 225:251.

Scott R, Cobba A, McQueary F, et al. Unicompartmental knee arthroplasty: Eight to 12 year follow-up evaluation with survivorship analysis. Clin Orthop 1991; 271:96.

Siegel M. The Maquet osteotomy: A review of the risks. Orthopedics 1987; 10:1073.

Wright J, Ewald FC, Walker PS, et al. Total knee arthroplasty with the kinematic prosthesis. Results after five to nine years: A follow up note. J Bone Joint Surg 1990; 72A:1003.

HEMOPHILIC ARTHROPATHY OF THE KNEE

A. The knee is the most common site of arthropathy and most likely to result in orthopedic disability. Recurrent intra-articular hemorrhage in hemophilic patients results in a progressive and disabling arthropathy. Radiographic changes progress over time and are usually diagnostic (Fig. 1). The radiographic changes include osteoporosis, irregularity of the subchondral surface, cyst formation, erosions, and joint space changes and narrowing. Osteophyte formation is uncommon.

B. Treat acute bleeding into the joint by infusion of the missing clotting factor, usually factor VIII. An increase of plasma levels to 25% to 30% is sufficient. Use ice packs and splinting for 2 days to reduce the swelling. Patient should begin active movement as soon as pain subsides and undertake intensive muscle strengthening.

C. When the intra-articular bleed is large enough to cause a tense effusion, aspirate the joint, but only after giving adequate factor replacement. Aspirate early, before the blood has extravasated into the surrounding soft tissues.

D. Chronic proliferative synovitis results from repeated hemorrhage. Platelet derived growth factor is a potent stimulus for proliferation of mesenchymal synovial cells. Iron appears to stimulate proteinase biosynthesis by synovial fibroblasts. The proliferative destructive synovitis is caused by the blood and not by any immune mechanism. There is damage to the articular cartilage from the synovitis, and loss of subchondral support as the destructive process continues.

E. Several roentgenographic classifications have been proposed. The most useful is that by Greene et al (Table 1). Four categories are listed: (1) irregularity of the subchondral surface, (2) narrowing of the joint space, (3) erosion of the joint margin, and (4) incongruity of the joint surfaces. A scoring system for each category helps determine the severity of the disease. Scores of less than 4 are indicative of mild disease, whereas higher scores show severe disease.

F. Do synovectomy for recurrent bleeding with synovitis. Removal of the vascular and villous synovial tissue reduces its vulnerability to minor trauma. Patients with a persistent boggy synovitis benefit the most, provided they still have a good range of knee motion and articular damage is not severe. Patients with early synovial fibrosis, contracture, and subluxation are not candidates for synovectomy. Chemical synovectomy has been used in Europe and is not available in the United States. The use of radioactive yttrium appears to be beneficial in some patients without severe joint damage.

G. Once advanced joint destruction is present, arthroplasty may be the only therapy to prevent additional disability. Many patients are young (average age 35 years). The surgery is technically more demanding and potential complications are formidable. A preoperative flexion contracture is the most frequently seen deformity and may require extensive release at the time of knee replacement. Contracture of the quadriceps may prevent adequate range of motion. Advanced hemophilic arthropathy accompanied by quadriceps contracture may require a quadriceps-plasty as well as extensive mobilization of the tissues around the knee. Patients undergoing total knee arthroplasty require continuous infusion of factor VIII, which may increase the cost of treatment to between $80,000 and $100,000.

TABLE 1 Roentgenographic Categories and Seven-point Classification of Hemophilic Arthropathy

Roentgenographic Category	Points
1 Subchondral irregularity:	
Absent	0
Mild	1
(≤ 50 percent of the joint surface)	
Pronounced	2
2 Narrowing of the joint space:	
Absent	0
≤ 50 percent	1
>50 percent	2
3 Erosion of the joint margin:	
Absent	0
Present	1
4 Incongruity of the joint surfaces:	
Absent	0
Mild	1
Pronounced	2

Adapted from Greene WB, Yankaskas BC, Guilford WB. Roentgenographic classifications of hemophilic arthropathy. J Bone Joint Surg 1989; 71A:237-244; with permission.

HEMOPHILIC ARTHROPATHY OF THE KNEE

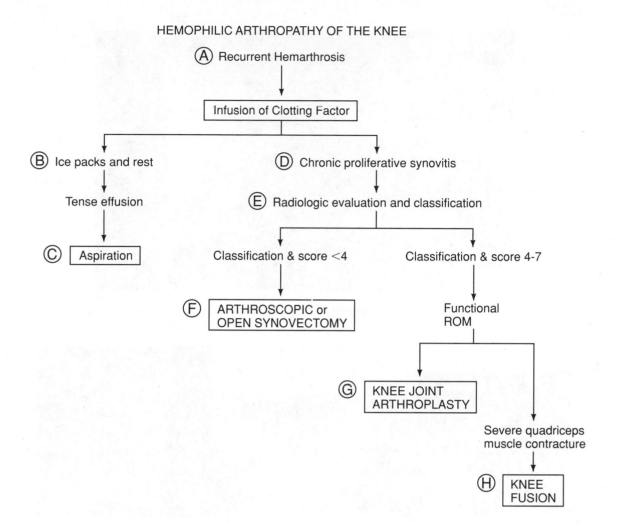

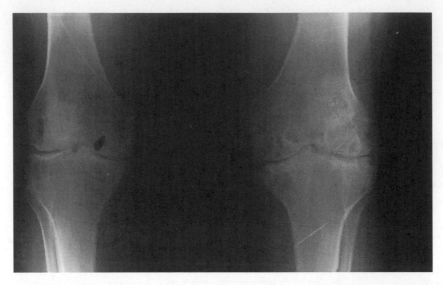

Figure 1 Radiograph of the knees showing loss of joint space, erosion, and lytic areas in the bone.

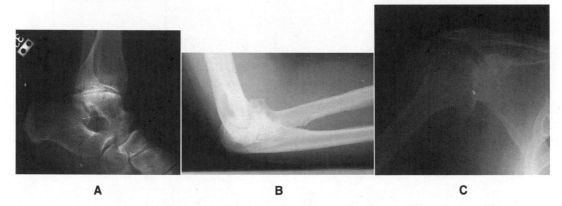

A   B   C

Figure 2 Radiographs of the ankle **(A),** elbow **(B),** and shoulder **(C)** of a hemophilic patient with severe knee problems, showing the involvement of those joints in association with the knee arthropathy.

H. In some patients, a knee fusion can provide good pain relief and function. This procedure should be considered if the knee is ankylosed and the quadriceps muscles are fibrosed.

References

Figgie MP, Goldberg VM, Figgie HE, et al. Total knee arthroplasty for the treatment of chronic hemophilic arthropathy. Clin Orthop 1989; 248:98.

Gilber M, Greene W, eds. Musculoskeletal problems in hemophilia. Proceedings. The National Hemophilia Foundation, March, 1989.

Greene WB, Yankaskas BC, Guilford WB. Roentgenographic classifications of hemophilic arthropathy. J Bone Joint Surg 1989; 71A:237.

Lachiewicz PF, Inglis AE, Insall JN, et al. Total knee arthroplasty in hemophilia. J Bone Joint Surg 1985; 67A:1361.

Luck JV, Kasper CK. Surgical management of advanced hemophilic arthropathy. Clin Orthop 1989; 242:60.

McCollough NC, Enis JE, Lovitt J, et al. Synovectomy or total replacement of the knee in hemophilia. J Bone Joint Surg 1979; 61A:69.

Montane I, McCollough NC, Lian EC. Synovectomy of the knee for hemophilic arthropathy. J Bone Joint Surg 1986; 68A:210.

Pettersson H, Ahlberg A, Nilsson IM. A radiologic classification of hemophilic arthropathy. Clin Orthop 1980; 149:153.

PAINFUL TOTAL KNEE REPLACEMENT

Pain following total knee replacement may occur soon after surgery or at any time in the long-term postoperative phase. Question the patient about episodes of injury, possible sources of infection, types of activity that could predispose to loosening, and pertinent information regarding medical problems. Signs of swelling, redness, or heat suggest possible infection. The presence of a limp, laxity, instability and muscle weakness may be associated with minor trauma or loosening of the components (Fig. 1). Development of a deformity (valgus or varus) implies component loosening or fracture (Fig. 2). Radiographs, blood tests, and bone scans should be done to help with the diagnosis.

A. Distal femur fracture near the femoral component is usually associated with a sudden traumatic episode. Deformity may be present with the swelling. Radiographs often confirm the diagnosis. Surgery may be a revision of the femoral component or an appropriate form of internal fixation. Rigid stabilization of the fracture is important. Nonoperative treatment such as bracing or traction most often leads to an unsatisfactory outcome.

B. Acute pain without a history of trauma is most often caused by infection, usually seeded from a bacteremia. The most common organism is usually gram-positive staphylococci, but gram negative infections are not infrequent. Aspiration of the knee may confirm the presence of infection. Special investigations such as bone scans or activity tests (erythrocyte sedimentation rate and C reactive protein) are of little help in the acute postoperative phase. If infection is diagnosed within 2 weeks of the onset of symptoms, a one-stage operation to debride the knee may be possible. Any delay in diagnosis or treatment should be managed by a two-stage procedure.

C. A traumatic episode may result in acute knee pain. Soft tissue disruption may involve the extensor mechanism or the collateral ligaments. Provided the knee is stable and the extensor mechanism is intact, nonoperative treatment may be appropriate. This includes bracing and physical therapy.

D. Soft tissue disruption resulting in an unstable knee requires repair. If the extensor mechanism is torn, appropriately repair the patella tendon or quadriceps tendon. The patient should wear a brace for several months to allow healing. Mobilization of the knee should be done under the supervision of a physical therapist.

E. Deep vein thrombosis after total knee replacement has been reported in up to 40% of patients in the early postoperative phase. Presence of the thrombosis either below, at, or above the knee should be confirmed by B-mode ultrasound or venogram. Treatment consists of appropriate anticoagulation and when necessary, an elastic support of the limb.

F. Chronic pain following total knee replacement may have several causes. A careful history and physical may provide sufficient information to exclude infection or a soft tissue problem, such as instability related to muscle or ligaments. Symptoms of pain with activity suggest mechanical loosening, whereas pain at rest may indicate chronic infection. Special investigations include blood tests and evaluation of the sedimentation rate and C reactive protein. Technetium, Gallium, and Indium labeled white cell scans may be needed to diagnose infection. Evidence of loosening of the implants should be managed surgically.

G. Treat infection with a two-stage operation whereby the components are removed and the knee debrided at the initial procedure. Then place an antibiotic impregnated spacer and several weeks later place the new components. Treat mechanical loosening by standard revision.

H. Mechanical loosening of components requires revision surgery. If bone loss is not severe and the components can be easily removed, and revision components inserted, satisfactory results can be obtained. In some patients bone graft of the tibia and or femur may be necessary. Chronic subluxation of the patella is difficult to treat. Patella realignment may be done in selected patients. Patellectomy is of value if functional impairment is severe.

PAIN AFTER TOTAL KNEE REPLACEMENT

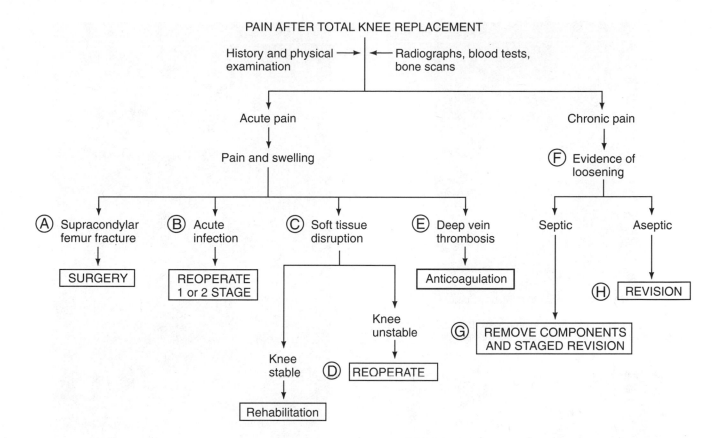

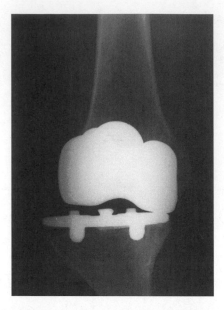

Figure 1 Radiograph showing loosening of the tibial component and loss of polyethylene thickness on the medial side.

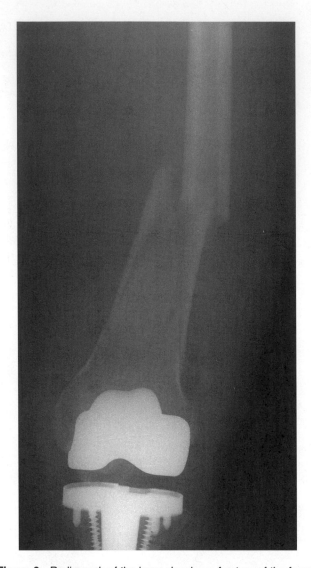

Figure 3 Radiograph of the knee showing a fracture of the femur proximal to the femoral component.

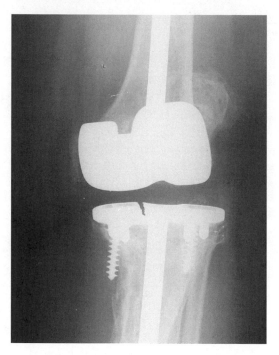

Figure 2 Radiographs of the left knee showing fracture of the tibial tray and deformity of the polyethylene.

References

Burger RR, Basch T, Hopson CN. Implant salvage in infected total knee arthroplasty. Clin Orthop 1991; 273:105.

DiGioia AM, Rubash HE. Periprosthetic fractures of the femur after total knee arthroplasty: A literature review and treatment algorithm. Clin Orthop 1991; 271:135.

Donley BG, Mathews LS, Kaufer H. Arthrodesis of the knee with an intramedullary nail. J Bone Joint Surg 1991; 73A:907.

Greene KA, Wilde AH, Stulberg BN. Preoperative nutritional status of total joint patients. J Arthroplasty 1991; 6:321.

Hodge WA. Prevention of deep vein thrombosis after total knee arthroplasty. Clin Orthop 1991; 271:101.

Leblanc J. Patellar complications in total knee arthroplasty. Orthop Review 1989; 18:296.

Pritchett JW, Mallin BA, Mathews AC. Knee arthrodesis with a tension-band plate. J Bone Joint Surg 1988; 70A:285.

Rand JA. Total knee arthroplasty. New York: Raven, 1993.

Rosenberg AG, Andriacchi TP, Barden R, Galante JO. Patellar component failure in cementless total knee arthroplasty. Clin Orthop 1988; 236:106.

Wilson MG, Kelley K, Thornhill TS. Infection as a complication of total knee replacement arthroplasty: Risk factors and treatment in sixty-seven cases. J Bone Joint Surg 1990;72A:878.

Windsor RE, Insall JN, Urs WK. Two-stage reimplantation for the salvage of total knee arthroplasty complicated by infection: Further follow-up and refinement of indications. J Bone Joint Surg 1990; 72A:272.

CHRONIC ANKLE PAIN

A. Post-traumatic arthrosis after ankle fractures may cause disabling pain and discomfort (Fig. 1). Loss of joint space is noted on radiographs and loss of ankle motion occurs as the joint deteriorates. Displacement of the talus by a few millimeters alters the joint congruity and loading leads to degenerative changes. Initial treatment is nonoperative and includes anti-inflammatory medication and ankle foot orthoses. A rocker bottom shoe helps reduce stress across the ankle joint during walking. Osteonecrosis of the body of the talus results in collapse of the dome and degenerative changes. Ankle motion may be limited and function severely impaired. Nonoperative treatment includes bracing and a rocker sole.

B. Persistent pain and failure to respond to nonoperative treatment is an indication for ankle arthrodesis. Several methods of stabilization are available, all using the principle of rigid fixation. Ankle fusion should be at neutral flexion, 5° of valgus, and 5° to 10° of external rotation. Posterior displacement of the talus under the tibia tends to produce a more normal gait pattern. Functionally, tibiotalar arthrodesis produces good long-term results.

C. Repeated ankle sprain with chronic lateral ligament disruption is a common cause of chronic ankle pain (Fig. 2). Radiographic stress views show significant talar tilt. Nonoperative treatment includes strengthening exercises, bracing, and anti-inflammatory medication. Physical therapy includes wobble board exercises, ice, and ultrasound to help reduce discomfort and increase strength around the ankle. Tendon subluxation or displacement of the peroneus brevis or longus may not respond to conservative treatment. A hinged ankle foot orthosis may be sufficient to reduce symptoms in these patients.

D. If symptoms persist, and instability of the ankle has not responded to nonoperative treatment, ligament reconstruction should be done. Repair of the anterior talo-fibular ligament and the calcaneo-fibular ligament with or without additional soft tissue augmentation may resolve the problem. Other types of ligament reconstruction use some or all of the peroneus brevis, peroneus longus, or fasciae latae.

E. Overuse syndrome is common in athletes. Tendinitis of tibialis anterior or tibialis posterior may occur as part of an overuse syndrome. Crepitus is noted along the course of the tendon and a localized swelling may be present. Peroneal tendinitis may occur in isolation or with chronic ankle instability. Achilles tendinitis is the most common form seen in athletes (Fig. 3). Initial treatment in all these situations is rest, ice, ultrasound, and anti-inflammatory medication. Splinting may be necessary as an initial treatment in severe cases.

F. Symptoms recalcitrant to nonoperative treatment may require surgical intervention. Tendon decompression or displacement may be indicated. Excise bony protuberances impinging on soft tissue.

G. Inflammatory diseases such as rheumatoid arthritis may cause bony and soft tissue problems. Radiographs show diffuse joint space narrowing with erosions on either side of the ankle joint. Swelling around the ankle may be present. Hemophilic arthropathy of the ankle occurs after repeated intra-articular bleeds and ultimately results in a painful ankylosis.

H. Joint involvement may result in significant functional impairment because of pain and discomfort and loss of motion. Ankylosis of the ankle is noted in patients with rheumatoid arthritis and hemophilia. Nonoperative treatment consists of bracing and use of rocker bottom shoes to reduce stress across the joint. Consider arthroscopy after all nonoperative treatments have failed. Indications for arthroscopy include synovitis, arthrofibrosis, loose bodies, and osteochondral lesions. Synovitis or soft tissue excision may be amenable to arthroscopic treatment.

I. Ankle fusion relieves pain and discomfort and obviates the need for a brace (Fig. 4). A rocker bottom shoe improves the patient's gait.

J. Soft tissue involvement usually results in deformity. Rupture of the tibialis posterior occurs commonly in rheumatoid arthritis if the associated tendinitis is not controlled. Pes planus and instability with pain and discomfort occur around the ankle. Nonoperative treatment includes anti-inflammatory medication and bruising.

K. Unstable deformity of the ankle with joint changes may require tibiotalar arthrodesis or subtalar fusion. In severe rheumatoid arthritis a pan-talar fusion may be indicated. Tendon reconstruction or transfer has a limited place and is indicated if deformity is correctable and the inflammation is well controlled medically. Manage painful pes planus resulting from a rupture of the tibialis posterior by triple arthrodesis.

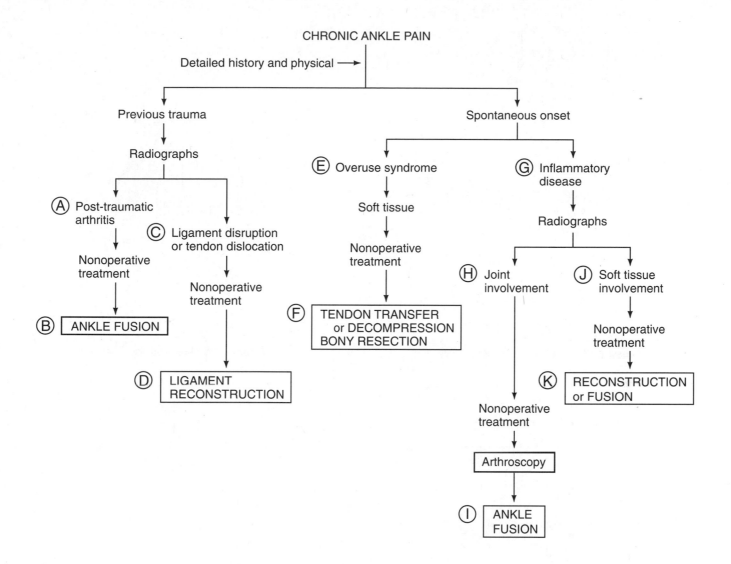

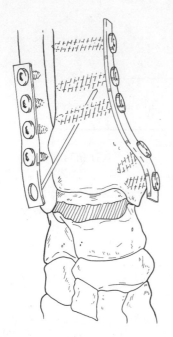

Figure 1   Traumatic arthrosis of the ankle.

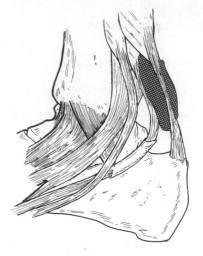

Figure 3   Achilles tendinitis.

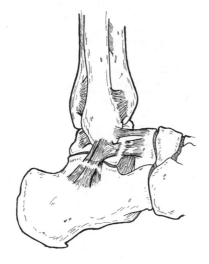

Figure 2   Disruption of the calcaneo-fibular ligament and talo-fibular ligament.

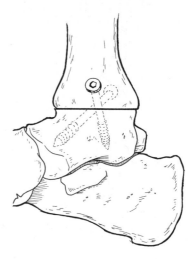

Figure 4   Ankle fusion using two oblique screws.

References

Buck P, Morrey BF, Chao EYS. The optimum position of arthrodesis of the ankle. J Bone Joint Surg 1987; 69A:1052.

Cass JR, Morrey BF, Katoh Y, et al. Ankle instability: Comparison of primary repair and delayed reconstruction after long term follow up study. Clin Orthop 1985; 198:110.

Ferkel RD, Scranton PE. Arthroscopy of the ankle and foot. J Bone Joint Surg 1993; 75A:1233.

Gamble JG, et al. Arthropathy of the ankle in haemophilia. J Bone Joint Surg 1991; 73A:1008.

Harrington KD. Degenerative arthritis of the ankle secondary to long-standing lateral ligament instability. J Bone Joint Surg 1979; 61A:354.

Kannus P, Renstrom P. Current Concepts review: treatment for acute tears of the lateral ligaments of the ankle. J Bone Joint Surg 1991: 73A:305.

Karlsson J, Bergsten T, Lansinger O, et al. Lateral instability of the ankle treated by the Evans procedure. J Bone Joint Surg 1988; 70B:476.

Lachiewicz PF, Inglis AE, Ranawat CS. Total ankle replacement in rheumatoid arthritis. J Bone Joint Surg 1984; 66A:340.

Moran CG, et al. Ankle arthrodesis in rheumatoid arthritis. Acta Orthop Scand 1991; 62:538.

Morrey BF, Wiedman GP. Complications and long-term results of ankle arthrodeses following trauma. J Bone Joint Surg 1980; 62A:777.

Sammarco GJ. Foot and ankle manual. Philadelphia: Lea and Febiger, 1991.

Snook GA, Chrisman OD, Wilson TC. Long term results of the Chrisman-Snook operation for reconstruction of the lateral ligaments of the ankle. J Bone Joint Surg 1985; 67A:1.

MEDIAL ARCH PAIN

A. The physical loading of high impact activities such as running in place increases forces on the foot and may cause medial arch pain at several different sites. Elicit a history to evaluate the chronicity of symptoms as well as the relationship of pain to activity and foot wear. Note any asymmetry or increase in foot deformity. Clinical evaluation should focus on the overall foot alignment as well as the localization of tenderness. Examine the foot with the patient both seated and standing. Inspection of the shoe for wear pattern and gait adds information about the dynamic forces imparted on the foot. Weight-bearing radiographs help assess alignment and may reveal degenerative changes to the talonavicular or subtalar joint as well as a tarsal coalition.

B. A recent increase in activity (e.g., in athletes, military recruits) may produce a stress fracture of the navicular, which is often missed. A bone scan or computed tomography (CT) helps to confirm the diagnosis. Healing after immobilization may occur, but results are often unpredictable. Open reduction and internal fixation (ORIF) is performed early.

C. Assess foot alignment and determine the location of the predominant deformity (Fig. 1). Forefoot abduction may be primary from breakdown at the midfoot, or may follow a hindfoot deformity.

D. The posterior tibial tendon (PTT) runs posterior to the medial malleolus as it inserts on the plantar surface of the navicular, cuneiforms, and bases of 2nd and 3rd metatarsals. Its function as an inverter of the hindfoot and dynamic stabilizer of the medial arch is opposed by the peroneus brevis. The tendon may become inflamed, attenuated, or may progress to a complete rupture. Clinical signs of PTT dysfunction include swelling and tenderness along the course of the tendon beginning just distal to the medial malleolus. Consider a seronegative inflammatory disease with younger patients or with multiple site involvement. A collapse of the medial longitudinal arch with hindfoot valgus and forefoot abduction is a late sign indicating failure of the PTT. Functional testing with a single stance heel raise is a sensitive indicator for PTT competence (Fig. 2). Anteroposterior radiographs may show divergence of the talocalcaneal angle, and lateral radiographs may reveal breakdown at the midfoot as the deformity progresses. A sag may occur at the talonavicular, naviculocuneiform, or tarsometatarsal (TMT) joints. Magnetic resonance imaging (MRI) may reveal inflammatory changes to the PTT. Nonsurgical treatment consists of rest and shoe wear modification for extremely mild cases, or a trial of immobilization in a walking cast. If symptoms persist, or if deformity is significant, surgical intervention is warranted. Surgical options are based on the degree of PTT insufficiency, which is graded as follows: Stage I—tenosynovitis; Stage II—attenuation or early disruption of the tendon with a passively correctable deformity; Stage III—progressive deformity that does not correct completely, with or without degenerative changes to the subtalar, or talonavicular joints. Debridement of the PTT is indicated with stage I. Stage II requires tendon transfers, such as flexor digitorum longus (FDL) to the navicular to help offset the unopposed pull of the peroneus brevis. Stage III deformities require a limited arthrodesis, or a triple arthrodesis for advanced arthrosis.

E. Tarsal tunnel syndrome is a compressive neuropathy of the posterior tibial nerve as it passes through a fibroosseous sheath posterior to the medial malleolus. It is characterized by dysesthesias along the plantar surface of the foot in the distribution of the medial and lateral plantar nerves, terminal branches of the posterior tibial nerve. Symptoms are worsened by activity and night pain is not uncommon. The etiology is most often idiopathic, however, it may be associated with inflammatory or post-traumatic conditions. Clinical findings include sensory changes, which are variable, and a positive Tinel's sign posterior to the medial malleolus. EMGs and nerve conduction studies may confirm the diagnosis. Treatment is initially conservative, consisting of nonsteroidal anti-inflammatory drugs (NSAIDs), orthotics, and activity modification. Surgical release is reserved for patients with persistent symptoms after a minimum of 6 months of treatment (Fig. 3).

F. Tarsal coalition is a source of recurrent ankle pain, but may also cause a rigid flatfoot with medial arch pain. Calcaneonavicular coalitions are followed by talocalcaneal bars in frequency and may be bilateral in 40%–60% of patients. Examination reveals markedly decreased subtalar motion. The presence of peroneal spasm is variable. A union spanning the calcaneus and navicular is best revealed by 45° oblique views, and axial (Harris) views demonstrate a bony bridge of the middle and posterior facets of the talocalcaneal joint. CT is indicated when clinical suspicion is high and radiographs fail to show a coalition. Initial treatment of mild symptoms include orthotics and activity modification. Attempt a trial of immobilization for 3 weeks in a short leg walking cast in patients with more significant symptoms. In the absence of degenerative changes, surgical treatment of a calcaneonavicular coalition includes resection of the bar with soft tissue interposition. When degenerative changes are present a triple arthrodesis is performed.

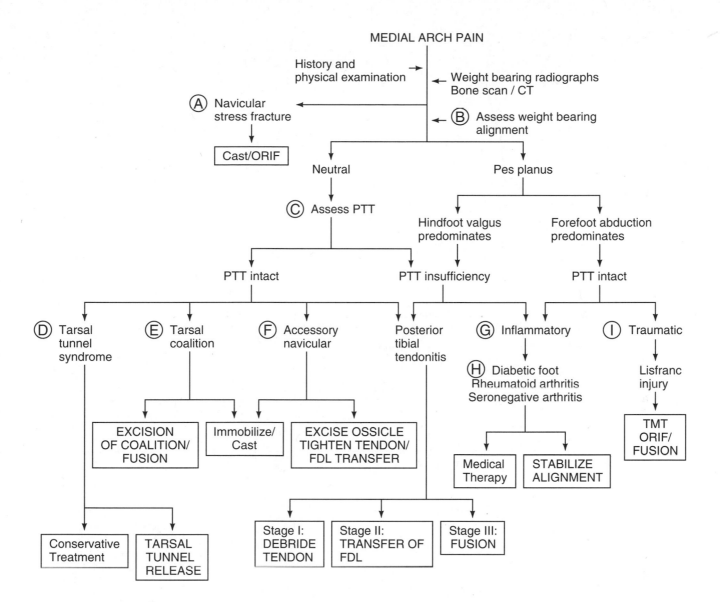

MEDIAL ARCH PAIN

History and physical examination → ← Weight bearing radiographs Bone scan / CT

(A) Navicular stress fracture

← (B) Assess weight bearing alignment

Cast/ORIF

Neutral

Pes planus

(C) Assess PTT

Hindfoot valgus predominates

Forefoot abduction predominates

PTT intact

PTT insufficiency

PTT intact

(D) Tarsal tunnel syndrome

(E) Tarsal coalition

(F) Accessory navicular

Posterior tibial tendonitis

(G) Inflammatory

(I) Traumatic

(H) Diabetic foot Rheumatoid arthritis Seronegative arthritis

Lisfranc injury

EXCISION OF COALITION/ FUSION

Immobilize/ Cast

EXCISE OSSICLE TIGHTEN TENDON/ FDL TRANSFER

Medical Therapy

STABILIZE ALIGNMENT

TMT ORIF/ FUSION

Conservative Treatment

TARSAL TUNNEL RELEASE

Stage I: DEBRIDE TENDON

Stage II: TRANSFER OF FDL

Stage III: FUSION

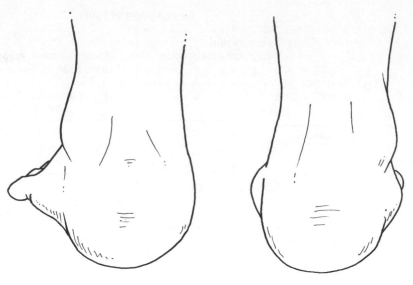

Figure 1 The "too many toes" sign is seen in the posterior tibial tendon deficient foot from the posterior view. This represents forefoot abduction, which is seen in conjunction with hindfoot valgus.

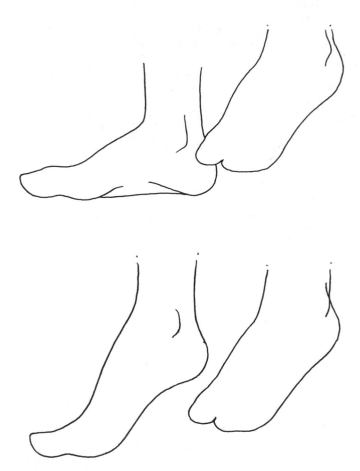

Figure 2 The patient with posterior tibial tendon deficiency is unable to perform a single stance heel rise on the affected foot. With a partial deficiency the heel rises to a lesser degree and does not invert.

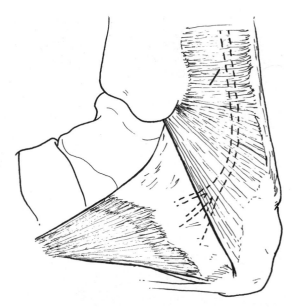

Figure 3 Tarsal tunnel release includes flexor retinaculum and abductor hallucis fascia.

G. Patients with an accessory navicular may complain of medial arch pain as well as bony prominence and difficulty with shoe fit. Perform a careful evaluation to confirm the accessory navicular is the true cause of symptoms. Radiographs may reveal an accessory navicular or a navicular beak. Conservative treatment, including shoe wear and activity modification and casting, is attempted initially. Surgical treatment, initially described by Kidner, consists of excising the ossicle and advancing the PTT, repairing it to the undersurface of the navicular. When PTT insufficiency is present, an FDL transfer is considered.

H. An inflammatory arthropathy due to rheumatoid or a seronegative arthritis, as well as diabetes mellitus affects the entire foot. The diabetic foot often presents with midfoot collapse and destruction, with or without hindfoot valgus or forefoot abduction (see p 184). Foot involvement is eventually present in 90% of patients with rheumatoid arthritis. Changes to the midfoot include pes planus as a result of ligamentous laxity of the longitudinal arch and accommodative changes to hindfoot deformity. Treatment is initially conservative with optimization of medical management and accommodative footwear such as an extra depth shoe with Plastizote inserts or orthotics to help contain the foot. Surgical reconstructive procedures are performed for pain relief and correction of deformity and instability. Options include a selective arthrodesis of the hindfoot, a triple arthrodesis, or a pantalar fusion.

I. Frank dislocation and fracture dislocations of the TMT joint are usually obvious, high-energy injuries associated with multiple trauma. A more subtle injury to the Lisfranc joint is often missed initially and given the diagnosis of a "foot sprain" in the emergency department. Initial injury is usually associated with severe midfoot pain and swelling and inability to bear weight. Later, patients present with persistent medial arch pain as well as tenderness over the TMT joints. Abduction of the forefoot elicits pain and decreased resistance. Radiographic findings include associated avulsion fractures, displacement of the metatarsals, a discontinuity between the medial borders of the second metatarsal and middle cuneiform, or between the medial borders of the fourth metatarsal and cuboid. Initial treatment of the acute and delayed Lisfranc injury includes anatomic reduction with rigid screw fixation, with subsequent removal after 3 months. In late cases when degenerative changes are present, fusion of the 1st, 2nd, and 3rd TMT joints is performed.

References

Cimino WR. Tarsal tunnel syndrome: Review of the literature. Foot Ankle 1990; 11:47.

Cowell HR, Elener V. Rigid painful flatfoot secondary to tarsal coalition. Clin Orthop 1983; 177:54.

Fitch KD, Blackwell JB, Gilmour WN. Operation for nonunion of stress fracture of the tarsal navicular. J Bone Joint Surg 1989; 71B:105.

Funk DA, Cass JR, Johnson KA. Acquired adult flat foot secondary to posterior tibial-tendon pathology. J Bone Joint Surg 1986; 68A:95.

Gonzalez P, Kumar SJ: Calcaneonavicular coalition treated by resection and interposition of the extensor digitorum brevis muscle. J Bone Joint Surg 1990; 72A:71.

Inglis G, Buxton RA, Macnicol MF. Symptomatic calcaneonavicular bars. J Bone Joint Surg 1986; 68B:128.

Johnson KA. Tibialis posterior tendon rupture. Clin Orthop 1983; 177:140.

Mann RA, Thompson FM. Rupture of the posterior tibial tendon causing flat foot. J Bone Joint Surg 1985; 67A:556.

McClain III EJ, Gruwn GA, Hansen ST. Fracture-Dislocation of the Tarsometatarsal Joint. Perspect Orthop Surg 1991; 2:35.

Myerson M. The diagnosis and treatment of injuries to the Lisfranc joint complex. Orthop Clin North America 1989; 20:655.

Myerson M, Solomon G, Shereff M. Posterior tibial tendon dysfunction: Its association with seronegative inflammatory disease. Foot Ankle 1989; 9:219.

Ray S, Goldberg VM. Surgical treatment of the accessory navicular. Clin Orthop 1983; 177, 61.

Torg JS, Pavlov H, et al. Stress fractures of the tarsal navicular. J Bone Joint Surg 1982; 64A:700.

HEEL PAIN

Heel pain is a common complaint with numerous etiologies (Fig. 1). Localization of the pain is often the key to diagnosis. Initial evaluation should include examination of the entire lower extremity. Observe the overall foot type and gait, and obtain weight-bearing radiographs, with attention to the lateral view. An axial or Harris view may also be helpful. Obtain a technetium-99 bone scan when a stress fracture is suspected in light of normal radiographs or when localization is difficult. Consider systemic causes of heel pain such as rheumatoid arthritis and the seronegative arthropathies when symptoms are bilateral or other joints are involved.

A. Pain is most often on the plantar surface, and localization along the plantar surface helps in diagnosis. Plantar fasciitis presents with pain that is localized to the medial tuberosity of the os calcis where the plantar aponeurosis originates. The onset is usually insidious and symptoms tend to be worse with the first steps taken in the morning, or after a period of rest. Pain tends to subside with gradual walking, however, it may worsen with prolonged activity. A flexible planus foot places the plantar fascia under increased stress, and a sudden increase in activity may also contribute to the onset of symptoms. An acute onset may indicate a complete or partial rupture of the plantar fascia. A bone spur seen on a lateral radiograph arises from the attachment of the flexor digitorum brevis, and is not the source of pain. Initial treatment is conservative, consisting of modification of activity, Achilles tendon stretching, nonsteroidal anti-inflammatory drugs (NSAIDs), and heel cups. Orthotics may be helpful in those with pes planus to help control the medial arch, reducing stretch or tensile stress over the plantar fascia. Injection with a local corticosteroid produces a variable amount of relief. Surgical release is considered for patients who have at least 12 months of symptoms that are refractory to conservative therapy.

B. Compression neuropathy at various sites may cause subcalcaneal pain. Typically the pain is neuritic, with radiation proximal or distally. Findings of tarsal tunnel syndrome include lack of localized tenderness over the medial aspect of the heel, and a positive Tinel's sign posterior to the medial malleolus. Entrapment of the medial calcaneal nerve may also cause heel pain. Baxter and others have proposed that the nerve to abductor digiti quinti (ADQ), the first branch of the lateral plantar nerve, is a common etiology for heel pain. It is important to realize that the local inflammation from a plantar fasciitis may cause compression of the nerve with both processes being responsible for the pain. EMG and nerve conduction studies may assist in localization of compression and may document a double crush syndrome. Treatment is initially conservative and is similar to treatment for plantar fasciitis. Surgical decompression is reserved for patients who have not responded after a minimum of 6–12 months.

C. Inflammatory arthritis may also be a source of heel pain. Reiter's syndrome typically produces an inflammatory response posteriorly at the insertion of the Achilles. Radiographic findings include spur formation as well as erosion (see p 176). Hindfoot involvement is frequently seen in rheumatoid arthritis. Heel pain from various sources is a cause for disability. Etiologies include an enthesopathy as described above in the seronegative arthropathies, as well as rheumatoid nodules over the heel pad and tarsal tunnel syndrome. Primary treatment is pharmacologic control of the inflammatory component as well as foot wear modification and orthotics to help cushion and control the hind foot.

D. Localized pain and tenderness present centrally over the os calcis indicates intrinsic heel pad pathology. Heel pad atrophy is seen in rheumatoid arthritis and advanced age. Treatment includes use of heel cups to cushion the heel. Any mass within the heel pad should be evaluated. Most tumors are benign and include lipomas, fibromas, and vascular tumors. Magnetic resonance imaging (MRI) is helpful to evaluate the extent of the mass. Biopsy is performed to confirm the diagnosis. Symptomatic masses are excised.

E. Haglund's deformity or retrocalcaneal bursitis is a source of posterosuperior heel pain. Its etiology and treatment are discussed on p 176. Localized pain in the region of the retrocalcaneal bursa typically worsens with increased activity and with rigid shoes that increase local irritation. A swollen bursa may be palpable. Radiographs reveal an increased pitch to the calcaneus. Conservative treatment includes padding or modifying the heel counter, heel lifts, Achilles stretching, NSAIDs, and activity modification. Steroid injections may cause tendon rupture and should be avoided. Surgical management involves excising the offending tubercle, but if the prominence is located at the tendo Achilles insertion choices include a collapsing wedge osteotomy or a direct trans-Achilles approach with excision of the prominence.

F. Posterior heel pain may also be due to impingement of an os trigonum or an enlarged posterior talar process. An os trigonum may also fracture and a fibrous union may lead to chronic symptoms. Tenderness is localized to the os trigonum and pain with motion of the flexor hallucis longus may be present. Pain is elicited by passively plantarflexing the foot, reproducing the impingement (Fig. 2). Lateral radiographs reveal an os trigonum. A bone scan reveals whether the os trigonum is inflamed. Surgical excision with exploration of the flexor hallucis longus tendon should be reserved for cases that are refractory to conservative management.

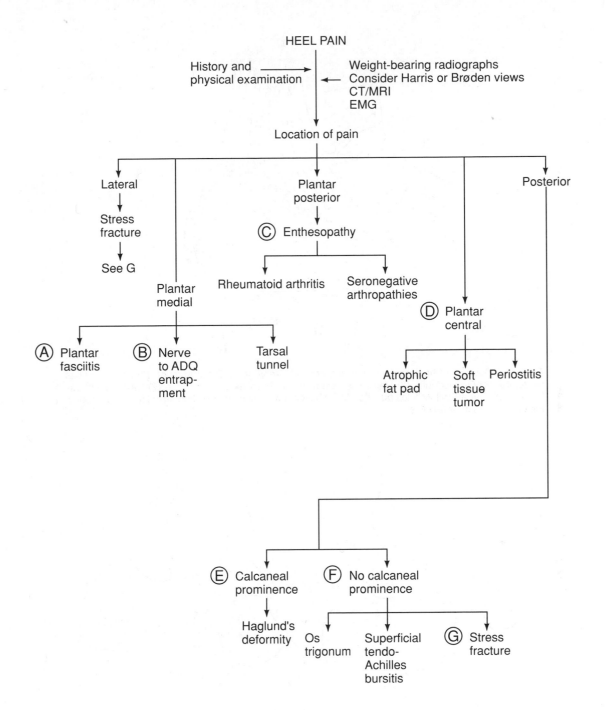

HEEL PAIN

History and
physical examination → ← Weight-bearing radiographs
Consider Harris or Brøden views
CT/MRI
EMG

Location of pain

Lateral

Stress
fracture

See G

Plantar
medial

(A) Plantar
fasciitis

(B) Nerve
to ADQ
entrap-
ment

Tarsal
tunnel

Plantar
posterior

(C) Enthesopathy

Rheumatoid arthritis

Seronegative
arthropathies

(D) Plantar
central

Atrophic
fat pad

Soft
tissue
tumor

Periostitis

Posterior

(E) Calcaneal
prominence

Haglund's
deformity

(F) No calcaneal
prominence

Os
trigonum

Superficial
tendo-
Achilles
bursitis

(G) Stress
fracture

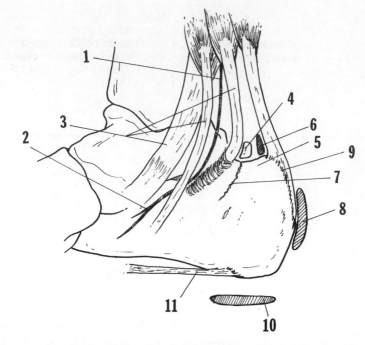

Figure 1 Sources of heel pain. (1) Tarsal tunnel. (2) Nerve to ADQ entrapment. (3) Posterior tibial tendonitis. (4) Os trigonum. (5) Haglund's deformity. (6) Retrocalcaneal bursitis. (7) Calcaneal stress fracture. (8) Superficial Achilles bursitis. (9) Enthesopathy at Achilles insertion. (10) Heel pad atrophy/ tumors. (11) Plantar fasciitis.

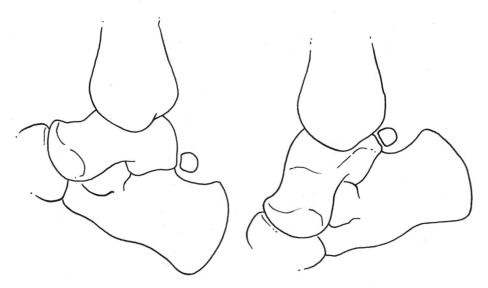

Figure 2 The posterior impingement test for a symptomatic os trigonum is performed by plantarflexing the ankle and pushing up on the heel.

G. Stress fractures are a source of heel pain and present with posterior or lateral pain. They typically do not cause pain on the plantar surface. A lateral radiograph and a Harris view may reveal the stress fracture. A bone scan is helpful to confirm the diagnosis when radiographs are normal. Treatment includes rest, which varies from activity modification to immobilization in a short leg walking cast.

References

Baxter D, Pfeffer G, Thigpen M. Chronic heel pain: Treatment rationale. Orthop Clin North Am 1989; 20:563.

Baxter D, Thigpen M. Heel pain—Operative results. Foot Ankle 1984; 5:16.

Bordelon L. Subcalcanel pain: A method of evaluation and plan for treatment. Clin Orthop 1983; 177:49.

Chand Y, Johnson K. Foot and ankle manifestations of Reiters syndrome. Foot Ankle 1980; 1:167.

Graham C. Painful heel syndrome: Rationale of diagnosis and treatment. Foot Ankle 1983; 3:261.

Heneghan J, Pavlov H. The Haglund painful heel syndrome. Experimental investigation of cause and therapeutic implications, Clin Orthop 1984; 187:228.

Leach R, DiIorio E, Harney R. Pathologic hindfoot conditions in the athlete. Clin Orthop 1983; 177:116.

Quirk R. In: Myerson, M, ed. Current Therapy in Foot and Ankle Surgery. St. Louis: Mosby-Year Book, 1993.

Radin E. Tarsal tunnel syndrome. Clin Orthop 1983; 181:167.

Schon L, Glennon T, Baxter D. Heel pain syndrome: Electrodiagnostic support for nerve entrapment. Foot Ankle 1993; 14:129.

ACHILLES TENDINITIS

There are several potential sites of pain about the Achilles tendon insertion. The history and physical examination should focus on chronicity of symptoms, the specific location of pain, and the relationship of the pain to activity and shoewear. Radiographs of the ankle and hindfoot are obtained routinely. Consider an inflammatory work up in cases with bilateral involvement, rest pain, or erosive changes to the posterior os calcis on radiographs.

A. The location of pain and tenderness is a guide to diagnosis. Tenderness is appreciated in one of three distinct locations (Fig. 1). An enthesopathy and retrocalcaneal bursitis occur distally at the insertion. Inflammation of the Achilles tendon and its sheath occurs at the relatively avascular region from 2–6 cm proximal to the insertion. The musculotendinous junction is a common site for strains and partial ruptures.

B. Enthesopathy at the Achilles tendon insertion is a common presentation of the seronegative inflammatory disorders such as Reiter's syndrome, psoriatic arthritis, and ankylosing spondylitis. Those affected are generally younger adults, who have a history of a previous enthesopathy, an inflammatory process in multiple locations, and a family history of psoriasis or other inflammatory disorder. Lateral radiographs of the calcaneus reveal erosive changes at the bone-tendon junction. Treatment includes medical management with nonsteroidal anti-inflammatory drugs (NSAIDs) or other appropriate "second line" medications such as gold compounds, antimalarials, or methotrexate. Temporary splinting or use of orthotics may provide symptomatic relief. Local steroid injection predisposes the tendo Achilles to rupture, and should be avoided.

C. Retrocalcaneal bursitis, a source of posterosuperior heel pain, is a result of inflammation in the subfascial bursa. It is found deep and anterior to the Achilles insertion and can occur in conjunction with Achilles tendon inflammation. Initial treatment is nonoperative, and most patients show improvement within 6 months. Surgical treatment is reserved for rare refractory cases and includes relieving the superoposterior prominence of the os calcis, and excising the inflamed bursa. The bony prominence is aggressively osteotomized, noting that the Achilles tendon inserts not superiorly, but in the middle one third of the tuberosity of the os calcis. Occasionally, the prominence is posterior to the insertion site. A dorsally-based closing wedge osteotomy collapses the prominence anteriorly (Fig. 2).

D. A spectrum of pathology is seen in the patient with subacute or chronic pain to the Achilles tendon. The tendo Achilles is surrounded by a peritenon, not by a true synovial sheath, giving rise to the classification as noted by Puddu et al. They may represent a continuum of the same inflammatory process; however, peritendinitis may occur independently of tendino-

sis, likewise with an isolated tendinosis without inflammation of the peritenon. A ruptured Achilles tendon may or may not have preceding symptoms or findings of degeneration. There is some overlap in the clinical presentation. Magnetic resonance imaging (MRI) is helpful in determining the presence of degenerative or inflammatory changes within the Achilles tendon.

E. Peritendinitis presents with significant pain and swelling over the distal Achilles tendon. This occurs subacutely or insidiously most often in runners. Examination reveals a warm, tender, swollen, and boggy Achilles. An MRI obtained for persistent symptoms shows an inflammation surrounding the Achilles, without degenerative changes to the tendon. Initial treatment is nonoperative and includes a period of relative rest in athletes. NSAIDs tend to be less effective, which is attributable to the lack of a true tenosynovium. Surgical exploration and debridement of the inflamed peritenon is reserved for refractory cases.

F. The presence of tendinosis along with peritendinitis may be difficult to detect by examination when there is significant inflammation. However, one may appreciate thickening or nodules within the tendon. The initial treatment is as outlined for peritendinitis. Degenerative changes, such as a yellowish coloration, thickening, or nodules, are found upon exploration. Surgical treatment includes excision of the peritenon and debridement of the involved tendon, using vertical incisions. This prevents weakening of the tendon and allows for proliferation of new vessels, promoting healing.

G. Tendinosis is a source of a low grade discomfort and tightness to the Achilles and can be seen without inflammation of the peritenon. Chronic inflammatory changes and partial tears are seen, and may be considered a precursor to rupture. Exploration and debridement of involved tendon is performed when symptoms persist despite conservative therapy.

H. Complete rupture of the Achilles tendon occurs acutely with forced dorsiflexion of the ankle. Some patients note antecedent symptoms of Achilles tendon pathology. Clinically, there is acute pain and inability to ambulate without assistance. Upon examination, there is a palpable gap in the avascular zone, with variable tenderness. Weak active plantarflexion is possible with tendons of the deep posterior compartment. However, there is little or no plantarflexion upon squeezing the calf. Hyperdorsiflexion of the ankle is also appreciated (Fig. 3). Treatment of the young, active patient consists of primary repair of the Achilles tendon. There are several techniques, including augmentation with the plantaris tendon, or a gastrocnemius fascial turndown. In the less active adult, or an incomplete tear, treatment includes a gravity equinus cast initially, gradually bringing the foot to neutral. Some studies report an increased recurrence

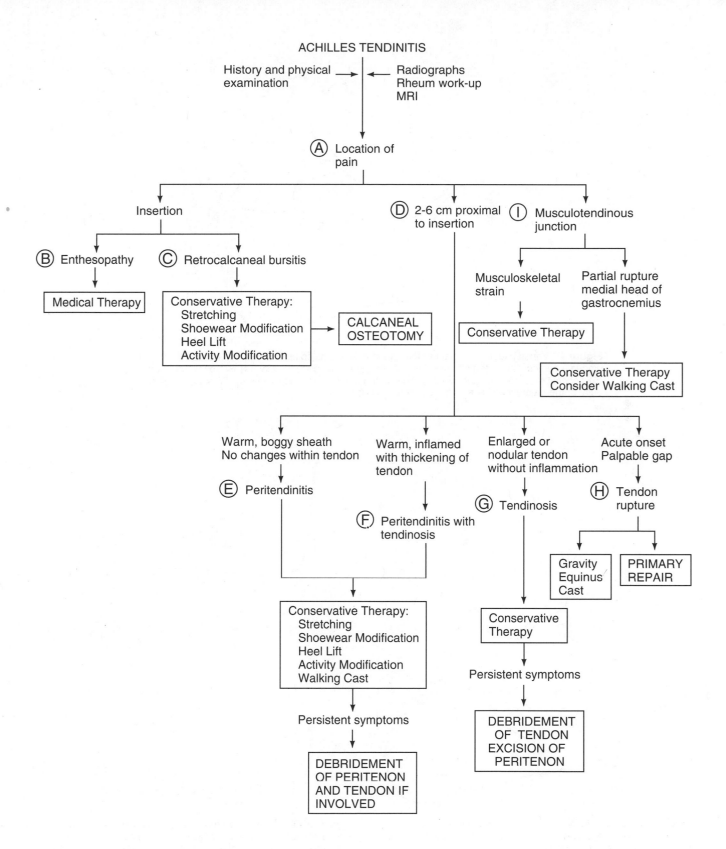

ACHILLES TENDINITIS

History and physical examination → ← Radiographs / Rheum work-up / MRI

(A) Location of pain

Insertion

(B) Enthesopathy

Medical Therapy

(C) Retrocalcaneal bursitis

Conservative Therapy:
Stretching
Shoewear Modification
Heel Lift
Activity Modification
→ CALCANEAL OSTEOTOMY

(D) 2-6 cm proximal to insertion

(I) Musculotendinous junction

Musculoskeletal strain

Conservative Therapy

Partial rupture medial head of gastrocnemius

Conservative Therapy
Consider Walking Cast

Warm, boggy sheath
No changes within tendon

(E) Peritendinitis

Warm, inflamed with thickening of tendon

(F) Peritendinitis with tendinosis

Enlarged or nodular tendon without inflammation

(G) Tendinosis

Acute onset
Palpable gap

(H) Tendon rupture

Gravity Equinus Cast

PRIMARY REPAIR

Conservative Therapy:
Stretching
Shoewear Modification
Heel Lift
Activity Modification
Walking Cast

Persistent symptoms

DEBRIDEMENT OF PERITENON AND TENDON IF INVOLVED

Conservative Therapy

Persistent symptoms

DEBRIDEMENT OF TENDON EXCISION OF PERITENON

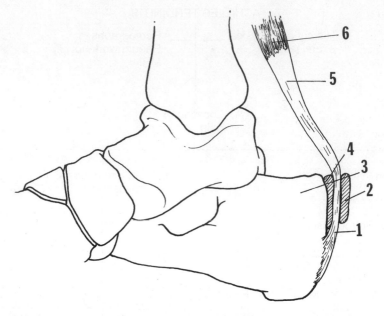

Figure 1 Various sources of pain in the region of the Achilles tendon. (1) Enthesopathy at the tendinous insertion. (2) Superficial Achilles bursitis. (3) Haglund's deformity. (4) Retrocalcaneal bursitis. (5) Tendinitis, tendinosis, and rupture occur at the relative avascular zone. (6) Rupture of the medial belly of the gastrocnemius at the musculotendinous junction.

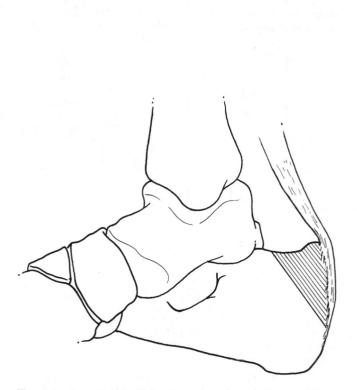

Figure 2 An osteotomy of the posterosuperior prominence of Haglund's deformity is reserved for refractory cases. An aggressive osteotomy is performed to prevent recurrence.

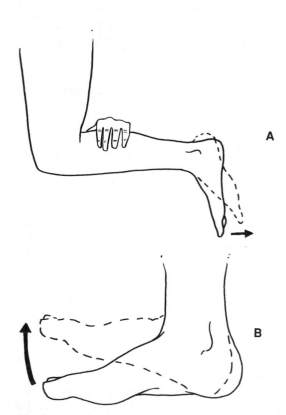

Figure 3 A, Signs of Achilles tendon competency include the Thompson test. Passive plantarflexion should be symmetric with the unaffected leg when the gastrocnemius muscle is squeezed. **B,** Hyperdorsiflexion of the foot is a sign of Achilles tendon rupture.

rate with conservative treatment, but this is offset by the decreased risk of skin slough and infection seen with surgical treatment.

I. A partial tear of the medial head of the gastrocnemius occurs at the musculotendinous junction. It is seen in the adult athlete, who may give a history of prodromal symptoms. Clinically a tearing sensation is noted posteriorly during forced dorsiflexion of the ankle with a near fully extended knee. There is an immediate onset of pain. Some are unable to ambulate without assistance. The medial calf is tender and swollen but the Achilles mechanism is intact. Treatment is nonoperative, ranging from rest, ice, NSAIDs, and a heel lift to brief immobilization with a short leg walking cast. This is followed by a program of stretching and strengthening both Achilles, since bilateral involvement is not uncommon. The diagnosis of plantaris tendon rupture, a popular label for acute medial calf pain, is based more on anecdotes than established fact, and has not been clearly established.

References

Beskin J, Sanders R, et al. Surgical repair of Achilles tendon ruptures. Am J Sports Med 1987; 15:1.

Fox J, Blazina M, et al. Degeneration and rupture of the Achilles tendon. CORR 1975; 107:221.

Gould N, Korson R. Stenosing tenosynovitis of the pseudosheath of the tendo Achilles. Foot Ankle 1980; 1:179.

Inglis A, Scott W, et al. Ruptures of the tendo Achilles. J Bone Joint Surg 1976; 58A:990.

Leach R, James S, Wasilewski S. Achilles tendinitis. Am J Sports Med 1981; 9:94.

Miller W. Rupture of the musculotendinous juncture of the medial head of the gastrocnemius muscle. Am J Sports Med 1977; 5:191.

Myerson M, Solomon G, Shereff M. Posterior tibial tendon dysfunction: Its association with seronegative inflammatory disease. Foot Ankle 1989; 9:219.

Nistor LO. Surgical and non-surgical treatment of Achilles tendon rupture. J Bone Joint Surg 1981; 63A:394.

Plattner P, Mann R. Disorders of tendons, In: Mann RA, Coughlin MJ, eds. Surgery of the Foot and Ankle, 6th Ed. St. Louis: Mosby—Year Book, 1993.

Puddu G, Ippolito E, et al. A classification of Achilles tendon disease. Am J Sports Med 1976; 4:145.

Schepsis A, Leach R. Surgical management of Achilles tendinitis. Am J Sports Med 1987; 15:308.

Shields C, Redix L. Acute tears of the medial head of the gastrocnemius. Foot Ankle 1985; 5:186.

Weinstabl R, Stiskal M, et al. Classifying calcaneal tendon injury according to MRI findings. J Bone Joint Surg 1991; 73B:683.

METATARSALGIA

Metatarsalgia is pain related to the metatarsal heads and should be considered a symptom rather than a true disease entity. It is usually related to the distribution of weight across the metatarsal heads. However, the term is frequently used to describe generalized pain in the forefoot. Metatarsalgia should first be differentiated from other etiologies of generalized pain, then further narrowed before a treatment plan is implemented.

A. The initial assessment includes evaluation of the standing alignment of the foot, documenting any transfer lesions, and inspecting the shoe for abnormal wear patterns. Obtain weight bearing anteroposterior (AP), lateral, and oblique radiographs. The location and quality of pain determined from the history and physical direct one toward the proper diagnosis. Pain that is not localized to the metatarsal heads, not related to weight bearing or shoe wear and present at night suggests a nonmechanical etiology.

B. Pain radiating into the third and fourth toes suggests Morton's neuroma (Fig. 1). Conservative treatment with accommodative foot wear, metatarsal pads, and corticosteroid injection may be helpful, but excision is often necessary. Burning pain across the forefoot and plantar aspect of the foot suggests tarsal tunnel syndrome. Physical examination reveals plantar tenderness and a positive Tinel's sign. Distinguish between a plantar wart and keratosis (Fig. 2). When shaved, plantar warts are studded with small black dots.

C. The painful metatarsal head of the hallux may be further differentiated. A structural etiology from a relatively long or plantar flexed first ray may increase the relative weight bearing and may predispose to a painful first metatarsal head. Hallux rigidus also presents with limited motion at the metatarsophalangeal (MTP) joint, and radiographic changes that include flattening of the head and dorsal osteophytes. Conservative treatment such as modified shoe wear with a steel shank is used to limit MTP motion during toe off. Surgical options include dorsal cheilectomy (Fig. 3), arthrodesis, and arthroplasty. First MTP joint pain secondary to hallux valgus usually is medial, not plantar, and related to shoe wear. Owing to the dynamics of the deformity there tends to be less weight bearing on the first ray and more on the second metatarsal head, which may predispose to transfer keratoses.

D. For sesamoid pain obtain tangential sesamoid radiographs and bone scan. Symptoms may be due to degenerative joint disease (DJD) at the articulation between the sesamoid and metatarsal head. A prominent sesamoid may become symptomatic from increased weight bearing. The prominence is appreciated by exam with associated intractable plantar keratoses, and may be confirmed by radiographs. Other etiologies include avascular necrosis (AVN), traumatized bipartite sesamoid, and symptomatic fibrous union. Pressure under the sesamoid may be relieved by a steel shank in the shoe with a rocker bottom sole. Reserve partial or complete excision of one sesamoid for refractory cases. Excision of both sesamoids may create a cock-up deformity to the hallux and should be avoided.

E. Weight-bearing alignment is helpful in making the diagnosis when evaluating metatarsalgia of the lesser metatarsals. The location of a keratosis or transfer lesions should help to identify the source. The etiology is usually biomechanical, with changes in normal load bearing across the metatarsal heads. This may be developmental due to a shortened or hypermobile first ray or in the cavus foot as mentioned below. Iatrogenic causes are also common.

F. The changes seen in the rheumatoid foot, including cock-up toes and related metatarsal head prominence with distal migration of the plantar fat pad, may also be seen with other inflammatory arthropathies and may predispose to metatarsalgia. Treatment includes medical treatment of the underlying condition as well as accommodative shoe wear such as an extra depth shoe with a Plastizote insert. Surgical treatment may include isolated or multiple metatarsal head resection.

G. Freiberg's disease, or "infraction," is thought to be due to AVN of the metatarsal head, though some support a traumatic etiology. It most frequently occurs in adolescents and young adults, affecting the second metatarsal head. Clinically, pain and stiffness of the affected MTP joint are present. In addition, a warm, swollen joint is appreciated, suggestive of a synovitis. Radiographically, there may be a progression of findings, from no changes, to sclerosis, to late collapse with degenerative changes (Fig. 4). A bone scan demonstrates increased uptake at the metatarsal head. Magnetic resonance imaging (MRI) shows an increased signal on T2 weighted images.

Early treatment consists of accommodative shoe wear with a steel shank or other orthosis to relieve force over the metatarsal head; however, there is no evidence that this will halt disease progression. Surgical options include excision of the metatarsal head, Keller procedure of the base of the proximal phalanx, or a dorsiflexion osteotomy of the metatarsal neck.

H. A stress fracture, which is more common in the second and third metatarsals, may be present in those who have recently increased their activity, such as military recruits or athletes, but is also seen in those with metabolic disease. Radiographs may be negative early but later show signs of callus formation. A bone scan is helpful in providing an early diagnosis. Treatment includes reduction of activity, a rigid soled shoe, and, in certain causes, a short leg walking cast.

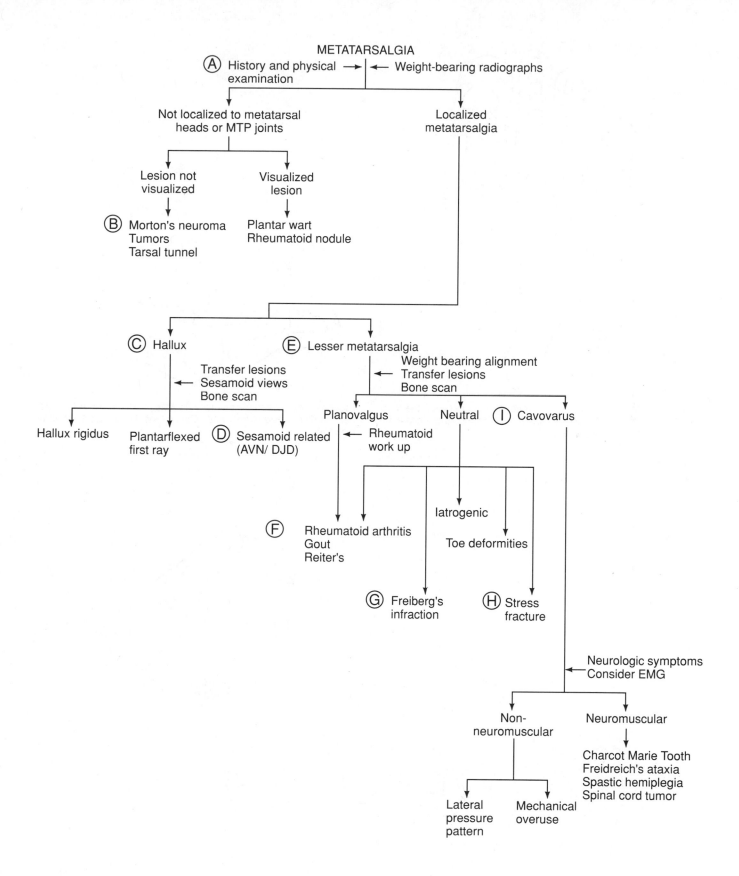

METATARSALGIA

Ⓐ History and physical examination → ← Weight-bearing radiographs

Not localized to metatarsal heads or MTP joints

Localized metatarsalgia

Lesion not visualized

Visualized lesion

Ⓑ Morton's neuroma
Tumors
Tarsal tunnel

Plantar wart
Rheumatoid nodule

Ⓒ Hallux

Ⓔ Lesser metatarsalgia

Transfer lesions
← Sesamoid views
Bone scan

Weight bearing alignment
← Transfer lesions
Bone scan

Hallux rigidus

Plantarflexed first ray

Ⓓ Sesamoid related (AVN/ DJD)

Planovalgus

Neutral

Ⓘ Cavovarus

← Rheumatoid work up

Iatrogenic

Toe deformities

Ⓕ Rheumatoid arthritis
Gout
Reiter's

Ⓖ Freiberg's infraction

Ⓗ Stress fracture

Neurologic symptoms
← Consider EMG

Non-neuromuscular

Neuromuscular

Lateral pressure pattern

Mechanical overuse

Charcot Marie Tooth
Freidreich's ataxia
Spastic hemiplegia
Spinal cord tumor

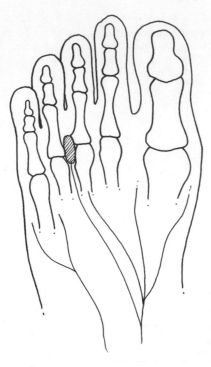

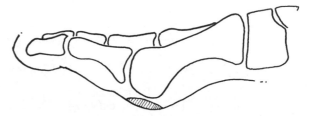

Figure 1 Morton's neuroma most often occurs between the third and fourth toes. Tenderness is localized to the webspace and a Tinel's sign is frequently present.

Figure 2 An intractable plantar keratosis results when the weight-bearing distribution is abnormal. Causes include a plantarflexed or long ray.

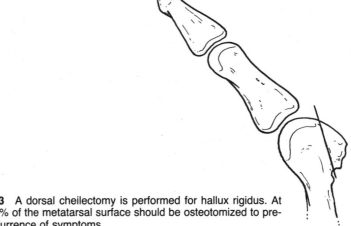

Figure 3 A dorsal cheilectomy is performed for hallux rigidus. At least 30% of the metatarsal surface should be osteotomized to prevent recurrence of symptoms.

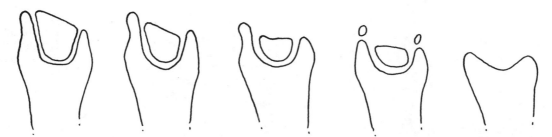

Figure 4 Smille's classification of Freiberg's infraction ranges from early fracture to advanced collapse and flattening.

I. A cavovarus deformity predisposes the foot to increased stresses over the metatarsal heads. The forces are concentrated laterally over the fifth ray and increase if hindfoot varus is progressive or rigid. The etiologies may be developmental, traumatic, or neuromuscular. A thorough neurologic evaluation should be performed on all patients with a cavus foot and a high index of suspicion should be maintained for either a peripheral or central neuropathy. A well-molded orthosis, which distributes the force throughout the foot, provides symptomatic relief. Stretching exercises may help keep the foot supple. For supple deformities that continue to be symptomatic, soft tissue procedures are performed. Bony procedures of the forefoot and hindfoot are reserved for rigid deformities and may be combined with soft tissue transfers to achieve a plantigrade foot.

DIABETIC FOOT

Diabetes is a progressive tissue perfusion disease that affects all organ systems. The feet are the most commonly affected end organ and a frequent source of morbidity. From 50% to 70% of lower extremity nontraumatic amputations occur in diabetics, most resulting from foot lesions.

Patient education and early recognition of lesions are the hallmark of diabetic foot treatment. Make the patient part of the treatment team early. Patients responsible for their care have improved continuity of care. Common problems complicating patient self-evaluation are peripheral vascular disease and neuropathy. The small vessel disease of diabetes is most likely related to altered basement membrane permeability, not to obstructive lesions of the microcirculation. Neuropathy causes lack of sweating leading to dry skin and callous formation, which can cause pressure points.

The initial work-up for the diabetic foot includes a history and physical examination, weight-bearing radiographs of the feet, laboratory tests, and a vascular evaluation. Loss of protective sensation is caused by neuropathy and measured using Semmes-Weinstein filaments. Selective nuclear medicine studies sometimes help in distinguishing between osteopathy and osteomyelitis.

A. The goal of treatment is the prevention of mal perforans and its sequelae. Malalignment and bony deformities such as hammer toe, bunions, pes cavus, and bunionettes make the foot susceptible to perforating ulcers. Treatment is accomplished primarily through patient education, behavior modification, and self-examination. Teach patients that they have a propensity to develop ulcers and are susceptible to thermal and penetrating injuries. Smoking increases their risk of developing foot lesions. Instruct them to wear properly fitted footwear, to trim nails properly, and to avoid temperature extremes. Train patients to look for keratoses and other pressure points.

B. Treat diabetic foot ulcers aggressively. Assess the healing potential with physical and vascular examinations. An arterial brachial index (ABI) indicates the severity of extremity ischemia. An ABI of at least 0.45 is needed for healing. Poor local tissue perfusion can be compounded by large vessel disease, which is correctable. Refer the patient to a vascular surgeon for correction of large vessel perfusion deficiencies. Ulcers often heal after bypass surgery. Follow Wagner's classification, which is based on extent of soft tissue and bone involvement, to make treatment decisions (Fig. 1). The goal of treating mal perforans of the diabetic foot is to heal the ulcer and to avoid recurrence.

C. In evaluating the hot swollen foot for infection, determine if a portal of entry exists. Typical portals of entry are ingrown toenails, nail punctures, maceration due to fungal infections, or mal perforans. A common dilemma is distinguishing between Charcot foot and infection. The decision is based on clinical judgment. Absence of systemic signs rules out infection.

D. Osteopathy progresses through three stages: inflammation, fragmentation, and consolidation. Inflammation is characterized by bony resorption and soft tissue edema. Fragmentation is characterized by destructive changes around joints leading to deformity. Consolidation is the resolution of the destructive process. The resulting foot shape and alignment are fixed. The goal of treatment is a plantar grade ambulatory foot that can be accommodated by footwear (Fig. 2).

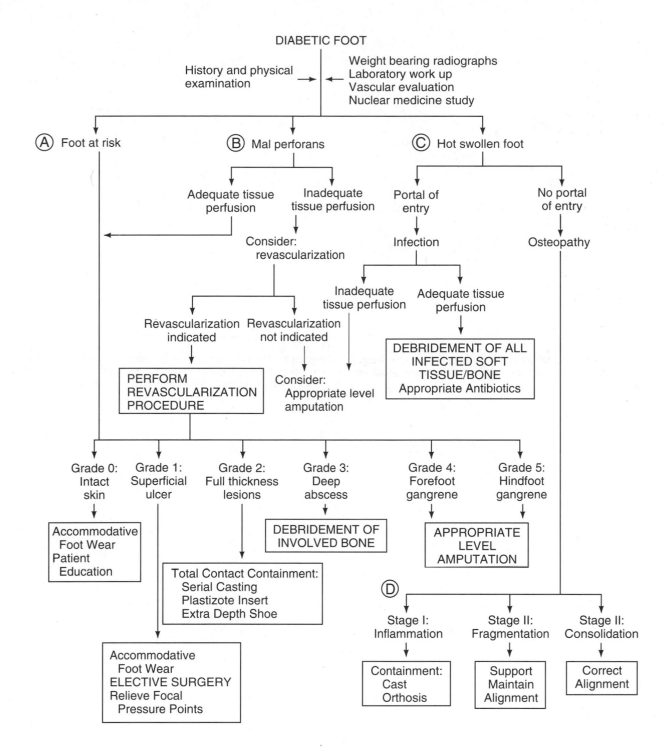

DIABETIC FOOT

History and physical examination → ← Weight bearing radiographs
Laboratory work up
Vascular evaluation
Nuclear medicine study

(A) Foot at risk

(B) Mal perforans

(C) Hot swollen foot

Adequate tissue perfusion

Inadequate tissue perfusion

Consider: revascularization

Portal of entry

No portal of entry

Infection

Osteopathy

Revascularization indicated

Revascularization not indicated

Inadequate tissue perfusion

Adequate tissue perfusion

PERFORM REVASCULARIZATION PROCEDURE

Consider: Appropriate level amputation

DEBRIDEMENT OF ALL INFECTED SOFT TISSUE/BONE
Appropriate Antibiotics

Grade 0: Intact skin

Grade 1: Superficial ulcer

Grade 2: Full thickness lesions

Grade 3: Deep abscess

Grade 4: Forefoot gangrene

Grade 5: Hindfoot gangrene

Accommodative Foot Wear
Patient Education

DEBRIDEMENT OF INVOLVED BONE

APPROPRIATE LEVEL AMPUTATION

Total Contact Containment:
Serial Casting
Plastizote Insert
Extra Depth Shoe

(D)

Accommodative Foot Wear
ELECTIVE SURGERY
Relieve Focal Pressure Points

Stage I: Inflammation

Stage II: Fragmentation

Stage II: Consolidation

Containment:
Cast
Orthosis

Support Maintain Alignment

Correct Alignment

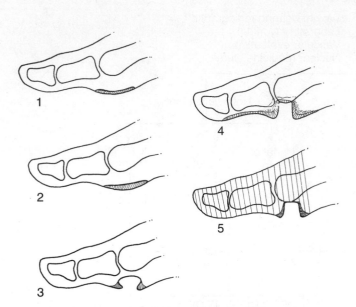

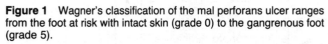

Figure 1 Wagner's classification of the mal perforans ulcer ranges from the foot at risk with intact skin (grade 0) to the gangrenous foot (grade 5).

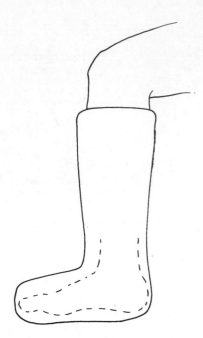

Figure 2 The total contact cast provides hydraulic containment of the foot and ankle. It is well padded at areas of prominence and extends distally to cover the metatarsal heads and toes.

References

Berquist TH. Radiology of the foot and ankle. New York: Raven Press, 1989:377.

LoGerfo FW, Coffman JD. Vascular and microvascular disease of the foot in diabetes. New Engl J Med 1984; 311:1615.

McDermott JE. The diabetic foot: Diagnosis and prevention. Instructor Course Lecture 1993; 42:117.

Wagner F, William MD. The diabetic foot: Orthopedics 1987; 10(1):163.

HALLUX VALGUS

Hallux valgus is a common disorder affecting the great toe. It is characterized by a progressive valgus deformity at the first metatarsophalangeal (MTP) joint, with increased varus at the first ray.

There are intrinsic, hereditary factors as well as extrinsic factors involved in the etiology of hallux valgus. Shoes are major contributors to the deformity and the symptoms associated with hallux valgus. Shoes worn by adults are frequently too small for the foot, and modification of shoewear is a major part of the initial treatment.

A. Initially, it is important to obtain a thorough assessment of the chief complaint as well as the patient's short- and long-term expectations. Many technically good postoperative results are seen in disappointed patients with unrealistic expectations, since it may take 6 months to achieve an end result. Physical examination is performed with the patient seated and standing. The overall orientation of the foot is assessed with the patient standing. Standing may reveal a worsening of the deformity, pes planus, as well as overlap with the second toe. A pronated foot, forefoot abduction, hindfoot valgus, and tightness of the Achilles tendon contribute to the hallux valgus deformity, and should be noted. With the patient seated, the motion of the MTP joint and the first metatarsal cuneiform joint is assessed. Standard anteroposterior (AP), lateral, and oblique weight-bearing radiographs are obtained. The degree and location of the surgical correction are planned based on the intermetatarsal (IM) angle (Fig. 1). The distal metatarsal articular angle (DMMA) and hallux valgus (HV) angle are measured and any signs of arthritis in the MTP joint evaluated.

B. Significant degenerative joint disease is uncommon in the patient with hallux valgus. More commonly it is associated with hallux rigidus.

The patient with advanced arthritis complains of stiffness and pain involving the MTP joint in addition to the characteristic pain over the medial eminence seen in hallux valgus. Range of motion is limited, especially in dorsiflexion. Radiographs reveal joint space narrowing, subchondral sclerosis, and osteophyte formation most prominent on the dorsal surface. A cheilectomy is performed when hallux rigidus predominates.

When advanced arthrosis is present in the patient with hallux valgus, arthrodesis of the MTP joint will correct the deformity, relieve pain, and preserve stability of the hallux during gait. A Keller arthroplasty, consisting of resection of the base of proximal phalanx and removal of the medial eminence is technically less demanding than fusion, requires a shorter recovery period, and relieves pain in the elderly patient. However, active plantarflexion of the hallux is greatly reduced, leaving the patient with an apropulsive gait; thus this procedure should not be considered in a younger, more active adult.

A standard bunionectomy will not relieve dorsal impingement pain and may further reduce motion in a joint that is already stiff. A Silastic implant is seldom used for hallux valgus today, because it may fail given the higher demands of an otherwise healthy patient, and may produce joint problems related to a silicone synovitis.

C. The management of the adolescent, adult, and physiologically older patient with hallux valgus differs. Compliance and recurrence are specific issues in the adolescent. In addition, many adolescents with hallux valgus are asymptomatic and have unrealistic expectations of treatment goals and outcome. The concerns of the parents as well as the patient need to be addressed.

In many adolescents, conservative treatment alleviates the symptoms. Shoewear modification with a widened toe box accommodates the forefoot. An orthotic insert is used in patients with a pronated foot.

Though the patient with a mild deformity may be treated nonoperatively, surgical treatment is indicated when the symptoms and deformity become more severe. Because there is a tendency to progress, a more aggressive surgical approach is warranted. There are numerous procedures described in the literature. The timing of surgery in the skeletally immature individual can be delayed until the physes are closed. Surgical complications include recurrence and nonunion. In the authors experience there is an increased incidence of wound problems in the adolescent bunion.

D. The adolescent with hallux valgus typically has an increased IM angle and in those with a more severe deformity, there is often an increased obliquity of the first metatarsal cuneiform joint. A modified Lapidus is performed on patients with a more severe deformity. When strict attention is paid to the position of the metatarsal and dorsiflexion is avoided, this procedure corrects the deformity, and recurrence is seen less often.

In patients with a lesser deformity, a proximal metatarsal osteotomy will reduce the IM angle and correct the deformity without excessive shortening. A chevron osteotomy, which is less technically demanding, has been performed on adolescents with a good subjective result (Fig. 2). Neither procedure addresses the increased obliquity and hypermobility as well as the Lapidus, contributing to a higher rate of recurrence.

E. The adult patient is assessed as described above. Initial treatment is conservative. Shoes with a wider toe box accommodate the medial prominence and alleviate symptoms in many cases. The goal of surgery is to achieve a foot that is comfortable in properly fitted shoes. Postoperatively, patients should be instructed that wearing of high heeled shoes with a narrow toe box postoperatively is not recommended and may contribute to recurrence of the problem. The patient who needs to wear narrower shoes for professional reasons should realize that it may be 3—6 months

HALLUX VALGUS

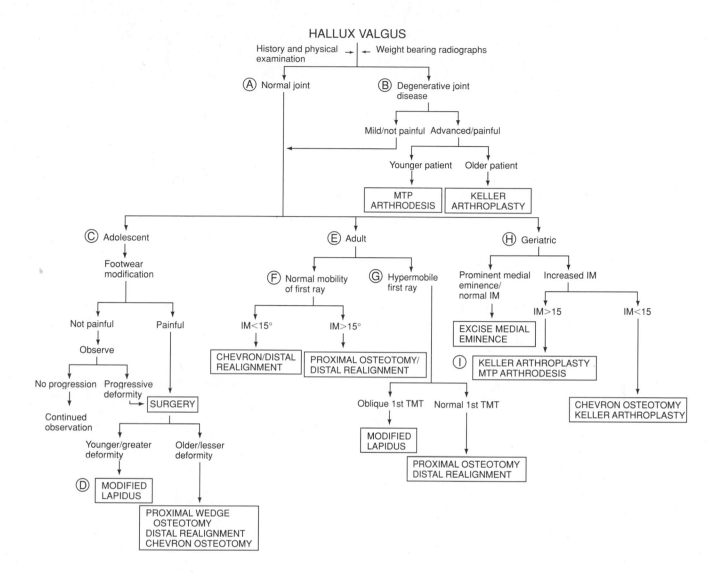

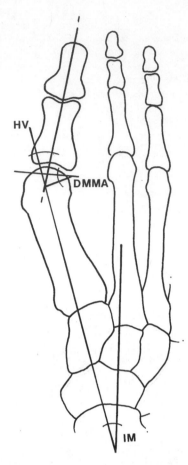

Figure 1 Angular measurements, which define the bunion deformity, are made on the AP weight-bearing radiographs. The first metatarsophalangeal or hallux valgus (HV) angle is less than 15°. The normal intermetatarsal (IM) angle measures less than 9°. DMMA = distal metatarsal articular angle.

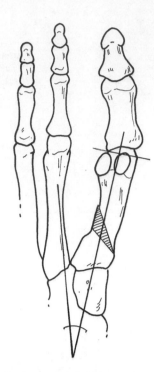

Figure 3 A proximal metatarsal osteotomy is combined with a distal soft tissue procedure to achieve greater correction of the increased IM angle.

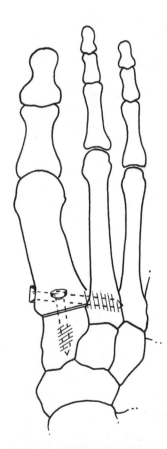

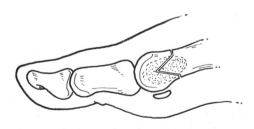

Figure 2 A chevron osteotomy is combined with soft tissue release. The metatarsal head is displaced laterally 30%-50% of the shaft width to achieve the appropriate correction.

Figure 4 A Lapidus or tarsometatarsal arthrodesis corrects both the IM angle and position of the metatarsal in saggital plane. The two screws provide compression and rotational stability of the fusion site.

postoperatively before fashionable shoes may be comfortably worn for brief periods.

F. Most patients have normal mobility of the first tarsometatarsal (TMT) joint and the selected procedure is based on the location and severity of the deformity. Patients with a lesser deformity typically have an IM angle <15°, and a chevron osteotomy of the distal metatarsal metaphysis and soft tissue realignment is performed. In patients with a greater deformity, correction may not be sufficient with a distal osteotomy. In these patients a proximal metatarsal osteotomy with distal soft tissue realignment is performed (Fig. 3).

G. A hypermobile first ray is seen in some young adults and adolescents with hallux valgus and is associated with a higher postoperative recurrence rate. The mobility of the first ray should be assessed. Criteria for hypermobility include greater dorsiflexion than plantar flexion of the first ray at the TMT joint as well as lack of a firm end point upon dorsiflexion. The presence of a transfer lesion beneath the second metatarsal head should also raise suspicion of a hypermobile first ray. Radiographs commonly reveal an increased IM angle with an obliquely oriented metatarsal cuneiform joint.

A proximal osteotomy combined with a distal soft tissue realignment is performed in patients when the first metatarsal cuneiform joint is <30°. When the first metatarsal cuneiform joint is more obliquely oriented, a modified Lapidus procedure provides the best chance to prevent recurrence (Fig. 4). This is a technically unforgiving procedure that requires precise positioning and rigid internal fixation of the metatarsal cuneiform joint to prevent a dorsiflexed first ray, and nonunion. The Akin procedure, a closing wedge osteotomy of the proximal phalanx, is performed when hallux valgus interphalangeus predominates.

H. The geriatric patient is defined as the physiologically older, sedentary patient with low physical demands. Specific concerns in this patient population includes vascular perfusion and skin problems. A vascular evaluation should be performed in patients with decreased peripheral pulses or physical signs of vascular insufficiency.

I. In the older patient with a normal IM angle and symptoms related to a prominent medial eminence, simple excision of the medial eminence can be performed if symptoms persist despite nonsurgical care with shoe wear modification and local padding. When hallux valgus is present, a chevron bunionectomy, arthrodesis, or Keller arthroplasty is performed based on the degree of the deformity and needs of the patient. A chevron bunionectomy performed on an older patient is associated with an increased prevalence of symptoms of joint stiffness. An arthrodesis performed on elderly patients provides symptomatic relief but is associated with a higher rate of nonunion and requires a longer period of postoperative immobilization. The Keller is less technically difficult and has a shorter recuperation period. However, it leaves the patient with a apropulsive gait.

References

Austin D, Leventen E. A new osteotomy for hallux valgus. Clin Orthop 1981; 157:25.

Frey C, Thompson F, et al. American orthopedic foot and ankle society women's shoe survey. Foot Ankle 1993; 14:78.

Geissele A, Stanton R.Surgical treatment of adolescent hallux valgus. J Pediat Orthop 1990; 10:642.

Johnson K, Cofield R, Morrey B. Chevron osteotomy for hallux valgus. Clin Orthop Rel Research 1979; 142:44.

Mann R. Decision-making in bunion surgery. Instructional course lectures. AAOS 1990; 39:3.

Mann R. The great toe. Orthop Clin North Am 1989; 20:519.

O'Doherty D, Lowrie P, Gregg P. The management of the painful first metatarsophalangeal joint in the older patient. J Bone Joint Surg 1990; 72B:839.

Richardson EG, Graves S, McClure JT, Boone RT. First metatarsal head-shaft angle: A method of determination. Foot Ankle 1993; 14:181.

Richardson EG. Keller resection arthroplasty. Orthopaedics 1990; 13:1049.

Sangeorzan B, Hansen S. Modified Lapidus procedure for hallux valgus. Foot Ankle 1989; 9:262.

Zimmer T, Johnson K, Klassen R. Treatment of hallux valgus in adolescents by the chevron osteotomy. Foot Ankle 1989; 9:190.

FOCAL BONE LESION

The evaluation of the patient presenting with a focal bone lesion can be problematic and present the clinician with diagnostic uncertainty. The evaluation should be orderly and methodical, including, in turn, the history, the physical examination, followed by pertinent and appropriate laboratory studies and, finally, directed imaging studies designed to provide the greatest information for the expense.

A. The history should include details as to how the lesion was discovered. Was it discovered accidentally in the course of radiographs taken for another reason? For example, is it a distal tibia non-ossifying fibroma noted incidentally on ankle x-ray films for ankle trauma or an incidental "hot" spot noted on technetium bone scan obtained for another reason? If the lesion was noted as the result of a directed examination, what were the initial complaints? Is pain present? If so, the nature of the pain, its duration, and variation in the pain are all important aspects of the history. A history of trauma may be of questionable association to the actual lesion, except that the regional trauma may draw attention to the pre-existing condition. Other medical conditions in the individual as well as family history are important in consideration of genetic or neoplastic factors.

Physical findings are important to determine local tenderness, swelling, mass, warmth, erythema, as well as any effect on range of motion of adjacent joints. Document any joint effusion. Perform and record evaluations of neurovascular function and regional lymphatic drainage. Perform a complete physical examination, especially in that population, typically over 40 years of age, who are at greatest risk for having their bone lesion be the initial manifestation of a cancer that has metastasized. This should include a thyroid examination, breast examination in women, and prostate examination in men.

Laboratory studies usually are of little value in the evaluation of patients with solitary bone lesions discovered accidentally and having a benign or latent appearance. They may be of greater value in the evaluation of patients who have symptomatic bone lesions. Complete blood count with erythrocyte sedimentation rate (ESR) may show anemia or elevated ESR seen in chronic disease such as neoplasia or infection. Serum chemistries can help differentiate metabolic from nonmetabolic conditions as well as give an idea of local bone metabolism. Laboratory studies on patients presenting with possible metastatic lesions should be directed at identifying the tissue of origin. Included in these studies are thyroid function studies, urinalysis, serum and urine immunoelectrophoresis, and prostate specific antigen.

B. Imaging studies should be appropriate, deliberate, and problem focused to provide essential information in a sequence that will have the greatest benefit in determining future imaging studies in a cost-appropriate fashion. Begin with high quality orthogonal radiographs that include the adjacent joint (Fig.1, A). The radiographs should be sufficient to judge cortical and endosteal involvement, periosteal reactions, subtle erosions, and soft tissue mineralizations. From the plain radiographs, decisions on further imaging studies will be based. "Benign" radiographic findings in asymptomatic patients may be observed for interval change on regular follow-ups. Symptomatic lesions or lesions with worrisome radiographs deserve further evaluation.

C. After plain radiographs have been obtained, nuclear medicine bone scan is the next appropriate study. The triple phase scan provides information about the vascularity of the lesion, venous pooling, metabolic activity, and an overall skeletal screen of the patient to assess for other asymptomatic lesions such as polyostotic conditions or metastases. Further imaging is dependent on clinical decisions made based on the bone scan.

D. Suspicious lesions on radiographs with abnormal bone scans should undergo either magnetic resonance imaging or computed tomography (CT), depending on whether the lesion is primarily cortical or endosteal and how much if any soft tissue is involved. Often both imaging studies are necessary to fully evaluate the process.

E. Based on the history and physical, plain radiographs, and bone scan, a preliminary differential diagnosis can be developed to direct further imaging. Chest radiograph, chest CT, and abdominal CT are useful in establishing the presence or absence of metastatic disease from a primary bone malignancy or in identifying the site of origin in the case of skeletal metastases.

F. Only after all imaging is complete is the biopsy performed, which may be open or closed depending on the previous information gained. Open biopsies are usually preferred for skeletal lesions in order to obtain adequate tissue for diagnosis as well as chromosomal analysis, which is becoming increasingly important. Always take cultures, and perform frozen section for adequacy of tissue.

G. Treatment decisions regarding surgery, chemotherapy, and radiation are made after establishing the diagnosis and stage (Fig. 1, B and C). Therapeutic decisions are best made in collaboration with medical and radiation oncology when malignancies are involved.

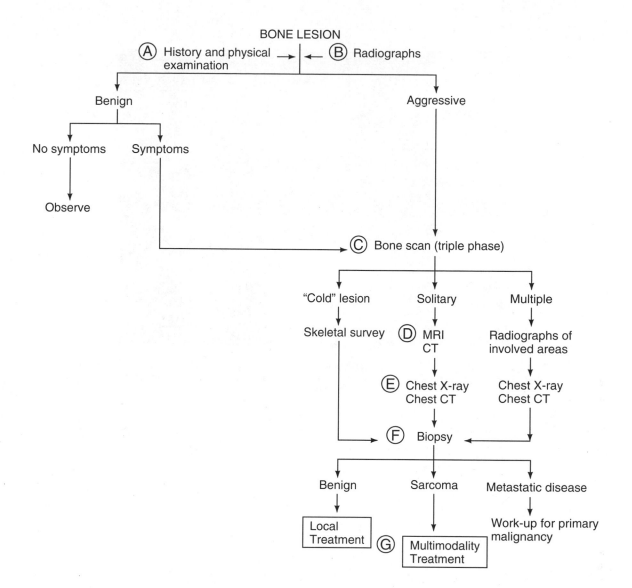

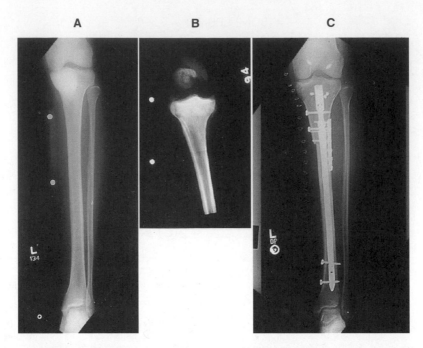

Figure 1 **A,** Radiograph showing a high-grade osteosarcoma of proximal tibia. **B,** Osteoarticular allograft. **C,** Postoperative radiograph following resection and osteoarticular allograft reconstruction.

References

Brage ME, Simon MA. Metastatic bone disease, evaluation, prognosis, and medical treatment considerations of metastatic bone tumors. Orthopedics 1992; 15:589.

Brostrom LA, Harris MA, Simon MA, et al. The effect of biopsy on survival of patients with osteosarcoma. J Bone Joint Surg 1979; 61.

Dalinka MK, Zlatkin MB, Chao P, et al. The use of magnetic resonance imaging in the evaluation of bone and soft-tissue tumors. Radiol Clin North Am 1990; 28:461.

Enneking WF, Spanier SS, Goodman MA. A system for the surgical staging of musculoskeletal sarcoma. Clin Orthop 1980; 153:106.

Gold RI, Seeger LL, Bassett LW, Steckel RJ. An integrated approach to the evaluation of metastatic bone disease. Radiol Clin North Am 1990; 28:471.

Joyce ML, Mankin HJ. Caveat arthroscopos: Extra-articular lesions of bone simulating intra-articular pathology of the knee. J Bone Joint Surg 1983; 65A.

Lewis MM, ed. Musculoskeletal oncology: A multidisciplinary approach. Philadelphia: WB Saunders, 1992.

Madewell JE, Ragsdale BD, Sweet DE. Radiologic and pathologic analysis of solitary bone lesions. Radiol Clin North Am 1981; 19:715.

Mankin HJ, Lange TA, Spanier SS. The hazards of biopsy in patients with malignant primary bone and soft-tissue tumors. J Bone Joint Surg 1982; 64A.

Moore TM, Meyers MH, Patzakis MJ, et al. Closed biopsy of musculoskeletal lesions. J Bone Joint Surg 1979.

Orthopaedic Knowledge Update 3. Chicago: American Academy of Orthopaedic Surgeons, 1990.

Simon MA, Biermann JS. Biopsy of bone and soft tissue lesions. J Bone Joint Surg 1993; 75A:616.

Simon MA. Current concepts review: Biopsy of musculoskeletal tumors. J Bone Joint Surg 1982; 64A:1253.

SOFT TISSUE MASS

A. The history of a patient presenting with a soft tissue mass is important in evaluating how long the mass has been present or noticed, an interval history of growth, presence or absence of pain, association with trauma or injury, fluctuation in size, associated warmth or erythema, and interference with normal activities. Incorporate a general overall history, paying attention to previous history of neoplastic disease in the individual or in the family.

B. The physical examination should define the size of the mass, differentiating between those <5 cm and those >5 cm. Location of the mass with respect to the superficial fascia is important; those deep to the fascia are of greater concern than those superficial to that structure. Physical examination should evaluate presence or absence of tenderness, warmth, bruit, and fixation to adjacent structures (skin, fascia, bone, etc.). Range of motion of adjacent joints and presence or absence of effusion are important to note. A survey of the regional lymphatics also should be performed.

C. Small, superficial, asymptomatic lesions, whether cystic or solid, can be observed at regular intervals (initially at 3–4 months), and then at longer intervals if no change is noted. Symptomatic lesions that are small, superficial, and cystic may be aspirated or excised. Symptomatic lesions that are small and solid may be biopsied in an excisional fashion with a cuff of normal tissue, with all tissue submitted for pathologic study to include margins. Frozen section analysis of the tissue may be performed at the time of surgery to ensure adequacy of margins.

D. Small lesions that are deep to the superficial fascia are of more concern and deserve greater evaluation. Each should undergo radiographic evaluation to assess the presence or absence of soft tissue mineralization or associated skeletal changes. Magnetic resonance imaging (MRI) is useful in delineating the homogeneity of the lesion, the presence or absence of inflammation, and association with adjacent structures (e.g., bone, neurovascular, joint). Those that are reasonably accessible in the extremity can undergo either incisional or excisional biopsy depending on location and adjacent structures. Frozen section should be performed on incisional biopsies to ensure adequate tissue for diagnosis and on excisional biopsies to evaluate adequacy of margins. Inaccessible lesions (in spine or pelvis) can undergo needle biopsy under fluoroscopic control.

E. Larger lesions (>5 cm) should undergo MRI evaluation as a general rule (Fig. 1, A). Those that are cystic and superficial can be aspirated utilizing ultrasound if necessary, with the fluid submitted for cytology, culture, and cell count. Large superficial lesions of a solid nature should undergo an incisional or needle biopsy (Fig. 1, B), with further therapeutic decisions based on frozen section analysis. Large lesions deep to the superficial fascia are likely to be malignant and should therefore undergo further staging prior to biopsy, including chest radiograph, chest computed tomography (CT), and triple phase bone scan evaluation, with consideration given to CT examination with contrast of the lesion. These evaluations will help better define the exact nature of the lesion, its association with adjacent structures, and the best route for biopsy with the ultimate resection of the lesion kept in mind (Fig. 1, C).

SOFT TISSUE MASS

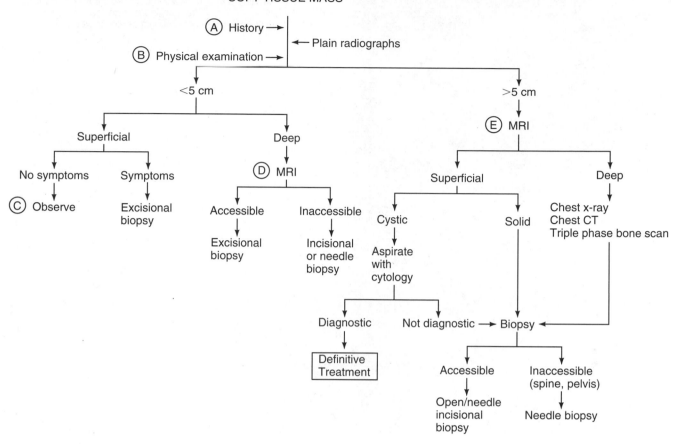

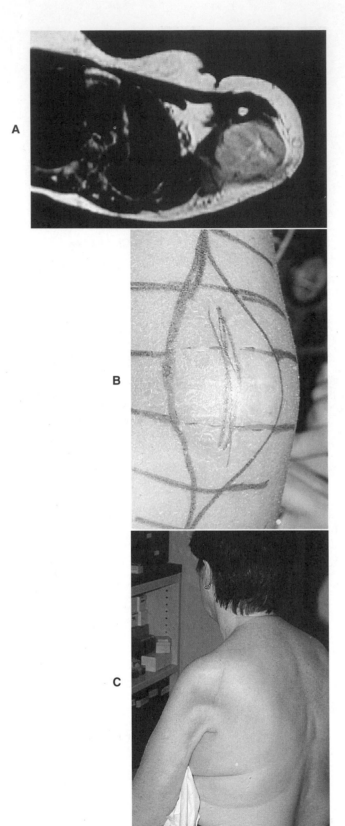

Figure 1 **A,** High-grade liposarcoma of proximal arm. **B,** Biopsy site and incision outline. Wide margins around the incisional biopsy rear are obtained. **C,** Postoperative clinical photograph.

References

Brage ME, Simon MA. Metastatic bone disease, Evaluation, prognosis, and medical treatment considerations of metastatic bone tumors. Orthopedics 1992; 15:589.

Brostrom LA, Harris MA, Simon MA, et al. The effect of biopsy on survival of patients with osteosarcoma. J Bone Joint Surg 1979; 61B.

Dalinka MK, Zlatkin MB, Chao P, et al. The use of magnetic resonance imaging in the evaluation of bone and soft-tissue tumors. *Radiol Clin North Am* 1990; 28:461.

Eilert RE, ed. AAOS Instructional Course Lectures XLI. Chicago: American Academy of Orthopaedic Surgeons, 1992.

Enneking WF, Spanier SS, Goodman MA. A system for the surgical staging of musculoskeletal sarcoma. Clin Orthop 1980; 153:106.

Gold RI, Seeger LL, Bassett LW, Steckel RJ. An integrated approach to the evaluation of metastatic bone disease. Radiol Clin North Am 1990; 28:471.

Joyce ML, Mankin HJ. Caveat Arthroscopos: Extra-articular lesions of bone simulating intra-articular pathology of the knee. J Bone Joint Surg 1983; 65A.

Lewis MM, ed. Musculoskeletal oncology: A multidisciplinary approach. Philadelphia: WB Saunders, 1992.

Mankin HJ, Lange TA, Spanier SS. The hazards of biopsy in patients with malignant primary bone and soft-tissue tumors. J Bone Joint Surg 1982; 64A.

Moore TM, Meyers MH, Patzakis MJ, et al. Closed biopsy of musculoskeletal lesions. J Bone Joint Surg 1979.

Orthopaedic Knowledge Update 3. Chicago: American Academy of Orthopaedic Surgeons, 1990.

Sim FH: Diagnosis and management of metastatic bone disease. New York: Raven Press, 1988.

Simon MA, Biermann JS: Biopsy of bone and soft tissue lesions. J Bone Joint Surg 1993; 75A:616.

Simon MA. Current concepts review: Biopsy of musculoskeletal tumors. J Bone Joint Surg 1982; 64-A:1253.

METASTATIC LESIONS OF BONE

The patient with metastatic skeletal disease may present a clinical challenge for treatment depending on many factors, including his or her age, performance status, known primary disease, physiologic status, and life expectancy.

A. The patient with a known primary malignancy presenting with a bone lesion cannot automatically be assumed to have metastatic disease though it is statistically most likely. Careful history and physical examination are important. Evaluation includes laboratory studies to determine elevations in tumor markers or serum chemistries. Imaging studies are important to evaluate extent of disease systemically and in the individual bones involved (Fig. 1, A).

   Patients with known malignancy who have new pain referable to the musculoskeletal system require full staging in order to assess the systemic involvement with metastatic disease and the amount of skeletal involvement in particular. The amount of metastatic disease, projected survival, and performance status affect the surgical options. Assess at the outset the number of skeletal metastatic lesions requiring fixation so that operating room resources can be coordinated effectively.

B. Following plain radiographs, nuclear medicine bone scan is the most efficient and sensitive skeletal screening for metastatic disease. Leukemia, lymphoma, and myeloma are unpredictably seen on bone scans; patients with these diseases should have a skeletal survey.

C. Cross sectional imaging is useful in certain anatomic areas, especially the spine and pelvis, to assess the full extent of involvement. Computed tomography (CT) is predictably more reliable at assessing cortical integrity whereas magnetic resonance imaging (MRI) is superior at defining intraosseous and extraosseous extent of disease (Fig. 1, B). Both modalities may be indicated in some patients.

D. Solitary lesions, especially with a significant interval between the treatment of a known primary malignancy and the identification of the lesion, should undergo biopsy. Needle biopsy under fluoroscopic control is helpful to confirm the metastatic nature of the lesion.

E. In patients without a known primary, evaluation and treatment are tailored to the patient and the degree of skeletal involvement. With fractures or impending fractures, perform prompt evaluation to assess other bones at risk. A triple phase bone scan can be expeditiously arranged and will provide valuable information about the amount of local bone involvement, the vascularity of the lesion, and the extent of skeletal disease. Prior to definitive fixation, perform an incisional biopsy to confirm the metastatic nature of the lesion. If confirmatory, proceed with stabilization. If questionable, confirm adequate tissue for diagnosis. Protect patient postoperatively to guard against fracture.

F. For patients not at immediate risk, seek the primary lesion by means of thorough history and physical examination, chest and abdominal CT, and directed laboratory studies. Identification and management of the primary and metastatic lesions may obviate the need for immediate skeletal fixation, depending on the response of the tumor to local or systemic therapy.

G. Techniques for stabilization of impending pathologic fractures depend on the primary tumor, the location, the patient's age and performance status. The responsiveness of the primary malignancy may dictate whether use of polymethylmethacrylate (PMMA) is indicated. Intramedullary fixation may be preferred to plate fixation because of less surgical dissection, less blood loss, faster procedures, and improved fixation. Interlocked intramedullary fixation with or without PMMA may provide the best stability in appropriate diaphyseal metastatic lesions. Metaphyseal lesions often require adjunctive PMMA in addition to plate or plate and compression screw fixation. Cemented endoprosthetic replacement of proximal femoral and proximal humeral metastatic lesions is a sound approach to rapidly addressing the patient's disease and mobilizing the shoulder shortly after surgery (Fig. 1, C). Multiple skeletal metastases may be addressed during the same anesthetic episode depending on the patient's physiologic status and intraoperative stability. Once the impending lesions have been satisfactorily addressed, the patient may begin rehabilitation in addition to other local and systemic therapies. Close follow up of skeletal metastasis needs to be performed on a routine basis in order to address lesions before they threaten the patient's activities of daily living.

METASTATIC DISEASE

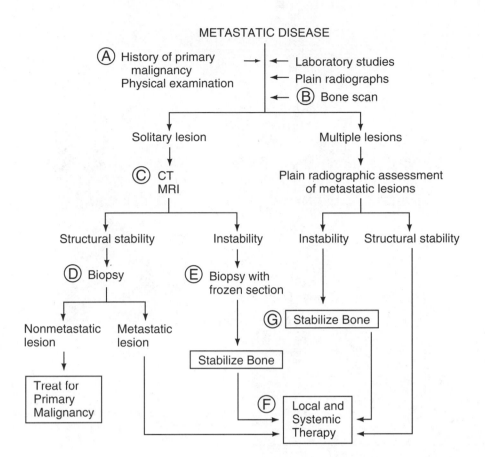

(A) History of primary
malignancy
Physical examination

→ ← Laboratory studies
← Plain radiographs
← (B) Bone scan

Solitary lesion

Multiple lesions

(C) CT
MRI

Plain radiographic assessment
of metastatic lesions

Structural stability   Instability

Instability   Structural stability

(D) Biopsy

(E) Biopsy with
frozen section

(G) Stabilize Bone

Nonmetastatic
lesion

Metastatic
lesion

Stabilize Bone

Treat for
Primary
Malignancy

(F) Local and
Systemic
Therapy

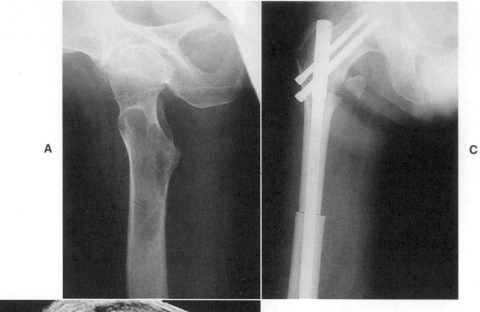

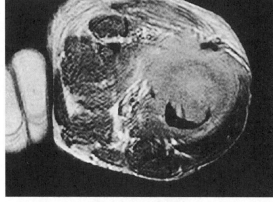

Figure 1   Lung cancer metastasis to the proximal femur. **A,** Radiograph. **B,** MRI. **C,** Postoperative radiograph following intercalary allograft reconstruction.

References

Brage ME, Simon MA. Metastatic bone disease, Evaluation, prognosis, and medical treatment considerations of metastatic bone tumors. Orthopedics 1992; 15:589.

Brostrom LA, Harris MA, Simon MA, et al. The effect of biopsy on survival of patients with osteosarcoma. J Bone Joint Surg 1979; 61B.

Dalinka MK, Zlatkin MB, Chao P, et al. The use of magnetic resonance imaging in the evaluation of bone and soft-tissue tumors. Radiol Clin North Am 1990; 28:461.

Eilert RE (ed). AAOS Instructional Course Lectures XLI. Chicago: American Academy of Orthopaedic Surgeons, 1992.

Enneking WF, Spanier SS, Goodman MA. A system for the surgical staging of musculoskeletal sarcoma. Clin Orthop 1980; 153:106.

Gold RI, Seeger LL, Bassett LW, Steckel RJ. An integrated approach to the evaluation of metastatic bone disease. Radiol Clin North Am 1990; 28:471.

Joyce ML, Mankin HJ. Caveat arthroscopos: Extra-articular lesions of bone simulating intra-articular pathology of the knee. J Bone Joint Surg 1983; 65A.

Lewis MM, ed. Musculoskeletal oncology: A multidisciplinary approach. Philadelphia: WB Saunders, 1992.

Mankin HJ, Lange TA, Spanier SS. The hazards of biopsy in patients with malignant primary bone and soft-tissue tumors. J Bone Joint Surg 1982; 64A.

Moore TM, Meyers MH, Patzakis MJ, et al. Closed biopsy of musculoskeletal lesions. J Bone Joint Surg 1979;

Orthopaedic Knowledge Update 3. Chicago: American Academy of Orthopaedic Surgeons, 1990.

Sim FH. Diagnosis and management of metastatic bone disease. New York: Raven Press, 1988.

Simon MA. Current concepts review biopsy of musculoskeletal tumors. J Bone Joint Surg 1982; 64A:1253.

Simon MA, Biermann JS. Biopsy of bone and soft tissue lesions. J Bone Joint Surg 1993; 75A:616.

CHILDREN'S ORTHOPAEDICS

Growth Plate Injuries
Fractures of the Proximal Humerus in Children
Fractures of the Distal Humerus in Children
Elbow Fractures and Dislocations in Children
Fractures of the Femoral Shaft in Children
Fracture of the Distal Femur in Children
Neck Deformity/Restriction of Motion
Torticollis
Klippel-Feil Syndrome
Foot Deformity
Clubfoot Deformity
Metatarsus Adductus
Cavus Foot
Flatfoot Deformity
Tarsal Coalition
Vertical Talus
Congenital Leg Deformity
Congenital Pseudarthrosis of the Tibia
Proximal Femoral Focal Deficiency
Tibial Hemimelia
Fibular Hemimelia
Legg-Calve-Perthes Disease
Slipped Capital Femoral Epiphysis
Limb Length Inequality
Developmental Dysplasia of the Hip Before 6 Months of Age
Developmental Dysplasia of the Hip After 6 Months of Age
Spinal Deformity
Idiopathic Scoliosis
Congenital Scoliosis
Neuromuscular Scoliosis
Spondylolysis/Spondylolisthesis
Scheuermann's Kyphosis
Angular Deformity
Infantile Blount's Disease
Adolescent Blount's Disease
Partial Physeal Arrest

GROWTH PLATE INJURIES

A. Injuries to the growth plate occur in approximately 18% of pediatric fractures, producing very specific fracture patterns. Although several authors have described these lesions, the work of Salter and Harris has been adopted as the standard classification system. The five injury patterns described can be separated into extra-articular fractures, intra-articular fractures, and plate destruction. All epiphyseal fractures occur through the hypertrophic zone of the plate (Fig. 1), but may extend into the metaphysis or into the adjacent joint. The extra-articular fractures include Salter-Harris I and Salter-Harris II lesions (Fig. 2). The Type I fractures are pure epiphyseal plate fractures; while the Type II fractures have extension into the adjacent metaphysis. Both these fractures can be undisplaced or displaced. Undisplaced Salter-Harris I fractures are diagnosed from the history and a physical finding of tenderness at the epiphyseal plate, as the radiographs will not show any bony lesion. These occur commonly in pediatric athletes.

B. Displaced extra-articular fractures usually require closed reduction. In children, a thick periosteal hinge on the side of displacement may tether the distal fragment and needs to be taken into account during reduction. Anatomic reduction, although desired, is not necessary as these injuries have been shown to remodel. Inability to obtain a closed reduction occurs rarely but suggests interposition of soft tissue, often periosteum. Unstable reductions are held with percutaneous smooth pins for 2 to 4 weeks until stable.

C. Salter-Harris III and Salter-Harris IV injuries (Fig. 3) have extensions into the adjacent joint—thereby becoming intra-articular fractures. The Salter-Harris III lesions have a fracture through the growth plate with an extension into the joint. Salter-Harris IV lesions have the fracture through the growth plate and concomitant extensions into both the metaphysis and the joint. These injuries may be undisplaced, minimally displaced, or displaced.

D. As these injuries extend into the joint, it is crucial to determine if they have any deformity at the joint surface. Although tomograms are helpful, computed tomography (CT) scans with sagittal reconstructions (particularly if smaller cuts have been used) best define the fracture anatomy. Injuries that have no step off at the joint surface and less than 2-mm gap between the articular fragments are deemed minimally displaced and treated with closed reduction and immobilization.

E. Initial immobilization should be noncircumferential to accommodate for postinjury swelling. A significant number of these injuries are at risk for compartment syndromes because they occur at or distal to either the elbow or the knee. However, plaster splint or split cast still needs to be molded to counteract the periosteal hinge that displaces the distal fragment. This hinge is always on the side to which the distal fragment displaced, or opposite an opening in the cortex.

F. At 7 to 10 days, place the fracture in a well-molded cast. As cancellous bone is involved in these injuries, the fractures are clinically united in 6 to 8 weeks. Because of the significant potential for displacement of the distal fragment by the intact periosteal hinge, mold all casts in the opposite direction.

G. Intra-articular fractures that are displaced require open reduction and fixation. Open reduction must respect the vascular supply of the involved epiphysis as well as the growth plate integrity. Fixation that remains entirely within the bony epiphysis may be either threaded or nonthreaded. Any fixation crossing an open epiphyseal plate, however, must be as small as possible for the size of the fragment and nonthreaded. Any trauma to the germinal cells of the growth plate (Fig. 1) that occurred at time of injury can be increased by surgical manipulation or inappropriate fixation. Long-term results of well treated intra-articular and extra-articular fractures tend to be good.

H. The Salter-Harris V injury results in arrest of at least part of the growth plate (Fig. 4). Initial radiographs do not usually reveal an injury, and the lesion must be suspected from a history of high velocity trauma, burns, or frostbite. In the past, the suspected lesions were followed radiographically until a bony bar was visualized. Recent research suggests that the magnetic resonance imaging (MRI) unit may identify these lesions earlier than was previously possible. Other than immobilization until symptom-free, there is no initial treatment available for these injuries.

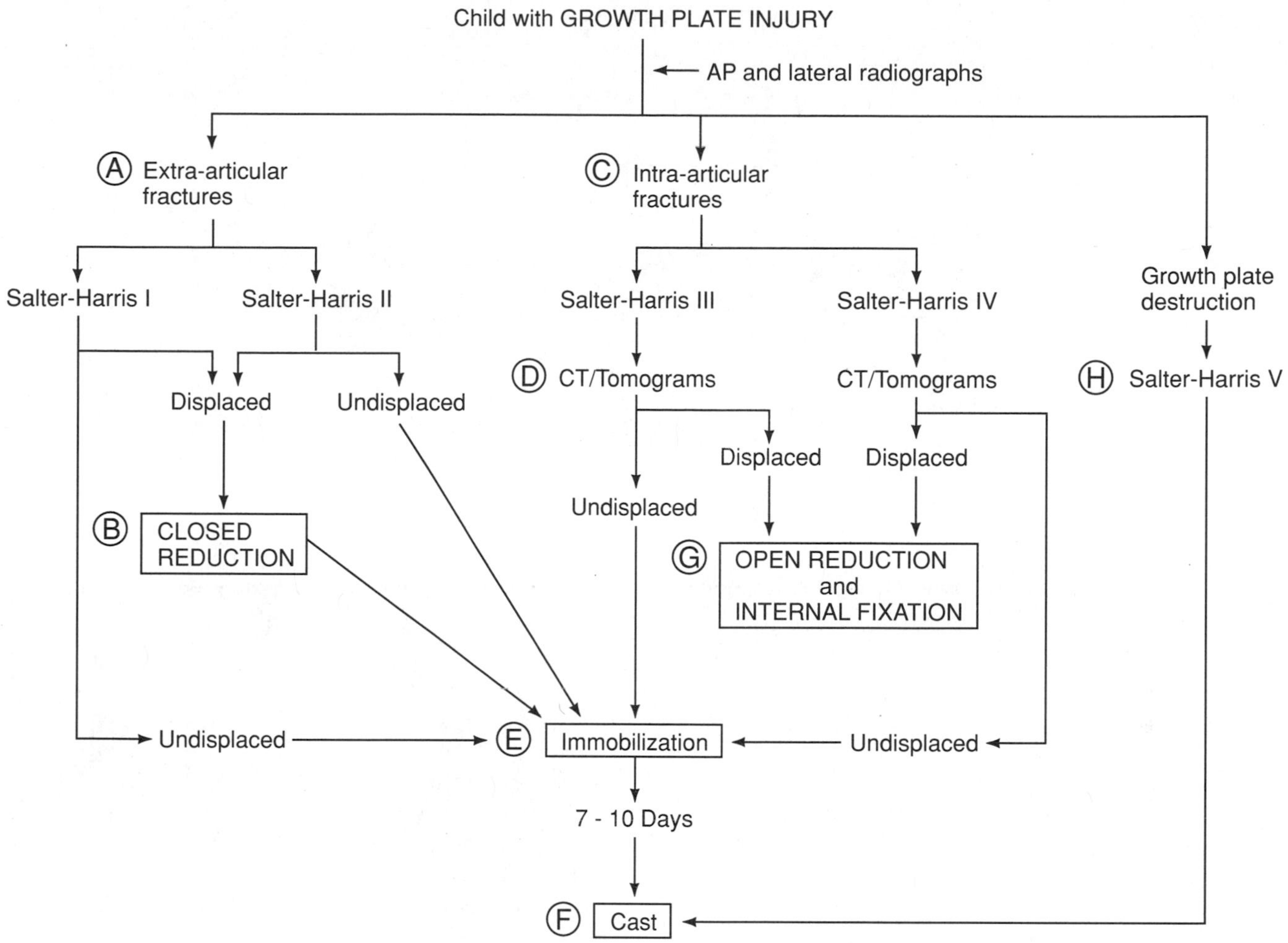

Child with GROWTH PLATE INJURY

← AP and lateral radiographs

(A) Extra-articular fractures

(C) Intra-articular fractures

Growth plate destruction

Salter-Harris I

Salter-Harris II

Salter-Harris III

Salter-Harris IV

(H) Salter-Harris V

Displaced

Undisplaced

(D) CT/Tomograms

CT/Tomograms

Displaced

Displaced

Undisplaced

(B) CLOSED REDUCTION

(G) OPEN REDUCTION and INTERNAL FIXATION

Undisplaced → (E) Immobilization ← Undisplaced

7 - 10 Days

(F) Cast

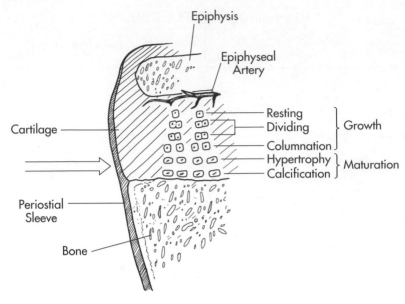

Figure 1 A representative growth plate is demonstrated. Epiphyseal fractures occur through the zone of hypertrophy (*arrow*).

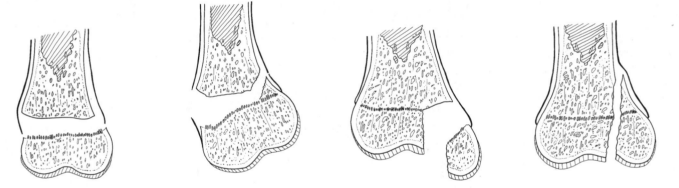

Figure 2 Salter-Harris fractures, Types I and II.

Figure 3 Salter-Harris fractures, Types III and IV.

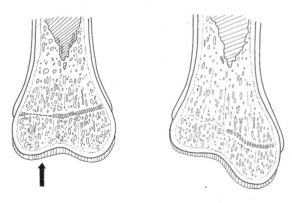

Figure 4 Salter-Harris fracture, Type V.

References

Arkin AM, Katz JF. The effects of pressure on epiphyseal growth: The mechanism of plasticity of growing bone. J Bone Joint Surg 1956; 38A:1056.

Beals RK. Premature closure of the physis following diaphyseal fractures. J Pediatr Orthop 1990; 10:717.

Bigelow DR, Ritchie GW. The effects of frostbite in childhood. J Bone Joint Surg 1963; 45B:122.

Bright RW, Burstein AH, Elmore SM. Epiphyseal plate cartilage: A biomechanical and histological analysis of failure modes. J Bone Joint Surg 1974; 56A:688.

Chadwick CJ, Bentley G. The classification and prognosis of epiphyseal injuries. Injury 1987; 18:157.

Evans EB, Smith JR. Bone and joint changes following burns. J Bone Joint Surg 1959; 41A:785.

Hresko MT, Kasser JR. Physeal arrest about the knee associated with nonphyseal fractures in the lower extremity. J Bone Joint Surg 1989; 71A:698.

Jaramillo D, Shapiro F, Hoffer FA, et al. Post-traumatic growth plate abnormalities: MR imaging of bony-bridge formation in rabbits. Radiology 1990; 175:767.

Landin LA, Danielson LG, Jonsson K, Pettersson H. Late results in 65 physeal ankle fractures. Acta Orthop Scand 1986; 57:530.

Larson RL. Epiphyseal injuries in the adolescent athlete. Orthop Clin North Am 1973; 4:839.

Mendez AA, Bartal E, Grillot MB, Lin JJ. Compression (Salter-Harris Type V) physeal fracture: An experimental model in the rat. J Pediatr Orthop 1992; 12:29.

Mizuta T, Benson WM, Foster BK, et al. Statistical analysis of the incidence of physeal injuries. J Pediatr Orthop 1987; 7:518.

Peterson HA, Burkhart SS. Compression injury of the epiphyseal growth plate: Fact or fiction? J Pediatr Orthop 1981; 1:377.

Salter RB, Harris WR. Injuries involving the epiphyseal plate. J Bone Joint Surg 1963; 45A:587.

Wilson-MacDonald J, Houghton GR, Bradley J, Morscher E. The relationship between periosteal division and compression or distraction of the growth plate. J Bone Joint Surg 1990; 72B:303.

FRACTURES OF THE PROXIMAL HUMERUS IN CHILDREN

A. Obstetric shoulder "dislocation" is not infrequently a Salter-Harris (S-H) I fracture of the proximal humerus. As less than a quarter of newborns have a visible ossific nucleus in the proximal humeral epiphysis, the differential diagnosis is difficult. These children usually present with a pseudoparalysis of the involved extremity and radiographs demonstrating displacement of the shaft in relation to the glenoid. An arthrogram demonstrates the relationship of the proximal humeral epiphysis to the glenoid. A single gentle attempt at reduction with the arm in 90° flexion and 90° abduction may be warranted. Further or more aggressive reductions are not advised as this lesion will usually remodel. Humerus varus, a potential complication of the initial injury, also may be potentiated with aggressive manipulation.

B. Children < 5 years old usually sustain Salter-Harris I injuries of the proximal humerus. These are frequently displaced but remodel extensively. Numerous authors have reviewed clinical series of proximal humeral epiphyseal injuries and have unanimously concluded that injuries in the younger child remodel well and should not be manipulated unless the deformity involves >70° angulation or >50% displacement. Fractures that require manipulation and are unstable after the procedure may be held in position by either percutaneous pinning (Fig. 1) or overhead traction for 7 to 10 days.

C. Because of the growth pattern of the proximal humerus, children between the ages of 5 and 10 years are most likely to sustain a metaphyseal fracture. These are rarely displaced because of the force needed to do so and can be treated in a Velpeau sling.

D. Proximal humeral epiphyseal injuries are common in adolescents, particularly those actively involved in sports. Overuse in throwing sports can produce an epiphysiolysis that resolves with rest and does not require surgical treatment. More commonly, and usually in contact sports, a Salter-Harris II injury is produced (Fig. 2). The need for reduction depends on the remodeling potential of the patient; a factor that is usually age related. Older adolescents with less growth potential require a more anatomic reduction than the younger ones. Salter-Harris III and IV lesions are extremely rare and require open reduction and internal fixation (ORIF).

E. Attempted closed reduction of these fractures produces three outcomes. In the first instance, the fracture is reducible and is stable with the arm at the patient's side—these do well in a Velpeau sling. More commonly, the fracture is reducible with the arm in 90° abduction but displaces as the arm is brought to the side of the patient. These can be treated either in a shoulder spica in the "salute" position or with percutaneous pinning (see Fig. 1). Not infrequently the fracture is irreducible, either because the long head of the biceps is caught between the fracture fragments or because the shaft has buttonholed through the periosteum (Fig. 3). Both of these require an open reduction and stabilization at that time is recommended.

F. Glenohumeral dislocations associated with proximal humeral epiphyseal fractures are rare but serious injuries. The epiphyseal injuries are frequently Salter-Harris III or IV intra-articular fractures. ORIF is the treatment of choice; nonthreaded, removable pins are recommended in the younger child to retain as much postinjury growth as possible.

Child with PROXIMAL HUMERAL FRACTURE

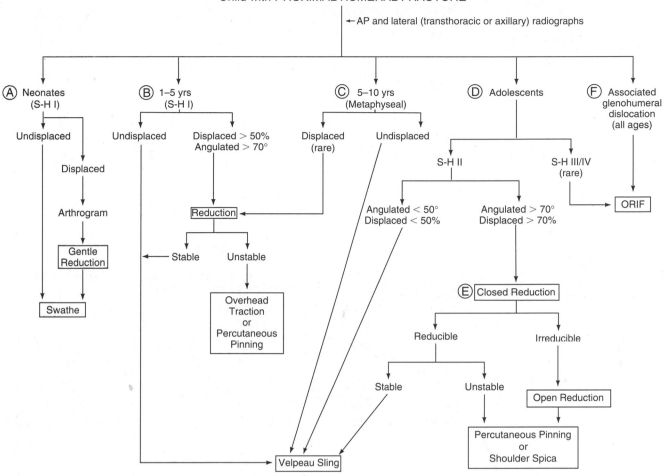

← AP and lateral (transthoracic or axillary) radiographs

Ⓐ Neonates (S-H I)
Undisplaced
Displaced
Arthrogram
Gentle Reduction
Swathe

Ⓑ 1–5 yrs (S-H I)
Undisplaced
Displaced > 50% Angulated > 70°
Reduction
Stable
Unstable
Overhead Traction or Percutaneous Pinning

Ⓒ 5–10 yrs (Metaphyseal)
Displaced (rare)
Undisplaced

Ⓓ Adolescents
S-H II
S-H III/IV (rare)
Angulated < 50% Displaced < 50%
Angulated > 70° Displaced > 70°
Ⓔ Closed Reduction
Reducible
Irreducible
Stable
Unstable
Open Reduction
Percutaneous Pinning or Shoulder Spica

Ⓕ Associated glenohumeral dislocation (all ages)
ORIF

Velpeau Sling

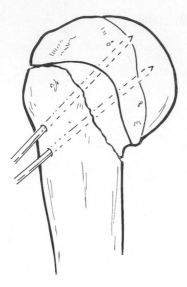

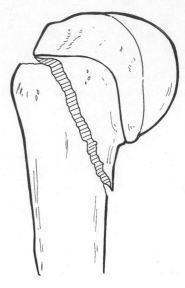

Figure 1 Unstable Salter-Harris I or II fractures can be stabilized with percutaneous non-threaded pins. These are usually left outside the skin and removed in the office at three to four weeks.

Figure 2 A common adolescent shoulder injury is a Salter-Harris II fracture of the proximal humerus.

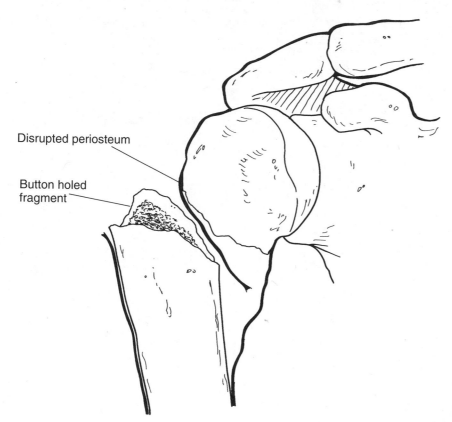

Disrupted periosteum

Button holed fragment

Figure 3 Irreducible fractures are usually secondary to soft tissue entrapment between the two fragments, either periosteum or the long head of the biceps.

References

Barnett LS. Little league shoulder syndrome: Proximal humeral epiphysiolysis in adolescent baseball pitchers. J Bone Joint Surg 1985; 67A:495.

Baxter MP, Wiley JJ. Fractures of the proximal humeral epiphysis: Their influence on humeral growth. J Bone Joint Surg 1986; 68B:570.

Beaty J. Fractures of the proximal humerus and shaft in children. Instructional Course Lectures 1992; XLI:369.

Cahill BR, Tullos HS, Fain RH. Little league shoulder. J Sports Med 1974; 2:150.

Curtis RJ. Operative management of children's fractures of the shoulder region. Orthop Clin North Am 1990; 21:315.

Dameron TB, Reibel DB. Fracture involving the proximal humeral epiphyseal plate. J Bone Joint Surg 1969; 51A:289.

Fraser RL, Haliberton RA, Barber JR. Displaced epiphyseal fractures of the proximal humerus. Can J Surg 1967; 10:427.

Gardner E. The prenatal development of the human shoulder joint. Surg Clin North Am 1963; 43:1465.

Gilchrist D. A Stockinette-Velpeau for immobilization of the shoulder girdle. J·Bone Joint Surg 1967; 49A:750.

Howard NJ, Eloesser L. Treatment of fractures of the upper end of the humerus: An experimental and clinical study. J Bone Joint Surg 1934; 16:1.

Jeffrey CC. Fracture separation of the upper humeral epiphysis. Surg Gynecol Obstet 1953; 96:205.

Kohler R, Trilland JM. Fracture and fracture-separation of the proximal humerus in children: Report of 136 cases. J Pediatr Orthop 1983; 3:326.

Larsen CF, Kiaer T, Lindequist S. Fractures of the proximal humerus in children: Nine year follow-up of 64 unoperated on cases. Acta Orthop Scand 1990; 61:255.

Neer CS, Horwitz BS. Fractures of the proximal humeral epiphyseal plate. Clin Orthop 1965; 41:24.

Scaglietti O. The obstetrical shoulder trauma. Surg Gynecol Obstet 1938; 66:868.

Sheek HH, Probst C. Fractures of the proximal humeral epiphysis. Orthop Clin North Am 1975; 6:401.

FRACTURES OF THE DISTAL HUMERUS IN CHILDREN

A. Extra-articular fractures of the distal humeral epiphysis are an uncommon but distinct entity. Although usually seen in infants and young children, they have been reported in children as old as 8 years. These injuries are frequently confused with elbow dislocations; however, identifying the relationship of the radius and ulna to the capitellum and/or trochlea (Fig. 1) helps distinguish between the two. Treatment, unlike the diagnosis, is usually straightforward. Displaced fractures reduce easily and then are immobilized for the appropriate period of time depending on the child's age.

B. Infants and young children in whom the distal humeral epiphysis has not yet ossified are the most likely to sustain this injury and the most difficult to diagnose. An index of suspicion should be aroused with swelling and crepitus around the elbow in children under 2 years of age. The cause is birth trauma in neonate and often child abuse in the infant. Diagnosis is established by an elbow arthrogram or magnetic resonance imaging (MRI), which will demonstrate the relationship of the radius and ulna to the cartilaginous epiphysis. Treatment is the same as in the older child.

C. Supracondylar fractures of the distal humerus in children are one of the most common pediatric injuries. The history of injury is usually a fall on an outstretched arm. The extremity should be splinted in the position that it lies and neurovascular examination recorded. Neurologic injuries are common and resolve spontaneously over 6 to 8 weeks. Injury to the anterior interosseous nerve is frequently missed and requires examination of the flexor profundus to the index finger. Vascular injury is not uncommon secondary to the location of the brachial artery in relation to the fracture. Treatment for undisplaced or minimally displaced fractures includes initial placement in a posterior slab in as much flexion as is tolerated. This is followed by circumferential immobilization once the swelling has decreased for a total treatment time of 6 weeks.

D. Fractures that are displaced require closed reduction and stabilization. Radiographs taken at time of reduction are critical. Figure 2, *A*, demonstrates the effect of humeral rotation on reduction. Varus–valgus tilt predicts those fractures most likely to develop angular deformities. Figure 2, *B*, demonstrates two methods of visualizing the reduction on the anteroposterior (AP) film for estimation of tilt. Once reduction has been obtained, stability of the reduction is determined under fluoroscopy. Most fractures that were initially displaced are unstable and require percutaneous pinning. Two common methods of pinning are demonstrated in Fig. 3. If crossed pinning is chosen, blunt dissection to bone is recommended on the medial side to avoid injury to the ulnar nerve. Occasionally closed reduction and stabilization is not possible and traction is an option. Dunlop traction is the most commonly used form of traction for supracondylar fractures.

E. A small percentage of these injuries will present with diminished peripheral circulation. If closed reduction restores flow, the fracture is treated as described above. If flow is not restored, an open vascular exploration is required. If arteriography is easily accessible, it is an option; but do not delay treatment significantly for an arteriogram. Once the degree of vessel damage has been assessed, stabilize the fracture, usually with crossed pins, prior to vessel repair. Assess the need for fasciotomies at the time of repair and perform fasciotomies if there are concerns.

F. In adolescents, the pattern of injuries to the distal humerus changes. Although supracondylar fractures may occur, the T-condylar pattern is more common. As these fractures usually have a vertical fracture line extending into the elbow joint, internal fixation is required. For the minimally displaced fractures, screw fixation, percutaneous or open, will usually hold the intra-articular fracture anatomically. Fractures not amenable to minimal fixation will require open reduction and internal fixation (Fig. 4).

Child with DISTAL HUMERAL FRACTURE

← AP and true lateral radiographs

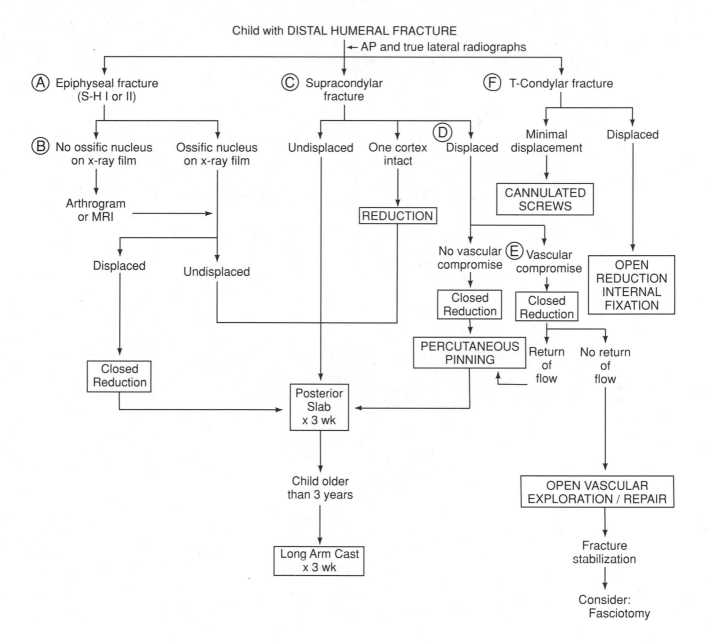

Ⓐ Epiphyseal fracture (S-H I or II)

Ⓑ No ossific nucleus on x-ray film

Ossific nucleus on x-ray film

Arthrogram or MRI

Displaced

Undisplaced

Closed Reduction

Ⓒ Supracondylar fracture

Undisplaced

One cortex intact

Ⓓ Displaced

REDUCTION

No vascular compromise

Ⓔ Vascular compromise

Closed Reduction

Closed Reduction

PERCUTANEOUS PINNING

Return of flow

No return of flow

Posterior Slab x 3 wk

Child older than 3 years

Long Arm Cast x 3 wk

Ⓕ T-Condylar fracture

Minimal displacement

Displaced

CANNULATED SCREWS

OPEN REDUCTION INTERNAL FIXATION

OPEN VASCULAR EXPLORATION / REPAIR

Fracture stabilization

Consider: Fasciotomy

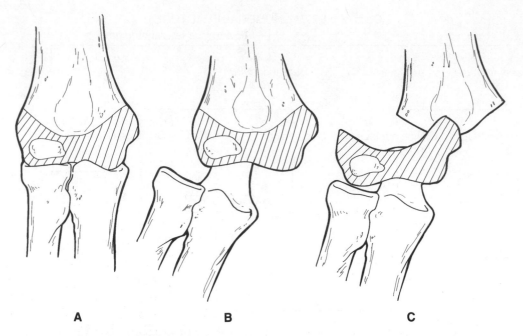

A   **B**   **C**

Figure 1 The relationship of the proximal radius and olecranon to the distal humeral epiphysis is key in distinguishing between fractures and dislocations. **A,** Normal elbow alignment. **B,** Dislocation of the elbow joint with the distal humeral epiphysis remaining with the humerus. **C,** Salter-Harris I fracture of the distal humerus. Displacement occurs through the growth plate, while the proximal radius and olecranon are aligned with the epiphysis.

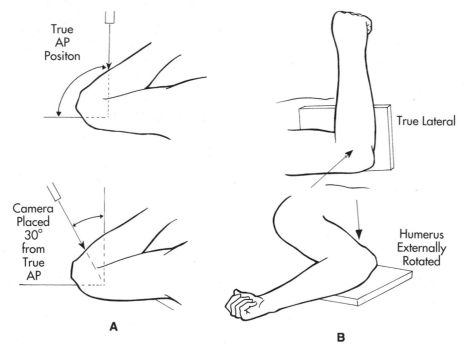

Figure 2 **A,** Rotation of the humerus for lateral radiographs frequently displaces the fracture. True lateral films with the humerus in neutral are preferred. **B,** AP radiographs following fracture reduction require the elbow to be in flexion. A second AP film shot 30° from the true AP outlines the distal humerus without overlap of the radius and ulna.

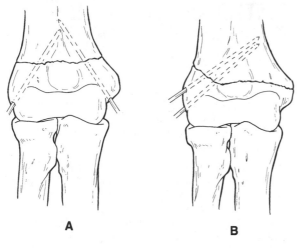

Figure 3 Percutaneous pinning of supracondylar fractures can be accomplished in two ways: crossed pins **(A)** or two lateral pins **(B)**.

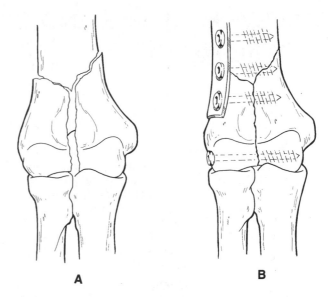

Figure 4 The T-condylar fracture **(A)** seen commonly in adolescents. Internal fixation is required. Minimally displaced fractures with no extension to the cortex may only require a supra-articular screw; more complicated fractures require standard internal fixation **(B)**.

References

Abraham E, Powers T, Witt P, Roy RD. Experimental hyperextension supracondylar fractures in monkeys. Clin Orthop 1982; 171:309.

Aronson DD, Prager BI. Supracondylar fractures of the humerus in children: A modified technique for closed pinning. Clin Orthop 1987; 219:174.

Basom WC. Supracondylar and transcondylar fractures in children. Clin Orthop 1953; 1:43.

Bosanquet JS, Middleton RW. The reduction of supracondylar fractures of the humerus in children treated by traction in extension. Injury 1983; 14:373.

Dameron TB. Transverse fractures of the distal humerus in children. Instr Course Lect 1981; 30:224.

DeLee JC, Wilkins KE, Rogers LF, Rockwood CA. Fracture separation of the distal humeral epiphysis. J Bone Joint Surg 1980; 62A:46.

Dunlop J. Transcondylar fractures of the humerus in childhood. J Bone Joint Surg 1939; 21:59.

Flynn JC, Matthews JD, Benoit RL. Blind pinning of displaced supracondylar fractures of the humerus in children: A sixteen year experience with longterm follow-up. J Bone Joint Surg 1974; 56A:263.

Haddad RJ, Saer JK, Riordan DC. Percutaneous pinning of displaced supracondylar fractures of the elbow in children. Clin Orthop 1970; 71:112.

Jarvis JG, D'Astous JL. The pediatric T-supracondylar fracture. J Pediatr Orthop 1984; 4:697.

Lipscomb PR, Burleson RJ. Vascular and neural complications in supracondylar fractures of the humerus in children. J Bone Joint Surg 1955; 37A:487.

McGraw JJ, Akbania BA, Hanel DP, et al. Neurological complications resulting from supracondylar fractures of the humerus in children. J Pediatr Orthop 1986; 6:647.

McIntyre WM, Wiley JJ, Charette RJ. Fracture separation of the distal humeral epiphysis. Clin Orthop 1984; 188:98.

Nacht JL, Ecker ML, Chung SM, et al. Supracondylar fractures of the humerus in children treated by closed reduction and percutaneous pinning. Clin Orthop 1983; 177:203.

Papavasilian VA, Beslikas TA. T-Condylar fractures of the distal humerus during childhood: An analysis of six cases. J Pediatr Orthop 1986; 6:302.

Spinner M, Schreiber SN. Anterior interosseous nerve palsy as a complication of supracondylar fractures of the humerus in children. J Bone Joint Surg 1969; 51A:1584.

Worlock PH, Coltan C. Severely displaced supracondylar fractures of the humerus in children: A simple method of treatment. J Pediatr Orthop 1987; 7:49.

ELBOW FRACTURES AND DISLOCATIONS IN CHILDREN

A. Radiographic evaluation and understanding the radiologic anatomy are crucial in pediatric elbow injuries. Due to the variance in epiphyseal ossification at different ages, comparison views of the uninjured elbow should be taken to help in outlining normal and abnormal anatomy for a given age. The fat pad sign (Fig. 1) is also a key component of the x-ray examination, but is not always pathognomonic. Review the pediatric elbow films in a systematic fashion. Viewing the bony components as forming a circle or outline, starting at a given point and progressing around the circle, most pathology should be picked up.

B. The distal humerus contributes four components to the elbow—two epicondyles and two condyles. The condyles form the articular surface but often, particularly in younger children, have not yet fully ossified. A small metaphyseal flake, either undisplaced or displaced, may be the only clue to a fracture of the physis; check the relationship of the condyle to the distal humerus. Lateral condylar fractures (Fig. 2) are far more common than medial (Fig. 3), but the treatment is the same. Undisplaced fractures require rigid splinting and close monitoring for further displacement. Fractures that are displaced < 2 mm require closed reduction followed by splinting and monitoring as above. Percutaneous pinning is an option for the minimally displaced lateral condyle.

C. Unsuccessful closed reduction or original displacement > 2 mm requires open reduction and internal fixation (ORIF). Soft tissue stripping is minimal to avoid injury to the blood supply of the trochlea. Reduction of the articular surface is anatomic. Perform fixation with unthreaded pins, sized to provide adequate stability, for minimal growth plate damage (Fig. 4).

D. The two epicondyles of the distal humerus serve as origins for major muscle groups; fractures usually indicate significant soft tissue injury as seen in a dislocation. In contrast to the condylar injuries, medial epicondylar fractures (Fig. 5, A to C) are more common than lateral (Fig. 5, D). Treat undisplaced fractures with initial splinting. Fractured epicondyles that have displaced into the joint require ORIF. Treatment of displaced fractures that remain extra-articular is controversial. In these instances, joint stability is critical. An unstable elbow with a displaced epicondylar fracture requires reduction and fixation. However, the same injury in a stable elbow may do very well treated with immobilization.

E. Isolated olecranon fractures in children, unlike adults, are usually minimally displaced, frequently reduce in extension, and are usually treated with casting. Diagnosis of an olecranon fracture requires careful documentation of the radial head to rule out a Monteggia injury. In teenage athletes, the olecranon epiphysis may sustain a stress fracture, especially with throwing sports.

F. Monteggia fractures—radial head dislocations associated with olecranon fractures (Fig. 6)—are common in children. Most of these injuries are treated successfully with closed reduction. Those that are not closed reduced usually only require open reduction of the olecranon fracture to produce spontaneous reduction of the radial head. Neurologic examination in these children should document posterior interosseous nerve function, because this nerve is at risk.

G. Fractures of the proximal radius in children routinely involve the radial neck. Infrequently these fractures are completely displaced and require open reduction. Far more commonly, they are angulated (Fig. 7, A to C). Those angulated < 30° are splinted. Those angulated > 60° require attempted reduction. Treatment of fractures between 30° and 60° is debated, but most clinicians recommend attempted closed reduction over 45°. Any fracture that is angulated < 60° after closed reduction is treated conservatively.

H. Radial neck fractures angulated > 60° do not function as well after healing. However, the precarious blood supply to this small disc has resulted in equally poor results with open reduction. As demonstrated in Fig. 7, D, percutaneous reduction using a Steinmann pin may be the best compromise.

I. Dislocations are not uncommon in the pediatric elbow and usually have an associated fracture, commonly either the medial epicondyle or the coronoid process. The most common is the humeral-radioulnar dislocation. However, this can be associated with dislocation of the proximal radioulnar joint (Fig. 8, A and B), the divergent dislocation. Both simple and divergent dislocations usually reduce with manipulation. Failure of reduction of the radial head signifies an unrecognized divergent dislocation and requires a repeat closed reduction or possible open reduction. Neither congenital radial head dislocation nor recurrent pulled elbows produce a unilateral radial head dislocation.

J. Incomplete reductions are secondary to either interposition or transposition (Fig. 8, C and D) during reduction. In children, interposition following reduction can be the median nerve, emphasizing the need for neurologic re-examination after reduction. Translocations occur when hyperpronation during injury causes reversed positioning of the proximal radius and ulna. Closed reduction may continue the reversed positioning; the few cases reported suggest a need for open reduction but a potentially poor outcome.

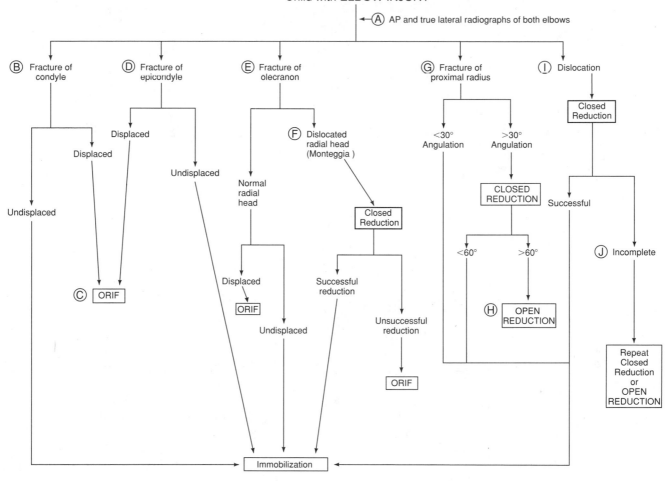

Child with ELBOW INJURY

(A) AP and true lateral radiographs of both elbows

(B) Fracture of condyle
(D) Fracture of epicondyle
(E) Fracture of olecranon
(G) Fracture of proximal radius
(I) Dislocation

Displaced
Undisplaced
Displaced
Undisplaced
(F) Dislocated radial head (Monteggia)
Normal radial head
<30° Angulation
>30° Angulation
Closed Reduction

Closed Reduction
CLOSED REDUCTION
Successful

Undisplaced
(C) ORIF
Displaced
ORIF
Successful reduction
Undisplaced
<60°
>60°
(J) Incomplete

Unsuccessful reduction
(H) OPEN REDUCTION

ORIF
Repeat Closed Reduction or OPEN REDUCTION

Immobilization

References

Aitken AP, Childress HM. Intraarticular displacement of the internal epicondyle following dislocation. J Bone Joint Surg 1938; 20:161.

Badelon O, Bensahel H, Mazda K, Vie P. Lateral humeral condylar fractures in children: A report of 47 cases. J Pediatr Orthop 1988; 8:31.

Bensahel H, Csukonyi A, Badelon O, Badaoui S. Fractures of the medial condyle of the humerus in children. J Pediatr Orthop 1986; 6:430.

Foster DE, Sullivan JA, Gross RH. Lateral humeral condylar fractures in children. J Pediatr Orthop 1985; 5:16.

Fowles JV, Kassab MT. Observations concerning radial neck fractures in children. J Pediatr Orthop 1986; 6:51.

Green NE. Entrapment of the median nerve following elbow dislocation. Case report. J Pediatr Orthop 1983; 3:384.

Harvey S, Tchelebi H. Proximal radio-ulnar translocation. Case report. J Bone Joint Surg 1979; 61A:447.

Hines RF, Herndon WA, Evans JP. Operative treatment of medial epicondyle fractures in children. Clin Orthop 1987; 223:170.

Holbrook JL, Green NE. Divergent pediatric elbow dislocation: Case report. Clin Orthop 1988; 234:72.

Letts M, Locht R, Wiens J. Monteggia fracture: Dislocations in children. J Bone Joint Surg 1985; 67B:724.

MacSween WA. Transposition of the radius and ulna associated with dislocation of the elbow in a child. Injury 1979; 10:314.

Mardam-Rey T, Ger E. Congenital radial head dislocation. J Hand Surg 1979; 4:316.

Matthews JG. Fractures of the olecranon in children. Injury 1980; 12:207.

Morey BF, An K-N. Articular and ligamentous contributions to the stability of the elbow joint. Am J Sports Med 1983; 11:315.

Murphy WA, Siegel MJ. Elbow fat pads with new signs and extended differential diagnosis. Radiology 1977; 124:659.

Rutherford A. Fractures of the lateral humeral condyle in children. J Bone Joint Surg 1985; 67A:851.

Sovio OM, Tredwell SJ. Divergent dislocation of the elbow in a child. Case report. J Pediatr Orthop 1986; 6:96.

Steinberg EL, Golamb D, Salama R, Weintroub S. Radial head and neck fractures in children. J Pediatr Orthop 1988; 8:35.

Tibone JE, Stoltz M. Fractures of the radial head and neck in children. J Bone Joint Surg 1981; 63A:100.

Torg JS, Moyer RA. Nonunion of a stress fracture through the olecranon epiphyseal plate observed in an adolescent baseball pitcher. A case report. J Bone Joint Surg 1977; 59A:264.

Wiley JJ, Pegington J, Horwich JP. Traumatic dislocation of the radius at the elbow. J Bone Joint Surg 1974; 56B:501.

Wiley JJ, Galey JP. Monteggia injuries in children. J Bone Joint Surg 1985; 67B:728.

Wilkins KE. Fractures and dislocations of the elbow region. In Rockwood CA, Wilkins KE, King RE, eds. Fractures in Children. Philadelphia: JB Lippincott, 1991.

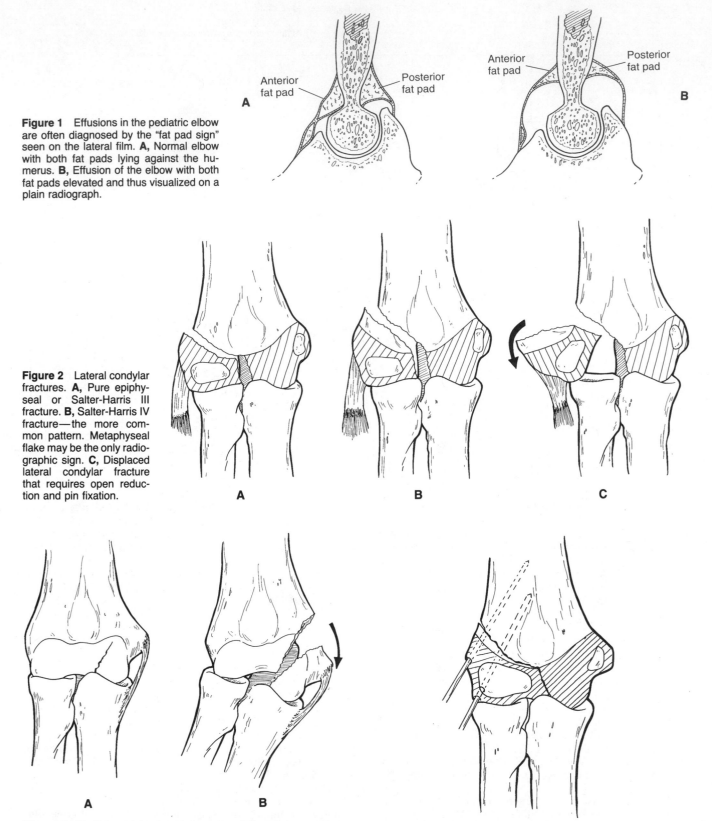

Figure 1 Effusions in the pediatric elbow are often diagnosed by the "fat pad sign" seen on the lateral film. **A,** Normal elbow with both fat pads lying against the humerus. **B,** Effusion of the elbow with both fat pads elevated and thus visualized on a plain radiograph.

Figure 2 Lateral condylar fractures. **A,** Pure epiphyseal or Salter-Harris III fracture. **B,** Salter-Harris IV fracture—the more common pattern. Metaphyseal flake may be the only radiographic sign. **C,** Displaced lateral condylar fracture that requires open reduction and pin fixation.

Figure 3 Medial condylar fractures are much less common. Frequently the fracture starts at the articular surface **(A).** If it becomes displaced **(B),** then it requires open reduction and fixation.

Figure 4 Two pin fixation following anatomic reduction is usually stable. Nonthreaded pins are required.

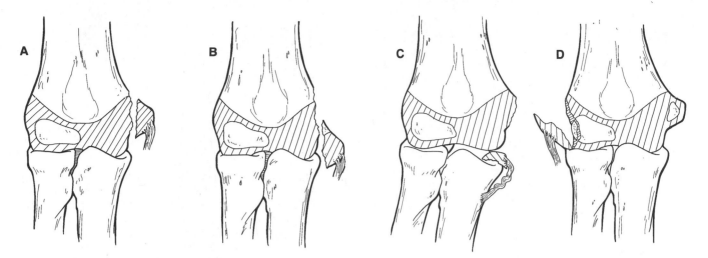

Figure 5 Epicondylar fractures occur most commonly on the medial side. The fragment may be minimally displaced **(A)**, at the joint line **(B)**, or lying in the joint **(C)**. Lateral epicondylar fractures **(D)** are less common.

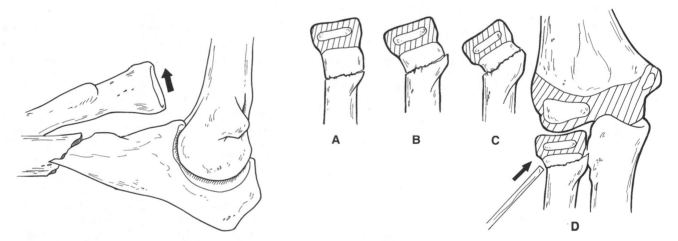

Figure 6 Monteggia fracture/dislocations occur when the angulation of the proximal ulnar fracture is severe enough to force the radial head to dislocate. The direction of the radial head corresponds to the apex of angulation of the ulnar fracture.

Figure 7 Proximal radial fractures usually involve the radial neck. These can be angulated less than 30° **(A)** less than 60° **(B)** and more than 60° **(C)**. If closed reduction fails, use of a Steinmann pin percutaneously **(D)** as a joystick to push the fragment back in place is recommended. Open reduction is rarely required.

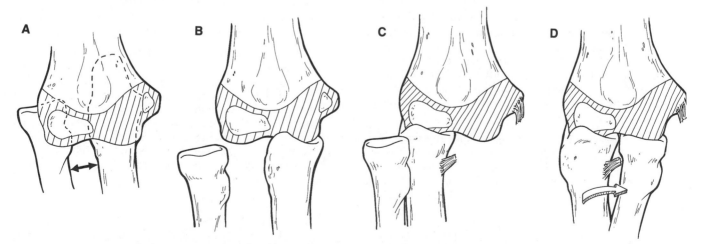

Figure 8 Complex dislocations of the elbow. **A,** At the time of humeral-radioulnar dislocation, the proximal radioulnar joint is also disrupted. **B,** The radial head remains dislocated following closed reduction. These divergent dislocations can be managed by repeat reduction if identified early; otherwise an ulnar osteotomy may be required. **C,** Transposition occurs when the elbow is partially reduced leaving the olecranon articulating with the lateral condyle. **D,** A rotational force applied with further attempted reduction may articulate the radial head with the medial condyle.

FRACTURES OF THE FEMORAL SHAFT IN CHILDREN

A. At initial assessment, include radiographic views of the ipsilateral hip and knee. Review the fracture pattern in light of the history to rule out child abuse because this is a common fracture in the battered child. In general, infants not yet walking do not usually sustain spiral diaphyseal fractures and children of walking age do not usually sustain transverse fractures in household falls.

B. The method of treatment for pediatric femoral fractures is determined mainly by age and weight. The fracture pattern may also influence treatment choice, particularly in the more proximal or distal shaft fractures. For instance, the commonly flexed, adducted proximal fragment of a subtrochanteric fracture is best reduced with 90°/90° traction. Severity of associated trauma also affects the decision making.

C. Bryant's traction (Fig. 1) is the recommended method of traction in children under 2 years or 20 pounds. Traction is applied to both legs with enough weight to elevate the sacrum just off the mattress. Volkmann's ischemia is a potential complication of this traction. Monitor the child closely. When tenderness at the fracture site has diminished, place the child in a hip spica.

D. Immediate spica for children under 2 who are otherwise stable has had good results. For children from 2 to 7 years closed reduction under general anesthetic followed by application of the spica is recommended. Close follow-up monitoring is required and the cast frequently needs wedging. Shortening in the cast always occurs. A period of traction to allow for reduction in muscle spasms prior to early casting has therefore been proposed. Cast application must be meticulous as pressure sores and nerve palsy can occur.

E. Traction can be applied through either the skin or a skeletal pin. Skin can only tolerate up to 10 pounds of weight; increase in weight necessitates a pin. Self-adhesive skin traction that does not require the use of benzoin decreases blister formation. Pad all bony prominences. Distal femoral pins are recommended over proximal tibia pins because they are less likely to cause growth plate injuries.

F. Single leg traction can be set up in three ways. The method chosen depends on the size of the child and/or the location of the fracture. Straight leg traction with skin tapes is ideal for midshaft fractures (Fig. 2). One can use 90°/90° for all shaft fractures, but it is ideal for subtrochanteric and proximal third fractures (Fig. 3). Use the split Russell method with either skin or pin traction (Fig. 4).

G. Do not include the foot on the fractured limb in the hip spica cast so as to decrease the chance of shortening. Include the opposite leg at least to the knee to stabilize the pelvis and avoid malunion. Total length of treatment (in weeks) from day of injury is generally the child's age (until adolescence) plus 3 weeks. Expect femoral overgrowth. This is more likely in the younger child and in simple fractures not associated with the growth plate. Post spica rehabilitation is rarely necessary. Encourage children to progress activities at their own rate.

H. In the 2 to 12 year age group, traction is sometimes either not appropriate or not effective. Vascular injury, severe head trauma with associated spasm, and/or "floating knees" may require more stable and more rapid fixation. Generally, angulation of more than 15° or shortening of more than 2 cm is unacceptable. However, the most important malalignment is rotation because this is less likely to correct with growth. Rotational alignment should be within 10° of the uninjured limb.

I. Fixation used in the 2 to 12 year age group does not have the same time and strength demands on it as does adult fixation. This has allowed increasing use of "flexible" fixation such as stacked rods and external fixators. Avoidance of injury to the growth plate is essential.

J. The large physical size and labile emotions of adolescents has made prolonged traction difficult. The use of either flexible fixation or intramedullary rods is increasing in this age group. Plates have been used successfully to treat femoral fractures in children, but because of the potential post-treatment complications, this has not become commonplace.

K. Special considerations need to be made when undertaking intramedullary rodding in children. The pediatric femoral canal is narrow and rods as small as 9 mm may be needed even in a large adolescent. Epiphyseal plates need to be respected. Distal fragment reaming should be careful and the distal epiphysis avoided. Trochanteric arrest, resulting in a valgus femoral neck, has been reported in children under 10 years of age. It is recommended that the entrance portal be placed lateral to the neck.

Child with FEMORAL SHAFT FRACTURE

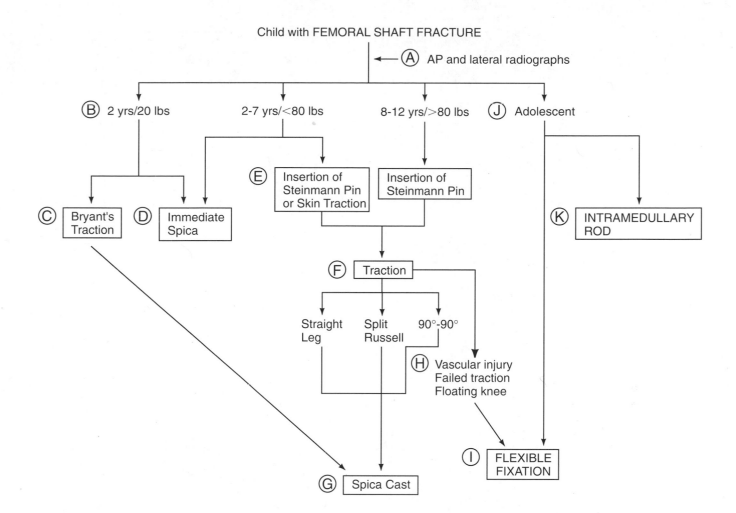

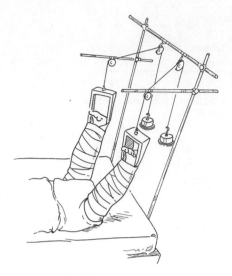

Figure 1 Bryant's traction.

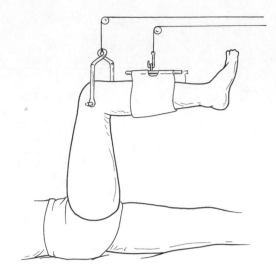

Figure 3 90°-90° traction.

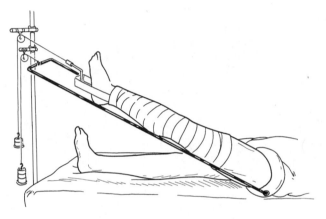

Figure 2 Straight leg traction.

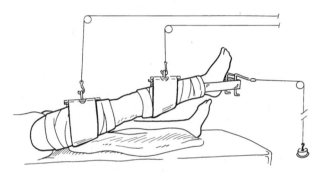

Figure 4 Split Russell traction.

References

Aronson DD, Singer RM, Higgins RF. Skeletal traction for fractures of the femoral shaft in children. J Bone Joint Surg 1987; 69A:1435.

Griffin PP, Anderson M, Greet WT. Fractures of the shaft of the femur in children. Orthop Clin North Am 1972; 3:213.

Henderson OL, Morrissey RT, Gerdes MH, McCarthy RE. Early casting of femoral shaft fractures in children. J Pediatr Orthop 1984; 4:16.

Herndon WA, Mahnken RF, Ynge DA, Sullivan JA. Management of femoral shaft fractures in the adolescent. J Pediatr Orthop 1989; 9:29.

Holmes SJK, Sedgwick DM, Scobie WG. Domiciliary gallows traction for femoral shaft fractures in young children. J Bone Joint Surg 1983; 65B:288.

Irani RN, Nicholson JT, Chung SMK. Long term results in the treatment of femoral shaft fractures in young children by immediate spica immobilization. J Bone Joint Surg 1976; 58A:945.

Kirschenbaum D, Albert MC, Robertson WW, Davidson RS. Complex femur fractures in children: Treatment with external fixation. J Pediatr Orthop 1990; 10:588.

Letts M, Vincent N, Gouw G. The "floating knee" in children. J Bone Joint Surg 1986; 68B:442.

Ligier JN, Metaizeau JP, Prévot J, Lascombes P. Elastic stable intramedullary nailing of femoral shaft fractures in children. J Bone Joint Surg 1988; 70B:74.

Litchman HR, Duffy J. Lower extremity balanced traction: A modification of Russell traction. Clin Orthop 1969; 66:144.

Mann DC, Weddington J, Davenport K. Closed Ender nailing of femoral shaft fractures in adolescents. J Pediatr Orthop 1986; 6:651.

McCarthy RE. Method of early spica cast application in treatment of pediatric femoral shaft fractures. J Pediatr Orthop 1986; 6:89.

Ogden JA. In Skeletal injury in the child. Philadelphia: W.B. Saunders, 1990.

Reeves RB, Ballard RI, Hughes JL. Internal fixation versus traction and casting of adolescent femoral shaft fractures. J Pediatr Orthop 1990; 10:592.

Reynolds DA. Growth changes in fractured long bones. J Bone Joint Surg 1981; 63B:83.

Staheli LT. Femoral and tibial growth following femoral shaft fracture in childhood. Clin Orthop 1962; 55:159.

Staheli LT, Sheridan GW. Early spica cast management of femoral shaft fractures in young children. Clin Orthop 1977; 126:162.

Stephens MM, Hsu LCS, Leong JCY. Leg length discrepancy after femoral shaft fractures in children. J Bone Joint Surg 1989; 71B:615.

Sugi M, Cole W. Early plaster treatment for fractures of the femoral shaft in childhood. J Bone Joint Surg 1987; 69B:743.

Ward WT, Levy J, Kaye A. Compression plating for child and adolescent femur fractures. J Pediatr Orthop 1992; 12:626.

Weiss AC, Schenk RC, Sponseller PD, Thompson JD. Peroneal nerve palsy after early cast application for femoral fractures in children. J Pediatr Orthop 1992; 12:25.

FRACTURE OF THE DISTAL FEMUR IN CHILDREN

A. In children, as in adults, high velocity injuries around the knee are predisposed to vascular injuries because of proximity of the vessels to the joint as well as relative "tethering" of the popliteal vessels by the adjacent muscle attachments and collateral circulation. All patients with suspected distal femoral injuries need a thorough neurovascular exam and tibial compartment assessment.

B. Undisplaced extra-articular physeal injuries may be missed if not suspected. These fall into the Salter-Harris (S-H) Classifications I and II (see p 206). Obstetric trauma may produce a S-H I injury. Low-velocity athletic injuries in adolescents that traditionally produce collateral ligament injuries will frequently yield S-H II fractures of the distal femur. Examination reveals swelling often proximal to the joint and tenderness to palpation may be more localized horizontally along the growth plate than vertically along the ligament. Stress radiographs are *not* recommended as the potential exists to displace the fracture.

C. Intra-articular fractures (S-H III and IV) need precise evaluation of the fracture at the joint surface. A gap at the joint surface of more than 2 mm or any step-off requires anatomic reduction. Either a computed tomography (CT) scan with sagittal or 3-D reconstruction or anteroposterior (AP) and lateral tomograms usually provide the needed information.

D. Immobilization requires some understanding of the mechanism of injury, because force in the wrong direction could allow fracture displacement. The metaphyseal fragment of the S-H II fractures is on the side of intact periosteum and opposite the disrupted periosteum (Fig. 1). Molding of the cast should push the distal part of the limb towards the unstable side to prevent displacement by the thick intact periosteum. As this is epiphyseal plate and metaphyseal bone, healing occurs rapidly—3 weeks for obstetric injuries and 6 to 8 weeks for the adolescent athlete. Even in low velocity injuries, growth disturbances occur and these children need to be followed to maturity, assessing leg length as well as varus and valgus deformity.

E. Displaced fractures, either intra-articular or extra-articular, suggest higher velocity injury to the plate and thus are at risk for growth injuries. All displaced intra-articular fractures require open reduction to restore an anatomic joint surface. A large percentage of the displaced extra-articular distal femoral physeal fractures will reduce by closed means. Irreducibility usually signifies entrapment of periosteum or muscle in the fracture site, and necessitates open reduction.

F. Decision making on the preferred internal fixation for these injuries needs to take into account both type of fracture and the child's age. Nonthreaded fixation across the plate is mandatory unless the plate has already started to close as documented radiographically in the contralateral noninjured limb. However, lag screws within the epiphyseal bone (Fig. 2) allow good compression of the fracture and maintenance of the joint surface reduction. In young children with small bony epiphysis and in extra-articular fractures, small smooth pins provide adequate fixation during healing (Fig. 3).

G. Extra-articular fractures that were initially displaced and could be reduced will be either stable or unstable following reduction. Using the principles of intact/disrupted periosteum (Fig. 1) for molding the cast, reduction can be easily maintained in the stable fractures. Unfortunately, a good number of the adolescent athletic injuries are unstable following reduction and require percutaneous pinning to hold the reduction during healing (Fig. 3).

H. Those distal femoral physeal fractures associated with vascular injuries require a different approach. It is essential that the vascular injury be suspected. Because children have active collateral circulation, weak pulses or pulses present with Doppler may mask a significant injury. Arteriograms and a vascular surgery consult should be obtained if there are any suspicions. In order to protect the vascular repair, all these fractures require stabilization. Lag screws in combination with smooth pins will usually suffice.

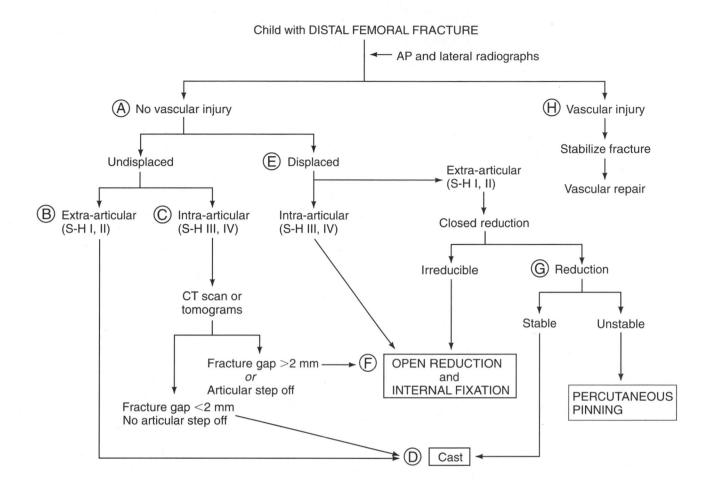

Child with DISTAL FEMORAL FRACTURE

AP and lateral radiographs

(A) No vascular injury

(H) Vascular injury

Stabilize fracture

Vascular repair

Undisplaced

(E) Displaced

Extra-articular
(S-H I, II)

Closed reduction

(B) Extra-articular
(S-H I, II)

(C) Intra-articular
(S-H III, IV)

Intra-articular
(S-H III, IV)

Irreducible

(G) Reduction

CT scan or
tomograms

Stable

Unstable

Fracture gap >2 mm
or
Articular step off

(F)

OPEN REDUCTION
and
INTERNAL FIXATION

PERCUTANEOUS
PINNING

Fracture gap <2 mm
No articular step off

(D) Cast

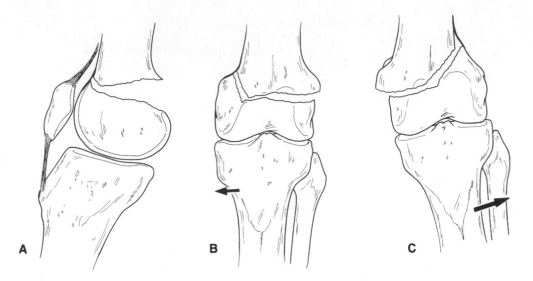

Figure 1 Intact periosteum attached to the metaphyseal fragment. **A,** Periosteum intact anteriorly; reduction accomplished with posterior force and flexion. **B,** Medial periosteum intact. **C,** Lateral periosteum intact.

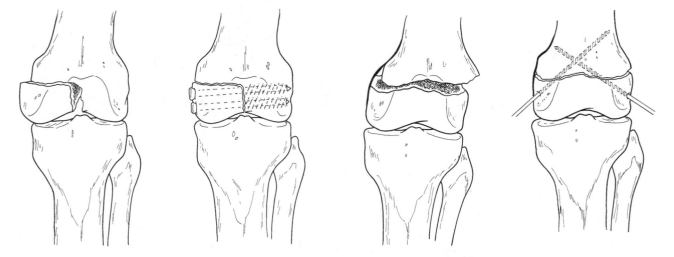

Figure 2 Intra-articular fracture treated with lag screws in the epiphysis.

Figure 3 Salter-Harris II fracture stabilized with crossed non-threaded Steinmann pins.

References

Abbott LC, Gill GG. Valgus deformity of the knee resulting from injury to the lower femoral epiphysis. Journal Bone Joint Surg 1942; 24:97.

Burman MS, Langsam MJ. Posterior dislocation of the lower femoral epiphysis in breech delivery. Arch Surg 1939; 38:250.

Cassebaum WH, Patterson AH. Fractures of the distal femoral epiphysis. Clin Orthop 1965; 41:79.

Criswell AR, Hand WL, Butler JE. Abduction injuries of the distal femoral epiphysis. 1976; 115:189.

Ford LT, Key JA. A study of experimental trauma to the distal femoral epiphysis in rabbits. J Bone Joint Surg 1956; 38A:84.

Lombardo SJ, Harvey JP. Fractures of the distal femoral epiphysis. Factors influencing prognosis: A review of thirty-four cases. J Bone Joint Surg 1977; 59A:742.

Neer CS. Separation of the lower femoral epiphysis. Am J Surg 1960; 99:756.

Ogden J. Femur in skeletal injury in the child. In: Ogden J, ed. Philadelphia: W.B. Saunders, 1990.

Riseborough EJ, Barret IR, Shapiro F. Growth disturbance following distal femoral physeal fracture—separations. J Bone Joint Surg 1983; 65A:885.

NECK DEFORMITY/RESTRICTION OF MOTION

A. Plain radiographs of the neck include anteroposterior and lateral views of the cervical spine and open mouth view of the odontoid. Appropriate additional ancillary investigations could include computed tomography (CT) of specific regions of bony anomaly evident on plain films, CT myelogram for lesions of encroachment upon the spinal cord, magnetic resonance imaging (MRI), technetium bone scan, and laboratory investigations in suspected cases of juvenile arthritis.

B. Congenital fusions of the cervical spine generally cause some restriction of motion. An exception may be a single level fusion in the lower cervical spine which may be completely asymptomatic. Any congenital fusion of the cervical spine with or without other anomaly is termed *Klippel-Feil syndrome*. Most fusions produce a combination of obvious restriction of motion and the appearance of a short neck. For more thorough discussion, see page 238.

C. Torticollis may be due to congenital muscular torticollis with contracture of the sternocleidomastoid muscle, congenital cervical spinal anomaly, extraocular muscle palsy, posterior fossa tumor, and other rare causes. These will need to be investigated fully. See page 234.

D. Congenital elevation of the scapula (actually a failure of descent of the scapula from the cervical spine to the posterior thorax during embryologic development) is termed *Sprengel's deformity* (Fig. 1). Patients with Sprengel's deformity may have other congenital anomalies, including congenital spinal and intrathecal anomalies, and should be evaluated for the same. Patients with unacceptable cosmetic deformity may be candidates for the Woodward or related procedure, which is mobilization of the scapula and reduction in a more normal position on the posterior thorax.

E. Patients with neck deformity or restriction of motion after an injury must be considered to have an acutely unstable bone and/or soft tissue injury of the cervical spine until proved otherwise. The first investigation should be a cross-table lateral radiograph to determine whether any significant dislocation or instability exists. If the cross table lateral radiograph is normal, a flexion-extension lateral radiograph should be obtained to further rule out instability. If instability is identified by either investigation, the patient's neck should be stabilized and treated appropriately. If the plain radiographs are normal, technetium bone scan, CT scan, or MRI should be performed as clinically indicated based on the severity and nature of the patient's symptoms.

F. Examples of atraumatic painful lesions of the cervical spine in children include aneurysmal bone cyst, eosinophilic granuloma, osteoid osteoma, acute calcific discitis, and other rare infectious and neoplastic causes.

G. If the patient's radiographs and clinical examination reveal torticollis, a CT scan of C1-2 should be obtained to determine whether fixed rotatory subluxation has occurred (Figs. 2 and 3). Right and left-looking horizontal studies should reveal the fixed rotational displacement of C1 on 2. See page 234.

NECK DEFORMITY/ RESTRICTION OF MOTION

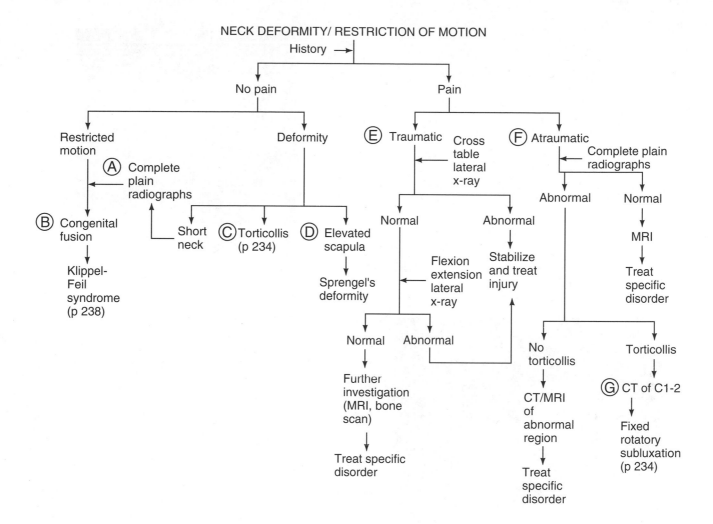

History →

No pain

Restricted motion

Ⓐ Complete plain radiographs

Ⓑ Congenital fusion

Klippel-Feil syndrome (p 238)

Deformity

Short neck

Ⓒ Torticollis (p 234)

Ⓓ Elevated scapula

Sprengel's deformity

Pain

Ⓔ Traumatic

Cross table lateral x-ray

Normal

Flexion extension lateral x-ray

Normal

Further investigation (MRI, bone scan)

Treat specific disorder

Abnormal

Abnormal

Stabilize and treat injury

Ⓕ Atraumatic

Complete plain radiographs

Abnormal

No torticollis

CT/MRI of abnormal region

Treat specific disorder

Torticollis

Ⓖ CT of C1-2

Fixed rotatory subluxation (p 234)

Normal

MRI

Treat specific disorder

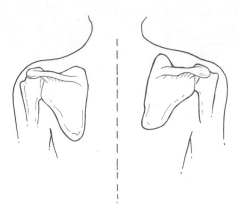

Figure 1 Sprengel's deformity is characterized by congenital elevation of the scapula. Radiographs of the spine will be necessary to rule out associated scoliosis or other congenital vertebral anomaly.

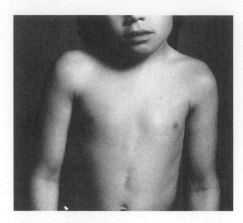

Figure 3 Child with right-sided torticollis. The etiology of the deformity will require investigation.

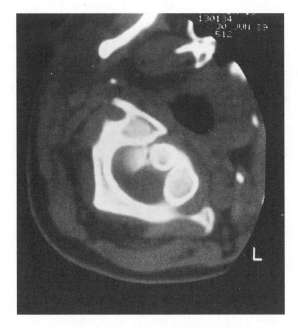

Figure 2 CT scan of fixed rotatory subluxation of C1 on C2. The fixed nature of the deformity is determined by absence of mobility of these segments on cinefluoroscopy or right and left look CT scan.

References

Bradford DS, Hensinger RM. The Pediatric Spine. New York: Thieme, 1985.

Canale ST, Griffin DW, Hubbard CN. Congenital muscular torticollis: A long-term follow-up. J Bone Joint Surg 1982; 67A:1356.

Carson WG, Lovell WW, Whitesides TE Jr. Congenital elevation of the scapula: Surgical correction by the Woodward procedure. J Bone Joint Surg 1981; 63A:1199.

Dubousset J. Torticollis in children caused by congenital anomalies of the atlas. J Bone Joint Surg 1986; 68:178.

Leibovic SJ, Ehrlich MG, Zaleske DJ. Sprengel deformity. J Bone Joint Surg 1990; 72A:192.

Mathern GW, Batzdorf V. Grisel's syndrome: Cervical spine clinical, pathologic, and neurologic manifestations. Clin Orthop 1989; 244:131.

Morrissy RT. Lovell and Winter's Pediatric Orthopaedics. Philadelphia: JB Lippincott, 1990.

Tachdjian MO. Pediatric Orthopedics. Philadelphia: WB Saunders, 1990.

Weinstein SL. The Pediatric Spine: Principles and Practice. New York: Raven Press, 1994.

TORTICOLLIS

A. The most common cause of torticollis in an infant is congenital muscular torticollis. When the sternocleidomastoid muscle (SCM) is contracted the ear is flexed towards and the chin rotated away from the affected side (Fig. 1). Other potential causes of torticollis are usually not seen in this age group but should be considered (see below).

B. Classically, infants with congenital muscular torticollis develop a firm palpable mass or nodule within the body of the affected SCM within the first few weeks of life. This mass resolves spontaneously. The presence of this mass or history of it having been present confirms the diagnosis of congenital muscular torticollis. The etiology of the mass is unknown.

C. Infants with a congenital muscular torticollis should be encouraged to actively stretch the tight SCM by looking up and over the shoulder towards the affected side (Fig. 2). Cribs and hanging toys should be situated to encourage the infant to look in this direction. In addition, parents can be taught to gently passively stretch the muscle by rotating the chin into a neutral position or beyond (i.e., towards the shoulder on the affected side) and tilting the head away from the affected side. Examine the hips carefully to rule out developmental dysplasia of the hip (DDH) as there is an association between congenital muscular torticollis and DDH. Obtain an ultrasound study or radiographs of the hips if there is any doubt.

D. If there is persistent SCM tightness after age 2 that is deemed cosmetically unacceptable to the family and physician, SCM lengthening is indicated. Clinically the SCM is lengthened in a modified V-Y fashion (Fig. 3) at the distal pole. Unusually tight SCMs should also be released at their origin on the occiput. Proximal release from the occiput requires careful protection of the spinal accessory nerve.

E. Patients who have no history of SCM mass with fixed deformities should have anteroposterior (AP) and lateral radiographs of the spine. Seek a specific vertebral anomaly. The most common ones to produce an impression of torticollis include occiput-C1-C2 anomaly such as C1 hemivertebra; other congenital asymmetric deformities in the lower cervical spine, and congenital cervicothoracic anomalies. In these patients the SCM typically is not tight on rotation. Evaluate patients with congenital cervical spinal anomalies as for Klippel-Feil syndrome and other congenital spine anomalies (see pp 238 and 310). Assess the patient for evidence of associated instability, followed by sequential radiographs to rule out progressive deformity requiring fusion.

F. Patients with no history of an SCM mass, no shortening of the SCM on physical examination, and a flexible deformity must be carefully investigated for evidence of an extraocular muscle palsy or posterior fossa tumor. Patients with strabismus on ocular movement testing require referral to an ophthalmologist. Patients with other neurologic findings require an MRI of the brain and spinal cord. Patients with uncertain findings should have one or both investigations.

G. Patients who present with an acute torticollis without evidence of bony anomaly can be presumed to have acute muscular torticollis. The etiology is usually unknown. Grisel's syndrome (acute muscular torticollis associated with an upper respiratory tract infection, and thought to occasionally lead to fixed rotatory subluxation of C1-2) is one known cause. Patients are treated symptomatically with a collar, light skin cervical traction, sedation, and analgesics until symptoms resolve. Symptoms that do not resolve within a few weeks should be investigated as to other causes (extraocular muscle palsy, posterior fossa tumor, or fixed rotatory subluxation of C1-2).

H. Fixed rotatory subluxation of C1-2 can occur spontaneously, after trauma, or after acute upper respiratory tract infection (Grisel's syndrome). There is radiographic evidence of C1-2 rotational deformity: in the AP open mouth view, the lateral masses of C1 are asymmetric, and eccentrically centered on the dens, while on the lateral radiograph there is a variable amount of C1-2 translation. Cinefluoroscopy evaluation of the cervical spine or right and left CT views demonstrate the fixed rotational deformity of C1 or C2. Patients with <3 months of symptoms are treated with traction (either skin or skeletal). If reduction is achieved, the patient is immobilized in a halo for 6–8 weeks, then periodically reassessed for evidence of recurrence or C1-2 instability. If the patient cannot be reduced or if there is C1-2 instability, C1-2 fusion is required.

I. Other potential causes of torticollis include aneurysmal bone cyst, acute calcific discitis of the cervical spine, and other rare lesions.

TORTICOLLIS

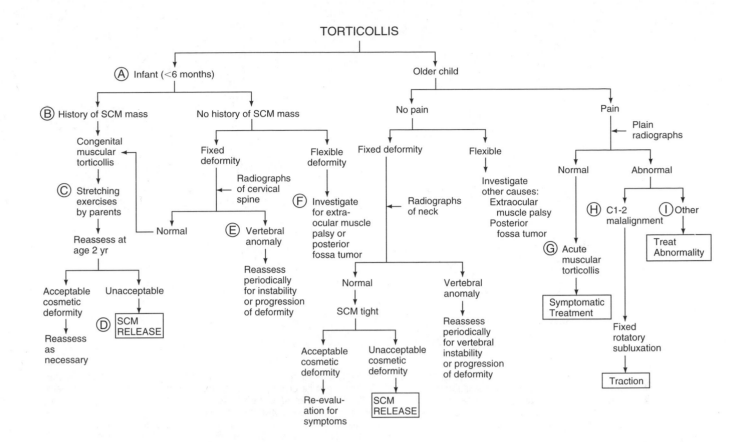

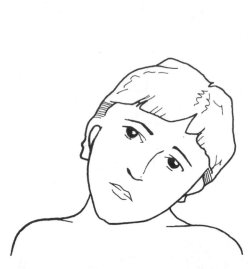

Figure 1 In patients with congenital muscular torticollis the sterno-cleidomastoid (SCM) muscle is contracted *(in this illustration, on the left).* This contracture produces lateral flexion of the head to the affected side, and rotation of the chin and face away from the affected side. Usually there is associated slight hypoplasia of the face on the affected side.

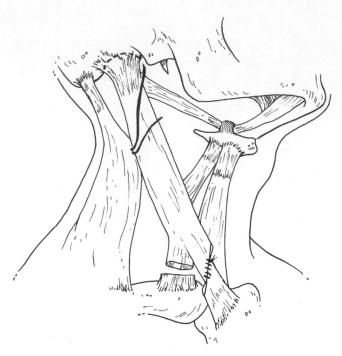

Figure 3 Surgical release of a tight SCM muscle is typically performed at its distal pole. The clavicular portion of the SCM muscle is released and the sternal portion lengthened obliquely. The sternal portion is sutured side-to-side in a lengthened fashion to preserve the outline of the SCM muscle in the neck. In extreme situations the muscle may also be removed from its insertion in the occiput *(dashed line).*

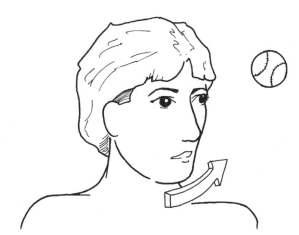

Figure 2 Gentle passive stretching exercises to reduce this deformity can be prescribed. Alternatively, objects of interest to the infant can be placed in a way to encourage the child to look actively against the deformity. In this case, with a tight left SCM muscle, these objects should be placed to the left and slightly behind the child to encourage rotation of the face towards the contracture.

References

Canale ST, Griffin DW, Hubbard CN. Congenital muscular torticollis: A long-term follow-up. J Bone Joint Surg [Am] 1982; 67:1356.

Chen JC, Au AW. Infantile torticollis: A review of 624 cases. J Pediatr Orthop 1994; 14:802.

Davis JR, Wenger DR, Mubarak SJ. Congenital muscular torticollis: Sequelae of intrauterine or perinatal compartment syndrome. J Pediatr Orthop 1993; 13:141.

Dubousset J. Torticollis in children caused by congenital anomalies of the atlas. J Bone Joint Surg [Am] 1986; 68:178.

Ferkel RD, Westin GW, Dawson EG, Oppenheim WL. Muscular torticollis: A modified surgical approach. J Bone Joint Surg [Am] 1983; 65:894.

Hummer DC Jr, MacEwen GD. The coexistence of torticollis and congenital dysplasia of the hip. J Bone Joint Surg [Am] 1972; 54:1255.

Mathern GW, Batzdorf V. Grisel's syndrome: Cervical spine clinical, pathologic, and neurologic manifestations. Clin Orthop 1989; 244:131.

Minamitani K, Inoue A, Okuno T. Results of surgical treatment of muscular torticollis for patients >6 years of age. J Pediatric Orthop 1990; 10:754.

Morrissy RT. Lovell and Winter's Pediatric Orthopaedics. Philadelphia: JB Lippincott, 1990.

Phillips WA, Hensinger RN. The management of rotatory atlanto-axial subluxation in children. J Bone Joint Surg [Am] 1989; 71:664.

Tachdjian MO. Pediatric Orthopedics. Philadelphia: WB Saunders, 1990.

KLIPPEL-FEIL SYNDROME

A. Klippel-Feil syndrome is defined as any congenital fusion of the cervical spine. Radiographic and clinical deformities vary from incidental radiographic finding of two lower cervical vertebrae fused together with no clinical signs, to a very short, webbed neck with severe restriction of neck motion (Fig. 1), and radiographic signs of multiple joint fusions and instability of the remaining few mobile segments (Fig. 2). General physical examination should determine the degree of neck instability, any evidence of neurologic dysfunction, and any associated anomalies such as scoliosis or Sprengel's deformity. Patients with Klippel-Feil syndrome have an increased incidence of congenital renal anomalies, congenital vertebral anomalies in the thoracic lumbar spine, and congenital intrathecal anomaly such as diastematomyelia or tethered cord. In addition, some patients are hearing impaired while others show subtle neurologic disorders such as mirror image movements. These signs have no implications in the management of Klippel-Feil itself. Patients should also have additional screening with anteroposterior and lateral radiographs of the spine and flexion-extension lateral radiographs of the spine to identify instability in the remaining mobile segments (Fig. 3).

B. Patients with Klippel-Feil syndrome are at some risk for developing symptomatic instability of the remaining mobile segments. This is relatively unlikely to occur with short segment, lower cervical fusions, but is more likely with upper cervical or multiple fusions. Any question regarding instability based on plain films should be further investigated by cinefluoroscopy, flexion-extension computed tomography (CT), or flexion-extension magnetic resonance imaging (MRI).

C. Patients who have no symptoms and acceptable deformity are re-evaluated once yearly with flexion extension radiographs during growth to confirm that no instability develops.

D. Patients with multiple level Klippel-Feil syndrome may have a short neck (essentially an untreatable condition), asymmetric neck deformity such as torticollis or cervical scoliosis, or webbing of the neckline. If cervical deformity is deemed unacceptable and surgical correction is being considered, the patient should first undergo MRI scan to rule out underlying intrathecal anomaly. If the sole symptom is unacceptable cosmesis due to webbing of the neck, plastic surgical Z-plasty may ameliorate those symptoms.

E. If a patient has a clinically unacceptable fixed head tilted due to asymmetric vertebral anomalies, consider correcting the head tilt by gradual skeletal traction and in situ fusion in a corrected position. Obviously, range of motion would be lost to the potential benefit of a more symmetric appearance, which should be taken into careful consideration.

F. Patients with Klippel-Feil syndrome undergoing surgical traction are at some risk for developing either cranial nerve or spinal cord dysfunction. While in traction they must be carefully monitored for this. If no neurologic dysfunction occurs and the head is gradually brought into an acceptable position, in situ posterior fusion and immobilization in a halo vest is carried out until the fusion is solid.

G. If cranial nerve or spinal cord dysfunction occurs, abandon traction. Observe the patient for progression over time; if progression occurs, perform in situ fusion.

H. If no specific anomalies are noted on MRI scan, treat the patient symptomatically with anti-inflammatory medication, analgesics, and soft surgical collar on an as-needed basis. If symptoms are resolved with this protocol, follow the patient periodically during growth with repeat flexion-extension radiographs or for resumption of symptoms.

I. If symptoms persist despite conservative care, consider in situ fusion of a symptomatic mobile segment. It is not always easy to determine which segment is causing discomfort, and further investigation including CT scan or local injections may be required. Loss of limited flexibility against the gain of decreased pain must be considered.

J. If radiographic instability of mobile segments is noted on flexion extension lateral radiographs the patient will likely require spinal fusion to stabilize the segment. Obtain flexion-extension MRI of the cervical spine to confirm that the reduced position relieves pressure on the spinal cord. If this is the case, carry out in situ fusion (usually posterior) of the unstable segment. If there is spinal cord compression in all positions, decompression and spinal fusion are required.

SUSPECTED KLIPPEL-FEIL SYNDROME

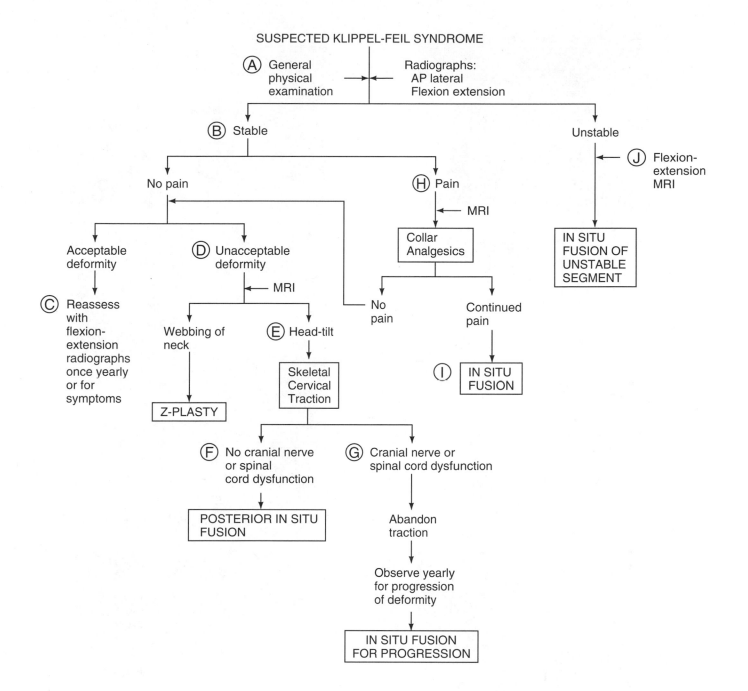

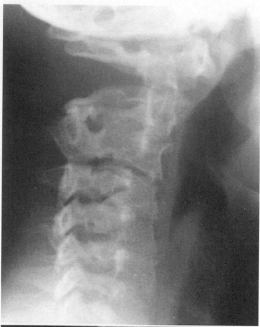

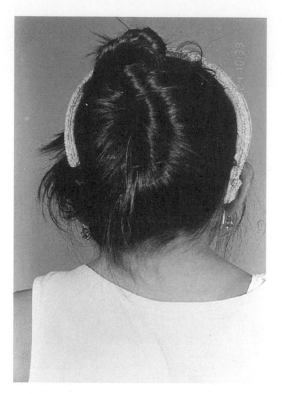

Figure 1 Klippel-Feil syndrome. Patients with significant congenital cervical fusions show restricted range of motion and a short webbed neck.

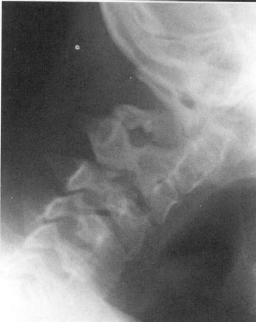

Figure 3 Flexion-extension lateral films of the cervical spine should be taken in patients with Klippel-Feil syndrome to rule out instability of the remaining mobile segments. In this example instability at C1-2 with fusions below is documented.

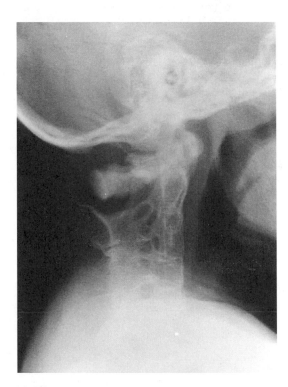

Figure 2 Radiographic appearance of Klippel-Feil syndrome. Congenital fusion of two or more cervical vertebral segments is characteristic.

References

Bradford DS, Hensinger RN. The Pediatric Spine. New York: Thieme, 1985.

Hensinger RN. Congenital anomalies of the cervical spine. Clin Orthop 1991; 264:16.

Hensinger RN, Lang JE, MacEwen GD. Klippel-Feil syndrome: A constellation of associated anomalies. J Bone Joint Surg 1974; 56A:1246.

Pizzutillo PD, Woods MW, Nicholson L. Risk factors in Klippel-Feil syndrome. Orthop Trans 1987; 11:473.

Weinstein SL. The Pediatric Spine: Principles and Practice. New York: Raven Press, 1994.

Winter RB, Moe JH, Lonstein JE. The incidence of Klippel-Feil syndrome in patients with congenital scoliosis and kyphosis. Spine 1984; 9:363.

FOOT DEFORMITY

A. The majority of foot deformities (e.g., metatarsus adductus [Fig. 1], clubfoot [Fig. 2], flatfoot) occur in otherwise healthy infants. However, most generalized neurologic disorders such as spina bifida, spinal dysraphism, and arthrogryposis frequently have associated foot disorders. Therefore the first component of examination of a child with a foot deformity is a general neuromuscular assessment including an evaluation of the spinal column. Any abnormalities should be investigated further.

B. A flexible equinovarus foot is very common postural deformity of the neonate. Emphasis is placed on the term *flexible* (i.e., both the forefoot adductus and hindfoot varus are easily, readily, and completely correctable to a normal position). Complete, spontaneous resolution of this postural deformity should be expected without treatment. Occasionally a child has a more severe deformity than average, or one with somewhat equivocal flexibility. These patients should be treated with serial casts and re-evaluation. Persistence or accentuation of the deformity should prompt re-evaluation of the child's neurologic status.

C. Fixed hindfoot equinus associated with a neutral or valgus forefoot which is also fixed is indicative of congenital vertical talus. Patients with vertical talus frequently have a known disorder such as spina bifida or arthrogryposis, or an occult spinal cord abnormality. Please see the chapter on Vertical Talus (p. 266).

D. Calcaneovalgus deformity of the foot can be seen as an anomaly associated with posteromedial bow of the tibia. The bowing of such tibial deformities is typically in the lower third of the tibia, with apex posteromedial. There is always some associated tibial shortening although this may not be readily apparent at initial evaluation. Although the calcaneovalgus deformity will resolve and the bowing deformity usually resolves, periodic re-evaluation is required to quantify progressive limb length inequality. Please see the chapter on Congenital Leg Deformity (p. 270).

E. Postural calcaneovalgus foot deformity can be a dramatic deformity characterized by marked dorsiflexion of the forefoot (Fig. 3). It is important to rule out associated neurologic abnormality, which is usually easy to do based on physical examination. Congenital vertical talus deformity is superficially similar; however, careful examination of the hindfoot will differentiate the two. In postural calcaneovalgus foot deformity the hindfoot is in calcaneus whereas in vertical talus the hindfoot is in equinus. The tibia should be palpated, and if necessary radiographs of the leg taken, to differentiate between simple calcaneovalgus foot deformity and that associated with posteromedial bow of the tibia.

F. Postural calcaneovalgus foot deformity in an otherwise healthy child without other anomaly can be expected to resolve spontaneously prior to walking age without treatment. Persistent deformity requires re-evaluation of the neurologic status of the child. A true equinocavus foot deformity is almost always associated with spinal cord abnormality such as lipoma, tethered cord from other causes, or spina bifida. If a specific neurologic abnormality is not known, a cause should be sought. If the deformity is interfering with function, surgery to restore a plantigrade foot is required. Soft tissue and/or bony procedures as appropriate for the child's age, severity of deformity, and the underlying diagnosis will need to be performed.

G. Cavovarus feet are characterized by forefoot plantiflexion with secondary dorsiflexion of the hindfoot to accommodate the forefoot deformity. Thus on clinical examination dorsiflexion appears to be limited, but this is because the hindfoot is already dorsiflexed maximally to accommodate the forefoot deformity. This is readily apparent on radiographs. Cavovarus foot deformity is usually associated with an identifiable neuromuscular cause, and specific diagnosis should be sought in addition to treating the deformity itself. Please see the chapter on Cavus Foot (p. 254).

FOOT DEFORMITY

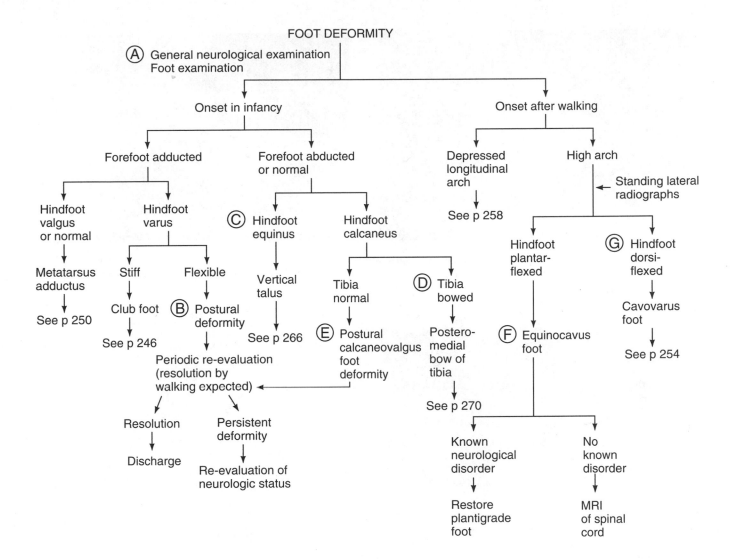

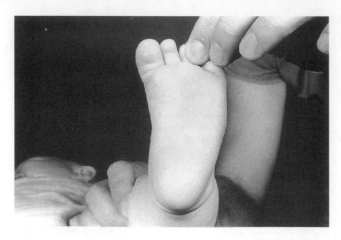

Figure 1 Metatarsus adductus. The forefoot is adducted relative to the hindfoot, which is in normal alignment or valgus.

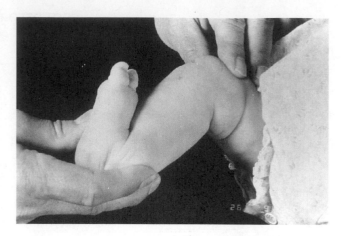

Figure 3 Calcaneovalgus foot. The foot is markedly dorsiflexed, with no underlying tibial deformity. Examination will reveal a limitation of plantarflexion.

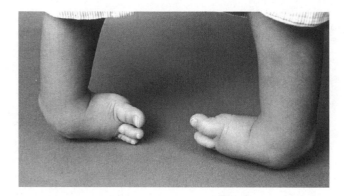

Figure 2 Clubfoot deformity. There is marked equinovarus of the foot, with forefoot adductus and supination. The foot deformity is resistant to passive correction.

References

Bensahel H, Catterall A, Dimeglio A. Practical applications in idiopathic clubfoot: A retrospective multicentric study in EPOS. J Pediatr Orthop 1990; 10:186-188.

Bleck EE. Metatarsus adductus: Classification and relationship to outcomes of treatment. J Pediatr Orthop 1983; 3:2.

Carroll NC. Congenital clubfoot: Pathoanatomy and treatment. Instr Course Lect 1987; 36:117.

Clark MW, D'Ambrosia RD, Ferguson AB. Congenital vertical talus. J Bone Joint Surg 1977; 59A:816.

Coleman SS. Complex Foot Deformity in Children. Philadelphia: Lea & Febiger, 1983.

Hensinger RN, Lang JE, MacEwen GD. Klippel-Feil syndrome: A constellation of associated anomalies. J Bone Joint Surg 1974; 56A:1246.

Morrissy RT. Lovell and Winter's Pediatric Orthopaedics. Philadelphia: JB Lippincott, 1990.

Mosier KM, Asher A. Tarsal coalition and peroneal spastic flatfoot: A review. J Bone Joint Surg 1986; 66A:976.

Tachdjian MO. The Child's Foot. Philadelphia: WB Saunders, 1985.

Tachdjian MO. Pediatric Orthopaedics. Philadelphia: WB Saunders, 1990.

Wenger DR, Mauldin D, Speck G, et al. Corrective shoes and inserts as treatment for flexible flatfoot in infants and children. J Bone Joint Surg 1989; 69A:800.

CLUBFOOT DEFORMITY

A. All patients with clubfoot deformity require a thorough general examination. Approximately 50% have bilateral deformities, often asymmetric in severity. These patients have an increased prevalence of developmental dysplasia of the hip (DDH). Specific associated neurologic or related disorders such as spina bifida and arthrogryposis must be ruled out. More subtle forms of spinal dysraphism may require radiographic evaluation of the spinal column or magnetic resonance imaging if tethered cord is suspected.

B. The fundamental management of congenital clubfoot deformity is passive manipulation of the foot into a corrected position, beginning as early as possible (Fig. 1). Manipulations first concentrate on eversion and abduction of the forefoot. Once completed, this is followed by dorsiflexion of the hindfoot. Between manipulation sessions, the foot must be held steady in some way. Most authors prefer casts, either short leg or long leg, but taping or splinting may be used if effective in the treating physician's hands.

C. Many clubfeet respond only partially to even vigorous passive manipulation and meticulous splinting or casting. Dorsiflexion lateral radiograph taken between the age of 3 and 4 months can allow the treating physician to evaluate the response of the clubfoot to manipulation (Fig. 2). On a dorsiflexion lateral radiograph, the axes of the talus and calcaneus normally converge at an angle of 20–40°. When there is resistant hindfoot deformity that axis is parallel. In addition, the absolute position of the calcaneus is reversed into an equinus position. Feet with persistent equinus and parallelism of the talus and calcaneus require surgical release. When the forefoot is dorsiflexed while the hindfoot is plantarflexed, a rocker bottom deformity is occurring. Discontinue casting with these findings.

   If the dorsiflexion lateral radiograph shows a converging talocalcaneal (T-C) angle (Fig. 3), conservative treatment may yet be successful. If the hindfoot is corrected, casting or other form of splinting should continue until walking age. Occasionally the dorsiflexion lateral radiograph is inconclusive. When this is the case serial manipulation and casting should continue. Repeat radiographs monthly until an evaluation can be made on either radiographic or clinical grounds.

D. There are two main approaches to surgical management of clubfoot. The posteromedial release described by Turco concentrates on the posterior, medial, and subtalar aspects of the deformity. Goldner and others have emphasized the posterolateral ligament complex of the tibia and fibula, and calcaneo-cuboid lateral release. Most series report 80%–90% clinically acceptable outcome irrespective of the surgical technique selected. The most likely untoward events are recurrence of the deformity, persistence of some aspect of the deformity (such as forefoot adductus, internal torsion of the entire foot) or overcorrection. Overcorrection produces a calcaneovalgus foot, which is both unsightly and weak. Ideal timing of surgery is controversial and has been recommended by various authors as between 6 weeks of age to after walking.

E. The most common complication of surgical release of clubfoot deformity is recurrence of the deformity. First rule out any underlying occult neurologic condition leading to muscle imbalance. Most truly recurrent deformities become apparent within 2 years after successful conservative management or surgery. Corrected clubfeet are several shoe sizes smaller than the normal contralateral foot, and the calf circumference is diminished, irrespective of the treatment modality.

F. Very occasionally there is gradual recurrence of forefoot deformity, which remains passively correctable. Split transfer of the tibialis anterior to the cuboid can correct this deformity.

G. If deformity recurs, soft tissue release can be repeated in patients up to age 8 years. The repeat release usually needs to be combined with some form of lateral column shortening (Lichtblau, cuboid decancellation, or cuboid wedge resection).

H. Severe multiply operated recurrent deformities in older patients may require triple arthrodesis to effect correction.

I. Prior to walking age there is a very strong propensity for clubfoot deformity to recur. Therefore the foot should be maintained in a corrected position with cast, splint, or corrective shoes until walking age.

J. In occasional clubfeet, the dorsiflexion lateral radiograph shows convergence of the T-C angle, but there is both radiographic and clinical evidence of mild equinus. In these circumstances percutaneous heelcord lengthening in the outpatient clinic can improve dorsiflexion. Casting is continued for 3–6 weeks after the heelcord lengthening followed by splinting until walking age.

K. Feet that remain plantigrade after conservative treatment should be re-examined periodically throughout growth for evidence of recurrence. Use of short leg braces to maintain the foot in a neutral position after walking age is controversial; recommendations vary from never using them to using them routinely until age 7. Most deformities that recur do so within 2 years of cessation of treatment.

CONGENITAL CLUBFOOT DEFORMITY

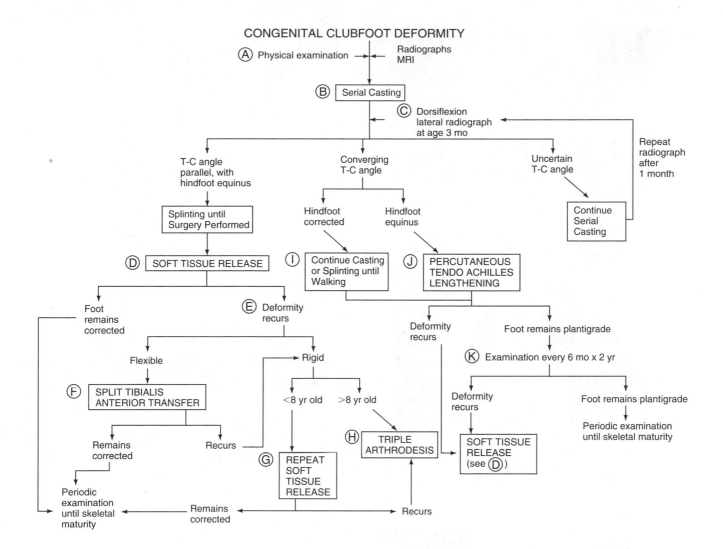

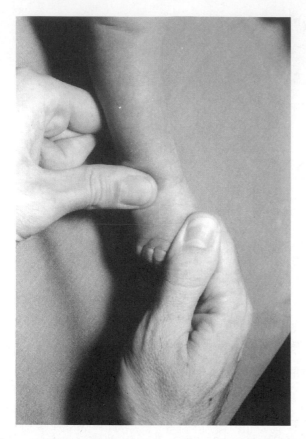

Figure 1 Initial conservative treatment consists of passive manipulation of the deformity, commencing with forefoot deformity. The foot is held in the corrected position between manipulations by splint or cast.

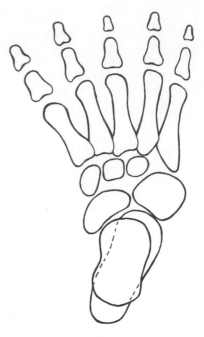

Figure 3 Schema of clubfoot deformity. The calcaneus is rotated underneath the talus rather than deviating laterally from it (reduced AP talocalcaneal angle). The forefoot is adducted relative to the hindfoot.

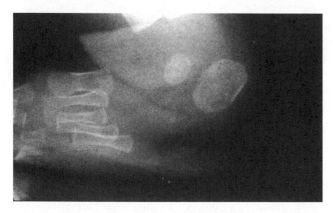

Figure 2 Typical lateral radiographic appearance of a resistant clubfoot with attempted dorsiflexion at age 3 to 4 months. The lateral talocalcaneal angle is reduced, the hindfoot remains in equinus, and secondary dorsiflexion occurs through the midfoot.

References

Bensahel H, Catterall A, Demeglio A. Practical applications in idiopathic clubfoot: A retrospective multicentric study in EPOS. J Pediatr Orthop 1990; 10:186.

Carroll NC. Congenital clubfoot: Pathoanatomy and treatment. Instr Course Lect 1987; 36:117.

Coleman SS. Complex Foot Deformity in Children. Philadelphia: Lea & Febiger, 1983.

Cowell JR, Wein BK. Genetic aspects of club foot. J Bone Joint Surg 1980; 62A:1381.

Crawford AH, Marxen JL, Osterfeld DL. The Cincinnati incision: A comprehensive approach for surgical procedures of the foot and ankle in childhood. J Bone Joint Surg 1982; 64A:1355.

Herzenberg J, Carroll N, Christofersen MR, et al. Clubfoot analysis with three-dimensional computer modeling. J Pediatr Orthop 1988; 8:257.

Kite JH. Principles involved in the treatment of congenital clubfoot: The results of treatment. J Bone Joint Surg 1973; 55A:1377.

Morrissy RT. Lovell and Winter's Pediatric Orthopaedics. Philadelphia: JB Lippincott, 1990.

Tachdjian MO. The Child's Foot. Philadelphia: WB Saunders, 1985.

Turco VJ. Resistant congenital clubfoot—one-stage posteromedial release with internal fixation: A follow-up report of a fifteen-year experience. J Bone Joint Surg 1971; 53A:447.

METATARSUS ADDUCTUS

A. Patients with metatarsus adductus typically present between birth and age 6 months. Most deformities seen in the neonatal nursery are quite flexible and resolve rapidly and spontaneously, requiring no treatment. Patients with persistent deformity or more severe or rigid deformity may require treatment. Serial casting is documented to be effective in patients up to 8 months of age.

B. While examining a child under 8 months of age, assess the flexibility of the lateral border of the foot (Fig. 1). If it is correctable to neutral or beyond with gentle pressure the parents may be taught passive stretching exercises and the patient reassessed after 6 weeks of such exercises. If there is resolution of the deformity, reassess the patient as necessary for recurrence. If there has been no improvement in the severity of the deformity, the patient should undergo serial casting.

C. If the lateral border of the foot is not passively correctable, treat the patient with serial short leg casts gradually abducting the forefoot for 6 to 8 weeks. After casting is discontinued the patient should be held in straight or reverse last shoes until walking independently. In most cases the deformity resolves and the patient can be reassessed as necessary for recurrence. If there is no resolution of the deformity, reassess the patient after age 5.

D. Children over 8 months of age are generally thought to be recalcitrant to conservative management such as serial casting or reverse last shoes. In the past, patients deemed to have sufficient deformity in this age group have undergone Heyman-Herndon metatarsal capsulotomy with postoperative cast correction. The long-term results of this procedure, however, are not satisfactory. Therefore patients in this age group should have neither conservative nor surgical treatment. Some patients show sufficient spontaneous resolution in this period that further treatment is not required. If, however, after age 5 there is persistent deformity, consider surgery.

E. Persistent metatarsus adductus in children over age 5 can be subdivided into major components of (1) dynamic adduction of the great toe only, (2) metatarsus primus varus, or (3) full metatarsus adductus. Patients who have clinical and radiographic evidence of normal alignment of the lateral rays of the foot and dynamic adduction of the great toe only can be considered for surgical lengthening of the adductor tendon and 6 to 8 weeks of cast immobilization.

F. Patients who have clinical and radiographic evidence of metatarsus primus varus only may be treated by surgical realignment of the first ray. The procedure to be performed is determined by the location of the deformity and the presence or absence of an open physis at the base of the first metatarsal. Correction of this deformity may be either accomplished by first metatarsal osteotomy (avoiding the physis at the base of the first metatarsal if open) or by the Fowler procedure (opening wedge first cuneiform-metatarsal joint arthrodesis with bone graft).

G. Patients who have a full metatarsus adductus involving all the rays of the foot and sufficient deformity to warrant surgical correction should undergo metatarsal osteotomy with cast immobilization for 6 to 8 weeks (Fig. 2). Osteotomy of the first metatarsal must avoid the physis at the base of the first ray; osteotomy may alternatively be replaced by first cuneiform-metatarsal joint capsulotomy. Occasionally medial and plantar soft tissue lengthening is required in addition to the osteotomy to fully correct the foot.

SUSPECTED METATARSUS ADDUCTUS

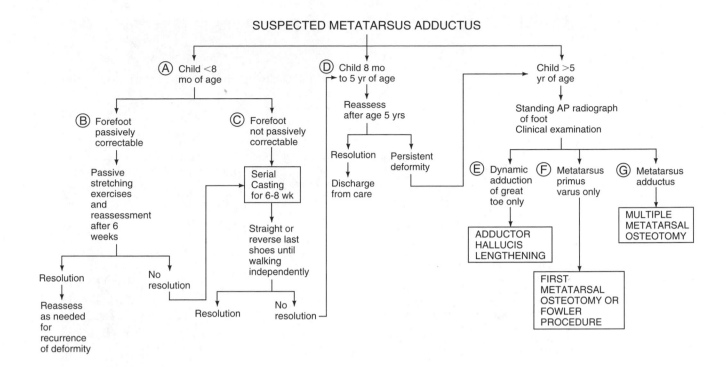

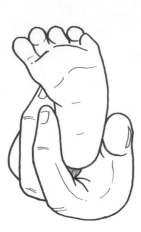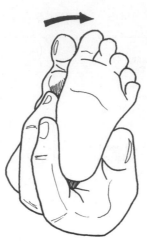

Figure 1 Metatarsus adductus is characterized by forefoot adduction relative to the hindfoot, best seen as rounding of the lateral border of the foot. Normally, the lateral border of the foot is straight. The severity of metatarsus adductus can be characterized by assessing the flexibility of the forefoot by abducting the forefoot with the hindfoot stabilized. Mild deformities easily correct to neutral or beyond, moderate deformities correct to neutral with pressure only, and severe deformities cannot be passively corrected.

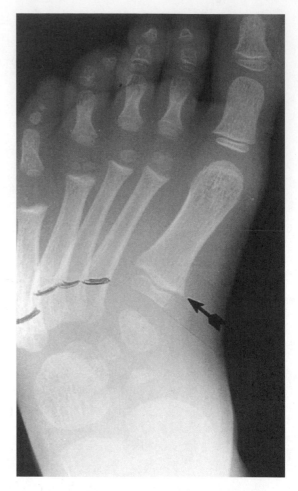

Figure 2 Radiograph of persistent metatarsus adductus deformity. Osteotomies may be performed at the base of the second through fifth metatarsals. Osteotomy of the first metatarsal must avoid the physis at its base *(arrow)*. Alternatively, the first cuneiform-metatarsal joint may be opened without performing an osteotomy.

References

Berg EE. A reappraisal of metatarsus adductus and skewfoot. J Bone Joint Surg [Am] 1986; 68:1185.

Bleck EE. Metatarsus adductus: Classification and relationship to outcomes of treatment. J Pediatr Orthop 1983; 3:2.

Coleman SS. Complex Foot Deformity in Children. Philadelphia: Lea & Febiger, 1983.

Farsetti P, Weinstein SL, Ponseti IV. The long-term functional and radiographic outcomes of untreated and non-operatively treated metatarsus adductus. J Bone Joint Surg [Am] 1994; 76:257.

Heyman CH, Herndon CH, Strong JM. Mobilization of the tar-sometatarsal and intermetatarsal joints for the correction of resistant adduction of the fore part of the foot in congenital club-foot or congenital metatarsus varus. J Bone Joint Surg [Am] 1958; 40:299.

Morrissy RT. Lovell and Winter's Pediatric Orthopaedics. Philadelphia: JB Lippincott, 1990.

Rushforth GF. The natural history of hooked forefoot. J Bone Joint Surg [Br] 1978; 60:530.

Stark JG, Johanson JE, Winter RB. The Heyman-Herndon tar-sometatarsal capsulotomy for metatarsus adductus: Results in 48 feet. J Pediatr Orthop 1987; 7:305.

Tachdjian MO. The Child's Foot. Philadelphia: WB Saunders, 1985.

CAVUS FOOT

A. Patients with a cavus foot must have a specific neurological diagnosis confirmed wherever possible, particularly when the deformity is unilateral. Often a known neurological disturbance such as documented cerebral palsy, spina bifida, or polio can be readily identified. Other common causes include Charcot-Marie tooth disease, Friedreich's ataxia, tethered cord, and other intrathecal anomalies such as lipoma or diastematomyelia. The diagnosis of idiopathic cavovarus feet is reserved for patients who cannot be identified as having one of the preceding diagnoses. Radiographs and magnetic resonance imaging of the spine, neurology consultation including nerve conduction velocities, electromyography, and muscle and/or nerve biopsies may be required to make the specific diagnosis.

B. Some patients have no symptoms associated with cavus feet. Evaluate the patient periodically for development of symptoms or progression of deformity that will require treatment.

C. Symptoms associated with cavus feet include local pressure phenomena of the toes, heel, or ball of the foot due to excessive weight bearing or ill fitting shoes; ankle sprains predisposed to by hindfoot varus; or pain in the calves from muscle weakness due to the underlying neurologic disorder. Conservative measures may be tried (when the patient has mild symptoms and deformity), including shoes with ample toe boxes for the deformed foot, custom-molded arch supports, ankle stirrup splints for instability, and ankle foot orthoses. These measures should be reserved for patients with mild deformity and mild symptoms, since they often are otherwise ineffective.

D. Patients with cavus feet are typically symptomatic and recalcitrant to conservative management. The basic deformity is forefoot plantarflexion and pronation (i.e., the first metatarsal is plantarflexed more than the lateral metatarsals) due to muscle imbalance from the underlying disorder. The plantar fascia contracts, and there is a variable amount of toe clawing. In stance, the hindfoot rolls into varus and dorsiflexes to accommodate the fixed forefoot deformity. The patient appears to have hindfoot equinus but lateral standing radiographs almost always confirm that the hindfoot is in a position of maximum dorsiflexion (Fig. 1). Surgical principles are to correct forefoot deformity and balance musculature by appropriate tendon transfer. The first preoperative assessment (after the specific etiologic diagnosis has been confirmed) is to determine the flexibility of the hindfoot deformity with the Coleman block test (Fig. 2). The patient stands with the heel and lateral border of the foot on a 1 to 2 cm block allowing the first ray to droop off the block to-

wards the floor. The block thus accommodates the plantarflexion pronation deformity of the first metatarsal. View the heel from behind to determine whether the hindfoot deformity is flexible or fixed.

E. When the hindfoot varus deformity is flexible the hindfoot has a normal valgus appearance with the Coleman block test. In such circumstances Dwyer osteotomy of the calcaneus or triple arthrodesis is usually not required.

F. The first stage of surgical treatment is plantar fascia release and first metatarsal or midfoot osteotomy to correct the forefoot plantarflexion, pronation deformity (Fig. 3). The second stage is creation of a balance in the musculature about the foot and ankle. The tendon transfer or combination performed is based on careful assessment of muscle strength about the foot. Posterior tibial tendon (PTT) transfer through the interosseous membrane to the dorsum of the foot will transform the plantarflexion-inversion force of the PTT into an ankle dorsiflexion-assisting motor. An alternative is peroneus longus transfer to the dorsum of the foot, removing the plantarflexion force on the first metatarsal and converting it into an ankle dorsiflexor. Other common tendon transfers include extensor digitorum and extensor hallucis longus transfers to the metatarsals in addition to interphalangeal (IP) joint fusion for symptomatic claw toes.

G. After corrective surgery symptoms may continue. These can be due to symptomatic claw toes, progression of the deformity or inadequate correction causing asymmetric weight bearing, or continued muscular pains due to the underlying neurologic diagnosis.

H. Claw toes are treated by IP joint fusion and transfer of the long-toe extensors to the metatarsals.

I. Patients with persistence of a symptomatic nonplantigrade foot should be converted to a triple arthrodesis with wedges in the hind and mid-foot calculated to correct the varus and forefoot deformities.

J. Patients with a plantigrade foot but muscular symptoms can be treated with a solid ankle foot orthosis (AFO).

K. If on Coleman block test the hindfoot does not correct, the varus deformity is fixed. In these circumstances a Dwyer osteotomy must be performed in conjunction with surgery and principles (see F), or alternatively triple arthrodesis performed. When triple arthrodesis is performed primarily the same considerations for muscle-balancing tendon transfers must be made.

SUSPECTED CAVUS FOOT DEFORMITY

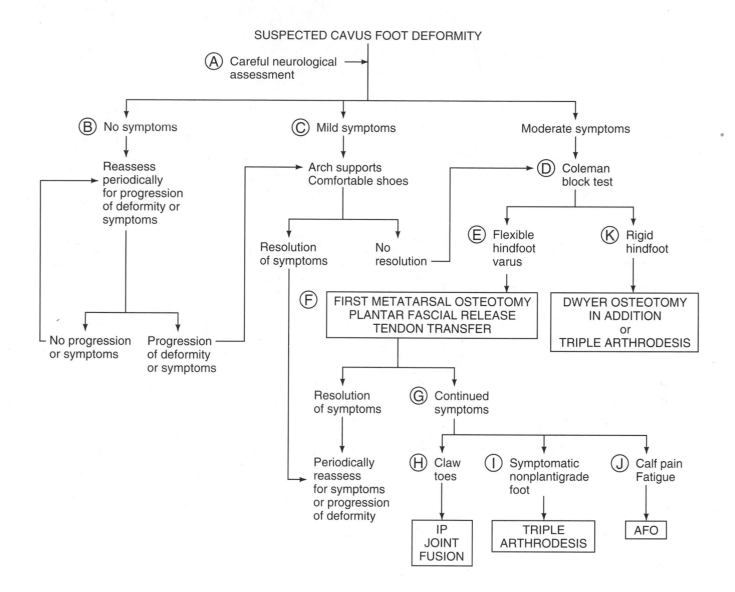

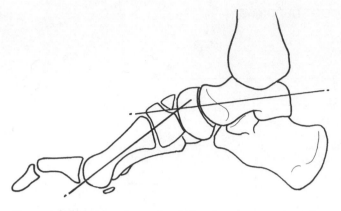

Figure 1 Lateral standing radiographs of a cavovarus foot show an increase in Meary's angle (the angle between the axis of the talus and the first metatarsal) due to plantarflexion of the forefoot. Lateral weight-bearing films generally demonstrate that the calcaneus is in dorsiflexion and that the talus is maximally dorsiflexed within the ankle mortise.

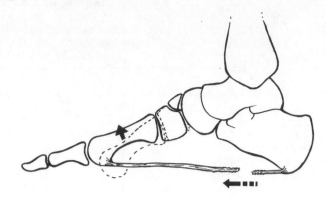

Figure 3 Surgical correction of cavus deformity. The plantar fascia should be divided, with dorsiflexion osteotomy of the first ray. If hindfoot varus is flexible, it will correct with the foot in this position. In this illustration the hindfoot varus is fixed.

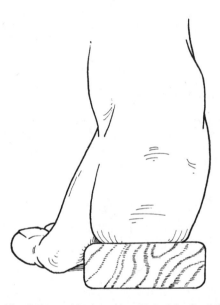

Figure 2 The Coleman block test is a test of the flexibility of hindfoot deformity. A block is placed under the lateral aspect of the heel and forefoot, thus accommodating the plantar flexion deformity of the first ray. If hindfoot varus is flexible, this deformity will be corrected with the foot in this position. In this illustration the hindfoot varus is fixed.

References

Bradley GW, Coleman SS. The treatment of the calcaneocavus foot deformity. J Bone Joint Surg [Am] 1981; 63:1159.

Coleman SS. Complex Foot Deformity in Children. Philadelphia: Lea & Febiger, 1983.

Coleman SS, Chesnut WJ. A simple test for hindfoot flexibility in the cavovarus foot. Clin Orthop 1977; 123:60.

Dwyer FC. Osteotomy of the calcaneus for pes cavus. J Bone Joint Surg [Br] 1959; 41:80.

Levitt RL, Canale ST, Cooke AJ, Gartland JJ. The role of foot surgery in progressive neuromuscular disorders in children. J Bone Joint Surg [Am] 1973; 55:1396.

Paulos LE, Coleman SS, Samuelson KM. Pes cavovarus: Review of a surgical approach using soft tissue procedures. J Bone Joint Surg [Am] 1980; 62:942.

Shapiro F, Bresnan MJ. Orthopaedic management of childhood neuromuscular disease. Part II: Peripheral neuropathies, Friedreich's ataxia and arthrogryposis multiplex congenita. J Bone Joint Surg [Am] 1982; 64:949.

Sherman FC, Westin GW. Plantar release in the correction of deformities of the foot in childhood. J Bone Joint Surg [Am] 1981; 63:1382.

Tachdjian MO. The Child's Foot. Philadelphia: WB Saunders, 1985.

Wukich DK, Bowen JR. A long-term study of triple arthrodesis for correction of pes cavovarus in Charcot-Marie-Tooth disease. J Pediatr Orthop 1989; 9:433.

FLATFOOT DEFORMITY

A. Patients presenting with the common complaint of flatfoot deformity (Fig. 1) with or without symptoms should have a general assessment of their mobility, strength, and lower extremity alignment. Occasionally patients with decreased muscle tone or generalized skeletal dysplasia present with a complaint of flatfoot deformity. Assess the foot carefully, including subtalar motion, ankle dorsiflexion and plantarflexion, and forefoot mobility. Check the condition of the longitudinal arch in the non−weight-bearing position. A flexible longitudinal arch may be ablated in the weight-bearing position and reconstituted in the non−weight-bearing position or when the patient is asked to walk on his toes. If subtalar motion and ankle dorsiflexion are normal and the longitudinal arch is reconstituted in the non−weight-bearing or toe-walking position (Fig. 2), the patient has a flexible flatfoot deformity. If there is a tight heelcord, limited subtalar motion or abnormal forefoot flexibility, or the longitudinal arch is not reconstituted in the non−weight-bearing or toe-walking position, the diagnosis is other than flexible flatfoot deformity.

B. The most common patient to present with parental complaint of flatfoot deformity is between the age of 2 and 5 years. This is due to the fact that the patients are flexible and have a physiologic valgus lower extremity alignment. In the weight-bearing position the longitudinal arch flattens, and reconstitutes in a non−weight-bearing position. If the patient has no symptoms and these physical findings, the parents can be reassured and no treatment recommended. The patient should be reassessed after age 5 (when physiologic valgus deformity should be resolving) for persistence of the deformity or for symptoms. Arch supports and other corrective measures are not indicated.

C. It is most unusual for patients under age 5 with flexible flatfoot deformity to have symptoms other than parental concern. True consistent symptoms should be carefully evaluated with appropriate investigation. These investigations include plain radiographs of the foot looking for bony anomaly (Fig. 3), erythrocyte sedimentation rate (ESR) to rule out inflammatory arthritis (which can present in the subtalar or talonavicular joint), technetium bone scan, and computed tomography (CT) or magnetic resonance imaging (MRI) to rule out specific local abnormality.

D. If the patient is over age 5 with flexible flatfoot deformity, lower extremity alignment should be assessed. Usually by this age the physiologic valgus deformity is resolved.

E. Patients over 5 who have symptomatic but apparently typical flexible flatfoot deformity should be further in-

vestigated, because consistent symptoms are unusual in patients with true flexible flatfoot. Investigations should be carried out as per C above. If a specific abnormality is identified, it is treated.

F. If test results are normal and the patient appears to have a truly symptomatic flexible flatfoot deformity he may be treated with an arch support for symptoms. Typically one or two sets of arch supports worn in regular shoes control symptoms. Caution the family that an effort is not being made to change the appearance of the foot but simply to control the symptoms.

G. In very rare circumstances patients with severe flexible flatfoot deformity cannot be symptomatically controlled with supports. In these rare circumstances surgical correction can be considered. Surgical options include Grice subtalar arthrodesis (to correct the hindfoot valgus), or lateral column lengthening calcaneal osteotomy with or without talonavicular joint capsulorrhaphy. The need for surgical correction is very rare.

H. Patients with flexible flatfoot deformity due to persistent genu valgum should be assessed to determine the cause of the persistent genu valgum.

I. Patients with decreased subtalar motion on physical examination should have anteroposterior lateral and oblique radiographs to assess any bony deformity.

J. Tarsal coalition can present as a peroneal spastic flatfoot with decreased subtalar motion and peroneal muscle spasm. Oblique radiographs demonstrate a calcaneonavicular bar. Subtalar coalition may require CT scan for adequate visualization.

K. Vertical talus presents as a rigid flatfoot deformity with decreased subtalar motion, hindfoot equinus, and forefoot valgus deformity. Dorsiflexion and plantarflexion radiographs confirm the diagnosis.

L. Heelcord contracture from any cause can lead to secondary flatfoot deformity due to breakdown of the longitudinal arch to compensate for the hindfoot equinus. Initial investigation is directed toward identifying the cause of heelcord contracture. Classically this is seen in association with static encephalopathy (cerebral palsy) readily identified by careful history and physical examination. More rarely, the contracture can be a subtle sign of tethered cord syndrome, determined by MRI. Treat the symptomatic patient with heel lift or ankle foot orthosis (AFO) accommodating the heelcord contracture. If this is inadequate, heelcord lengthening can be considered for symptomatic patients. Typically this will not improve the appearance of the foot, but allow the foot to be stabilized more effectively in an AFO.

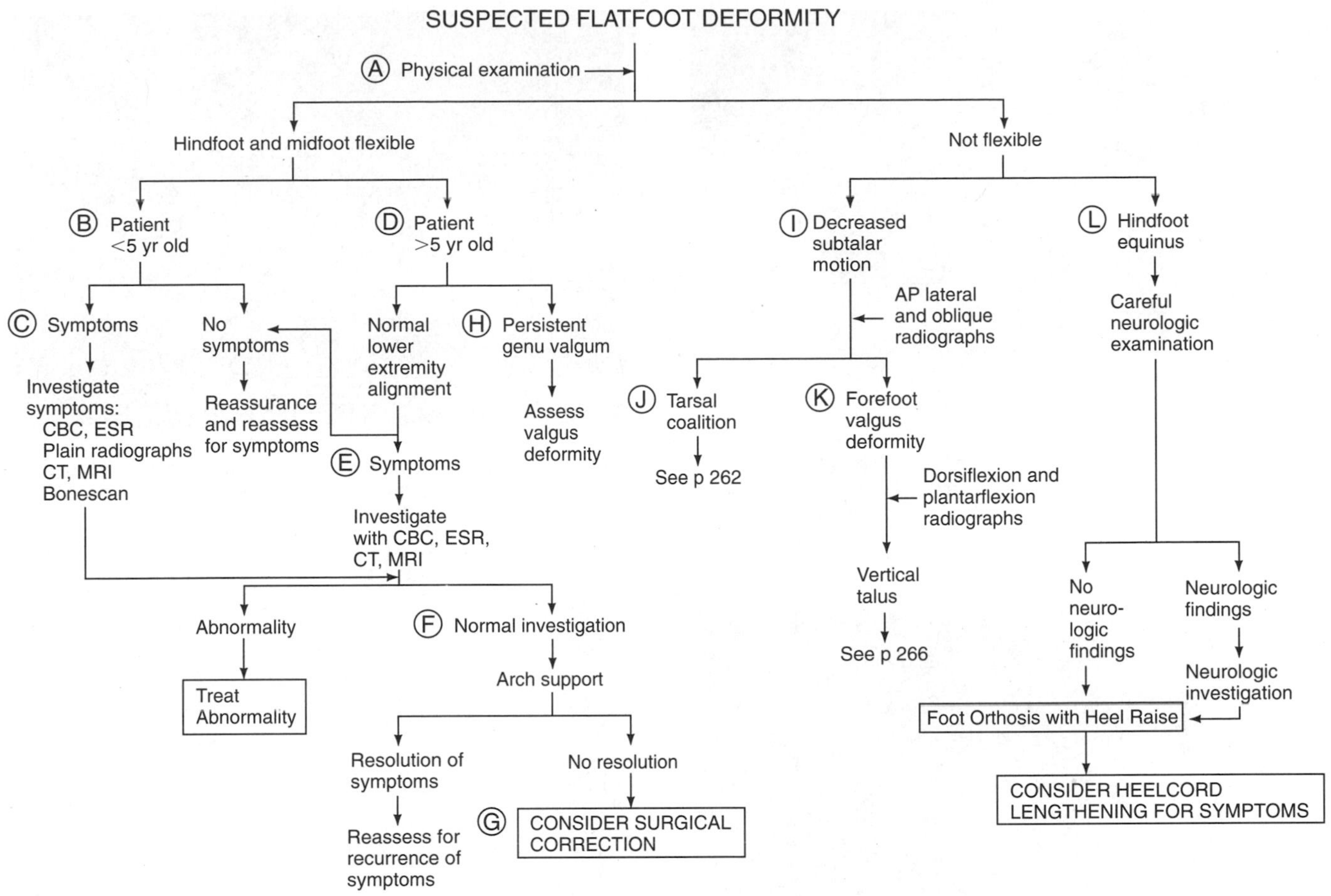

SUSPECTED FLATFOOT DEFORMITY

(A) Physical examination →

Hindfoot and midfoot flexible

(B) Patient <5 yr old

(C) Symptoms

Investigate symptoms:
CBC, ESR
Plain radiographs
CT, MRI
Bonescan

No symptoms

Reassurance and reassess for symptoms

(D) Patient >5 yr old

Normal lower extremity alignment

(E) Symptoms

Investigate with CBC, ESR, CT, MRI

(H) Persistent genu valgum

Assess valgus deformity

Abnormality

Treat Abnormality

(F) Normal investigation

Arch support

Resolution of symptoms

Reassess for recurrence of symptoms

No resolution

(G) CONSIDER SURGICAL CORRECTION

Not flexible

(I) Decreased subtalar motion

AP lateral and oblique radiographs

(J) Tarsal coalition

See p 262

(K) Forefoot valgus deformity

Dorsiflexion and plantarflexion radiographs

Vertical talus

See p 266

(L) Hindfoot equinus

Careful neurologic examination

No neurologic findings

Neurologic findings

Neurologic investigation

Foot Orthosis with Heel Raise ←

CONSIDER HEELCORD LENGTHENING FOR SYMPTOMS

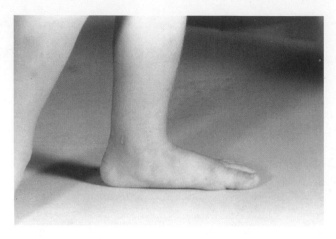

Figure 1 Typical clinical appearance of flexible flatfoot deformity. The child has mild physiologic genu valgum. The foot is flexible so that with weight bearing the longitudinal arch is depressed secondary to the genu valgum.

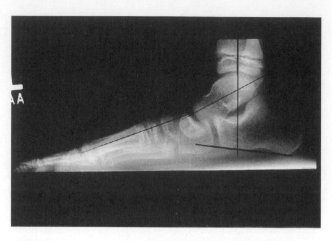

Figure 3 Lateral standing radiographic appearance of flexible flatfoot deformity. There is a reversal of Meary's angle but no dislocation of the navicular on the talus or hindfoot equinus.

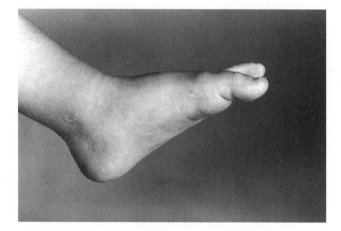

Figure 2 Same foot as in Figure 1, in non–weight-bearing position. The longitudinal arch is reconstituted.

References

Coleman SS. Complex Foot Deformity in Children. Philadelphia: Lea & Febiger, 1983.

Harris RI, Beath T. Hypermobile flat-foot with short tendo achillis. J Bone Joint Surg 1948; 30A:16.

Jones BS. Flatfoot. J Bone Joint Surg 1975; 57B:279.

Mosca VS. Calcaneal lengthening for valgus deformity of the hindfoot: Results in children who had severe, symptomatic flatfoot and skewfoot. J Bone Joint Surg 1995; 77A:500.

Staheli LT, Chew DE, Corbett M. The longitudinal arch. J Bone Joint Surg 1987; 69A:426.

Tachdjian MO. The Child's Foot. Philadelphia: WB Saunders, 1985.

Wenger DR, Mauldin D, Speck G, et al. Corrective shoes and inserts as treatment for flexible flatfoot in infants and children. J Bone Joint Surg 1989; 71A:800.

TARSAL COALITION

A. Patients with tarsal coalition typically present between the ages of 8 and 15 years with vague complaints of pain in the foot or lower leg. The pain is usually exercise induced. Physical examination usually reveals a depressed longitudinal arch, valgus appearance to the hindfoot, and pain or actual spasm in the peroneal tendons on forced inversion (so-called peroneal spastic flatfoot). Patients, however, may have none of these physical findings, and the diagnosis of tarsal coalition should be suspected solely on the basis of complaints of pain in the absence of other identifiable cause.

B. Anteroposterior and lateral radiographs of the foot typically do not reveal tarsal coalition. A coalition can be suspected based on the presence of a so-called "talar beak" on the talar side of the talonavicular joint. Oblique radiographs of the foot normally clearly identify a calcaneonavicular coalition (Fig. 1). If no coalition is identified on plain radiographs and the clinical history is suspicious, computed tomography (CT) of the foot should be carried out to specifically rule out the presence of subtalar or calcaneonavicular coalition. Other investigations, such as Harris axial view of the foot, technetium bone scan, and magnetic resonance imaging (MRI), can be used to help confirm the diagnosis; however, the vast majority of coalitions can be identified by plain radiographs and CT (Fig. 2). The most common types of tarsal coalition are calcaneonavicular and subtalar (usually middle facet). Patients can have a family history of tarsal coalition. Coalitions exist bilaterally in approximately 50% of patients but can be asymptomatic on one side, and do occur in association with some skeletal dysplasia syndromes.

C. In rare circumstances a patient presents with a peroneal spastic flatfoot but no coalition can be identified. Evaluate such patients for noncoalition conditions of peroneal spastic flatfoot: inflammatory arthritis, tethered cord or other intrathecal anomaly, and other rare causes such as tarsal bone or joint infection. Specific cause if identifiable should be treated. Patients without a diagnosis after this investigation are treated symptomatically with arch supports or ankle-foot orthoses (AFOs); very rarely triple arthrodesis is required.

D. Oblique radiographs of the foot or CT reveal the majority of the two most common types of tarsal coalition: calcaneonavicular and medial subtalar joint. When a coalition is identified, carefully assess the remaining joints radiographically to make sure that there is not another area of coalition, and the opposite foot as well to document an asymptomatic coalition.

E. Patients with severe pain in the foot or lower leg should be immobilized in a short leg walking cast or equivalent for approximately 6 weeks to control symptoms. In rare cases this completely ameliorates the symptoms. Reassess as necessary for resumption of symptoms. More commonly, moderate symptoms continue, requiring further definitive treatment.

F. On occasion, symptoms are moderate interfering only with certain vigorous activities. In these circumstances conservative treatment of arch support, AFO, limitation of activities, and anti-inflammatory medication may be tried. If these are unsuccessful after 6–12 weeks, consider surgery.

G. On occasion tarsal coalitions are identified on radiographs taken for other reasons or in an asymptomatic contralateral foot. In these circumstances no treatment is required. Reassess the patient as necessary for development of symptoms.

H. Patients requiring surgery for symptomatic tarsal coalition should be carefully assessed for the presence of more than one coalition in the same foot and signs of degenerative arthritis in other tarsal joints prior to determining the surgical management. The presence of talar beaking alone is not considered a sign of degenerative arthritis (Fig. 3); however, joint space narrowing or generalized osteophyte formation is. When degenerative changes are present and conservative treatment has failed, perform triple arthrodesis.

I. If the patient has continued symptoms without evidence of degenerative arthritis (excluding a talar beak), surgical management consists of resecting the coalition (calcaneonavicular, subtalar, or other rare coalition) with soft tissue interposition. The patient is immobilized in a short leg walking cast for 4 to 6 weeks postoperatively with gradual mobilization and resumption of activities thereafter.

J. If pain persists after resection of a tarsal coalition, re-evaluate the foot for signs of degenerative arthritis or recurrence of the coalition. If the coalition has reformed, consider repeat resection or triple arthrodesis based on the nature and severity of the symptoms. If there has been no recurrence of the coalition but no relief of symptoms, perform triple arthrodesis.

K. A patient with few or no symptoms after surgery can be reassessed periodically for recurrence of symptoms. Occasionally patients require 6 months or longer to become asymptomatic after resection of coalition. During this time part-time immobilization in ankle splints, AFO, or soft cast and modification of activity may be necessary.

SUSPECTED TARSAL COALITION

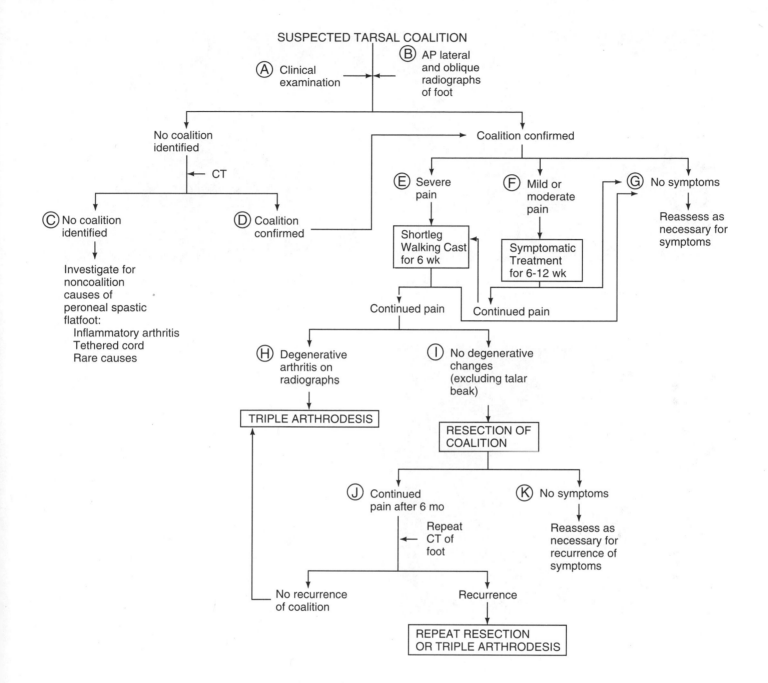

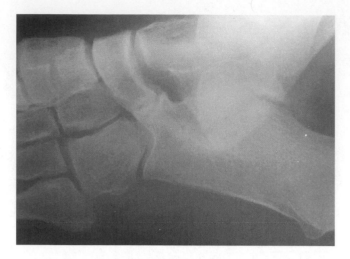

Figure 1 Calcaneonavicular coalition. This is the most common type of tarsal coalition, best seen on oblique radiographs of the foot.

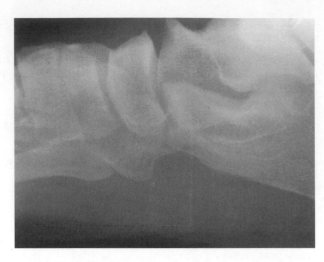

Figure 3 Lateral radiographs of a foot with tarsal coalition may show talar beaking. Provided there is no frank arthritis of contiguous joints, beaking is not a contraindication to coalition resection.

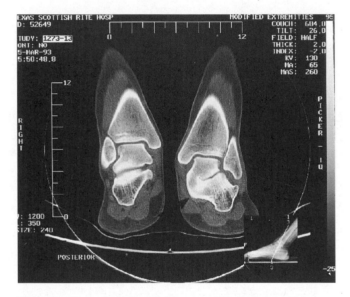

Figure 2 Computed tomographic scan of hindfoot demonstrates a coalition of middle facet of talocalcaneal joint.

References

Coleman SS. Complex foot deformity in children. Philadelphia: Lea & Febiger, 1983.

Cowell HR. Diagnosis and management of peroneal spastic flatfoot. Instr Course Lect 1975; 24:94.

Gonzalez P, Kumar SJ. Calcaneonavicular coalition treated by resection and interposition of the extensor digitorum brevis muscle. J Bone Joint Surg 1990; 72A:71.

Harris RI. Retrospect: Peroneal spastic flatfoot (rigid valgus foot). J Bone Joint Surg 1965; 47A:1657.

Harris RI, Beath T. Etiology of peroneal spastic flatfoot. J Bone Joint Surg 1948; 30B:624.

Mitchell GP, Gibson JMC. Excision of calcaneonavicular bar for painful spasmodic flat foot. J Bone Joint Surg 1967; 49B:281.

Mosier KM, Asher A. Tarsal coalition and peroneal spastic flatfoot: A review. J Bone Joint Surg 1986; 66A:976.

Olney BW, Asher MA. Excision of symptomatic coalition of the middle facet of the talocalcaneal joint. J Bone Joint Surg 1987; 69A:539.

Pineda C, Resnick D, Greenway G. Diagnosis of tarsal coalition with computed tomography. Clin Orthop 1986; 208:282.

Scranton PE. Treatment of symptomatic talocalcaneal coalition. J Bone Joint Surg 1987; 69A:533.

Swiontkowski MF, Scranton PE, Hansen S. Tarsal coalitions: Long-term results of surgical treatment. J Pediatr Orthop 1983; 3:287.

Tachdjian MO. The Child's Foot. Philadelphia: WB Saunders, 1985.

VERTICAL TALUS

A. True congenital vertical talus (convex pes valgus or rocker-bottom foot) is frequently associated with known generalized disorders such as arthrogryposis or spina bifida, or occult neurologic abnormality. Evaluate patients clinically for evidence of neurologic dysfunction in the lower extremity, including careful examination of the spine. True vertical talus is characterized clinically by forefoot dorsiflexion and valgus that is not passively correctable, and hindfoot equinus (Fig. 1). The diagnosis can be confirmed with plantarflexion and dorsiflexion lateral radiographs. In dorsiflexion the forefoot dislocation is noted, the projected outline of the navicular does not line up with the axis of the talus and first metatarsal because of the dorsal dislocation, and the hindfoot equinus is noted. On plantarflexion lateral radiographs the projected outline of the navicular again does not reduce on the talus, confirming the fixed nature of the dislocation (Fig. 2).

B. If plantarflexion radiographs show reduction of the projected outline of the navicular on the talus and the talus-first metatarsal axis align, the patient does not have a rigid fixed dorsal dislocation of the talonavicular joint.

C. If in addition the patient does not have clinical or radiographic evidence of a tight heelcord, the diagnosis is more likely oblique talus, which is a severe form of flexible flatfoot deformity. Treatment is not usually required.

D. If there is hindfoot equinus or clinically tight heelcord, midfoot breakdown is occurring in conjunction with the tight heelcord. Evaluate the patient to determine the etiology of the tight heelcord and treat appropriately.

E. If plantarflexion radiographs show no reduction of the navicular on the talus the patient has true congenital vertical talus deformity and fixed talonavicular dislocation. Surgical treatment almost always is required.

F. There is a very high incidence of associated disorders with congenital vertical talus. If one is not readily identifiable, carefully examine the spine including not only radiographs but also magnetic resonance imaging (MRI) to rule out lipoma or tethered cord. Orthopaedic treatment of the foot deformity is likely to be required in any case.

G. Conservative treatment of vertical talus is generally thought to be unsuccessful. Occasionally mild deformities are functional and asymptomatic and thus require no treatment. Such patients need to be observed until skeletal maturity to be certain that the deformity does not become progressive or symptomatic warranting surgery. The vast majority of patients require open reduction, which is a combination of talonavicular reduction with joint capsular reefing, posterior release of the equinus contracture, and lengthening of the long-toe extensors and peroneals, which are bowstrung across the ankle joint (Fig. 3). The foot is casted for 3 to 4 months postoperatively and then observed periodically throughout growth for evidence of recurrence.

H. Recurrent deformity of vertical talus requires repeat open reduction with Grice procedure to correct valgus deformity of the hindfoot or, alternatively, in an older child with more severe deformity, triple arthrodesis.

I. Patients >2–3 years old usually require the soft tissue release as described in G above and in addition require Grice subtalar arthrodesis to correct valgus deformity of the hindfoot. Postoperative immobilization and follow-up is as for soft tissue release.

J. Older patients or those whose deformity recurs require triple arthrodesis.

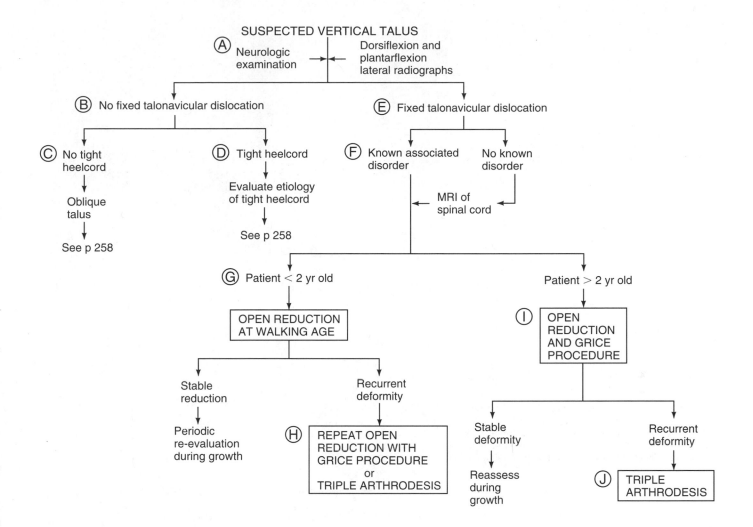

SUSPECTED VERTICAL TALUS

(A) Neurologic examination → ← Dorsiflexion and plantarflexion lateral radiographs

(B) No fixed talonavicular dislocation

(E) Fixed talonavicular dislocation

(C) No tight heelcord
↓
Oblique talus
↓
See p 258

(D) Tight heelcord
↓
Evaluate etiology of tight heelcord
↓
See p 258

(F) Known associated disorder

No known disorder

MRI of spinal cord

(G) Patient < 2 yr old
↓
OPEN REDUCTION AT WALKING AGE

Stable reduction
↓
Periodic re-evaluation during growth

Recurrent deformity
↓
(H) REPEAT OPEN REDUCTION WITH GRICE PROCEDURE or TRIPLE ARTHRODESIS

Patient > 2 yr old
↓
(I) OPEN REDUCTION AND GRICE PROCEDURE

Stable deformity
↓
Reassess during growth

Recurrent deformity
↓
(J) TRIPLE ARTHRODESIS

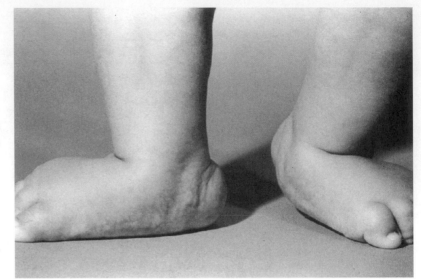

Figure 1 Clinical appearance of vertical talus. The hindfoot is in equinus, there is fixed flatfoot deformity, and the forefoot is in valgus.

Figure 2 **A,** Vertical talus in dorsiflexion. The talus is in marked plantarflexion; the calcaneus is in equinus. The navicular (not ossified) is dislocated dorsally on the talus. **B,** In plantarflexion the navicular remains dislocated dorsally on the talus, and the talus does not align with the first metatarsal.

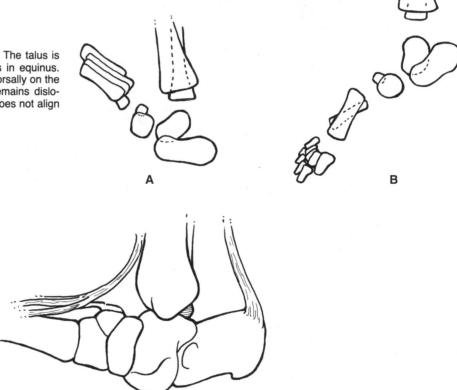

Figure 3 Open reduction of vertical talus deformity. The navicular must be reduced on the talus with talonavicular capsular plication, the achilles tendon lengthened, and the long-toe extensors and peroneal tendons lengthened.

References

Clark MW, D'Ambrosia RD, Ferguson AB. Congenital vertical talus. J Bone Joint Surg 1977; 59A:816.

Coleman SS. Complex Foot Deformity in Children. Philadelphia: Lea & Febiger, 1983.

Coleman SS, Martin AF, Jarret J. Congenital vertical talus: Pathomechanics and treatment. J Bone Joint Surg 1966; 48A:1442.

Dodge LD, Ashley RK, Gilbert RJ. Treatment of congenital vertical talus: A retrospective review of 36 feet with long-term follow-up. Foot Ankle 1987; 7:326.

Drennan JC, Sharrard WJW. The pathologic anatomy of convex pes valgus. J Bone Joint Surg 1971; 53B:455.

Hamanishi C. Congenital vertical talus: Classification with 69 cases and new measurement system. J Pediatr Orthop 1984; 4:318.

Herndon CH, Heyman CH. Problems in the recognition and treatment of congenital convex pes valgus. J Bone Joint Surg 1963; 45A:413.

Jacobsen ST, Crawford AH. Congenital vertical talus. J Pediatr Orthop 1983; 3:306.

Lloyd-Roberts GC, Spence AJ. Congenital vertical talus. J Bone Joint Surg 1958; 40B:33.

Oppenheim W, Smith CH, Christie W. Congenital vertical talus. Foot Ankle 1985; 5:198.

Seimon LP. Surgical correction of congenital vertical talus under the age of 2 years. J Pediatr Orthop 1987; 7:405.

Tachdjian MO. The Child's Foot. Philadelphia: WB Saunders, 1985.

CONGENITAL LEG DEFORMITY

A. When anteroposterior and lateral radiographs of the leg demonstrate antero-lateral bow, suspect congenital pseudarthrosis of the tibia variant. The severity of bowing and radiographic pathology vary. The tibia may have only a bow with preservation of the medullary canal; cyst at or near the apex of the deformity; sclerosis and tapering of the medullary canal at the apex of the deformity; or be fractured. These radiographic findings do not appear to have major prognostic significance. Approximately 50% of patients with congenital pseudarthrosis of the tibia have neurofibromatosis. A small percentage (particularly with cystic-type variant) have fibrous dysplasia. The fibula is often deformed in the same direction as the tibia and may be intact or fractured.

B. When the apex of the deformity is anteromedial, the limb is affected by some form of fibular hemimelia, varying from partial to absent. The fibula is hypoplastic or absent. The foot is usually in equinovarus. Dimpling of the skin over the apex of the tibial deformity is evident as well as a variable amount of shortening of the tibia. The medullary canal is preserved, and there is no propensity for pathologic fracture.

C. When the apex of tibial deformity is posteromedial, posteromedial bow deformity is the diagnosis. The foot is in a marked calcaneus position at birth. Less apparent but invariably present is shortening of the lower leg compared to the normal side. The natural history of this deformity is gradual resolution of the calcaneus deformity of the foot, and straightening of the tibial deformity. Very occasionally, a tibial deformity does not correct and requires osteotomy. Decision regarding osteotomy should be delayed at least several years. Even with spontaneous correction of the bowing and foot deformity, progressive limb length inequality due to growth inhibition of the affected tibia is certain. The patient must be examined on a regular basis for this inequality, and the projected ultimate limb length discrepancy treated appropriately. See page 298.

D. If radiographs demonstrate that the fibula is intact, but longer than the tibia, a variation of tibial hemimelia exists. The tibia may be completely absent, deficient proximally, or deficient distally. Associated foot deformity is usual.

E. If the tibia is shortened and the fibula deficient or absent, a variation of fibular hemimelia exists. Frequently, deformities of the femur are also present including hypoplasia of the proximal femur, shortening of the femur compared to the normal side, and valgus deformity at the knee. The lateral rays of the foot are often deficient, and the foot has a variable amount of equinovalgus deformity.

F. Femoral deformities usually are associated with shortening. In an infant, radiographs of the pelvis usually do not demonstrate hip anatomy. If deformity of the upper femur or hip joint is suspected, high resolution ultrasound of the hip should be performed. Congenital coxa vara is characterized by varus deformity of the upper femur, often with acetabular dysplasia. The patient is noted to have limited abduction mimicking fixed dislocation, but the femoral head is located. Congenital coxa vara may be seen as an isolated deformity, or in conjunction with generalized skeletal dysplasia such as cleidocranial dysostosis or Schmidt-type metaphyseal dysostosis. If the upper femur is deficient or absent, the deformity is proximal femoral focal deficiency. Femoral deformities may also be due to birth fractures such as seen with osteogenesis imperfecta.

CONGENITAL LEG DEFORMITY

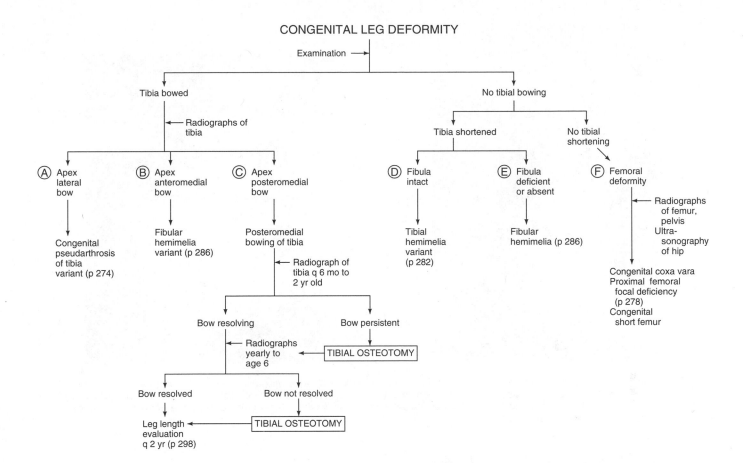

Examination →

Tibia bowed

← Radiographs of tibia

(A) **Apex lateral bow**

Congenital pseudarthrosis of tibia variant (p 274)

(B) **Apex anteromedial bow**

Fibular hemimelia variant (p 286)

(C) **Apex posteromedial bow**

Posteromedial bowing of tibia

← Radiograph of tibia q 6 mo to 2 yr old

Bow resolving

← Radiographs yearly to age 6

Bow resolved

Leg length evaluation q 2 yr (p 298) ←

Bow not resolved

TIBIAL OSTEOTOMY

Bow persistent

TIBIAL OSTEOTOMY →

No tibial bowing

Tibia shortened

(D) **Fibula intact**

Tibial hemimelia variant (p 282)

(E) **Fibula deficient or absent**

Fibular hemimelia (p 286)

No tibial shortening

(F) **Femoral deformity**

← Radiographs of femur, pelvis
Ultra-sonography of hip

Congenital coxa vara
Proximal femoral focal deficiency (p 278)
Congenital short femur

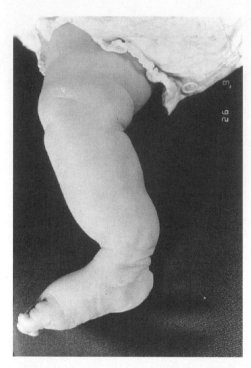

Figure 1 Clinical appearance of posteromedial bow of the tibia. There is an apex posterior and medial bow of the distal portion of the tibia. In infancy there is an associated calcaneovalgus foot deformity. This deformity resolves with growth.

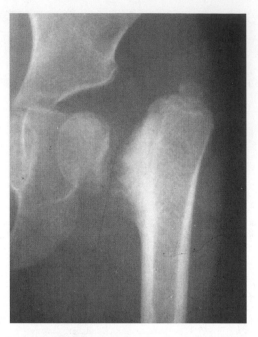

Figure 3 Anteroposterior radiograph of a patient with congenital coxa vara of the left hip. Associated shortening and limited abduction may mimic developmental dysplasia of the hip in infancy.

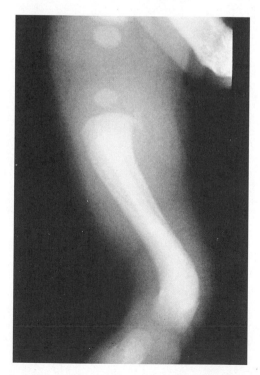

Figure 2 Lateral radiograph of an infant with posteromedial bow of the tibia. There is no propensity for the tibia to fracture. The angular deformity will usually resolve spontaneously.

References

Achterman C, Kalamchi A. Congenital deficiency of the fibula. J Bone Joint Surg 1979; 61B:133.

Aitken GT. Proximal femoral focal deficiency: Definition, classification and management. In: Aitken GT, ed. Proximal Femoral Focal Deficiency: A Congenital Anomaly. Washington, DC: National Academy of Sciences, 1969:1.

Anderson DJ, Schoenecker PL, Sheridan JJ, Rich MM. Use of an intramedullary rod for the treatment of congenital pseudarthrosis of the tibia. J Bone Joint Surg 1992; 74A:161.

Frantz CH, O'Rahilly R. Congenital skeletal limb deficiencies. J Bone Joint Surg 1961; 43A:1202.

Gillespie R, Tordoe IP. Classification and management of congenital abnormalities of the femur. J Bone Joint Surg 1983; 65B:557.

Hofmann A, Wenger DR. Posteromedial bowing of the tibia: Progression of discrepancy in leg lengths. J Bone Joint Surg 1981; 63A:384.

Jones D, Barnes J, Lloyd-Roberts GC. Congenital aplasia and dysplasia of the tibia with intact fibula. J Bone Joint Surg 1978; 60B:31.

Morrissy RT, Riseborough EJ, Hall JE. Congenital pseudarthrosis of the tibia. J Bone Joint Surg 1981; 63B:367.

Pappas AM. Congenital posteromedial bowing of the tibia and fibula. J Pediatr Orthop 1984; 4:525.

Tachdjian MO. The Child's Foot. Philadelphia: WB Saunders, 1985.

Westin GW, Sakai DN, Wood WL. Congenital longitudinal deficiency of the fibula. J Bone Joint Surg 1976; 58A:492.

CONGENITAL PSEUDARTHROSIS OF THE TIBIA

A. Approximately 50% of patients with congenital pseudarthrosis of the tibia (Fig. 1) have neurofibromatosis. Some patients present with a delayed variant of congenital pseudarthrosis of the tibia. Classically they have a fracture between age 3 to 5 after trivial trauma. These patients are treated as for more severe types of congenital pseudarthrosis of the tibia, but have a better prognosis for responding to surgical management.

B. The prognosis for congenital pseudarthrosis of the tibia does not appear to be influenced by the presence of neurofibromatosis. However, patients with neurofibromatosis are susceptible to other disorders of the musculoskeletal system such as local extremity gigantism, scoliosis, cutaneous lesions, and central nervous system (CNS) tumors. A family history can often be elicited.

C. If a fracture occurs in a patient with congenital pseudarthrosis of the tibia variant, treatment by conservative means rarely results in union. A fracture may be immobilized in either cast or brace until definitive treatment is carried out.

D. The most successful currently employed treatment of congenital pseudarthrosis of the tibia is Williams intramedullary rodding with or without electrical or electromagnetic stimulation (Fig. 2). The Williams rod is a smooth Steinmann pin with a threaded base for intramedullary insertion. At the time of surgery the pseudarthrosis must be resected, the fibula divided if intact, and the tibia and fibula rodded and bone grafted. The patient is immobilized in a spica cast for 3 months or longer followed by protective bracing. With severe deformities or small distal segments, the rod is left in the talus and calcaneus, thus fixing the ankle. With growth, the rod will migrate into the tibia. Until the rod has migrated beyond the ankle joint, protective bracing of the foot and ankle is obligatory. Multiple other surgical techniques incorporating internal fixation and grafting have been described with variable success. The most common problems are difficulty with fixation of the distal fragment, and persistent pseudarthrosis irrespective of the modality used.

E. If previous surgery has failed, then unless there are obvious technical reasons for that failure, the patient has a grim prognosis for subsequent healing and good function in the limb. Current salvage procedures include free vascularized fibular graft or use of the Ilizarov apparatus. The apparatus provides the option of secure distal fixation, incorporating the foot when necessary, and allows long-term immobilization.

F. Congenital pseudarthrosis of the tibia may be refractory to all forms of treatment. When an amputation should be performed as a final solution is controversial. If two major reconstructions such as Williams rod and free fibular transfer have been tried with persistent pseudarthrosis, amputation should be seriously considered. In children a Syme's amputation is usually the best choice. Maintenance of the distal tibial epiphysis will prevent overgrowth of the distal stump requiring revisions in the growing child. The pseudarthrosis will be immobilized in the prosthetic socket, but the stump will not be end bearing.

G. In general, if the tibia is intact no reconstruction should be undertaken because of the risk of nonunion after osteotomy of any type. Progressive deformity or pain may require reconstruction.

H. The role of protective bracing in the management of congenital pseudarthrosis of the tibia is not established. In general, if a medullary canal exists and there is neither deformity nor pain, protective braces are not used. In all other circumstances protective bracing is used. Short or long leg brace with or without an anterior shell for the tibia may be used.

I. The end of growth does not signal the end of problems as patients can fracture in adult life, with the prognosis as poor and treatment as difficult as it was during childhood.

CONGENITAL PSEUDARTHROSIS
OF TIBIA

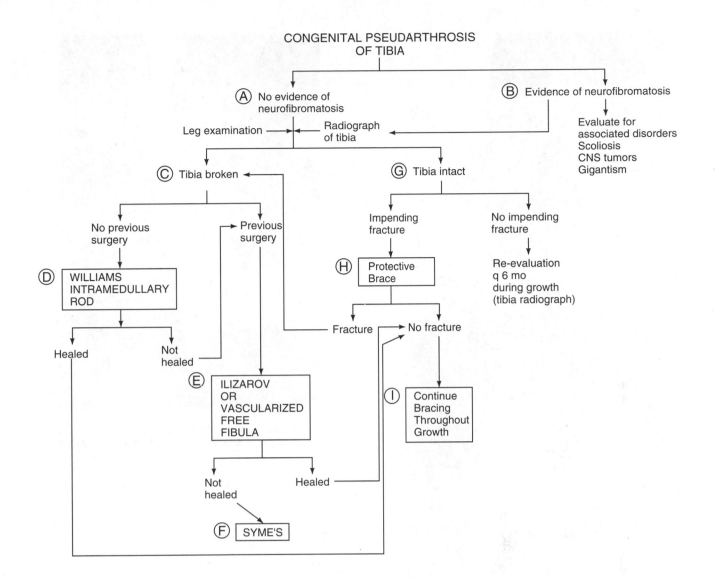

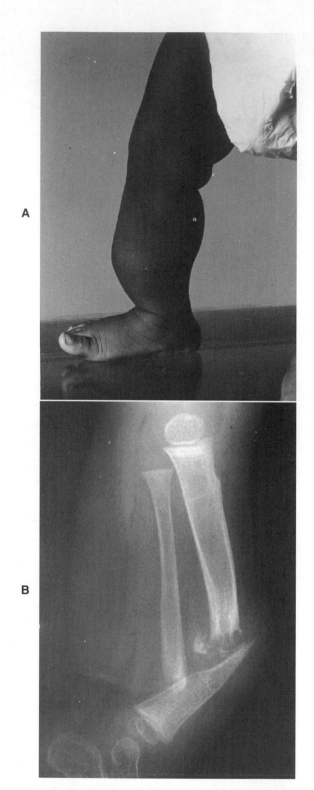

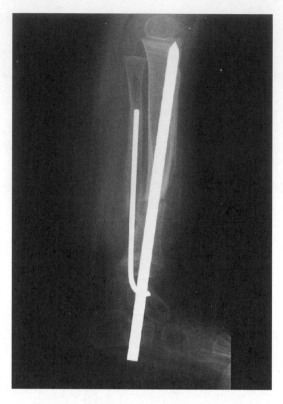

Figure 2 Williams rodding of the tibia. The smooth Steinmann pin is inserted through the foot and across the ankle joint into the tibia.

Figure 1 Congenital pseudarthrosis of the tibia. **A,** Clinical appearance of an infant. The angular deformity is apex anterior and lateral. **B,** Lateral radiograph.

References

Anderson DJ, Schoenecker PL, Sheridan JJ, Rich MM. Use of an intramedullary rod for the treatment of congenital pseudarthrosis of the tibia. J Bone Joint Surg 1992; 74A:161.

Baker JK, Cain TE, Tullos HS. Intramedullary fixation for congenital pseudarthrosis of the tibia. J Bone Joint Surg 1992; 74A:169.

Coleman SS, Coleman DA. Congenital pseudarthrosis of the tibia: Treatment by transfer of the ipsilateral fibula with vascular pedicle. J Pediatr Orthop 1994; 14:156.

Jacobsen ST, Crawford AH, Millar EA, Steel HH. The Syme amputation in patients with congenital pseudarthrosis of the tibia. J Bone Joint Surg 1983; 65A:533.

Morrissy RT, Riseborough EJ, Hall JE. Congenital pseudarthrosis of the tibia. J Bone Joint Surg 1981; 63B:367.

Paley D, Catagni M, Argnani F, et al. Treatment of congenital pseudoarthrosis of the tibia using the Ilizarov technique. Clin Orthop 1992; 280:81.

Paterson DC, Simonis RB. Electrical stimulation in the treatment of congenital pseudarthrosis of the tibia. J Bone Joint Surg 1985; 67B:454.

Paterson D. Congenital pseudarthrosis of the tibia: An overview. Clin Orthop 1989; 247:44.

Plawecki S, Capentier E, Lascombes P, et al. Treatment of congenital pseudarthrosis of the tibia by the Ilizarov method. J Pediatr Orthop 1990; 10:786.

Roach JW, Shindell R, Green NE. Late-onset pseudarthrosis of the dysplastic tibia. J Bone Joint Surg 1993; 75A:1593.

Uchida Y, Kojima T, Sugioka Y. Vascularized fibular graft for congenital pseudarthrosis of the tibia: Long-term results. J Bone Joint Surg 1991; 73B:846.

Umber JS, Moss SW, Coleman SS. Surgical treatment of congenital pseudarthrosis of the tibia. Clin Orthop 1982; 166:28.

Weiland AJ, Weiss AP, Moore JR, Tolo VT. Vascularized fibular grafts in the treatment of congenital pseudarthrosis of the tibia. J Bone Joint Surg 1990; 72A:654.

PROXIMAL FEMORAL FOCAL DEFICIENCY

A. Proximal femoral focal deficiency (PFFD) is a rare, very severe congenital limb deficiency characterized by a variable (usually severe) amount of femoral shortening, proximal deficiency varying from coxa vara to complete absence of the femoral head and acetabulum (Fig. 1). Quite frequently other lower extremity anomalies coexist such as tibial or fibular hemimelia aggravating the limb deformity. Clinical examination should determine upper extremity function, range of motion and stability of joints in the affected extremity, and the presence of associated lower leg anomalies. Radiographs of the tibia and femur document the severity of the shortening and the severity of hip dysplasia. Suspected lower leg deficiency also is confirmed on radiographs.

B. Approximately 15% of patients with PFFD have bilateral deformity. If the lower extremities are otherwise normal, the patient will have a short stature syndrome but no appreciable limb length inequality. Therefore no specific treatment is required during growth and the patient should be only assessed periodically during growth.

C. Associated lower extremity anomalies may interfere with a patient's mobility. Consideration should then be given towards lower extremity amputation to allow functional prosthetic fitting.

D. If there is any upper extremity deficiency, give very careful consideration to the potential for the use of any rudimentary lower extremity segment in a prehensile fashion in place of absent or deficient hands. If the foot or any remnant is being or could be used as a hand, under no circumstances should amputation be done for cosmetic or mobility purposes.

E. Patients with unilateral PFFD invariably show a severe degree of shortening (Fig. 2). Only in very rare circumstances is total limb shortening <20% of an opposite normal limb. Most such cases are thought to represent milder deformities such as congenital coxa vara or coxa vara with short femur rather than true PFFD.

F. If the patient has other lower extremity deformity, such as tibial or fibular hemimelia, appropriate amputation (e.g., Syme's) is carried out at walking age and the patient fitted with a below-knee prosthesis. This prosthesis is adjusted during growth as necessary.

G. If there are no other significant lower extremity anomalies, consider equalization of limb length by lengthening or epiphysiodesis (see p 298).

H. Much more typically patients show much greater than 20% shortening compared with the normal side. Because of the severity of the shortening and the congenital nature of the deformity lengthening is very rarely indicated.

I. If the patient has a deformed foot, a Syme's amputation should be performed at walking age followed by prosthetic fitting.

J. If the patient has a normal functional foot that is level to or below the opposite knee, consider Van Nes rotationplasty. In this procedure the foot is rotated 180° through a shortening tibial osteotomy (or knee fusion) to convert ankle plantarflexion and dorsiflexion into knee flexion and extension. The foot then acts as a short below-knee stump. While excellent functional results are reported with this procedure, parental refusal, derotation of the reconstruction during growth, and psychological disturbances are all reported. Consider surgical removal even of a normal foot as an alternative.

K. Patients with morphologically good hips function well in a prosthesis after the aforementioned corrections. However, hip function is frequently poor due to an unstable hip, a pseudarthrosis in the region of the subtrochanteric area, or a very short femur with a knee joint that cannot be stabilized in a prosthetic socket. Consider trying to improve hip function by one of the following procedures (L to N).

L. If the patient has a very short femoral remnant with either an unstable or absent hip, consider iliofemoral fusion. In this procedure the femoral remnant is fixed to the ilium in a 90° flexed position with the knee thereby being converted into a hip joint. Patient is then fitted as an above knee prosthesis wearer using the tibial segment.

M. If the patient has a short femur with an unstable or nonfunctional knee, because the knee cannot be stabilized in the prosthesis and provide adequate hip function, consider knee fusion (Fig. 3). This converts the femoral and tibial remnants into a single above knee remnant.

N. If the patient has adequate femoral head development and femoral length for prosthetic fitting with a subtrochanteric pseudarthrosis, internal fixation and bone grafting of the pseudarthrosis may be carried out.

SUSPECTED PROXIMAL FEMORAL FOCAL DEFICIENCY

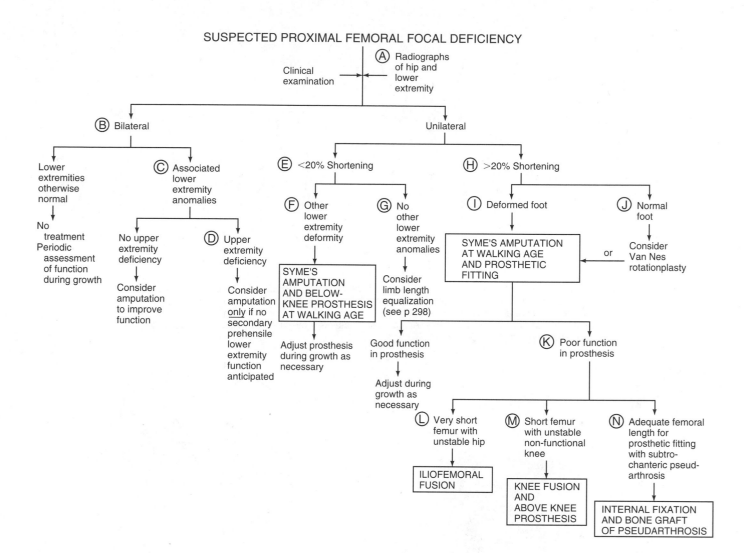

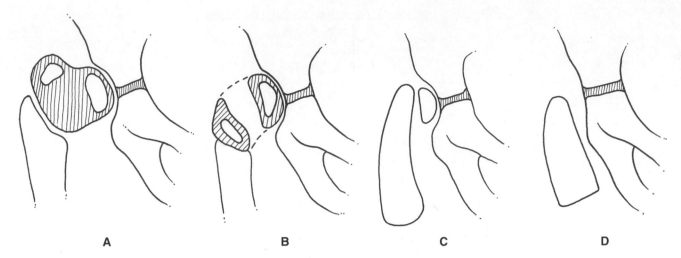

Figure 1 Aiken classification of proximal femoral focal deficiency (PFFD). **A,** Femoral head and acetabulum are present. Femur is short. Subtrochanteric varus angulation or pseudarthrosis is present. **B,** No osseous connection between femoral head and shaft. Acetabulum may be dysplastic. **C,** Absent femoral head or small ossicle only. Acetabulum is severely dysplastic. **D,** Femoral head and acetaulum absent. Femur may be extremely short.

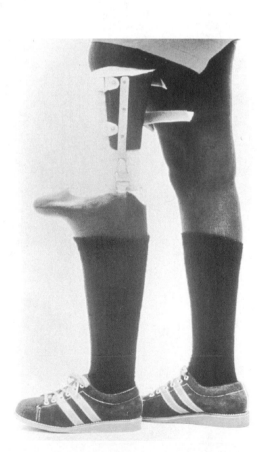

Figure 2 Sequelae of PFFD. Severe shortening of affected extremity will require extension orthosis for functioning in the older child.

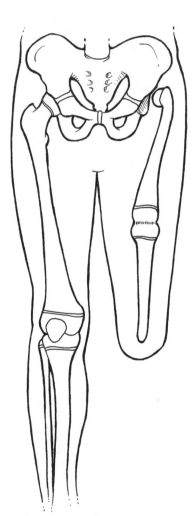

Figure 3 Deformity depicted in Figure 2 may be treated by knee fusion and Syme's amputation, creating an above knee or knee disarticulation limb.

References

Aitken GT. Proximal femoral focal deficiency: Definition, classification, and management. In: Aitken GT, ed. Proximal Femoral Focal Deficiency: A Congenital Anomaly. Washington, DC: National Academy of Sciences, 1969:1.

Bryant DD 3d, Epps CH Jr. Proximal femoral focal deficiency: Evaluation and management. Orthopedics 1991; 14:775.

Frantz CH, O'Rahilly R. Congenital skeletal limb deficiencies. J Bone Joint Surg 1961; 43A:1202.

Friscia DA, Moseley CF, Oppenheim WL. Rotational osteotomy for proximal femoral focal deficiency. J Bone Joint Surg 1989; 71A:1386.

Gillespie R, Torode IP. Classification and management of congenital abnormalities of the femur. J Bone Joint Surg 1983; 65B:557.

Kostuik JP, Gillespie R, Hall JE, Hubbard S. Van Nes rotational osteotomy for treatment of proximal femoral focal deficiency and congenital short femur. J Bone Joint Surg 1975; 57A:1039.

Kritter AE. Tibial rotation-plasty for proximal femoral focal deficiency. J Bone Joint Surg 1977; 59A:927.

Panting AL, William PF. Proximal femoral focal deficiency. J Bone Joint Surg 1978; 60B:46.

Pirani S, Beauchamp RD, Li D, Sawatzky B. Soft tissue anatomy of proximal femoral focal deficiency. J Pediatr Orthop 1991; 11:563.

Steel HH, Lin PS, Betz RR, et al. Iliofemoral fusion for proximal femoral focal deficiency. J Bone Joint Surg 1987; 69A:837.

Torode IP, Gillespie R. Rotationplasty of the lower limb for congenital defects of the femur. J Bone Joint Surg 1983; 65A:569.

Van Nes CP. Rotation-plasty for congenital defects of the femur: Making use of the ankle of the shortened limb to control the knee joint of a prosthesis. J Bone Joint Surg 1950; 32B:12.

TIBIAL HEMIMELIA

A. Tibial hemimelia is a very severe congenital limb deficiency (Fig. 1). The tibia may be completely absent, deficient proximally, deficient distally, or simply shortened with distal tibiofibular divergence (Fig. 2). There is usually severe varus foot deformity and ankle instability. The medial foot rays are often duplicated rather than deficient. Tibial hemimelia may be hereditary, bilateral, or associated with other limb deficiency syndromes. None of these factors influences decision-making in tibial hemimelia, with one important exception: if there is associated upper extremity deficiency, careful attention must be given to opportunity for the child to use the foot in place of a hand for tactile and prehensile purposes. If any question exists regarding use of the foot in place of a deficient upper limb, decision-making regarding amputation should be deferred.

B. The most important aspect of physical examination is whether or not active knee extension exists. Active knee extension is presumptive evidence for the presence of an intact quadriceps mechanism and a proximal tibial remnant. Occasionally the proximal tibial remnant is not ossified in infancy and thus not apparent on plain radiographs. The presence and size of an unossified proximal tibia remnant may be determined by ultrasound or magnetic resonance imaging (MRI) examination.

C. When the patient has active knee extension and a proximal tibial remnant, knee function should be preserved. If the patient has a tibial remnant that is long enough to allow prosthetic fitting, treatment should consist of Syme's amputation at cruising age and fitting of a Syme's or below-knee prosthesis.

D. A patient with active knee extension and a short tibial remnant is a candidate for surgical transfer of the fibula to the tibial remnant along with Syme's amputation (Fig. 3). This surgery should be deferred until the proximal tibial remnant has ossified sufficiently to allow some form of bony proximal tibial—fibular fixation. The effect is to provide a below-knee segment of adequate length for fitting with a below-knee or Syme's prosthesis. The foot may be preserved and centered on the distal fibula; however, this articulation is usually unstable, and significant shortening compared to the normal limb would persist. Theoretically the limb could be salvaged by lengthening of the fibular fragment and fusion of the foot to the distal fibula. In the majority of patients, however, this would be excessive treatment.

E. Patients with active knee extension but no proximal remnant are candidates for a Brown procedure. In this procedure the fibula is transferred into the femoral notch and the quadriceps mechanism attached to it. This procedure is combined with a Syme's amputation. The purpose of the Brown procedure is to provide active knee extension with a below-knee segment that can be fitted with a prosthesis. The likelihood of successful outcome is controversial, as often either the transfer is unstable or active knee extension does not remain functional.

F. Although the Brown procedure is a theoretically attractive option for preserving knee function, several series have indicated that the preservation of quadriceps function is inadequate to improve the functional status of the patient, or that the knee is sufficiently unstable that no functional benefit is gained. If after the Brown procedure no functional knee extension has been preserved or the knee remains unstable, and the preserved fibular segment presents an obstruction to effective fitting of a prosthesis, the patient should be converted to a knee disarticulation amputation.

G. The absence of active knee extension implies that neither a functional quadriceps mechanism nor a proximal tibial remnant (thus knee) is present. In such patients the outcome of segment preservation such as the Brown procedure (see E above) is universally poor. Best function is obtained by knee disarticulation at walking age and fitting the child with a knee disarticulation prosthesis.

TIBIAL HEMIMELIA

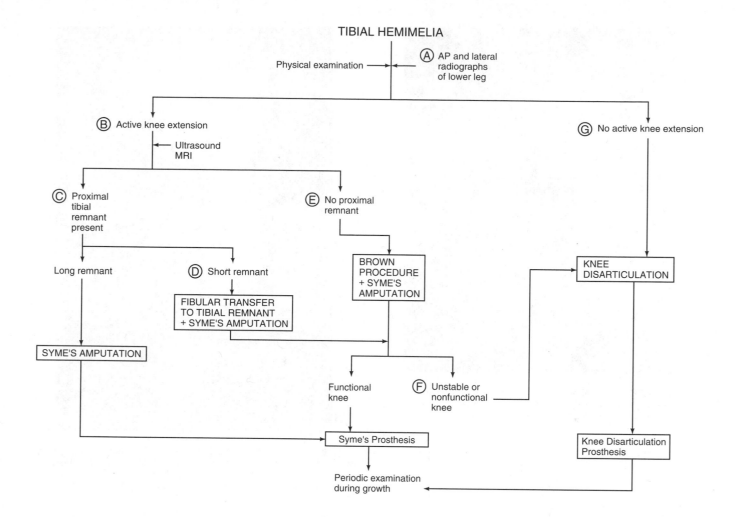

Physical examination ⟶ Ⓐ AP and lateral radiographs of lower leg

Ⓑ Active knee extension

Ultrasound MRI

Ⓒ Proximal tibial remnant present

Ⓔ No proximal remnant

Ⓖ No active knee extension

Long remnant

Ⓓ Short remnant

BROWN PROCEDURE + SYME'S AMPUTATION

KNEE DISARTICULATION

FIBULAR TRANSFER TO TIBIAL REMNANT + SYME'S AMPUTATION

SYME'S AMPUTATION

Functional knee

Ⓕ Unstable or nonfunctional knee

Syme's Prosthesis

Knee Disarticulation Prosthesis

Periodic examination during growth

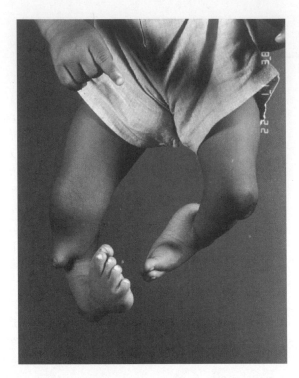

Figure 1 Bilateral tibial hemimelia. There is extreme shortening of the lower leg. The feet are in marked varus. There may or may not be active extension at the knee.

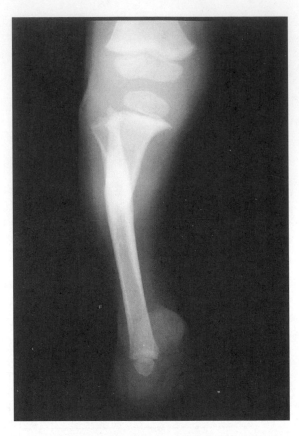

Figure 3 A variation of the Brown procedure involves transfer of the fibula to the proximal tibial remnant. This increases the length of the lower leg remnant and preserves knee function. This procedure is usually combined with Syme's amputation.

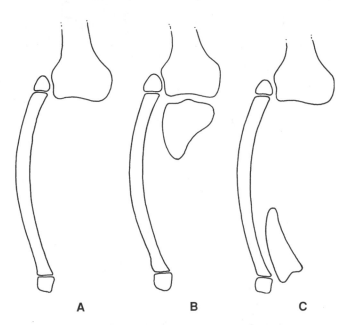

Figure 2 Classification of tibial hemimelia. **A,** The tibia may be completely absent. In these circumstances there is no true knee or ankle mortise. Knee disarticulation generally is required. Only occasionally is the Brown procedure (transportation of the fibula into the femoral notch) indicated. **B,** A proportion of proximal tibia may persist. In these cases quadriceps function is often preserved. The fibula should be transferred to the tibial remnant (usually combined with Syme's amputation), thus preserving knee motion. **C,** The tibia may be present distally. The absence of a functional knee, ankle instability, and the extreme shortening usually dictate knee disarticulation.

References

Brown FW. Construction of a knee joint in congenital total absence of the tibia (paraxial hemimelia tibia): A preliminary report. J Bone Joint Surg 1965; 47A:695.

Brown FW, Pohnert WH. Construction of a knee joint in meromelia tibia (congenital absence of the tibia): A 15-year follow-up study. J Bone Joint Surg 1972; 54:1333.

Grissom LE, Harcke HT, Kumar SJ. Sonography in the management of tibial hemimelia. Clin Orthop 1990; 251:266.

Jones D, Barnes J, Lloyd-Roberts GD. Congenital aplasia and dysplasia of the tibia with intact fibula. J Bone Joint Surg 1978; 60:31.

FIBULAR HEMIMELIA

Patients with fibular hemimelia have a variable amount of tibial shortening, fibular deficiency (from partial to complete), and foot deformity (Figs. 1 and 2). Foot deformity varies from mild equinovalgus to complete dislocation of the tibio-talar joint with extreme equinovalgus deformity. The lateral rays may be deficient. Subtalar or massive tarsal coalition is frequently present. Presumably due to the coalition older patients have a ball-and-socket tibio-talar joint in addition.

A. Appropriate management of fibular hemimelia is determined by the function of the foot and the overall shortening of the limb. A nonfunctional foot should undergo Syme's amputation. Serious consideration should be given to Syme's amputation of even a normal foot if the overall limb shortening is projected to be greater than 30% of the total limb length and/or there are significant other associated anomalies of the extremity.

B. Syme's amputation in a child is functionally an ankle disarticulation. Preservation of the distal epiphysis prevents diaphyseal overgrowth, a troublesome complication after midlong bone amputations in children. There appears to be no need to trim the malleoli in children. Some authors recommend Boyd or similar amputation to prevent posterior slipping of the heel pad. However, long-term studies of Syme's amputation for fibular hemimelia do not indicate that this becomes a functional problem. If Boyd is undertaken, the probable presence of a tarsal coalition should be kept in mind. Syme's amputation negates any requirement for limb length equalization and allows good prosthetic fitting. The procedure is normally performed when the child begins to stand.

C. If shortening of the tibia is greater than 30% of the opposite side, serious consideration should be given to performing a Syme's amputation, even if the foot itself is functional. A discrepancy of this severity requires major reconstruction including staged lengthenings. More effective external fixators employed with gradual distraction techniques undoubtedly extend the indications for limb reconstruction.

D. Fibular hemimelia, either partial or complete, is often associated with subtle deformity of the ipsilateral femur including mild shortening, distal femoral valgus deformity, and mild acetabular dysplasia. In general, most valgus deformities can be accommodated by a prosthetic socket. When this is not possible the deformity can be corrected in the skeletally immature patient by medial distal femoral and/or proximal tibial epiphysiodesis, with completion of epiphysiodeses on the lateral side when the limb is straightened. Alternatively, supracondylar varus osteotomy can be carried out in the skeletally mature patient or when too much growth remains to warrant epiphysiodesis.

E. Rarely is a projected limb length inequality in a patient with unilateral partial fibular hemimelia <2 cm and only occasionally is it <4 cm. Patients in that range should have an appropriately timed epiphysiodesis of the contralateral proximal tibia, distal femur, or both. In milder forms of partial fibular hemimelia there is a mild-to-moderate valgus of the distal femur that is generally asymptomatic. Similarly the ball-and-socket ankle joint associated with tarsal coalition is usually asymptomatic (Fig. 3).

F. Moderate partial fibular hemimelia has more significant discrepancy. When the predicted final discrepancy is 4–8 cm either epiphysiodesis of the contralateral limb or lengthening of the affected tibia can be carried out. It is preferable to delay lengthening until skeletal maturity whenever possible so that the absolute amount of discrepancy is known and there is no opportunity to dampen normal longitudinal growth by the effect of lengthening. Lengthening of the tibia tends to aggravate the valgus appearance of the knee and any foot malposition in addition to the usual potential complications. These considerations must be taken into account in determining which patient should undergo lengthening.

G. Typically, projected final discrepancies are often >8 cm. In these circumstances, more than a single lengthening will be required. There can be no hard and fast guidelines as to the timing and nature of the management of these patients, but in general a lengthening with an appropriately timed contralateral epiphysiodesis or alternatively two-stage lengthening can be carried out. Patients that require two-stage lengthening almost always have sufficient valgus of the distal femur to require treatment—osteotomy, osteotomy with lengthening, or medial epiphysiodesis.

H. Patients with bilateral fibular hemimelia do not have a problem with limb length inequality when the involvement is relatively symmetric, as is often the case. However, the foot deformity can be extreme; when this is the case, Syme's amputation is recommended.

I. Patients with bilateral fibular hemimelia should be periodically reevaluated throughout growth to detect progressive limb length inequality due to asymmetric shortening.

FIBULAR HEMIMELIA

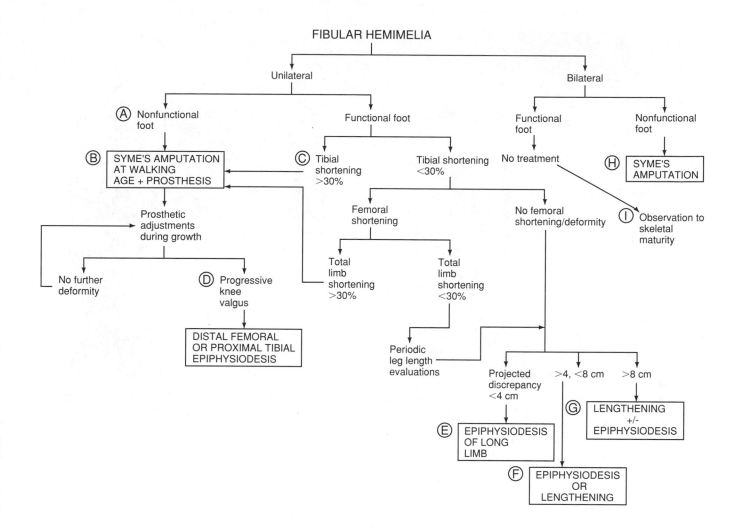

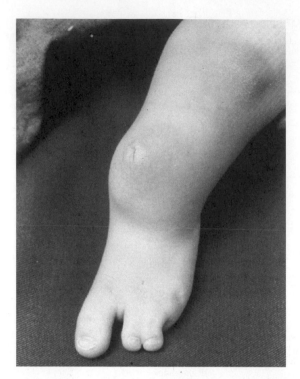

Figure 1 Fibular hemimelia. Severe forms show severe shortening of lower leg, anteromedial bowing of tibia, deficient lateral rays of foot, and equinovalgus of foot and ankle.

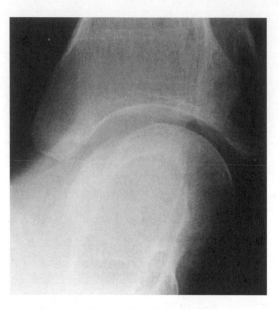

Figure 3 Ball-and-socket ankle joint is frequently present with fibular hemimelia because of associated tarsal coalition.

Figure 2 Classification of fibular hemimelia. **A,** Mild partial fibular hemimelia. There is an intact but short fibula and moderate tibial shortening. **B,** Moderate fibular hemimelia. There is more severe hypoplasia of fibula and tibia, often with angular deformity of the midshaft of the tibia, and formation of a ball-and-socket ankle joint. There is often associated mild distal femoral valgus deformity and a variable degree of femoral shortening. **C,** Severe fibular hemimelia. There is complete absence of the fibula, severe shortening, and angular deformity of the tibia. Typically, the foot and ankle are in marked equinovalgus or even completely dislocated.

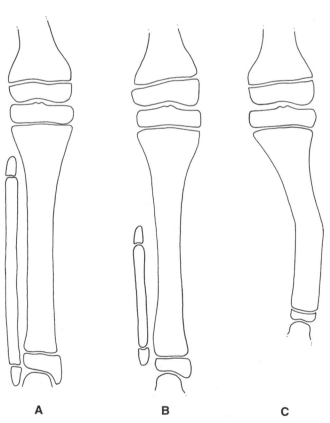

A   B   C

References

Achterman C, Kalamchi A. Congenital deficiency of the fibula. J Bone Joint Surg 1979; 61B:133.

Amstutz HC. Natural history and treatment of congenital absence of the fibula. J Bone Joint Surg 1972; 54A:1349.

Anderson L, Westin GW, Oppenheim WL. Syme amputation in children: Indications, results, and long-term follow-up. J Pediatr Orthop 1984; 4:550.

Catagni MA. Management of fibular hemimelia using the Ilizarov method. Instr Course Lect 1992; 41:431.

Catagni MB, Bolano L, Cattaneo R. Management of fibular hemimelia using the Ilizarov method. Orthop Clin 1991; 22:715.

Davidson WH, Bohne WHO. The Syme amputation in children. J Bone Joint Surg 1975; 57A:905.

Herring JA, Barnhill B, Gaffney C. Syme amputation: An evaluation of the physical and psychological function in young patients. J Bone Joint Surg 1986; 68A:573.

Kruger LM, Talbott RD. Amputation and prosthesis as definitive treatment in congenital absence of the fibula. J Bone Joint Surg 1961; 43A:625.

Westin GW, Sakai DN, Wood WO. Congenital longitudinal deficiency of the fibula. J Bone Joint Surg 1976; 58A:492.

LEGG-CALVE-PERTHES DISEASE

Legg-Calve-Perthes disease is an idiopathic avascular necrosis of the developing ossific nucleus of the immature hip. When a child presents with clinical and radiographic evidence of avascular necrosis of the femoral head, first rule out other causes such as post-traumatic or septic avascular necrosis, epiphyseal dysplasia, or Gaucher's disease. The last two are more likely if bilateral symmetric involvement of the hips is present, since Legg-Perthes typically involves only one hip. The natural history of Legg-Perthes disease is for the femoral ossific nucleus to pass through radiographic phases termed avascular, resorptive (so-called "fragmentation" phase) reossification, and "healed". Treatment of Legg-Perthes disease is of two types: symptomatic (crutches, traction) and definitive (ideally to promote spherical reconstitution of the femoral head). The influence of definitive treatment modalities to improve sphericity of femoral head remains controversial. Definitive treatment is reserved for hips of older patients with more extensive head involvement in the avascular and resorptive phases: after reossification has commenced only symptomatic treatment is indicated as necessary.

A. Initial radiographic evaluation of an affected hip should include anteroposterior (AP) and frog lateral films. If avascular or resorption phases of Perthes is identified, follow the treatment tree. Attempt to determine the extent of femoral head involvement. Catterall's classification (groups 1–4; Fig. 1), Herring classification (groups A, B, and C), and the Salter classification (more or less than half the femoral head) are used to quantify the extent of head involvement. The most important prognostic factor for ultimate sphericity of the head is the patient's age (see D). Perform careful clinical examination to document the range of motion (ROM) of the hip. Restricted ROM is considered to be >20° flexion contracture and <20° abduction on the affected side. In a patient with avascular or resorptive phase of the disease this requires treatment to improve motion.

   Occasionally patients present with symptoms and physical signs suggestive of Perthes disease and normal or equivocal radiographs. In these circumstances, technetium bone scan or magnetic resonance imaging (MRI) documents the avascular state of the femoral head. These investigations, however, do not quantify the extent of head involvement and thus cannot be used to predict the ultimate outcome.

B. ROM in an affected hip is virtually always restricted compared to normal. Consider traction for the purpose of improving ROM in the avascular or resorptive phases when the motion is <20° of abduction or flexion contracture >20°, particularly if the patient is symptomatic.

C. The purpose of traction is to rest the hip and gradually abduct and extend it to a more normal range. Balanced skin traction is used, and continued until the

motion has improved (to a maximum of 2 weeks). Traction may be reinstituted intermittently for either symptoms or recurrence of restricted ROM during the active stages. Traction does not influence the eventual sphericity of the femoral head.

D. Petrie casts are the original form of ambulatory abduction treatment for Perthes disease. They are long leg cast with the legs held abducted and internally rotated by connecting bars. If a patient has unrestricted ROM after a period in traction, he can be placed in Petrie casts as a temporary form of abduction treatment. If a restricted ROM persists under anesthetic after a period in traction, adductor and iliopsoas tenotomy may be required to improve motion, followed by application of the Petrie cast.

E. The single most important prognostic factor for the ultimate sphericity of the femoral head is the patient's age. Patients <6 years old may require symptomatic treatment during the active phases of the disease but have a good long-term prognosis. Patients over 6 have a less certain prognosis and therefore are considered candidates for definitive treatment.

F. After age, the next most significant prognostic factor is the extent of femoral head involvement. The three previously mentioned classifications are all plagued by inconsistencies in radiographic findings and significant inter-observer error. Thus, in general, unless the treating physician can be certain that there is less than half head involvement without lateral pillar collapse, more patients will be treated than ultimately prove to require it in retrospect.

G. Containment treatment for Perthes disease is any treatment that abducts the femoral head within the acetabulum. Theoretically, this protects the "soft" lateral portion of the femoral head during the avascular and resorption phases of the disease, which in turn allows more spherical reconstitution of the femoral head. "Containment" treatment is the only type of intervention considered definitive (i.e., to influence the ultimate sphericity of the femoral head). To what extent this actually does so, and whether one form of containment treatment is superior to any other, remains very controversial.

H. The Atlanta Scottish Rite abduction orthosis is the most popular conservative form of containment treatment for Perthes disease (Fig. 2). This hips are held abducted by the thigh cuffs connected to a pelvic band. Rotation is not controlled by this brace.

I. Salter osteotomy is containment treatment whereby the acetabulum is rotated over the femoral head. Theoretical advantages include the lack of need for permanent implant, and no aggravation of limb shortening frequently present in patients with Perthes.

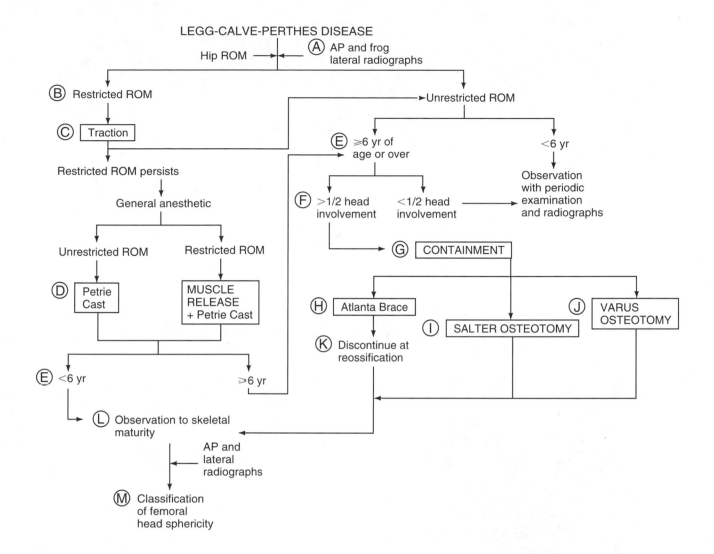

LEGG-CALVE-PERTHES DISEASE

(A) AP and frog lateral radiographs

Hip ROM →←

(B) Restricted ROM → (C) Traction → Restricted ROM persists → General anesthetic

Unrestricted ROM → (E) ≥6 yr of age or over

<6 yr → Observation with periodic examination and radiographs

(F) >1/2 head involvement   <1/2 head involvement

(G) CONTAINMENT

Unrestricted ROM → (D) Petrie Cast

Restricted ROM → MUSCLE RELEASE + Petrie Cast

(H) Atlanta Brace   (I) SALTER OSTEOTOMY   (J) VARUS OSTEOTOMY

(K) Discontinue at reossification

(E) <6 yr   ≥6 yr

(L) Observation to skeletal maturity

AP and lateral radiographs

(M) Classification of femoral head sphericity

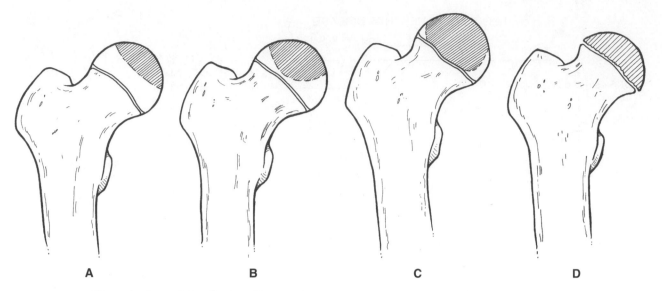

Figure 1 Catterall classification of Legg-Calve-Perthes disease. **A,** Group 1; anterior portion of femoral head only is affected. **B,** Group 2; anterior and lateral portions of femoral head are affected. **C,** Group 3; only posteromedial portion of femoral epiphysis is unaffected. **D,** Group 4; entire epiphysis is affected.

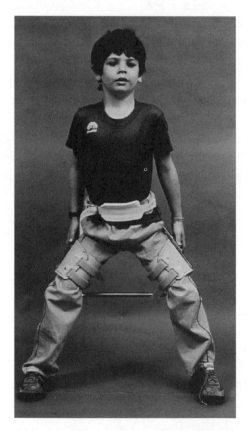

Figure 2 Atlanta brace for conservative treatment of Legg-Calve-Perthes disease. Joints in the brace allow the hips to flex and extend while maintaining abduction.

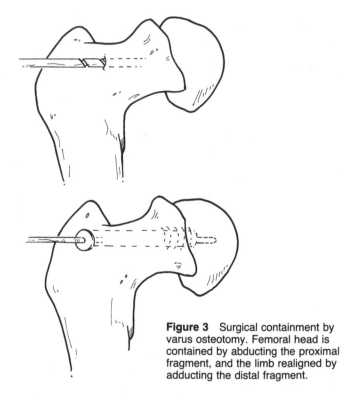

Figure 3 Surgical containment by varus osteotomy. Femoral head is contained by abducting the proximal fragment, and the limb realigned by adducting the distal fragment.

J. Varus rotational osteotomy contains the femoral head by virtue of abducting the proximal fragment (Fig. 3). Advantages are that the surgery is relatively easy to perform and has the most literature evidence to support its effectiveness over other forms of containment treatment. The main disadvantage is aggravation of any limb shortening.

K. The duration of susceptibility of the femoral head to deformation in the active stages of Perthes disease is not known. It is generally accepted, however, that this is the avascular and resorptive phases. Once reossification in the lateral portion of the femoral head is identified on an AP radiograph, the brace is discontinued. This generally occurs 12 to 18 months after onset of the disease.

L. Complete reconstitution of the femoral head radiographically takes 3 to 5 years. Symptoms, however, are generally limited to the first 12 to 18 months. Recurrence of Perthes disease is rare. Patients with persistent symptoms after completion of reossification are evaluated for possible osteochondritis dissecans of the femoral head (prevalence 3%) or early osteoarthritis. Involvement of the opposite hip is also rare. Its presence should initiate evaluation for systemic disorder.

M. Patients can be evaluated at skeletal maturity with AP and lateral radiographs and the femoral head sphericity classified according to the methods of Mose or Stulberg. The prognosis for the development of osteoarthritis after Perthes disease is directly related to the sphericity of the femoral head after skeletal maturity.

References

Brotherton BJ, McKibbon B. Perthes' disease treated by prolonged recumbency and femoral head containment: A long-term appraisal. J Bone Joint Surg 1977; 59B:8.

Catterall A. The natural history of Perthes' disease. J Bone Joint Surg 1971; 53B:37.

Chung SMK. The arterial supply of the developing proximal end of the human femur. J Bone Joint Surg 1976; 58A:961.

Coates CJ, Paterson JM, Woods KR, et al. Femoral osteotomy in Perthes' disease: Results at maturity. J Bone Joint Surg 1990; 72B:581.

Hardcastle PH, Ross R, Hamalainen M, Mata A. Catterall grouping of Perthes' disease: An assessment of observer error and prognosis using the Catterall classification. J Bone Joint Surg 1980; 62B:428.

Herring JA. The treatment of Legg-Calve-Perthes disease: A critical review of the literature. J Bone Joint Surg 1994; 76A:448.

Kelly FP, Canale ST, Jones RR. Legg-Calve-Perthes disease: Long-term evaluation of noncontainment treatment. J Bone Joint Surg 1980; 62A:400.

Lloyd-Roberts GC. The management of Perthes disease. J Bone Joint Surg 1982; 64B:1.

McAndrew MP, Weinstein SL. A long term followup of Legg-Calve-Perthes disease. J Bone Joint Surg 1984; 66A:860.

Mose K. Methods of measuring in Legg-Calve-Perthes disease with special regard to the prognosis. Clin Orthop 1980; 150:103.

Paterson DC, Leitch JM, Foster BK. Results of innominate osteotomy in the treatment of Legg-Calve-Perthes disease. Clin Orthop 1991; 266:96.

Petrie G, Bitenc I. The abduction weight bearing treatment in Legg-Perthes disease. J Bone Joint Surg 1971; 53B:54.

Purvis JM, Dimon JH III, Meehan PL, Lovell WW. Preliminary experience with the Scottish Rite Hospital abduction orthosis for Legg-Perthes disease. Clin Orthop 1980; 150:49.

Salter RB, Thompson GH. Legg-Calve-Perthes disease: The prognostic significance of the subchondral fracture and a two group classification of the femoral head involvement. J Bone Joint Surg 1984; 66A:479.

Stulberg SD, Cooperman DR, Wallenstein R. The natural history of Legg-Calve-Perthes disease. J Bone Joint Surg 1981; 63A:1095.

SLIPPED CAPITAL FEMORAL EPIPHYSIS

A. All patients with evidence of slipped capital femoral epiphysis (SCFE) (Fig. 1) require two particular evaluations: first, a general examination supplemented by laboratory studies as indicated to rule out generalized metabolic disease (specifically chronic renal failure, hypothyroidism, or more rare endocrinopathies such as panhypopituitarism); second, clinical and radiographic assessment of the opposite hip to rule out SCFE. Bilateral symptomatic slips in a younger child suggest that metabolic disease exists, and endocrinopathy should be vigorously excluded. Approximately 25% of adolescent patients will develop SCFE of the opposite hip.

B. Occasionally, with treatment of metabolic disorders such as chronic renal failure or hypopituitarism both clinical and radiographic findings of SCFE resolve. The surgeon may cautiously monitor the patient before proceeding with surgical treatment. If there is any doubt, once the metabolic condition has stabilized, surgical management of the slip should be undertaken.

C. Specifically caution patients to report any symptoms reminiscent of slip as soon as they occur. In addition, patients should be routinely radiographed approximately every 6 months until skeletal maturity to rule out occult development of SCFE in a previously unaffected hip.

D. Slipped epiphyses have been classified according to duration of symptoms as acute (<3 weeks of symptoms), chronic, or acute-on-chronic (an acute exacerbation of symptoms associated with radiographic evidence of both an acute slip and previous remodelling of a chronic slip). A more useful clinical and radiographic classification is to divide SCFE into "stable" and "unstable" types (i.e., the presence or absence of continued gross motion between the epiphysis and the femoral neck). In unstable slips the prevalence of avascular necrosis (AVN) is greatly increased, irrespective of the type of treatment carried out. Treatment regimens are the same as for a stable slip, but the likelihood of AVN is increased to approximately 30%.

E. The severity of SCFE is classified in several ways including the angle between the axis of the femoral neck and a perpendicular to the transverse axis of the epiphysis on the lateral radiograph (Fig. 2). The treatment modality selected tends to be the same irrespective of severity. Treatment options include spica immobilization, in situ pinning, and open epiphysiodesis. Most authors select in situ fixation with one or two cannulated screws to secure the epiphysis to the femoral neck. The purpose of this treatment is to prevent further slipping and enhance a fusion of the epiphysis to the femoral neck. Unstable slips are treated the same, but grossly unstable slips may be gently reduced by internal rotation of the limb, prior to pinning. This usually partially reduces the deformity. The postoperative management is partial weight bearing with crutches for 6 to 12 weeks, followed by regular examination and radiographs until the physis has fused.

F. Symptoms from slipped epiphysis should be expected to resolve within several days to several weeks after pinning. If the patient has persistent pain, vigorously re-evaluate the adequacy of pinning.

G. If symptoms persist and the physis is open, the pin should be reinserted if the pinning is inadequate, or alternatively an open epiphysiodesis carried out.

H. Chondrolysis is symptomatic narrowing of the cartilage space. This can occur spontaneously prior to any known treatment, or after in-situ pinning, open epiphysiodesis, or Southwick osteotomy. If any pins are in or near the hip joint, remove them. Patients should then be treated with crutches, active range of motion (ROM) exercises, and anti-inflammatory medications. Prognosis for recovery of joint motion is good as long as any intra-articular implant has been removed.

I. The other major complication of SCFE is AVN. AVN is specifically associated with unstable slips, injudicious efforts at closed reduction, open reduction, or osteotomies of the femoral neck. Segmental collapse is usually seen. The most common outcome is hip fusion or total joint arthroplasty. Initial management consists of removal of any implant that may damage the remaining articular surface with collapse of the femoral head. Occasionally, despite significant radiographic abnormality, the patient functions well with conservative management (restriction of activity, cane, anti-inflammatory medication). When conservative methods fail the patient must be considered for either hip fusion or total hip arthroplasty.

J. There is a tendency towards generalized improvement in symptoms of limp, muscle fatigue, and external rotation deformity during growth by remodeling of the upper portion of the femur. If, at the end of growth, there is symptomatic loss of flexion, or increased external rotation, subtrochanteric osteotomy as described by Southwick may be carried out.

SLIPPED CAPITAL FEMORAL EPIPHYSIS

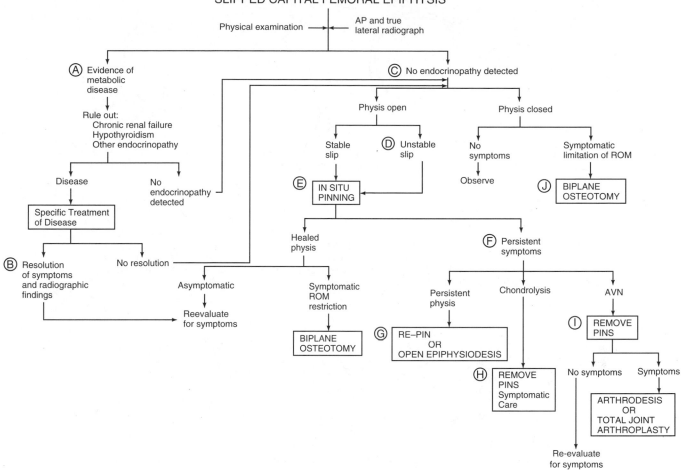

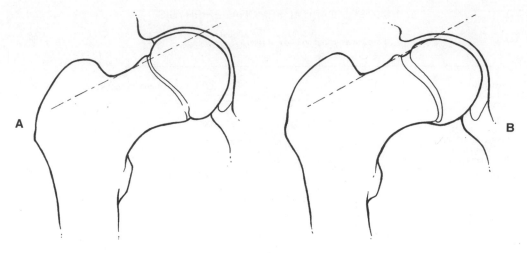

Figure 1 Appearance of normal and mild slipped capital femoral epiphysis on an anteroposterior radiograph. **A,** In a normal hip a small portion of femoral epiphysis lies lateral to a tangent (Klein's line) to the superior femoral neck. **B,** Because of posterior and medial displacement of the epiphysis, the entire epiphysis lies medial to Klein's line.

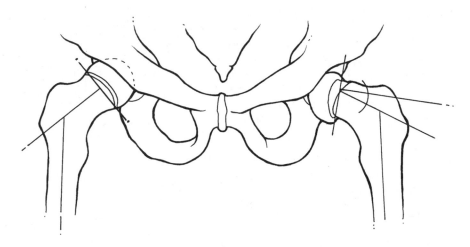

Figure 2 Slip angle. The severity of displacement of the capital femoral epiphysis on the femoral neck may be graded by measuring the angle between the axis of the femoral neck and a perpendicular to a tangent to the inferior portions of the capital femoral epiphysis. This angle is typically 0°. Mild slips are 0°-30°, moderate 31°-60°, and severe slips >60°.

References

Agamanolis DP, Weiner DS, Lloyd JK. Slipped capital femoral epiphysis: a pathological study: I—A light microscopic and histochemical study of 21 cases. J Pediatr Orthop 1985; 5:40.

Aronson DD, Carlson WE. Slipped capital femoral ephiphysis: a prospective study of fixation with a single screw. J Bone Joint Surg 1992; 74A:810.

Blanco JS, Taylor B, Johnston CE 2d. Comparison of single pin versus multiple pin fixation in treatment of slipped capital femoral epiphysis. J Pediatr Orthop 1992; 12:384.

Carney BT, Weinstein SL, Noble J. Long-term follow-up of slipped capital femoral epiphysis. J Bone Joint Surg 1991; 73A:667.

Crawford AH. The role of osteotomy in the treatment of slipped capital femoral epiphysis. Instr Course Lect 1989; 38:273.

Jones JR, Paterson DC, Hillier TM, Foster BK. Remodeling after pinning for slipped capital femoral epiphysis. J Bone Joint Surg 1990; 72B:568.

Melby A, Hoyt W, Weiner D. Treatment of chronic slipped capital femoral epiphysis by bone-graft epiphysiodesis. J Bone Joint Surg 1980; 62A:119

Morrissy RT. Principles of in situ fixation in chronic slipped capital femoral epiphysis. Instr Course Lect 1989; 38:257.

Morrissy RT. Slipped capital femoral epiphysis: Natural history and etiology in treatment. Instr Course Lect 1980; 29:81.

Salvati E, Robinson H, O'Dowd T. Southwick osteotomy for severe chronic slipped capital femoral epiphysis: Results and complications. J Bone Joint Surg 1980; 62A:561.

LIMB LENGTH INEQUALITY

A. Patients in the pediatric age group rarely complain of pain or other functional problems due to a limb length inequality of any cause. If such complaints occur, the patient should be thoroughly evaluated as to the exact etiology of the complaint. Typically the presenting complaint is trunk imbalance, tendency to toe walk, or other lower extremity posturing noted by the family. Clinical examination should concentrate on assessing the child's general health, neuromuscular status of the lower extremity, flexibility of joints, and the clinical estimation of the amount of limb length inequality. This can be accomplished by a tape measure or alternatively having the patient stand erect with blocks under the short side until the pelvis is levelled (Fig. 1). Radiographically, scanogram (a three exposure radiograph of the hip, knee, and ankle with a superimposed ruler) should be taken for an accurate documentation of the discrepancy (Figs. 2 and 3) as well as a hand and wrist film for bone age.

B. If clinical investigation with or without supplementary scanogram reveals a functional discrepancy due to joint contracture or neuromuscular disorder, correct those deformities based on their nature and severity.

C. Patients with a true limb length inequality who are skeletally mature are at no risk for progression of the discrepancy. Treatment should be undertaken solely for current functional complaints.

D. In general, patients who have <2 cm of discrepancy can be expected to be asymptomatic without any short- or long-term problems. In very rare circumstances there may be some functional complaints with these minor discrepancies, which can be treated by an appropriate size heel and shoe lift.

E. Patients with >2 cm of discrepancy may have functional complaints in the lower extremity or back. Consider correcting these larger discrepancies. Options include shoe lift, shortening of the appropriate segment on the long side, or, with larger discrepancies, lengthening.

F. Patients who are skeletally immature usually demonstrate a dynamic discrepancy. Obtain serial scanograms and bone age determinations every 6–12 months based on the child's age to determine these dynamics. In general, congenital anomalies maintain the same percentage length relative to the other leg; discrepancy due to physeal arrest from any cause has very predictable discrepancy based on the loss of growth of that involved physis; post-traumatic causes such as femoral shaft fracture may have a very variable course.

G. Three scanograms and a bone age taken ≥6 months apart usually provide excellent prediction of discrepancy at skeletal maturity using the Moseley straight line graph charting methods. If the projected discrepancy is <2 cm, no treatment is usually required and the patient can be discharged from care as skeletal maturity is approached.

H. Patients with projected discrepancy of 2–8 cm usually have some functional impairment. Consider an appropriately timed epiphysiodesis of the long limb, or, alternatively, lengthening. In general, consider lengthening if the patient requires osteotomy for angular deformity on the short side; simple osteotomy with appropriately timed epiphysiodesis on the opposite limb is an alternative. If there is no limb deformity, lengthening is generally reserved for patients with >4 cm of projected final discrepancy. Epiphysiodesis versus limb lengthening is a highly individualized decision based on underlying deformity, the degree of discrepancy, patient stature, and individual preference.

I. Patients with a projected discrepancy of 8–20 cm require treatment. In the pediatric population heel and sole lift or extension orthosis may be required temporarily to maximize function. Such orthotic correction certainly could be used permanently, but patients rarely accept this. Patients with >8 cm of discrepancy normally require more than one stage of treatment. The alternatives include lengthening of the short limb and appropriately timed contralateral epiphysiodesis for residual discrepancy, or, alternatively, two or three stages of lengthening for larger discrepancies. Staged lengthening requires a highly motivated patient with stable joints.

J. Patients with >20 cm of predicted ultimate discrepancy require an extension orthosis during growth to maximize lower extremity function. If there is difficulty fitting an orthosis, consider suitable amputation (such as a Syme's) and prosthetic fitting. Only rarely are staged lengthening and epiphysiodesis appropriate in patients with so severe a limb length inequality.

SUSPECTED LIMB LENGTH INEQUALITY

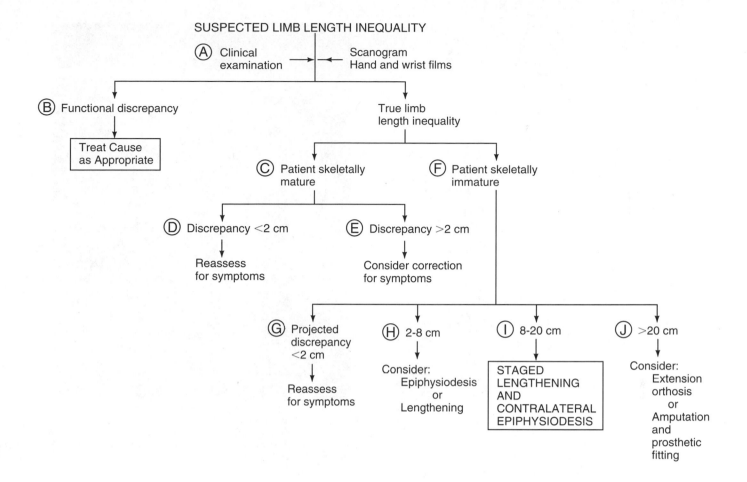

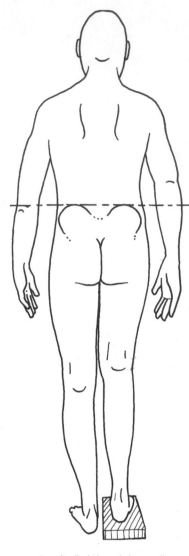

Figure 1 Lower extremity limb length inequality may be estimated by leveling the patient's pelvis with an appropriate-sized block under the shorter extremity. This leveling may be confirmed by a standing anteroposterior radiograph of the pelvis.

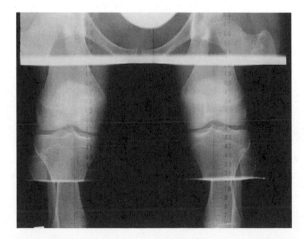

Figure 2 Plain radiographic scanogram. Three separate exposures of the hip, knee, and ankle are made from a single film over a ruler.

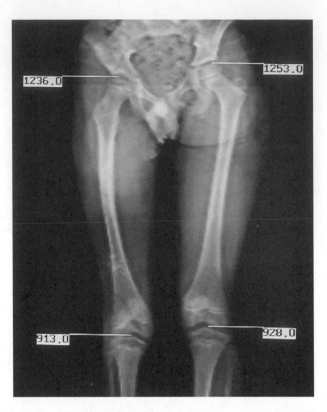

Figure 3 CT scanogram of the femurs. Direct measurement of the limb segment may be made from the scout radiograph. Flexion and/or abduction deformities must be taken into account by positioning limbs symmetrically for accurate measurements.

References

Altongy J, Harcke H, Bowen J. Measurement of leg length inequalities by microdose digital radiographs. J Pediatr Orthop 1987; 7:311.

Anderson M, Messner M, Green W. Distribution of lengths of the normal femur and tibia in children from one to eighteen years of age. J Bone Joint Surg 1964; 46A:1197.

Blount W. A mature look at epiphyseal stapling. Clin Orthop 1971; 77:149.

Canale S, Russel T, Holcomb R. Percutaneous epiphysiodesis: Experimental study and preliminary clinical results. J Pediatr Orthop 1986; 6:150.

Dal Monte A, Donzelli O. Comparison of different methods of leg lengthening. J Pediatr Orthop 1988; 8:62.

De Bastiani G, Aldegheri R, Renzi-Brivio L, et al. Limb lengthening by callus distraction (callotasis). J Pediatr Orthop 1987; 7:129.

Ilizarov GA. Transosseous Osteosynthesis. Berlin: Springer-Verlag, 1992.

Mosely C. A straight line graph for leg length discrepancies. J Bone Joint Surg 1977; 59A:174.

Shapiro F. Developmental patterns in lower-extremity length discrepancies. J Bone Joint Surg 1982; 64A:639.

Westh R, Menelaus M. A simple calculation for the timing of epiphyseal arrest: A further report. J Bone Joint Surg 1981; 63B:117.

Winquist R. Closed intramedullary osteotomies of the femur. Clin Orthop 1986; 212:155.

DEVELOPMENTAL DYSPLASIA OF THE HIP BEFORE SIX MONTHS OF AGE

A. The most important investigation to rule out developmental dysplasia of the hip (DDH) is a careful physical examination. If the first examination is inadequate or uncertain, the examination should be repeated later.

High resolution ultrasonography by virtue of visualizing the cartilaginous femoral head and acetabulum can aid in screening for DDH. It also is a way to monitor maintenance of reduction of the femoral head in the acetabulum. Ultrasound findings, however, must be correlated to physical examination.

B. DDH can occur in any child. The overall prevalence of neonatal hip instability is approximately one in 80 at birth, although spontaneous resolution in most cases reduces the prevalence to approximately one per thousand at 6 weeks of age. Known risk factors for DDH include first born birth order, female, breech presentation (irrespective of the form of delivery), and a positive family history. If any of these factors exist, ultrasound examination should supplement physical examination (particularly if examination has been unsatisfactory).

C. The role of long-term, part-time abduction splinting has not been documented, but is felt to be indicated for radiographic acetabular dysplasia. A variety of commercially available abduction orthoses are available. Their purpose is to hold the leg in a flexed, abducted position, which is felt to stimulate resolution of the acetabular dysplasia. Patients with persistent acetabular dysplasia beyond 4 or 5 years of age need to be considered for a pelvic osteotomy.

D. The severity of the hip pathology in an otherwise normal patient varies from subluxatable to fixed dislocation (Ortolani negative). Strictly speaking, an Ortolani-negative hip is not "unstable" by virtue of the fact that this is a fixed dislocation. Other classic signs of dislocation, however, usually are present, including shortening of the thigh, asymmetric thigh folds, limited abduction, and positive Galeazzi signs. The subluxatable hip is one in which the femoral head is resting in the acetabulum but there is a clinical and/or radiographic sense of subluxation of the femoral head. The dislocatable hip is one that is reduced in the resting position, but the femoral head can be displaced from the acetabulum by the Barlow maneuver. In such cases, the femoral head usually spontaneously reduces. The Barlow sign (Fig. 1) is normally lost within 6 weeks of birth. An Ortolani-positive hip is one in which the femoral head is dislocated in the resting position, but is reducible with the Ortolani maneuver. Generally, such a hip spontaneously redislocates after manual pressure is released. Normally, Ortolani positive hips will proceed to a fixed dislocation (i.e., the Ortolani sign will be lost).

E. With Ortolani-positive and Ortolani-negative hips, the physician must be certain that the projected femoral head points to the triradiate cartilage in the simulated Pavlik harness position as described in F below. If the projected femoral head points to the triradiate cartilage, most authors feel that the patient is a candidate for a trial of the Pavlik harness. The harness must be worn full-time until the hip has stabilized to repeated examination. If the femoral head does not point to the triradiate cartilage (it need not be reduced), then Pavlik harness use is contraindicated. Some authors feel that the lack of a concentric reduction from the onset is a contraindication for the Pavlik harness and that closed or open reduction should be performed.

F. Treatment for subluxatable and dislocatable hips and Ortolani-positive or negative hips in which the femoral head points to the triradiate cartilage is application of a Pavlik harness (Fig. 2). The diagnosis may be confirmed by ultrasound. Apply the Pavlik harness with the child's thigh flexed 100° or more, with abduction limited to within a few finger's breadth of midline. The harness should be worn full-time until hip instability has resolved. Check the patient once a week to ensure appropriate fit, to rule out the complication of femoral nerve palsy, and to monitor progress in the clinical examination. There should be a resting reduced position after 4 weeks in the Pavlik harness, or the Pavlik should be abandoned. The hip may maintain an instability (i.e., become Barlow positive or dislocatable), but the resting position must be reduced.

Weaning programs vary from several weeks to one and a half times the child's age at initiation of treatment. After the Pavlik harness has been removed, the child should have periodic radiographs every 3–6 months until acetabular dysplasia has completely resolved. This follow-up will normally take a minimum of 4 years.

G. If instability or dislocation persists after a trial of Pavlik harness wear, closed reduction under general anesthesia is indicated. If a stable closed reduction is obtained, the child is placed in a spica cast for 12–18 weeks. Re-evaluate every 6 weeks under general anesthetic including an arthrogram if necessary to confirm maintenance of a stable concentric reduction. After the spica cast is removed follow the child with periodic radiographs of the pelvis until complete resolution of the acetabular dysplasia is confirmed. If closed reduction fails or the hip does not stabilize after spica cast treatment, open reduction is indicated.

H. Ortolani-negative hips that do not point to the triradiate cartilage will require traction and attempted closed reduction as the initial form of treatment. If closed reduction fails, open reduction is required. In patients who are not yet walking, the surgeon may choose either anterior or medial open reduction.

DEVELOPMENTAL DYSPLASIA OF THE HIP (< 6 MO)

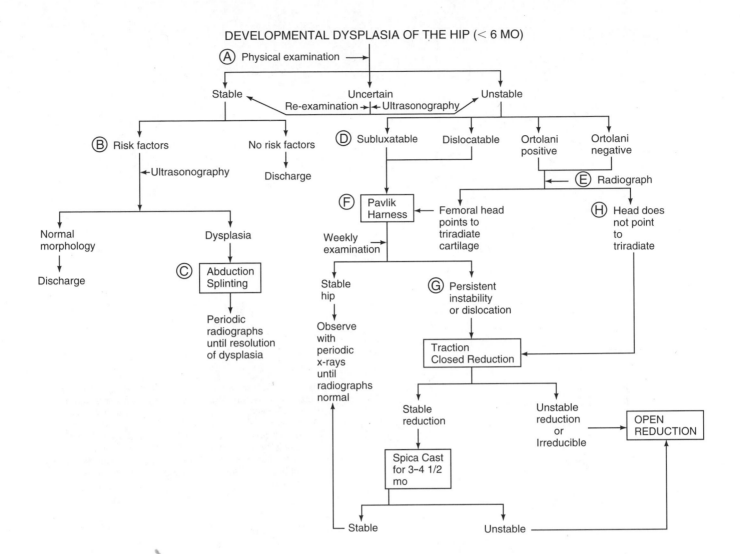

Ⓐ Physical examination

Stable — Uncertain — Unstable

Re-examination → ← Ultrasonography

Ⓑ Risk factors   No risk factors

Ⓓ Subluxatable   Dislocatable   Ortolani positive   Ortolani negative

← Ultrasonography

Discharge

Ⓔ Radiograph

Normal morphology   Dysplasia

Ⓕ Pavlik Harness   Femoral head points to triradiate cartilage   Ⓗ Head does not point to triradiate

Discharge

Ⓒ Abduction Splinting

Weekly examination

Periodic radiographs until resolution of dysplasia

Stable hip   Ⓖ Persistent instability or dislocation

Observe with periodic x-rays until radiographs normal

Traction Closed Reduction

Stable reduction   Unstable reduction or Irreducible   OPEN REDUCTION

Spica Cast for 3–4 1/2 mo

Stable   Unstable

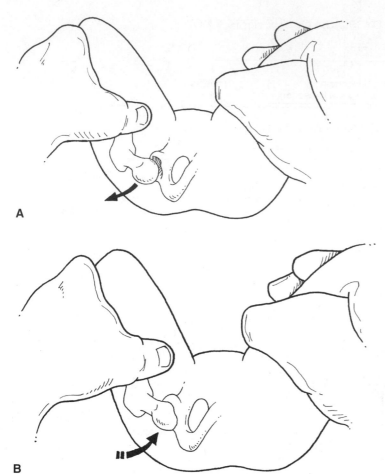

A

B

Figure 1   A, Barlow's sign is the examiner's sensation of dislocation of the femoral head from the acetabulum. This sign is elicited by adducting and posteriorly displacing the femur. The hip should be flexed approximately 90° and the hamstrings relaxed by knee flexion. The infant should be relaxed and warm. B, Relaxation of the adduction and posteriorly directed force will allow the femoral head to reduce spontaneously into the acetabulum in most cases.

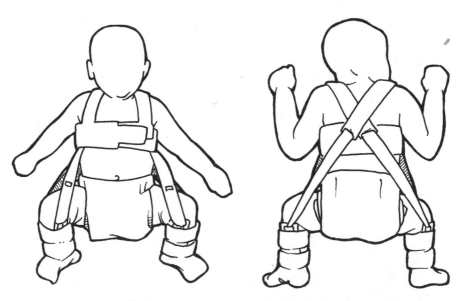

Figure 2   Positioniang in a Pavlik harness. The infant's thighs should be held symmetrically in the Pavlik harness in a position of 100° or more of flexion. The posterior strap should be adjusted to limit abduction to approximately neutral.

References

Barlow TC. Early diagnosis and treatment of congenital dislocation of the hip. J Bone Joint Surg [Br] 1962; 44:292.

Boeree NR, Clarke NM. Ultrasound imaging and secondary screening for congenital dislocation of the hip. J Bone Joint Surg [Br] 1994; 76:525.

Fleissner PR Jr, Ciccarelli CJ, Eilert RE, Chang FM, Glancy GL. The success of closed reduction in the treatment of complex developmental dislocation of the hip. J Pediatr Orthop 1994; 14:631.

Gabuzda GM, Renshaw TS. Reduction of congenital dislocation of the hip. J Bone Joint Surg [Am] 1992; 74:624.

Grill F, Bensahel H, Candell J, Dungel P, Matasovic T, Vizkelety T. The Pavlik harness in the treatment of the congenitally dislocating hip: Report on a multicenter study of the European Pediatric Orthopaedic Society. J Pediatr Orthop 1988; 8:1.

Harcke HT. Imaging in congenital dislocation and dysplasia of the hip. Clin Orthop 1992; 281:22.

Joseph K, MacEwen GD, Boos ML. Home traction in the management of congenital dislocation of the hip. Clin Orthop 1982; 166:83.

Kalamchi A, O'Connor J, MacEwen GD. Evaluation of the Pavlik harness in the treatment of congenital dislocation of the hip. Presented at the 45th Annual Meeting of the American Academy of Orthopaedic Surgeons, Dallas, 1978.

Lindstrom JR, Ponsetti IV, Wenger DR. Acetabular development after reduction in congenital dislocation of the hip. J Bone Joint Surg [Am] 1979; 61:112.

Morrissy RT. Lovell and Winter's Pediatrics Orthopaedics. 3rd ed. Philadelphia: JB Lippincott, 1990.

Tachdjian MO. Pediatric Orthopedics. Philadelphia: WB Saunders, 1990.

Tonnis D. Congenital Dysplasia and Dislocation of the Hip in Children and Adults. New York: Springer-Verlag, 1987.

DEVELOPMENTAL DYSPLASIA OF THE HIP
AFTER 6 MONTHS OF AGE

A. Children diagnosed with developmental dysplasia of the hip (DDH) after age 6 months are not candidates for use of the Pavlik harness (Fig. 1). In general, care of these children requires special expertise. Most experienced surgeons attempt closed reduction of the hip after traction as first treatment. If unsuccessful, open reduction is required. On physical examination patients generally show the typical stigmata of fixed dislocations (i.e., limited abduction, pistoning instability of the hip, Galeazzi sign, and, if walking, Trendelenburg gait). Rarely is true persistent unstable examination (either Barlow positive or Ortolani positive examination) present in these older children. If these signs are present, assess the patient carefully for evidence of generalized connective tissue disorders such as Larsen's or Ehlers-Danlos syndromes.

B. In general, achieving successful closed reduction by prolonged traction, or after a preliminary period of traction is much less likely in patients over 18 months of age. Extensive morphologic changes to both the upper femur and the acetabulum almost always require some bony procedure even after successful closed reduction in such patients. Therefore many surgeons choose this age as the upper limit for attempted closed reduction, preferring anterior open reduction for patients older than this. Preliminary traction may be used to relax the soft tissues. Femoral shortening performed simultaneously with open reduction is an effective alternative to preliminary traction. Pelvic osteotomy of the Salter or other type may also be required either at the time of open reduction, or secondarily for persist acetabular dysplasia.

C. Successful treatment protocols for management of DDH in children between 6 and 18 months vary from open reduction without preliminary traction to closed reduction by prolonged traction. Most surgeons attempt a closed reduction after preliminary traction under anesthesia in otherwise healthy children presenting with DDH in this age group. The purpose of preliminary traction is to relax the soft tissues, thereby increasing the likelihood of successful closed reduction at the end of traction, and decreasing the risk of avascular necrosis. Avascular necrosis is presumably caused by injury to the blood supply of the femoral head by either traumatic closed reduction, excessive pressure across the joint after reduction due to the constrictive soft tissues, or direct injury from open reduction. If attempted closed reduction is unsuccessful, open reduction will be required.

D. Patients weighing ≤30 lb are candidates for Bryant's traction. Alternatives include gradual abduction traction. With Bryant's traction the limbs are held straight in the air, with the knee fully extended and the hips flexed 90°. The feet must be examined regularly for evidence of (1) sciatic nerve palsy due to stretch or (2) vascular compromise due to either the elevated position of the feet or constriction by traction bandaging.

E. Patients >30 lb generally will not tolerate the elevated foot position of Bryant's traction. Balanced skin traction with the legs flexed <90° with a variable amount of abduction is generally used. Skin traction is usually sufficient and skeletal traction rarely required. The duration of traction will vary with the individual's preference, but should be for a minimum of 2–3 weeks followed by attempted closed reduction under anesthesia. Alternatively, traction may be used exclusively to attempt closed reduction in traction.

F. The purpose of preliminary traction is to relax the soft tissues increasing the likelihood of successful closed reduction and anesthesia, and reducing the likelihood of avascular necrosis (AVN). The duration of traction preceding closed reduction under general anesthesia varies with individual preference and circumstance, but should be a minimum of 2 weeks. Intraoperative arthrogram or ultrasound should be performed to confirm hip reduction. One of the circumstances as described in G, H, or I will be identified at the time of closed reduction and treatment continued accordingly.

G. A stable reduction is one in which the femoral head rests securely within the acetabulum with a broad safe zone as described by MacEwen et al. If a stable reduction is achieved and there is persistent tightness of the adductor longus, a tenotomy may be done to increase abduction, thereby increasing the stable arc of motion of the hip. The hip should be immobilized in a double hip spica cast from axilla to ankles in a position of moderate flexion (90° to 100°) abduction (maximum 60°), and rotation (usually neutral or slight internal rotation). Forced abduction or excessive internal rotation are to be avoided as these positions can induce AVN. Change the spica cast under anesthesia with arthrographic or ultrasound assessment of reduction as desired every 6 weeks. Casting is continued for 3–4½ months. After removal of the spica cast, evaluate the child every 6–12 months with physical examination and radiographs to confirm restitution of the morphology of the femoral head and acetabulum. Persistent deformity may require osteotomy in the future. AVN as consequence of treatment must be ruled out by these serial examinations.

H. The femoral head may be found to be marginally stable in the acetabulum. In this circumstance there is a more narrow range of motion through which the femoral head will remain in the acetabulum. The surgeon must decide whether there is a reasonable opportunity to hold the femoral head in the proper position in a cast without excessive force, specifically

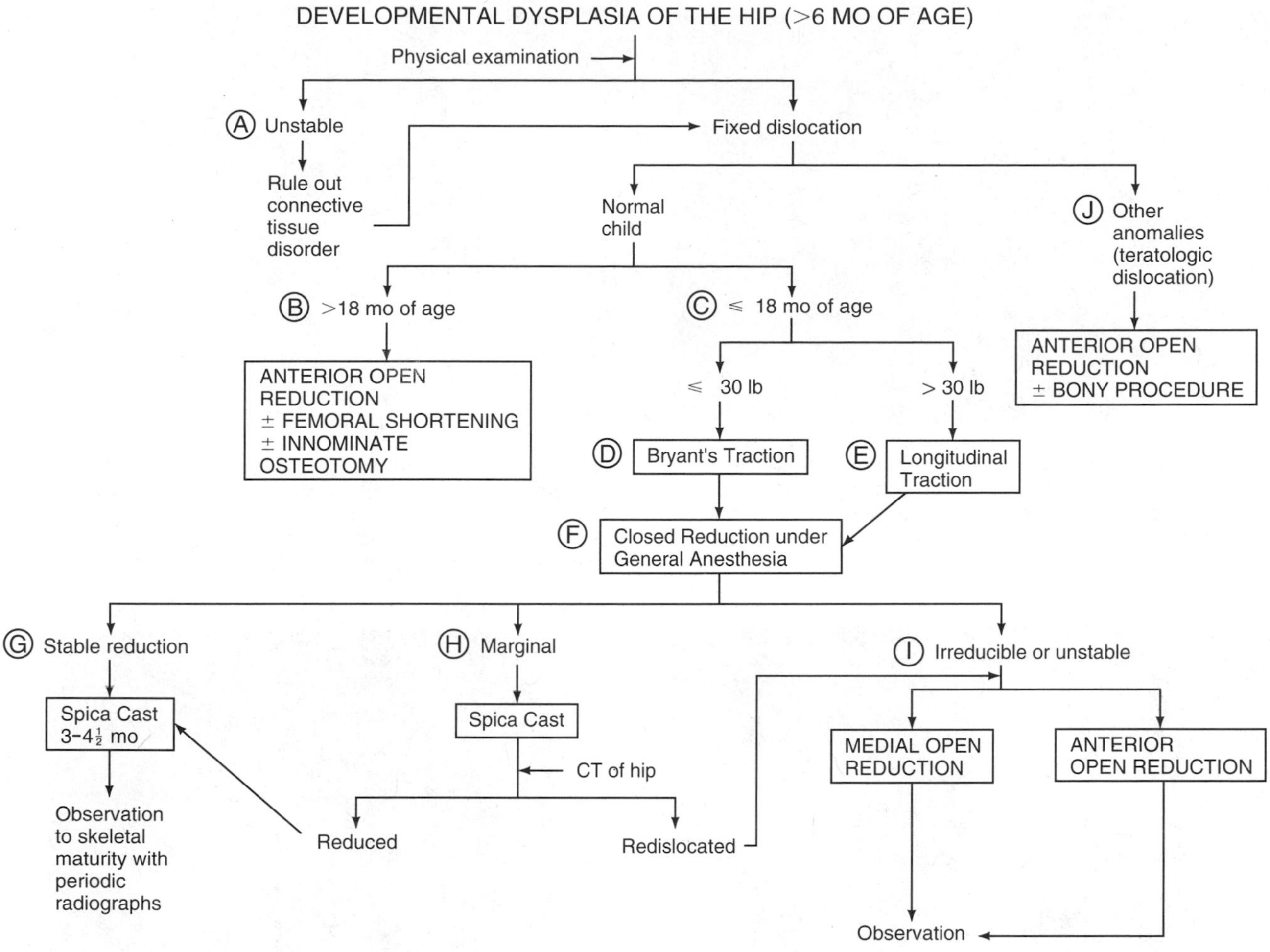

DEVELOPMENTAL DYSPLASIA OF THE HIP (>6 MO OF AGE)

Physical examination →

Ⓐ Unstable

Fixed dislocation

Rule out connective tissue disorder

Normal child

Ⓙ Other anomalies (teratologic dislocation)

Ⓑ >18 mo of age

Ⓒ ≤ 18 mo of age

ANTERIOR OPEN REDUCTION ± BONY PROCEDURE

ANTERIOR OPEN REDUCTION ± FEMORAL SHORTENING ± INNOMINATE OSTEOTOMY

≤ 30 lb

> 30 lb

Ⓓ Bryant's Traction

Ⓔ Longitudinal Traction

Ⓕ Closed Reduction under General Anesthesia

Ⓖ Stable reduction

Ⓗ Marginal

Ⓘ Irreducible or unstable

Spica Cast 3-4½ mo

Spica Cast

MEDIAL OPEN REDUCTION

ANTERIOR OPEN REDUCTION

Observation to skeletal maturity with periodic radiographs

← CT of hip

Reduced

Redislocated

Observation

307

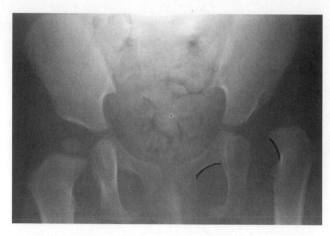

Figure 1 Anteroposterior radiograph of child with developmental dysplasia of the left hip. Shenton's line is broken. The femoral ossific nucleus is displaced laterally upward and is smaller than the opposite side.

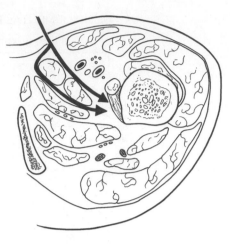

Figure 3 Medial approach to open reduction of a dislocated hip may proceed anterior to the adductor longus and brevis, or the interval between the adductor longus and brevis anteriorly and the pectineus posteriorly. Direct access to the iliopsoas tendon and medial capsular constriction is made via this approach.

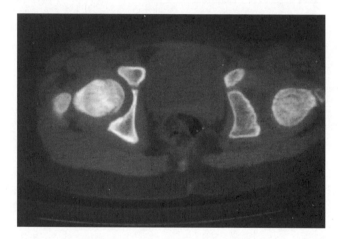

Figure 2 CT scan of the hip can be used to assess the adequacy of either closed or open reduction. In this case the left hip remains posteriorly dislocated.

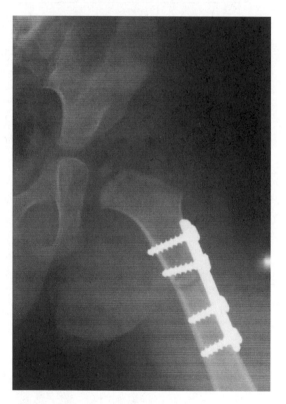

Figure 4 In older children requiring anterior open reduction of the hip, femoral shortening with internal fixation may be used to replace preliminary preoperative traction. Shortening of 1 to 1.5 cm is generally required.

abduction >60°. Adductor tenotomy may improve the stable arc of motion slightly. In the postoperative period the patient should have either computed tomography (CT) of the hips or ultrasound to confirm maintenance of reduction (Fig. 2). If the reduction is maintained, continue casting as per G. If the femoral head redislocates, open reduction is indicated.

I. The femoral head may be found to be grossly unstable in the acetabulum, or irreducible. In these circumstances open reduction is required. In patients <12 months of age, medial open reduction may be performed at the treating surgeon's preference (Fig. 3). Medial open reduction requires casting protocol as per closed reduction. In patients >12 months of age, or at the surgeon's preference, anterior open reduction with or without femoral shortening may be performed (Fig. 4). Postoperatively the patient is maintained with the hip in a stable position (in a 1½ spica cast), usually abduction, slight flexion, and neutral to slight internal rotation. Casting is continued for 8–12 weeks.

In all cases, patients must be observed regularly throughout growth at 6–12 month intervals for clinical examination and anteroposterior (AP) radiographs of the pelvis to document resolution of bony deformity of both the upper femur, acetabulum, and rule out evidence of avascular necrosis.

J. High riding fixed dislocations occurring in patients with other generalized disorders (spina bifida, arthrogryposis, etc.) are considered teratologic dislocations. In these patients, the dislocation has occurred in utero with major morphologic changes in the hip present from birth. Closed reductions in such hips are generally unsuccessful. Open reduction of the hip is indicated based on the child's mobility, and the treating surgeon's belief that the dislocated hip interferes with that mobility. Both anterior open reduction (usually with femoral shortening in place of traction) and medial open reduction have been employed successfully in these patients.

References

Galpin RD, Roach JW, Wenger DR, et al. One-stage treatment of congenital dislocation of the hip in older children including femoral shortening. J Bone Joint Surg 1989; 71A:734.

Kasser JR, Bowen JR, MacEwen GD. Varus derotation osteotomy in the treatment of persistent dysplasia in congenital dislocation of the hip. J Bone Joint Surg 1985; 67A:195.

Mankey MG, Arntz GT, Staheli LT. Open reduction through a medial approach for congenital dislocation of the hip: A critical review of the Ludloff approach in sixty-six hips. J Bone Joint Surg 1993; 75A:1334.

Powell EN, Gerrantana FJ, Gage JR. Open reduction for congenital hip dislocation: The risk of avascular necrosis with three different approaches. J Pediatr Orthop 1986; 6:127.

Salter RB, Dubos JP. The first fifteen years' personal experience with innominate osteotomy in the treatment of congenital dislocation and subluxation of the hip. Clin Orthop 1974; 98:72.

Schoenecker PL. Strecker WB. Congenital dislocation of the hip in children: Comparison of the effects of femoral shortening and of skeletal traction in treatment. J Bone Joint Surg 1984; 66A:21.

Tachdjian MO. Pediatric Orthopaedics. Philadelphia: WB Saunders, 1985.

Thomas IH, Dunin AJ, Cole WG, Menelaus MB. Avascular necrosis after open reduction for congenital dislocation of the hip: Analysis of causative factors and natural history. J Pediatr Orthop 1989; 9:525.

Tonnis D. Congenital Dysplasia and Dislocation of the Hip in Children and Adults. New York: Springer-Verlag, 1987.

Tonnis D. Surgical treatment of congenital dislocation of the hip. Clin Orthop 1990; 258:33.

Williamson DM, Glover SD, Benson MK. Congenital dislocation of the hip presenting after the age of three years: A long-term review. J Bone Joint Surg 1989; 71B:745.

SPINAL DEFORMITY

A. Scoliosis is most commonly identified by rotational deformity noted on examination of the back during forward bending (Fig. 1). The presence of rotational deformity is taken as presumptive evidence of scoliosis and investigation should continue. If the patient's pelvis is not level when asked to bend forward, the elevated side will show rotational deformity along the entire length of the spine. The most common causes for the pelvis not to be level on forward bending are true leg length discrepancy or functional discrepancies due to poor positioning, joint contracture, or other lower extremity deformity. Investigate and treat appropriately. Occasionally, lower extremity deformity and scoliosis co-exist. This can be ascertained by means of forward bending examination with the patient in a sitting position (i.e., with the lower extremity deformity neutralized).

B. Idiopathic scoliosis is a diagnosis of exclusion. Major identifiable causes of scoliosis include neuromuscular disorders, connective tissue disease, and congenital spinal abnormalities (Table 1). Careful history and physical examination with specific emphasis on evaluation of the integument for cutaneous abnormality (neurofibromatosis or spinal dysraphism) and neurologic function to rule out any neuromuscular disease are required. Idiopathic scoliosis is typically minimally symptomatic or totally asymptomatic. Significant pain symptoms require further evaluation as to cause. Investigate suspected nonidiopathic scoliosis as clinically appropriate with neurology consultation, magnetic resonance imaging (MRI), technetium bone scan, etc.

C. Pathologic versus physiologic kyphosis or postural round back deformity can be differentiated on physical examination by assessing the severity, sharp localization, and flexibility of kyphosis seen in the sagittal plane. Congenital and Scheuermann's kyphotic deformities are typically short, sharp, relatively inflexible deformities. Postural round back deformities have a gradual kyphotic deformity of the thoracic spine and are typically flexible (i.e., spontaneously correctable by the patient).

D. Congenital kyphosis is due to either a failure of segmentation or failure of formation. It requires thorough evaluation and management.

E. Scheuermann's kyphosis (Fig. 2) is characterized radiographically by excess thoracic kyphosis, vertebral end plate irregularity, and vertebral body wedging.

TABLE 1 Short List of Etiologic Causes of Scoliosis

Congenital
  Failure of formation
  Failure of segmentation
  Mixed
Connective Tissue Disorders
  Marfan's syndrome
  Ehlers-Danlos syndrome
  Neurofibromatosis
Neuromuscular Disorders
  Spinal cord injury
  Cerebral palsy
  Muscular dystrophy
  Spina bifida
  Poliomyelitis
  Intrathecal anomaly
    Lipoma
    Tight filum terminale
    Diastematomyelia
Other
  Osteoid osteoma
  Spondylolisthesis
  Scheuermann's kyphosis

F. Postural round back deformities are characterized by diffusely increased kyphosis on physical examination, easily reduced by asking the patient to hyperextend the thoracic spine. Lateral radiographs show no vertebra anomalies associated with either Scheuermann's kyphosis or congenital kyphosis. Postural round back deformity is usually neither progressive nor symptomatic and thus does not require treatment.

G. The presence of tight hamstrings when the patient is asked to bend forward is not in itself pathognomonic of a disease process. However, tight hamstrings are typically noted with spondylolisthesis, symptomatic spondylolysis, Scheuermann's kyphosis, and tethered cord. Investigate as clinically appropriate.

H. Patients demonstrating tight hamstrings with normal radiographs should be considered for the potential of having neurologic abnormality. Potential causes include any spasticity-producing disorder and tethered cord. Pursue investigation based on the nature and severity of symptoms.

SUSPECTED SPINAL DEFORMITY

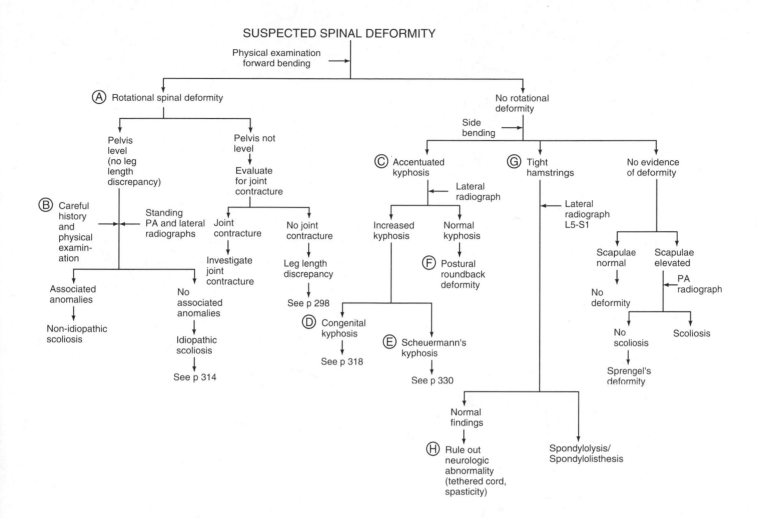

Physical examination forward bending

A Rotational spinal deformity

No rotational deformity

Pelvis level (no leg length discrepancy)

Pelvis not level

Side bending

C Accentuated kyphosis

G Tight hamstrings

No evidence of deformity

Evaluate for joint contracture

B Careful history and physical examination

Standing PA and lateral radiographs

Joint contracture

No joint contracture

Lateral radiograph

Lateral radiograph L5-S1

Increased kyphosis

Normal kyphosis

Investigate joint contracture

Leg length discrepancy

See p 298

Scapulae normal

Scapulae elevated

Associated anomalies

No associated anomalies

F Postural roundback deformity

PA radiograph

Non-idiopathic scoliosis

Idiopathic scoliosis

See p 314

D Congenital kyphosis

See p 318

E Scheuermann's kyphosis

See p 330

No deformity

No scoliosis

Scoliosis

Sprengel's deformity

Normal findings

H Rule out neurologic abnormality (tethered cord, spasticity)

Spondylolysis/ Spondylolisthesis

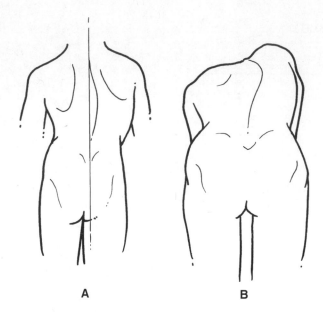

A   B

Figure 1 **A,** Scoliosis typically produces a number of visible deformities. In this illustration a right thoracic deformity results in elevation of the right shoulder and neckline, trunk shift to the right, and an asymmetric waist with the left leg appearing longer than the right. **B,** On forward bending prominence of the right posterior ribs is noted due to rotation of the spine.

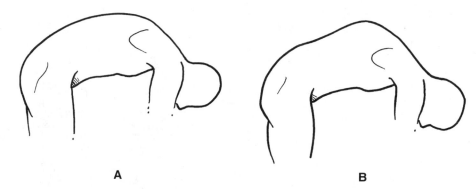

A   B

Figure 2 **A,** Viewed from the side, on forward bending the thoracic spine normally has a smooth, rounded appearance. **B,** With Scheuermann's and other forms of kyphosis there is a sharp area of increased kyphosis, with forward displacement or dropoff of the spine proximal to this. Typically this deformity is not flexible on further physical examination.

References

Asher M, Beringer G, Orrick J, Halverhout N. The current status of scoliosis in North America, 1986. Spine 1989; 14:652.

Bradford DS, Hensinger RM. The Pediatric Spine. New York: Thieme, 1985.

Bradford D, Lonstein J, Moe J, et al. Moe's Textbook of Scoliosis and Other Spinal Deformities. Philadelphia: WB Saunders, 1987.

Bunnell W. The natural history of idiopathic scoliosis before skeletal maturity. Spine 1986; 11:773.

Collis D, Ponseti I. Long-term follow-up of patients with idiopathic scoliosis not treated surgically. J Bone Joint Surg [Am] 1969; 51:425.

Hensinger RN. Spondylolysis and spondylolisthesis in children and adolescents. J Bone Joint Surg [Am] 1989; 71:1098.

Morrissy RT. Lovell and Winter's Pediatric Orthopaedics. Philadelphia: JB Lippincott, 1990.

Murray PM, Weinstein SL, Spratt KF. The natural history and long-term follow-up of Scheuermann kyphosis. J Bone Joint Surg [Am] 1993; 75:236.

Rogala E, Drummond D, Gurr J. Scoliosis: Incidence and natural history. J Bone Joint Surg [Am] 1978; 60:173.

Sachs B, Bradford D, Winter R, et al. Scheuermann kyphosis. J Bone Joint Surg [Am] 1987; 69:50.

Weinstein S. Adolescent idiopathic scoliosis: Prevalence and natural history. In: Barr J, ed. Instructional Course Lectures. Vol 38. Park Ridge, Ill.: American Academy of Orthopaedic Surgeons, 1989; 115-128.

Weinstein SL. The Pediatric Spine: Principles and Practice. New York: Raven Press, 1994.

IDIOPATHIC SCOLIOSIS

A. All skeletally immature patients with documented spinal deformity are at risk for progression of the deformity and require some type of intervention—regular observation to skeletal maturity, bracing, or spine fusion. Skeletal maturity characterized by the end of spinal growth is associated with a Risser IV or greater radiographic status (Fig. 1). Girls who are ≥2 years postonset of menses are usually skeletally mature. Idiopathic scoliosis is a diagnosis of exclusion (i.e., history and physical examination offer no evidence of an etiology for scoliosis and radiographs show no anomaly other than the curve itself). Idiopathic scoliosis is arbitrarily classified into three types based on age of onset of deformity: infantile (onset between birth and age 3), juvenile (onset between age 3 and 10), and adolescent (onset after age 10). Infantile scoliosis is a very rare disorder with a distinctly different therapeutic course and is not discussed here. Juvenile scoliosis is at much greater risk for progression than adolescent.

B. Periodic observation is required for patients who have documented spinal deformity (Fig. 2). The frequency and nature of that observation depend on the impression of the risk for progression. Young age, female sex, and larger curves (i.e., closer to 25°) are risk factors for progression; patients in these categories should have an examination and standing posteroanterior (PA) radiographs taken routinely every 4–6 months. Mild clinical and radiographic deformities can be evaluated by physical examination every 6 months, with radiographs repeated if progression appears to be occurring.

C. Patients with idiopathic scoliosis should be observed to skeletal maturity, i.e., until spinal growth is completed. If at that point stable deformity of <50° has been documented, routine re-evaluation is not required. Re-evaluate patients for symptoms or complaints of progression. Unstable progressive deformities or those >50° should be considered for spinal fusion (see K).

D. When the patient is skeletally immature and the curve measures between 25° and 45° bracing is indicated. The current specific recommendations of the Scoliosis Research Society are that bracing should be instituted in patients who are Risser II or less, 6 months postmenarchal or less, and who either have >25° curvature with 5° of documented progression, or 30°–45° of curvature. The actual effectiveness of bracing in preventing progression is controversial. Most studies suggest that spinal bracing reduces the likelihood of progression requiring spinal fusion. Milwaukee brace worn for 22–23 hours a day is considered the standard of care, although underarm custom molded plastic braces with shorter wearing times are more popular. The effectiveness of these alternative bracing methods over a Milwaukee brace worn essentially full-time is not established. In general, braces do not correct deformity, but simply maintain a curve at less than that which requires spinal fusion.

E. Patients undergoing brace treatment to try to control severe or progressive scoliosis should have PA radiographs taken of their spine out of brace every 4–6 months. If the curve remains stable and <45°, this protocol continues until skeletal maturity. Bracing at that point stops, and re-evaluation continues until curve stability is documented. If the curve progresses beyond 45° despite bracing, consider spinal fusion.

F. Spine fusion with instrumentation is indicated in skeletally immature patients with >45° curvature. The type of fusion is based on the location of the curve and the degree of skeletal maturation.

G. Single lumbar or thoracolumbar deformities usually are corrected most efficiently by anterior spinal fusion with instrumentation. Alternatives include posterior instrumentation with or without pedicle screws. The goal of all treatment, however, is stable fusion involving a minimum number of lumbar spinal segments and preserving a maximum amount of lumbar spinal mobility.

H. Patients who are quite immature (Risser 0 or less) are at risk for rotational growth and progressive deformity after posterior spinal fusion alone due to continued anterior growth. Patients who are more mature (i.e., Risser I or greater) are not generally considered at risk for substantial rotational anterior growth and posterior spinal fusion only is usually indicated.

I. Posterior spinal fusion of the deformed segment of the thoracic spine is carried out in conjunction with instrumentation to maintain internal stability. Patients must be followed for a minimum of 2 years after spinal fusion to document stable deformity without evidence of pseudarthrosis.

J. When the patient is Risser 0 or less, anterior spinal fusion of the deformed thoracic spine should be carried out in addition to posterior spinal fusion with instrumentation. The timing of anterior fusion at either the initial stage, simultaneous with posterior spinal fusion, or at a second stage is at surgeon's preference and based on the clinical situation. In all cases patients should be observed at regular intervals to skeletal maturity to confirm stable spinal deformity without evidence of progression or pseudarthrosis.

K. Skeletally mature patients with >50° of curvature are at risk for continued progression even as adults. The indications for spinal fusion in such cases are highly individual. At a minimum the patient should be observed periodically for evidence of significant progression and considered for spine fusion if this occurs.

IDIOPATHIC SCOLIOSIS

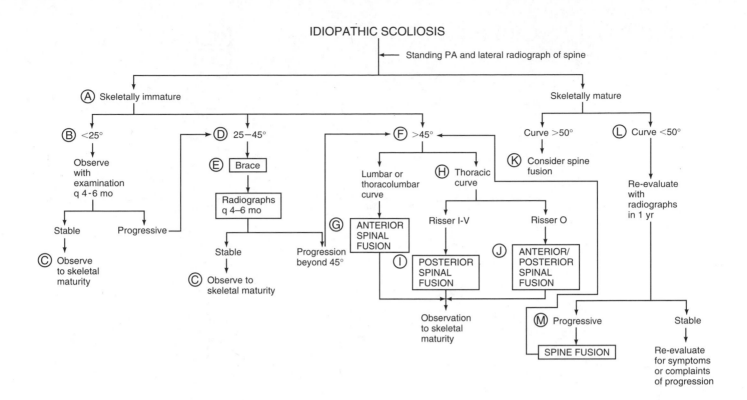

Standing PA and lateral radiograph of spine

Ⓐ Skeletally immature

Ⓑ <25°

Observe with examination q 4-6 mo

Stable

Progressive

Ⓒ Observe to skeletal maturity

Ⓓ 25−45°

Ⓔ Brace

Radiographs q 4–6 mo

Stable

Ⓒ Observe to skeletal maturity

Progression beyond 45°

Ⓕ >45°

Lumbar or thoracolumbar curve

Ⓖ ANTERIOR SPINAL FUSION

Ⓗ Thoracic curve

Risser I-V

Ⓘ POSTERIOR SPINAL FUSION

Risser O

Ⓙ ANTERIOR/ POSTERIOR SPINAL FUSION

Observation to skeletal maturity

Skeletally mature

Curve >50°

Ⓚ Consider spine fusion

Ⓛ Curve <50°

Re-evaluate with radiographs in 1 yr

Ⓜ Progressive

SPINE FUSION

Stable

Re-evaluate for symptoms or complaints of progression

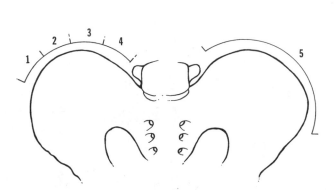

Figure 1 The Risser sign is an indication of relative spinal maturity. Risser 0 implies that no apophysis ossification is evident on the AP view of the pelvis. Risser I to IV occurs with progressive ossification of the apophysis. Risser V implies complete fusion of the apophysis to the iliac crest.

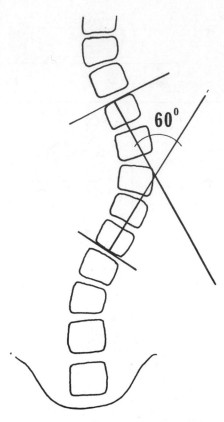

Figure 2 Scoliosis is a lateral (frontal plane) curvature of the spine. The Cobb method of estimating curve magnitude involves constructing perpendiculars to the vertebral end plates of the proximal-most and distal-most vertebral bodies deviated into the concavity of any particular curve, and measuring the angle between these perpendiculars.

L. Skeletally mature patients with <50° of spinal deformity are generally at low risk for subsequent clinically significant progression of the deformity. Yearly re-evaluation with radiographs should be undertaken until stable spine deformity is documented. Stable deformities of <50° do not require surgical management.

M. Curves that are progressive even after skeletal maturity should be considered for spinal fusion, taking into consideration the nature of the deformity as previously discussed, and the potential risk for complications based on treatment of an older population.

References

Ascani E, Bartolozzi P, Logroscino CA, et al. Natural history of untreated idiopathic scoliosis after skeletal maturity. Spine 1986; 11:784.

Bradford DS, Hensinger RM. The Pediatric Spine. New York: Thieme, 1985.

Bunnell WP. A study of the natural history of idiopathic scoliosis before skeletal maturity. Spine 1986; 11:773.

Dubousset J, Herring JA, Shufflebarger H. The crankshaft phenomenon. J Pediatr Orthop 1989; 9:541.

Lonstein JE, Carlson JM. The prediction of curve progression in untreated idiopathic scoliosis during growth. J Bone Joint Surg [Am] 1984; 66:1061.

Nachemson A. A long-term follow-up study of non-treated scoliosis. Acta Orthop Scand 1968; 39:446.

Nachemson AL, Peterson L. Effectiveness of treatment with a brace in girls who have adolescent idiopathic scoliosis. J Bone Joint Surg [Am] 1995; 77:815.

Peterson L, Nachemson AL. Prediction of progression of the curve in girls who have adolescent idiopathic scoliosis of moderate severity. J Bone Joint Surg [Am] 1995; 77:823.

Sponseller PD, Cohen MS, Nachemson AL, et al. Results of surgical treatment of adults with scoliosis. J Bone Joint Surg [Am] 1987; 69:667.

Weinstein SL. Adolescent idiopathic scoliosis: Prevalence and natural history. Instructional Course Lectures. Vol 38. Park Ridge, Ill.: American Academy of Orthopaedic Surgeons. 1989; 115-128.

Weinstein SL, Peterson K, Spoonamore M. Idiopathic scoliosis: Long term outcomes in untreated patients (50 year follow-up). J Bone Joint Surg 1993.

Weinstein SL. The Pediatric Spine: Principles and Practice. New York: Raven Press, 1994.

Westin SL, Ponseti IV. Curve progression in idiopathic scoliosis: Long-term follow-up. J Bone Joint Surg [Am] 1983; 65:447.

CONGENITAL SCOLIOSIS

A. Congenital spinal deformities are associated with renal or intrathecal anomalies in up to 15% of cases. Initial examination should include a careful neurologic exam to rule out neurologic disturbance. Obtain renal ultrasound studies to rule out renal abnormality.

B. Occult causes of neurologic abnormality include diastematomyelia, tethered cord, and direct impingement of the spinal cord or nerve roots by the spinal deformity. Magnetic resonance imaging (MRI) of the thoracolumbar spine, with neurosurgical evaluation as appropriate, is required.

C. Skeletally mature patients with an unacceptable deformity can be considered for spinal fusion after correction of the deformity. Correction of the deformity, however, is difficult because of the rigid bony nature of most such deformities and the risk of neurologic injury. Long-term traction effecting correction through mobile segments followed by spinal fusion and instrumentation can be performed in such circumstances. Alternatively, partial vertebrectomy or spinal osteotomy and instrumentation and fusion may be carried out. These procedures have substantial risk for neurologic injury and should be carried out only by very experienced surgeons and only when strongly indicated.

D. A patient with congenital spinal deformity who is skeletally immature is at risk for progression of the deformity. When such progression is documented, spinal fusion of the abnormal segment to prevent further progression is the standard of treatment. All patients with congenital anomaly should have sequential comparable standing posteroanterior (PA) and lateral radiographs of the spine every 6–12 months to document the degree of deformity. The risk of progression is based on the opportunity for the deformed segment to continue to grow in an abnormal way; in general that risk is indeterminate radiographically until progression has been documented. Unsegmented unilateral bars, particularly with well-developed hemivertebrae in their convexity are very high risk for progression and need to be observed carefully. Block and wedge vertebrae, however, have relatively little risk of progression. All congenital spinal anomalies, however, should be observed to skeletal maturity.

E. If no excessive kyphosis deformity is present on the initial standing lateral radiograph, observe the patient with repeat standing radiographs every 6–12 months, based on extent of deformity and presumed risk for progression. Continue observation until patient is skeletally mature. If kyphosis is present, determine whether it is due to failure of formation (Fig. 1) or failure of segmentation (Fig. 2). Failures of segmentation are usually mechanically stable deformities and in the absence of neurologic abnormality can be observed as other congenital spinal anomalies. Deformities due to failure of formation are potentially mechanically unstable. Gradual or acute neurologic compromise can occur. The risk for progression is high. Therefore upon identification of this deformity the patient usually requires anterior and posterior spinal fusion.

F. Theoretically any congenital spinal deformity can show evidence of progression radiographically at any point during a patient's growth. All patients should therefore be evaluated regularly both clinically and radiographically until skeletal maturity is reached. Routine re-evaluations after skeletal maturation are not required.

G. Documented 5°–10° progression of baseline deformity in a skeletally immature patient mandates spinal fusion to prevent further progression. Spinal braces to prevent progression are not indicated in patients with congenital scoliosis because of the bony, growth-related nature of the deformities. Patients being actively considered for spinal fusion should have an evaluation of the spinal cord including MRI. Frequently, instrumentation is used for stability, complicating subsequent evaluation of the spinal cord should it become necessary. Progression may be related to a subtle intrathecal anomaly. The presence of such an anomaly usually constitutes a contraindication to surgical correction of the deformity.

H. If the patient is Risser 0, there is substantial risk of rotational anterior growth (crankshaft phenomenon) with posterior spinal fusion only. Therefore in general in situ anterior and posterior spinal fusion are indicated. In young patients postoperative immobilization in a cast or brace is required until solid fusion has occurred. In older patients spinal instrumentation may be used to maintain the immobilization. Vigorous efforts to correct deformity with instrumentation are generally contraindicated because of the rigid bony nature of the deformity.

I. If the patient is Risser I or more, in situ posterior spinal fusion with or without instrumentation is generally adequate treatment.

J. If kyphosis is present, posterior spinal fusion alone even with instrumentation often is not adequate to obtain fusion. Anterior and posterior spinal fusion are usually indicated. Kyphosis places the child at significant risk for neurologic compromise with any efforts to correct the deformity, and in-situ fusion only is indicated.

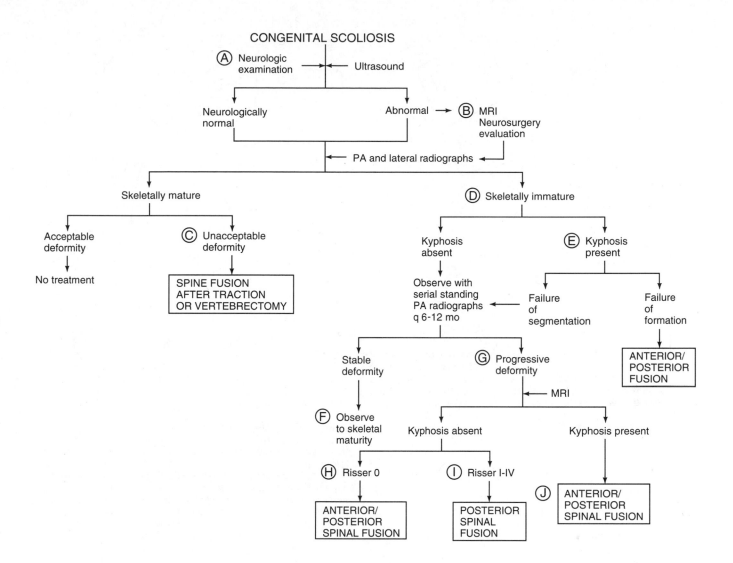

CONGENITAL SCOLIOSIS

(A) Neurologic examination ⟷ Ultrasound

Neurologically normal

Abnormal → (B) MRI Neurosurgery evaluation

PA and lateral radiographs

Skeletally mature

(D) Skeletally immature

Acceptable deformity

No treatment

(C) Unacceptable deformity

SPINE FUSION AFTER TRACTION OR VERTEBRECTOMY

Kyphosis absent

Observe with serial standing PA radiographs q 6-12 mo

(E) Kyphosis present

Failure of segmentation

Failure of formation

ANTERIOR/ POSTERIOR FUSION

Stable deformity

(G) Progressive deformity

MRI

(F) Observe to skeletal maturity

Kyphosis absent

Kyphosis present

(H) Risser 0

(I) Risser I-IV

(J) ANTERIOR/ POSTERIOR SPINAL FUSION

ANTERIOR/ POSTERIOR SPINAL FUSION

POSTERIOR SPINAL FUSION

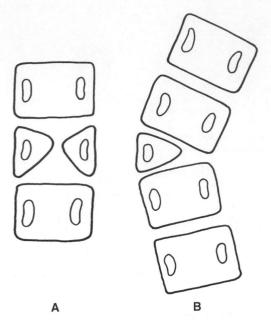

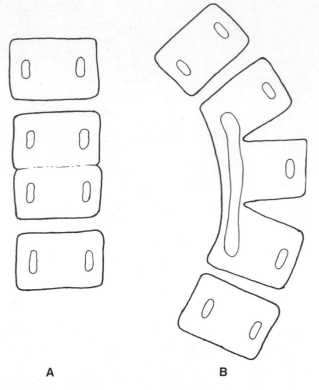

Figure 1 Congenital scoliosis: failure of formation. **A,** Common and usually benign form of failure formation is a pattern known as "butterfly" vertebra. **B,** Hemivertebrae are characterized by absence of formation in one half of the vertebra. The prognosis for the development of progressive scoliosis is determined by the degree of accommodation by the adjacent vertebral bodies and the growth potential of the end plates of the intact portion of the hemivertebra.

Figure 2 Congenital scoliosis: failure of segmentation. **A,** Block vertebrae are characterized by fusion of the vertebral bodies (and often posterior elements) without any intervertebral disk or end plate. Risk of development of progressive deformity is low with this malformation. **B,** Unsegmented bar. This deformity is characterized by failure of segmentation of the anterior and/or posterior elements on one side of two or more adjacent vertebral segments. Risk of progression can be high, determined by the growth potential of the vertebral elements in the convexity of the deformity.

References

Bradford DS, Boachie-Adjeci O. One-stage anterior and posterior hemivertebral resection and arthrodesis for congenital scoliosis. J Bone Joint Surg [Am] 1990; 72:536.

Bradford DS, Hensinger RM. The Pediatric Spine. New York: Thieme, 1985.

Bradford D, Lonstein J, Moe J, et al. Moe's Textbook of Scoliosis and Other Spinal Deformities. Philadelphia: WB Saunders, 1987.

Hall JE, Herndon WA, Levine CR. Surgical treatment of congenital scoliosis with or without Harrington instrumentation. J Bone Joint Surg [Am] 1981; 63:608.

Holte DC, Winter RB, Lonstein JE, Denis F. Excision of hemivertebrae and wedge resection in the treatment of congenital scoliosis. J Bone Joint Surg [Am] 1995; 77:159.

McMaster MJ, Ohtsuka K. The natural history of congenital scoliosis: A study of 251 patients. J Bone Joint Surg [Am] 1982, 64:1128.

Miller A, Guille JT, Bowen JR. Evaluation and treament of diastematomyelia. J Bone Joint Surg [Am] 1993; 75:1308.

Weinstein SL. The Pediatric Spine: Principles and Practice. New York: Raven Press, 1994.

Winter RB, Moe JH, Lonstein JE. Posterior spinal arthrodesis for congenital scoliosis: An analysis of 290 patients 5 to 19 years old. J Bone Joint Surg [Am] 1984, 66:1188.

NEUROMUSCULAR SCOLIOSIS

A. Neuromuscular scoliosis is typically seen in patients with static encephalopathy (cerebral palsy), spinal muscular atrophy, Duchenne muscular dystrophy (DMD), other muscular dystrophies, and myelomeningocele. Patients with myelomeningocele may have scoliosis secondary to congenital vertebral anomaly, which should be treated as for other congenital spinal anomalies (see p 310). Rapid unexplained progression in these patients also may be due to tethered cord or secondary hydromyelia; evaluate the patient for these conditions with magnetic resonance imaging (MRI). Because of frequent inability to ambulate, pelvic obliquity, and either functional or true limb length inequality, neuromuscular spinal deformity is best evaluated clinically and with an anteroposterior (AP) radiograph of the spine in a sitting position to make the radiographs more reproducible at sequential assessments.

B. Neuromuscular scoliosis <30° does not require treatment. However, patients who are skeletally immature require repeat radiographs every 6 months until skeletal maturity.

C. The natural history of neuromuscular scoliosis is in general not well documented in the adult population. However, deformities that appear to be stable at skeletal maturity are not thought to be progressive in adulthood unless quite severe.

D. Patients with curves of 30°–40° are more likely to progress and require treatment.

E. Once the curve reaches 30° in patients with DMD, progression is certain and can proceed quite rapidly. In addition, cardiopulmonary function will deteriorate as a general course of the disease. Therefore patients should almost always have posterior spinal fusion with segmental instrumentation recommended to them when the curve has reached 30° (Figs. 1 and 2).

F. Posterior spinal fusion with segmental instrumentation is recommended treatment for patients with DMD. Patients who have some pelvic obliquity should have the fusion extended to the pelvis (Fig. 3). There is some literature suggesting that fusion to L5 is adequate for patients who do not have functional pelvic obliquity at the time of surgery. If in doubt, it is wise to perform the fusion to the pelvis as treatment of secondary pelvic obliquity is usually quite difficult.

G. In patients with neurologic disorders other than DMD who are skeletally mature, significant progression is unlikely. Reassess the patient as needed.

H. Patients who are skeletally immature are at moderate risk for progression of scoliosis. Therefore obtain repeat radiographs every 6 months. The use of custom-molded thoracolumbosacral orthosis (TLSO) for neuromuscular scoliosis is in general controversial. The influence of orthotics on the natural history of the curve is uncertain. Some patients with spinal muscular atrophy have a curve onset at a young age and develop marked truncal imbalance and difficulty sitting. These patients may benefit from a TLSO to aid sitting balance and delay surgery. It is unlikely that the use of a TLSO prevents posterior spinal fusion, although adequate documentation is lacking.

I. For patients who have >40° of scoliosis consider spinal fusion. If there are no symptoms, the patient should be reassessed for symptoms only.

J. Skeletally mature patients who have difficulty with sitting balance and whose lifestyle can be enhanced by improved sitting balance should have posterior spinal fusion to the pelvis. If a patient's trunk cannot be levelled over the pelvis on preoperative bending films, consider anterior spinal release in addition to posterior spinal fusion to the pelvis. Every effort should be made to stabilize the trunk over the pelvis.

K. For skeletally immature patients who are nonambulatory and >10 years of age, consider posterior spinal fusion to the pelvis. Use anterior fusion in addition if there is concern about the potential for crankshaft phenomenon interfering with long-term results due to continued anterior growth, if the trunk cannot be adequately centered over the pelvis on preoperative bending films, or if there is a significant kyphotic component to the deformity that would compromise posterior spinal fusion and instrumentation.

L. Patients who have neuromuscular scoliosis and who are borderline ambulators should in general not have spinal fusion to the pelvis as the loss of lumbar sacral movement will often prevent them from regaining ambulation capability. Patients with moderately severe cerebral palsy or mid to upper lumbar level myelomeningocele are specific examples. In such patients make every effort to fuse the curve locally, preserving lumbosacral movement. Patients who are fused to the pelvis in these clinical circumstances must be warned that resumption of ambulation may be difficult or impossible after spinal fusion.

SUSPECTED NEUROMUSCULAR SCOLIOSIS

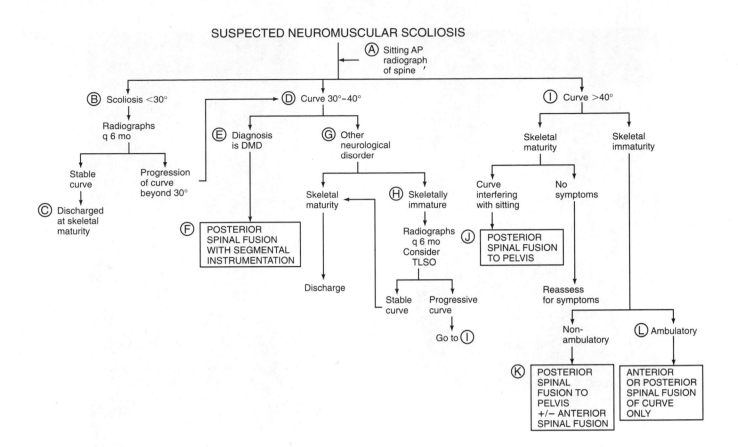

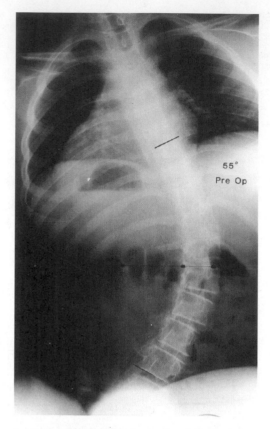

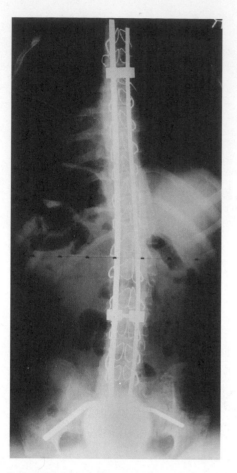

Figure 1 Anteroposterior radiograph of a patient with Duchenne's muscular dystrophy and scoliosis. Long, C-shape deformity with or without pelvic obliquity is typical of most neuromuscular scolioses.

Figure 2 Same patient as in Figure 1 after posterior spinal fusion and Luque instrumentation.

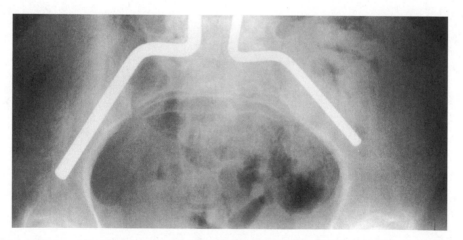

Figure 3 Most patients with neuromuscular scoliosis require posterior spinal fusion to the pelvis. The Luque-Galveston technique involves sublaminar wiring of the spine and extension of the rods across the sacroiliac joint into the iliac crest.

References

Allen BL, Ferguson RL. L-rod instrumentation for scoliosis in cerebral palsy. J Pediatr Orthop 1982; 2:87.

Bell DF, Moseley CF, Koreska J. Unit rod segmental spinal instrumentation in the management of patients with progressive neuromuscular spinal deformity. Spine 1989; 14:1301.

Boachie-Adjei O, Lonstein JE, Winter RB, et al. Management of neuromuscular spinal deformities with Luque segmental instrumentation. J Bone Joint Surg 1989; 71A5:48.

Bradford DS, Hensinger RN. The Pediatric Spine. New York: Thieme, 1985.

Broom MJ, Banta JV, Renshaw TS. Spinal fusion augmented by Luque-rod segmental instrumentation for neuromuscular scoliosis. J Bone Joint Surg 1989; 71A:32.

Dubousset J, Herring JA, Shufflebarger H. The crankshaft phenomenon. J Peditar Orthop 1989; 9:541.

Gersoff WK, Renshaw TS. The treatment of scoliosis in cerebral palsy by posterior spinal fusion with Luque-rod semental instrumentation. J Bone Joint Surg 1988; 70A:41.

Lonstein JE, Akbarnia A. Operative treatment of spinal deformities in patients with cerebral palsy or mental retardation. J Bone Joint Surg 1983; 65A:43.

Stanitski CL, Micheli LJ, Hall JE, Rosenthal RK. Surgical correction of spinal deformity in cerebral palsy. Spine 1982; 7:563.

Swank SM, Cohen DS, Brown JC. Spine fusion in cerebral palsy with L-rod segmental spinal instrumentation: A comparison of single and two stage combined approach with Zielke. Spine 1989; 14:750.

Weinstein SL. The Pediatric Spine: Principles and Practice. New York: Raven Press, 1994.

SPONDYLOLYSIS/SPONDYLOLISTHESIS

A. Patients with spondylolysis or spondylolisthesis (Fig. 1) may present with back pain or spinal deformity. In addition, occasional patients are noted to have spondylolysis or spondylolisthesis incidentally on radiographs obtained for other reasons. Physical examination in a symptomatic patient with spondylolysis typically reveals limited straight leg raising due to hamstring tightness. Neurologic disturbance of L5 or S1 nerve root or cauda equina is possible although rare but should be sought, particularly in patients with spondylolisthesis.

   Standing lateral radiographs centered on L5 and S1 normally show the anterior translation of the vertebral body L5 on S1. In spondylolysis the pars defect may be visible in this view, may require oblique views of L5-S1, or may require further investigation (see below). Rarely in the pediatric population is a pars defect noted above the L5 level or multiple levels, although this does occur occasionally.

B. Patients with persistent symptoms in the lumbosacral spine with or without neurologic findings should have a computed tomography (CT) scan of the lumbar spine specifically looking for defects of the pars interarticularis, central disc herniation, or other rare causes of back pain.

C. If no abnormality is noted on CT scan and the patient's symptoms warrant further investigation, order a technetium bonescan specifically to look for stress reaction (denoted by increased uptake) in the affected pars interarticularis. If increased uptake is noted, the diagnosis is usually stress reaction of the pars interarticularis. Treat symptomatically by activity reduction, low back exercise programs, and occasionally lumbosacral orthosis until symptoms resolve.

D. If radiographs, CT scan, and technetium bonescan are normal and the patient's symptoms or signs warrant further investigation, obtain magnetic resonance imaging (MRI) of the lumbar spine. Specific diagnoses being sought are: atypical disc herniation, tethered cord, other rare intra- or extra-thecal causes of the pain. If the MRI is normal and the approach is appropriate for the patient's symptoms, treat the patient symptomatically for low back pain from that point. Treat appropriately any abnormality detected on MRI.

E. If the CT scan shows pars defect (spondylolysis), institute symptomatic treatment. This consists of hamstring stretching exercises, abdominal and lumbar extensor muscle strengthening exercises, activity modification, and lumbosacral orthosis such as the Boston overlap brace.

F. If symptomatic treatment leads to resolution of symptoms, re-evaluate the patient during growth with standing lateral radiographs of the spine every 6 months to identify any progression of spondylolysis or spondylolisthesis, or alternatively for any resumption of symptoms (Fig. 2).

G. If the patient does not respond to a vigorous program of conservative management after 6–12 weeks, consider surgery of the pars defect. The options are direct pars interarticularis repair with bone grafting and internal fixation or L5-S1 posterolateral in situ fusion. Both procedures are documented to be effective.

H. Patients noted to have Grade II or less spondylolisthesis on standing lateral radiograph, no neurologic abnormalities, and no symptoms can be observed on a regular basis for progression of the spondylolisthesis. If a patient has local symptoms of back pain or hamstring tightness conservative treatment as per E can be instituted. If this leads to resolution of symptoms, patients may be subsequently evaluated as per I. If there is associated neurologic abnormality or there is no prompt resolution of the symptoms, the patient should undergo posterolateral in situ fusion from L4-S1.

I. Skeletally immature patients with Grade I or II spondylolisthesis are at some risk for gradual progression of the spondylolisthesis, even in the absence of exacerbation of symptoms. Therefore the skeletally immature patient should have standing lateral radiographs centered on L5-S1 every 6 months during growth. If the deformity remains stable and asymptomatic to skeletal maturity, the patient can be discharged from care at that time. If progression of deformity is identified or the patient develops intractable symptoms, perform posterolateral fusion from L4-S1.

J. Patients who present with or develop Grade III spondylolisthesis or greater are treated with in situ posterolateral spinal fusion from L4-S1. Solid fusion of the spondylolisthesis leads to improvement in the clinical deformity, hamstring tightness, and even radiculopathy. More severe associated neurologic symptoms, specifically cauda equina, that present preoperatively or develop acutely postoperatively require decompression. If symptoms persist after in situ fusion, evaluate for pseudoarthrosis or cauda equina compression.

   Anterior spinal fusion and reduction techniques with anterior, posterior, or both fusions are described. However, higher complication rates are noted. Excellent long-term studies indicate that in the pediatric population in situ fusion even for very severe spondylolisthesis produces quite acceptable long-term results.

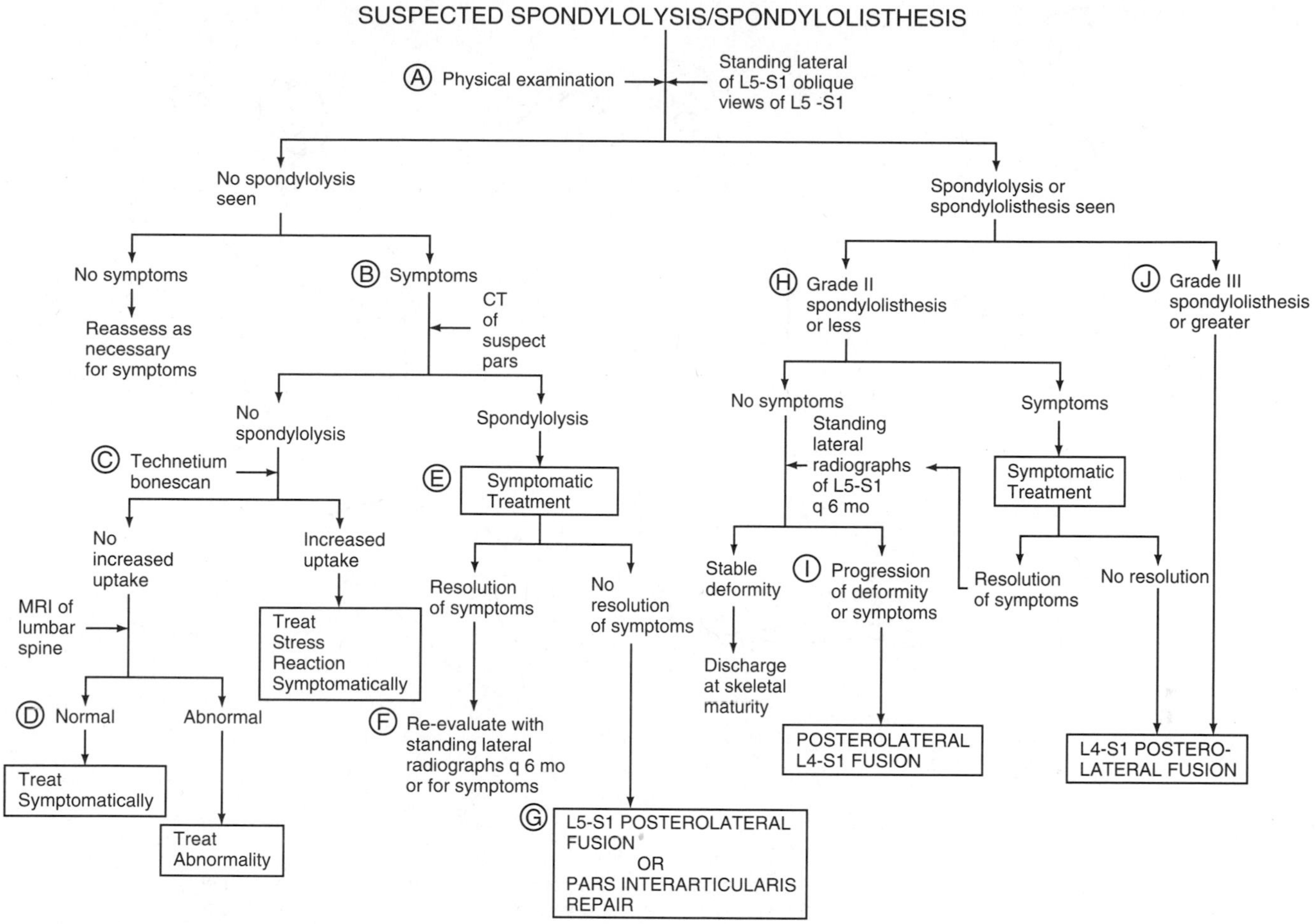

SUSPECTED SPONDYLOLYSIS/SPONDYLOLISTHESIS

(A) Physical examination → Standing lateral of L5-S1 oblique views of L5 -S1

No spondylolysis seen

No symptoms
↓
Reassess as necessary for symptoms

(B) Symptoms
← CT of suspect pars

No spondylolysis

(C) Technetium bonescan

No increased uptake
↓
MRI of lumbar spine →

Increased uptake
↓
Treat Stress Reaction Symptomatically

(D) Normal
↓
Treat Symptomatically

Abnormal
↓
Treat Abnormality

Spondylolysis
↓
(E) Symptomatic Treatment

Resolution of symptoms
↓
(F) Re-evaluate with standing lateral radiographs q 6 mo or for symptoms

No resolution of symptoms
↓
(G) L5-S1 POSTEROLATERAL FUSION OR PARS INTERARTICULARIS REPAIR

Spondylolysis or spondylolisthesis seen

(H) Grade II spondylolisthesis or less

No symptoms
Standing lateral radiographs of L5-S1 q 6 mo

Stable deformity
↓
Discharge at skeletal maturity

(I) Progression of deformity or symptoms
↓
POSTEROLATERAL L4-S1 FUSION

Symptoms
↓
Symptomatic Treatment

Resolution of symptoms

No resolution
↓
L4-S1 POSTERO-LATERAL FUSION

(J) Grade III spondylolisthesis or greater
↓
L4-S1 POSTERO-LATERAL FUSION

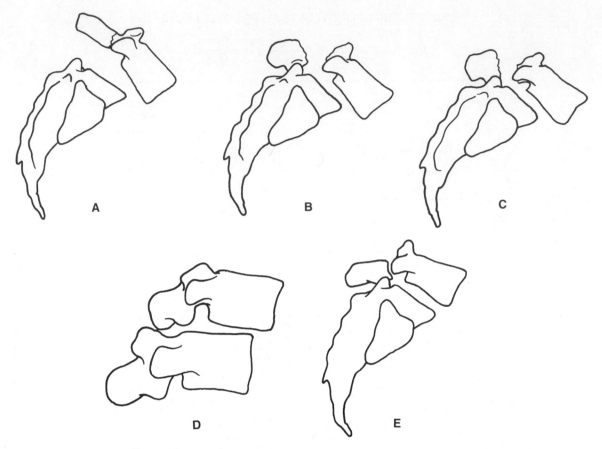

Figure 1 Wiltse classification of spondylolisthesis. **A,** Congenital. Malformation of posterior elements (such as sacral facets) allows anterior displacement of a vertebral body on the next lower adjacent body. **B,** Traumatic. Fracture of posterior elements other than the pars interarticularis allows spondylolisthesis. **C,** Isthmic. Defect in pars interarticularis (acquired secondary to other congenital anomalies, spinal deformities, or stress injury) produces a defect in the pars interarticularis with subsequent slipping of the vertebral body. **D,** Degenerative. Disk and posterior element changes allow instability between adjacent vertebral bodies. **E,** Pathologic. A generalized metabolic condition allows elongation or fracture of the pars interarticularis. Pathologic spondylolisthesis is most typically seen in osteogenesis imperfecta and Paget's disease of the bone.

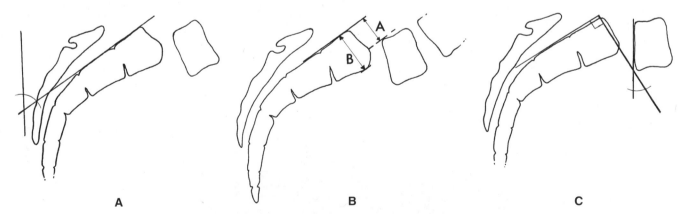

Figure 2 Methods of quantifying slip severity in spondylolisthesis. **A,** Sacral inclination. The angle between the vertical and a tangent to the posterior vertebral bodies of the upper sacrum. **B,** Slip grade. Fraction of anterior displacement of affected vertebral body on the subjacent body (usually S1). This fraction may be determined relative to either L5 or S1. Typically divided into Grade I (<25%), Grade II (26-50%), Grade III (51-75%), Grade IV (76-100%), and Grade V (apondyloptosis, or complete anterior and distal displacement of vertebral body on the subjacent body). **C,** Slip angle. A measurement of kyphotic deformity between the upper sacrum and the L5 vertebral body. It is the angle between a perpendicular to the posterior elements of the upper sacrum and the inferior end plate of L5. This angle is usually 0 to −5.

References

Bell DF, Ehrlich MG, Zaleske DJ. Brace treatment for symptomatic spondylolisthesis. Clin Orthop 1988; 236:192.

Boxall D, Bradford DS, Winter RB, Moe JH. Management of severe spondylolisthesis in children and adolescents. J Bone Joint Surg [Am] 1979; 61:479.

Bradford DS. Closed reduction of spondylolisthesis: An experience in 22 patients. Spine 1988; 13:580.

Bradford DS, Hensinger RM. The Pediatric Spine. New York: Thieme, 1985.

Frennered AK, Danielson BI, Nachemson AL. Natural history of symptomatic isthmic low-grade spondylolisthesis in children and adolescents: A seven-year follow-up study. J Pediatr Orthop 1991; 11:209.

Harris IE, Weinstein SL. Long-term follow-up of patients with grade III and IV spondylolisthesis. J Bone Joint Surg [Am] 1987; 69:960.

Hensinger RN. Spondylolysis and spondylolisthesis in children and adolescents. J Bone Joint Surg [Am] 1989; 71:1098.

Johnson GV, Thompson AG. The Scott wiring technique for direct repair of lumbar spondylolysis. J Bone Joint Surg [Br] 1992; 74:426.

Pizzutillo PD, Hummer CD 3d. Nonoperative treatment for painful adolescent spondylolysis or spondylolisthesis. J Pediatr Orthop 1989; 9:538.

Schoenecker PL, Cole HO, Herring JA, et al. Cauda equina syndrome after in situ arthrodesis for severe spondylolisthesis at the lumbosacral junction. J Bone Joint Surg [Am] 1990; 72:369.

Steiner ME, Micheli LJ. Treatment of symptomatic spondylolisthesis with the modified Boston brace. Spine 1985; 10:937.

Weinstein SL. The Pediatric Spine: Principles and Practice. New York: Raven Press, 1994.

Wiltse LL. Spondylolisthesis: Classification and etiology. In: Symposium on the Spine. Park Ridge, Ill.: American Academy of Orthopaedic Surgeons, 1969; 143.

SCHEUERMANN'S KYPHOSIS

A. Standing lateral radiographs of the spine in patients with suspected Scheuermann's kyphosis (Figs. 1 and 2) show increased thoracic kyphosis (>40°) and, by definition, >5° of wedging of three contiguous thoracic vertebrae with endplate irregularity. Alternative diagnoses include atypical Scheuermann's (less than the full radiographic criteria met, or endplate irregularities and back pain in the thoracolumbar or lumbar spine); postural roundback deformity where increased kyphosis is noted without other radiographic changes; or congenital kyphosis (see p 310 and 318).

B. Patients with 40°–70° of thoracic kyphosis generally are asymptomatic or minimally symptomatic, and have clinically acceptable deformity. The long-term natural history for Scheuermann's kyphosis is generally favorable for little or no increased incidence of back pain as an adult, with no propensity to cardiopulmonary problems. Therefore, unless the patient has uncontrollable symptoms or unacceptable clinical deformity or progressive deformity, treatment should be conservative.

C. Patients who are Risser III or greater are generally not considered bracing candidates to prevent further progression. The patient with an acceptable clinical deformity should have radiographs every 6 months until skeletal maturity. The patient with a stable, clinically acceptable deformity can be discharged after skeletal maturity. If, however, there is progression of deformity to clinically unacceptable levels, posterior spinal fusion is indicated.

D. Posterior spinal fusion is indicated for clinically unacceptable or progressive deformities in Scheuermann's kyphosis. In mild-to-moderate deformities (<70°) posterior spinal fusion only is usually adequate. Instrumentation with Harrington compression rod and multiple hooks, solid rods and multiple hooks, or Luque instrumentation have all been used successfully. When hooks are used take great care to keep the hooks outside the spinal canal as there are significant risks of displacement intrathecally, particularly at the apex of the deformity with three-point correction maneuvers.

E. Patients who are Risser II or less with moderate deformity may be modified Milwaukee brace candidates.

The brace is modified to push on the apex of the deformity thereby stabilizing and occasionally reducing the spinal deformity. Once fit, the patient should be examined and have lateral radiographs out of brace every 6 months. If the deformity progresses despite bracing, posterior spinal fusion may be indicated.

F. If the patient has a stable deformity in brace, discontinue bracing after 2 years. Re-examine the patient periodically to confirm that the deformity is stable. If there is progression of the deformity after discontinuation of the brace, consider posterior spinal fusion.

G. Patients with more severe deformity (>70°) are generally not good candidates for bracing, and are more likely to require posterior spinal fusion. Initial radiographic assessment of these more severe deformities includes a hyperextension lateral radiograph (a supine lateral film taken with patient hyperextended over a bolster placed at the apex of the thoracic deformity).

H. If the patient has acceptable clinical and radiographic reduction of the deformity (generally ≤50°) and is Risser II or less, consider a trial of modified Milwaukee brace. The likelihood of successful brace treatment is less than with less severe deformities, but if the deformity has enough flexibility to bring it into a clinically acceptable range this should be attempted. If the patient maintains a stable deformity that is clinically acceptable at skeletal maturity, no further assessment is necessary.

I. If deformity progresses despite bracing, consider posterior spinal fusion. Because the deformity is more severe, consider simultaneous anterior disc excision and fusion to improve the flexibility of the deformity and anterior bone graft to improve the likelihood of stable fusion.

J. Most patients who are Risser III or greater are not candidates for brace treatment. If there is a clinically unacceptable deformity that is flexible to ≤50°, consider posterior spinal fusion (see I).

K. If a patient does not demonstrate appreciable flexibility and has a clinically unacceptable deformity, carry out anterior spinal release and posterior spinal fusion with instrumentation (Fig. 3) (see D).

SUSPECTED SCHEUERMANN'S KYPHOSIS

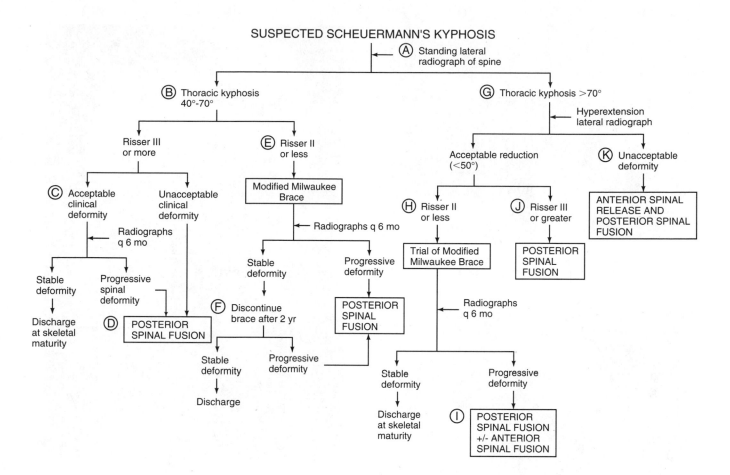

(A) Standing lateral radiograph of spine

(B) Thoracic kyphosis 40°-70°

(G) Thoracic kyphosis >70°

Hyperextension lateral radiograph

Risser III or more

(E) Risser II or less

Acceptable reduction (<50°)

(K) Unacceptable deformity

(C) Acceptable clinical deformity

Unacceptable clinical deformity

Modified Milwaukee Brace

(H) Risser II or less

(J) Risser III or greater

ANTERIOR SPINAL RELEASE AND POSTERIOR SPINAL FUSION

Radiographs q 6 mo

Radiographs q 6 mo

Trial of Modified Milwaukee Brace

POSTERIOR SPINAL FUSION

Stable deformity

Progressive spinal deformity

Stable deformity

Progressive deformity

Discharge at skeletal maturity

(D) POSTERIOR SPINAL FUSION

(F) Discontinue brace after 2 yr

POSTERIOR SPINAL FUSION

Radiographs q 6 mo

Stable deformity

Progressive deformity

Stable deformity

Progressive deformity

Discharge

Discharge at skeletal maturity

(I) POSTERIOR SPINAL FUSION +/- ANTERIOR SPINAL FUSION

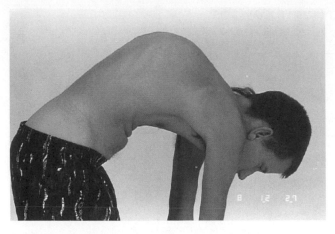

Figure 1 Scheuermann's kyphosis. The apex of increased kyphosis is typically in the middle or lower thoracic spine.

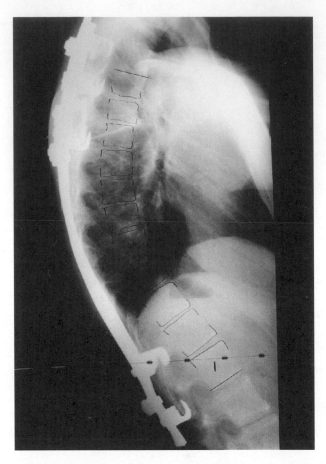

Figure 3 Progressive or unacceptable kyphosis may be treated with posterior spinal fusion and instrumentation. Anterior spinal release is often required in conjunction with posterior spinal fusion.

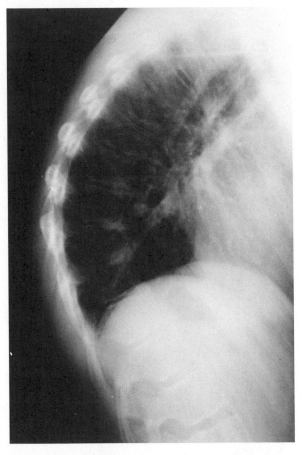

Figure 2 Radiographic criteria of Scheuermann's kyphosis. A diagnosis of Scheuermann's kyphosis requires increased thoracic kyphosis, vertebral end plate irregularity, and >5° wedging of three contiguous vertebrae.

332

References

Bradford DS, Hensinger RM. The Pediatric Spine. New York: Thieme, 1985.

Greene T, Hensinger R, Hunter L. Back pain and vertebral changes simulating Scheuermann's disease. J Pediatr Orthop 1985; 5:1.

Lowe TG. Current concept review: Scheuermann's disease. J Bone Joint Surg 1990; 72A:940.

Lowe TG, Kasten MD. An analysis of sagittal curves and balance after Cotrel-Dubousset instrumentation for kyphosis secondary to Scheuermann's disease: A review of 32 patients. Spine 1994; 19:1680.

Murray PM, Weinstein SL, Spratt KF. The natural history and long-term follow-up of Scheuermann kyphosis. J Bone Joint Surg 1993; 75A:236.

Otsuka NY, Hall JE, Mah JY. Posterior fusion for Scheuermann's kyphosis. Clin Orthop 1990; 251:134.

Sachs B, Bradford D, Winter R, et al. Scheuermann kyphosis. J Bone Joint Surg 1987; 69A:50.

Sturm PF, Dobson JC, Armstrong GW. The surgical management of Scheuermann's disease. Spine 1993; 18:685.

Taylor TC, Wenger DR, Stephen J, et al. Surgical management of thoracic kyphosis in adolescents. J Bone Joint Surg 1979; 61A:496.

Weinstein SL. The Pediatric Spine: Principles and Practice. New York: Raven Press, 1994.

ANGULAR DEFORMITY

A. The vast majority of angular deformities in the lower extremities are in the region of the knee (i.e., they occur primarily in the distal femur, proximal tibia, or both). Significant angular deformities elsewhere in the lower extremities are usually indicative of bone pathology requiring radiographs and treatment based on the nature of the problem. Obtain the following historical information when evaluating the patient with lower extremity varus or valgus angular deformity: age, general health, history of prior injury or infection in the limb, and progression of the deformity. Ascertain severity and symmetry of the deformity on physical examination.

B. Femoral-tibial varus is normal between birth and 18 months of age (Fig. 1). Therefore if the patient is less than 18 months of age, has mild-to-moderate varus deformity which is symmetric, and is healthy, a diagnosis of physiologic varus can be assumed. Radiographs are not generally indicated. The patient requires no treatment. Re-evaluate the patient if the deformity is progressive or persists after the age of 18 months.

C. Varus deformity which persists after the age of 18 months, is clearly asymmetric, or occurs in a patient with a history of prior injury, infection, or systemic disease (poor general health, short stature, evidence of multiple long bone or joint deformities) mandates anteroposterior (AP) radiographs of the lower extremities. These should be taken with the patient standing if possible. If radiographs show no abnormalities other than angular deformity and there is no evidence of systemic disease, the patient may be treated with observation as an asymmetric form of physiologic varus. Re-evaluate the patient periodically until the deformity resolves.

D. Patients with abnormal radiographic findings have non-physiologic varus. Differential diagnosis includes infantile Blount's disease (see p 338), epiphyseal dysplasia, metabolic bone disease (usually renal osteodystrophy secondary to chronic renal failure), or other rare disorders. They need to be treated on an individual basis.

E. Children between 18 months and 6 years of age typically show symmetric mild to moderate genu valgum (physiologic genu valgum). This deformity typically is maximal at age 3 to 4 years, and generally resolves spontaneously without treatment usually by age 6 to 7 years. Patients under 18 months of age or over 6 years of age should have an AP radiograph of the lower extremities. If that radiograph is normal and the child is otherwise healthy, observation to resolution is appropriate (see I below).

F. Pathologic valgus may result from metabolic bone disease (typically chronic renal failure; Fig. 2), physeal injury, proximal tibial metaphyseal overgrowth as a sequela of a proximal tibial metaphyseal fracture, epiphyseal dysplasia, or other rare causes. Treatment is on an individual basis.

G. Patients who present in the typical age range but with asymmetric deformity should have an AP radiograph of the lower extremities (Fig. 3). If that is normal and the patient is otherwise healthy, this may be treated expectantly as for physiologic valgus although it represents an atypical variation.

H. Other stigmata which may be identifiable on physical examination include short stature, deformities in other limb segments, or poor general health suggestive of metabolic bone disease.

I. Femoral-tibial valgus deformity can be physiologic between the age of 18 months and 6 years. This does not require treatment and can be expected to resolve spontaneously. If valgus deformity becomes asymmetric, accentuates after the age of 4 years, or persists after the age of 7 years, re-evaluation is required. Reassess the patient, including radiographic evaluation, to ascertain whether the initial diagnosis of physiologic valgus was correct.

J. Persistent valgus deformity, even if physiologic, may be distressing to patients as a cosmetic defect. If the deformity persists into the teenage years, consider correction by medial distal femoral or proximal tibial stapling, medial epiphysiodesis of these regions, or metaphyseal osteotomy of the deformed segment (usually the femur).

SUSPECTED ANGULAR DEFORMITY

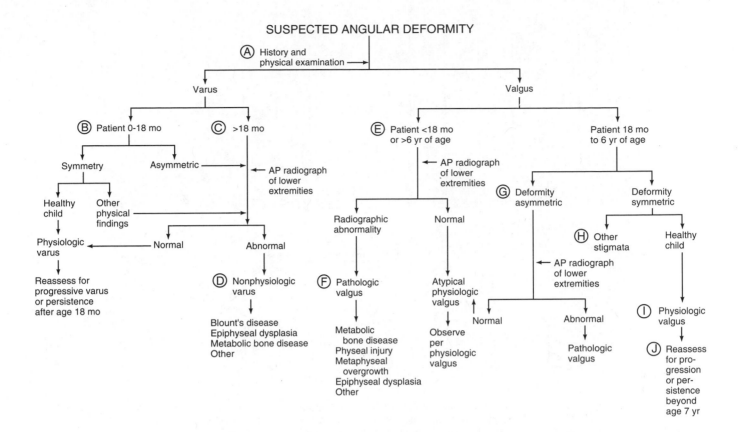

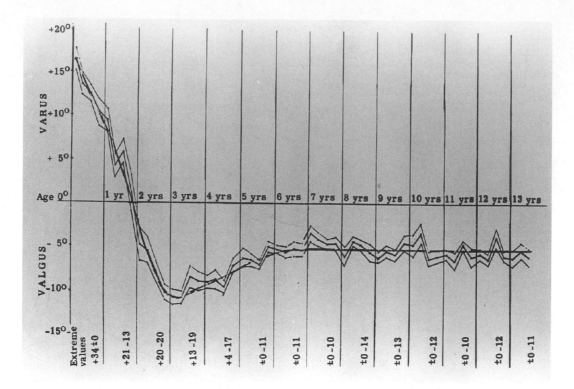

Figure 1 Evolution of frontal plane femoral-tibial angle. Between birth and 18 months the femoral-tibial angle on AP radiographs is typically in varus, between 18 months and 6 years in valgus, and from approximately 7 years of age onward is in 5° to 7° of valgus. (From J Bone Joint Surg.)

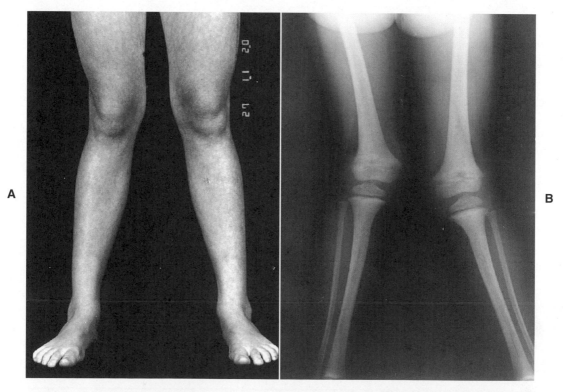

Figure 2 Bilateral symmetric genu valgum in an 8-year-old patient. At this point the legs should be in slight valgus or clinically neutral. **A,** Clinical photograph. **B,** AP radiograph of lower extremity shows generalized physeal widening. The diagnosis is renal osteodystrophy due to chronic renal failure.

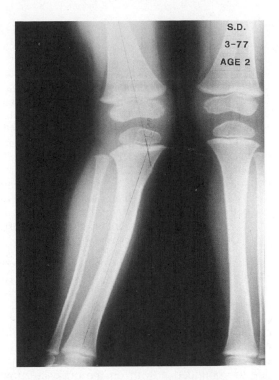

Figure 3 Asymmetric genu valgum evident on AP radiograph. The patient had previously experienced proximal tibial metaphyseal fracture. Medial proximal tibial overgrowth with valgus deformity is common after such fractures. These deformities usually resolve spontaneously.

References

Bowen JR, Leahey JL, Zhang Z, et al. Partial epiphysiodesis at the knee to correct angular deformity. Clin Orthop 1985; 198:184.

Engel GM, Staheli LT. The natural history of torsion and other factors influencing gait in childhood: A study of the angle of gait, tibial torsion, knee angle, hip rotation, and development of the arch in normal children. Clin Orthop 1974; 99:12.

Jordon SE, Alonso JE, Cook FF. The etiology of valgus angulation after metaphyseal fractures of the tibia in children. J Pediatr Orthop 1987; 7:450.

Levine AM, Drennan JC. Physiological bowing and tibia vara: The metaphyseal-diaphyseal angle in the measurement of bowleg deformities. J Bone Joint Surg 1982; 64A:1158.

Salenius P, Vanka E. The development of tibiofemoral angle in children. J Bone Joint Surg 1975; 57A:259.

Tachdjian MO. Pediatric Orthopedics. Philadelphia: WB Saunders, 1985.

Wenger DR, Mickelson M, Maynard JA. The evolution and histopathy of adolescent tibia vara. J Pediatr Orthop 1984; 4:78.

Zionts LE, MacEwen GD. Spontaneous improvement of post-traumatic tibia valga. J Bone Joint Surg 1986; 68A:680.

Zuege RC, Kempken TG, Blount WP. Epiphyseal stapling for angular deformity at the knee. J Bone Joint Surg 1979; 61A:320.

INFANTILE BLOUNT'S DISEASE

A. Patients <2 years of age rarely demonstrate clear radiographic evidence of Blount's disease according to the Langenskiold classification. Evaluate these patients clinically and radiographically every 3 months until either spontaneous resolution or progression of the deformity is documented. The rare patient with definite radiographic evidence of Blount's disease is treated as for older patients.

B. Patients >2 years of age typically demonstrate progressive angular deformity, characteristic radiographic abnormality of infantile Blount's disease, or both. Patients with progressive deformity after age 2 or with clear radiographic abnormality require treatment.

C. The Langenskiold classification of infantile Blount's disease defines six radiographic stages (Fig. 1). These stages are age related and demonstrate progressively severe disturbance of medial proximal tibial physeal growth. Langenskiold stage I, II, and III cases may show resolution (both clinical and radiographic) spontaneously or with treatment. The initial treatment for patients <4 years old with Langenskiold stage I, II, or III is a trial of long leg bracing.

D. Although the efficacy of long leg braces has not been clearly documented, they are considered the initial management of patients with infantile Blount's disease in whom conservative treatment is indicated. Their purpose is to effect a valgus moment at the knee. Braces are worn whenever the patient is weight bearing. Evaluate the patient clinically and radiographically every 3 months to rule out radiographic or clinical progression of the deformity. Discontinue bracing when clinical and radiographic resolution has occurred.

E. Langenskiold stage IV and V disease typically occurs in patients 4–8 years of age. These are more severe stages in which spontaneous resolution is unlikely. Recurrence of the deformity and persistence of radiographic abnormality can occur even after high tibial osteotomy. High tibial osteotomy is carried out beneath the growth plate with the varus deformity compensated for by overcorrection into valgus as much as clinically tolerable.

F. Langenskiold stage VI infantile Blount's disease is characterized by complete medial tibial physeal arrest (i.e., physeal bar or bony bridge). The deformity will recur after high tibial osteotomy in patients with this stage unless they are treated either by completion of the epiphysiodesis or successful physeal bar resection. Obtain scanogram and bone age determination to document the amount of existing limb length inequality as well as the presumed amount of growth remaining in the healthy proximal tibial physis. These determinations allow for appropriate decision making on the appropriate therapeutic modality.

G. If the patient has <2 cm of growth remaining, perform a high tibial osteotomy in the affected physis either above or below the tibial tubercle with completion of the epiphysiodesis on the affected side. Consideration will then need to be given to potential limb length discrepancy in patients with unilateral or asymmetric disease. The extent of shortening at maturity will be a combination of the pre-existing discrepancy and that due to continued growth on the opposite proximal tibial physis. No treatment, appropriately timed contralateral epiphysiodesis, or lengthening of the affected limb is undertaken, depending on the degree of shortening and patient motivation. For a more detailed description of the management of discrepancy, see p 342.

H. If the patient has >2 cm of growth remaining, treatment may be high tibial osteotomy (below the tibial tubercle) combined with partial physeal bar resection. Embed metallic markers in the metaphysis at the time of surgery to allow for early radiographic evaluation of resumption of growth, as well as early detection of cessation of growth after an initial resumption.

I. Resumption of growth after partial physeal bar resection is uncertain. Patients who have documented resumption of growth should be followed periodically with standing anteroposterior (AP) radiographs growth is completed. Patients who demonstrate recurrence of the deformity require completion of the epiphysiodesis combined with repeat high tibial osteotomy and lengthening as clinically indicated.

INFANTILE BLOUNT'S DISEASE

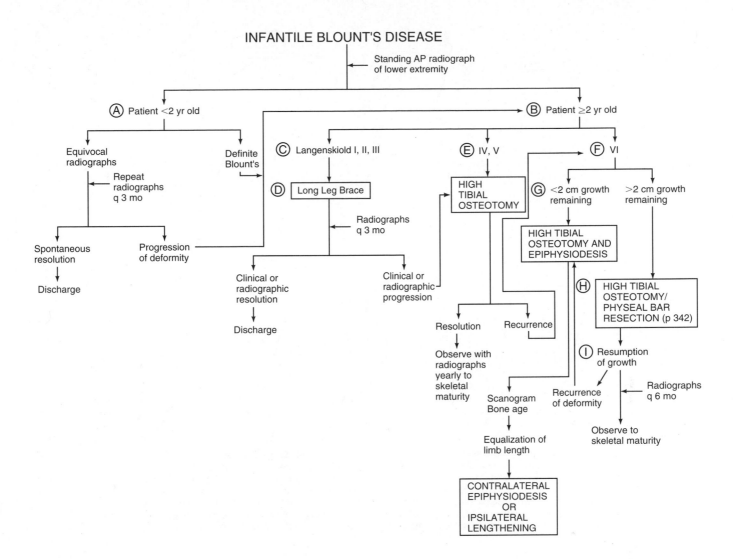

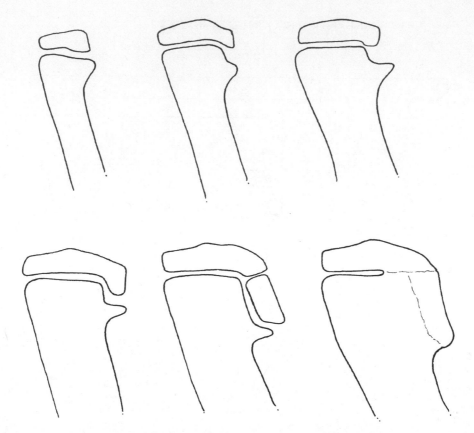

Figure 1 Langenskiold classification of infantile Blount's disease. Stage I *(upper left)* is characterized by irregularity of the medial proximal tibial epiphysis with varus deformity. Stage II *(upper center)* shows medial tapering of the epiphysis and metaphysis with a slight step in the metaphysis. Stage III *(upper right)* is characterized by a sharp angular step in the medial proximal tibial metaphysis. By Stage IV *(lower left)* ossification of the epiphysis into the medial metaphyseal step has occurred. Stage V *(lower center)* shows the appearance of the separate medial fragment in the depressed epiphysis. Stage VI *(lower right)* demonstrates complete medial physeal closure (bony bridge formation).

References

Beck CL, Burke SW, Roberts JM, Johnston CE 2d. Physeal bridge resection in infantile Blount disease. J Pediatr Orthop 1987; 7:161.

Blount WP. Tibia vara. Osteochondrosis deformans tibiae. J Bone Joint Surg 1937; 19:1.

Engel GM, Staheli LT. The natural history of torsion and other factors influencing gait in childhood: A study of the angle of gait, tibial torsion, knee angle, hip rotation, and development of the arch in normal children. Clin Orthop 1974; 99:12.

Ferriter P, Shapiro F. Infantile tibia vara: Factors affecting outcome following proximal tibial osteotomy. J Pediatr Orthop 1987; 7:1.

Foreman KA, Robertson WW Jr. Radiographic measurement of infantile tibia vara. J Pediatr Orthop 1985; 5:452.

Greene WB. Infantile tibia vara. Instructional Course Lectures, Vol 42. Park Ridge, Ill.: American Academy of Orthopaedic Surgeons, 1993; 525.

Greene WB. Infantile tibia vara. J Bone Joint Surg [Am] 1993; 75:130.

Hofmann A, Jones RE, Herring JA. Blount's disease after skeletal maturity. J Bone Joint Surg [Am] 1982; 64:1004.

Johnston CE 2d. Infantile tibia vara. Clin Orthop 1990; 255:13.

Langenskiöld A, Riska EB. Tibia vara (osteochondrosis deformans tibiae). J Bone Joint Surg [Am] 1964; 46:1405.

ADOLESCENT BLOUNT'S DISEASE

A. Adolescent Blount's disease is characterized by varus deformity of the proximal tibia, an essentially normal tibial epiphysis, and a widened medial tibial physis (Figs. 1 and 2). Deformity may be unilateral or bilateral. Frequently, subtle varus deformity of the distal femur coexists (frequently ignored in the management of this deformity). Evaluate patients with bilateral disease and extensive physeal changes for rickets or related disorders.

B. Decision making regarding the therapeutic management of skeletally immature patients with adolescent Blount's disease requires an estimation of the amount of growth remaining in the proximal tibial physis. This information is deduced by obtaining a scanogram and wrist films for bone age. Pre-existing limb length discrepancy in unilateral disease, percentile length of the tibia, and growth remaining based on skeletal age is then determined using the Green-Anderson growth-remaining charts. Since patients with adolescent Blount's disease often have an advanced skeletal age, calculations of growth remaining should not be made relying on chronologic age.

C. Patients with unacceptable deformity who are skeletally immature or have a clinically insignificant amount of growth remaining (<1 cm) should undergo tibial osteotomy for angular deformity correction. This osteotomy may be performed above or below the tibial tubercle based on surgeon's preference. If the deformity is unilateral, document limb length inequality, and consider lengthening the limb simultaneously if the discrepancy is ≥2 cm, based on patient motivation and the severity of the deformity.

D. Patients with bilateral disease generally do not have limb length inequality because of the symmetric nature of the disease. They can therefore be considered for either lateral epiphysiodesis or high tibial osteotomy at surgeon's preference.

E. Lateral epiphysiodesis of the proximal tibia and epiphysiodesis of the proximal fibula is carried out with the hope that the remaining medial proximal tibial physis growth will effect gradual correction of the angular deformity. Perform a 1-cm deep peripheral epiphysiodesis of the lateral proximal tibial physis in either open or closed fashion. This procedure produces relatively minor soft tissue disruption and maintains an intact bone, advantageous in these typically obese patients. The main disadvantage is the uncertain outcome. Series indicate that 50% of patients will show evidence of correction after this procedure.

F. Complete correction by lateral epiphysiodesis occurs in 50% or less of cases. If it does occur, a medial epiphysiodesis is required to prevent overgrowth into valgus. Assess the patient clinically and radiographically with a standing anteroposterior (AP) radiograph every 3 months until skeletal maturity.

G. Partial correction with lateral epiphysiodesis may occur. High tibial osteotomy can be considered after skeletal maturity.

H. Tibial osteotomy with acute correction and fixation is an alternative approach. The osteotomy may be performed above or below the tibial tubercle, based on surgeon's preference, because of the limited growth remaining. Either internal or external fixation may be used. Osteotomies should be corrected to a normal femoral-tibial angle without overcorrection.

I. Manage patients with unilateral Blount's disease not only for angular deformity but for limb length inequality resulting from asymmetric disease. Keep in mind the existing limb length inequality and subsequent limb length inequality that would result from epiphysiodesis.

J. For patients with >2 cm limb length inequality, consider angular correction and gradual lengthening with external fixation. The advantages of this approach are restoration of length and assessment of angular deformity correction in a functional weight-bearing position. The disadvantages are that the patient must be highly motivated and cooperative, and that treatment time to achieve correction is relatively prolonged.

K. High tibial osteotomy may be performed below the tibial tubercle, with either internal or external fixation (Fig. 3). Perform an appropriately timed epiphysiodesis of the opposite limb to normalize limb length inequality.

L. When there is <2 cm of limb length inequality, consider lateral epiphysiodesis as discussed in E. Because limb length inequality exists, the patient should undergo opposite limb epiphysiodesis to prevent progressive limb length inequality.

M. An alternative approach with <2 cm of limb length inequality is high tibial osteotomy below the growth plate. Either internal or external fixation may be used. The patient should then be observed to skeletal maturity to detect recurrence or progression of limb length inequality due to asymmetric disease.

ADOLESCENT BLOUNT'S DISEASE

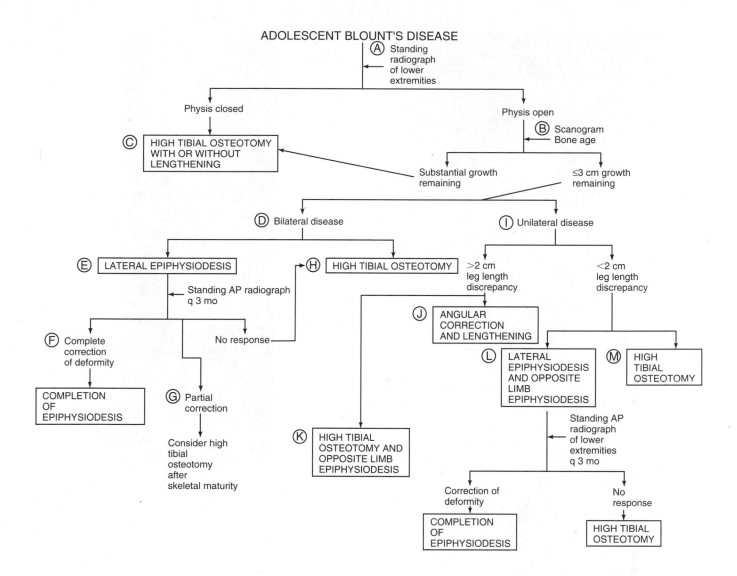

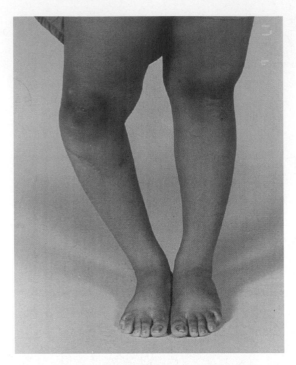

Figure 1 Varus deformity of adolescent Blount's disease. These patients are often obese. Deformity may be unilateral or bilateral

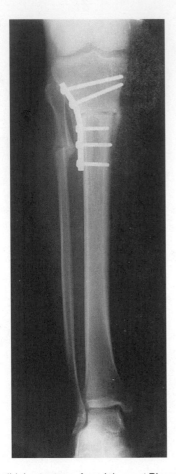

Figure 3 High tibial osteotomy for adolescent Blount's disease. Osteotomy may be performed above or below the tibial tubercle. Deformity should be corrected to anatomic alignment.

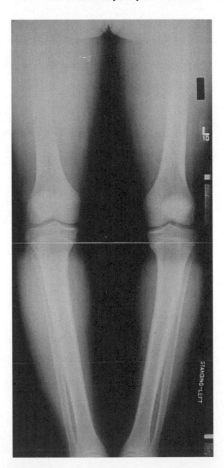

Figure 2 Radiographic appearance of adolescent Blount's disease. The medial physis is typically widened. The proximal tibial epiphysis is relatively unaffected in contradistinction to infantile Blount's disease.

References

Blount WP. Tibia vara: Osteochondrosis deformans tibiae. J Bone Joint Surg 1937; 19:1.

De Pablos J, Franzreb M. Treatment of adolescent tibia vara by asymmetrical physeal distraction. J Bone Joint Surg 1993; 75B:592.

Henderson RC, Kemp GJ, Greene WB. Adolescent tibia vara: Alternatives for operative treatment. J Bone Joint Surg 1992; 74A:342.

Henderson RC, Kemp GJ, Hayes PR. Prevalence of late-onset tibia vara. J Pediatr Orthop 1993; 13:255.

Kline SC, Bostrum M, Griffin PP. Femoral varus: An important component in late-onset Blount's disease. J Pediatr Orthop 1992; 12:197.

Loder RT, Schaffer JJ, Bardenstein MB. Late-onset tibia vara. J Pediatr Orthop 1991; 11:162.

Martin SD, Moran MC, Martin TL, Burke SW. Proximal tibial osteotomy with compression plate fixation for tibia vara. J Pediatr Orthop 1994; 14:619.

Thompson GH, Carter JR. Late-onset tibia vara (Blount's disease). Clin Orthop 1990; 155:24.

PARTIAL PHYSEAL ARREST

A. Insult to a portion of physis may result in the development of a bony bridge or bar connecting the metaphyseal and epiphyseal bone, thereby arresting normal longitudinal growth. Patients at risk are those with Salter Harris type 3 or 4 physeal fractures, fractures involving the distal femoral physis, severe infantile Blount's disease, or infections crossing the physis. At-risk patients should have clear anteroposterior (AP) and lateral radiographs of the affected part, as well as careful examination to detect angular deformity or shortening compared to the companion limb. Radiographic evidence of a partial physeal bar include visualization of the bar itself spanning the physis, Harris grow arrest line tapering to the bar, angular deformity, shortening, or tenting of the epiphysis all due to the disturbance of normal physeal growth.

B. In some patients a bar is suggested by limb length inequality and angular deformity without clear visualization of a bar on plain radiographs. This can be seen after severe metaphyseal-physeal injuries, infection, or radiation. Hypocycloidal axial tomography, computed tomography (CT), or magnetic resonance imaging (MRI) may be used to document or rule out discrete bar formation in such patients. If no discrete bar is documented, further treatment is based on the presence or absence of significant limb deformity. If there is minimal or no deformity, re-evaluate the patient periodically with radiographs as appropriate every 6 months until it is certain that normal growth is occurring or skeletal maturity is achieved.

C. Some patients without a clearly documentable physeal bar develop progressive deformity due to growth disturbance, as if a bar was present. Treat these patients as if they had an unresectable bar (see E). Such circumstances typically occur with post-irradiation physeal injury or growth disturbance due to enchondromata.

D. When a bar has been clearly documented, approximate the extent of surface area of physis affected. If >50% of the surface area is affected, the prognosis for resumption of growth after physeal bar resection is poor, and with rare exceptions the patient should be treated as if the physeal bar is unresectable.

E. If <50% of the surface area of the physis is affected, consider partial physeal bar resection. The next step is to determine how much growth remains in the equivalent normal physis. Obtain this information by documenting the bone segment percentile length and the bone age of the patient, and use this information to determine growth remaining from Green-Anderson growth-remaining charts.

F. If the patient has <2 years of growth remaining, in general physeal bar resection should not be entertained. More definitive, predictable procedures should be performed.

G. If <50% of the surface area of a particular physis is affected, and there is at least 2 years of growth remaining, consider physeal bar resection. At surgery remove the bony bar from the affected physis with as little damage to the remaining healthy physis as possible. Place interposition material within the defect to retard reformation of the bridge. Embed metallic markers in the metaphysis to allow documentation of restoration of growth and to monitor its progress. Although spontaneous correction of angular deformity and acceleration of normal growth to diminish a pre-existing limb length inequality are reported to occur, these events are erratic and uncertain. In most cases if a substantial angular deformity exists, osteotomy should be carried out simultaneously with surgical resection of the bar. Patients require clinical and radiographic evaluation at least every 6 months to document restoration of growth and monitor progress to skeletal maturity.

H. The likelihood of resumption of growth is uncertain. In general, well-isolated, post-traumatic, small bars have a good prognosis for resumption of growth, while more extensive lesions, particularly those due to non-traumatic causes, are less certain. If resumption of growth is documented, continue to observe the patient every 6–12 months including radiographs to identify recurrence of a bar if it should occur prior to skeletal maturity. Recurrence of a physeal bar after initial resumption of growth can be treated with the same considerations as when it was originally evaluated.

I. In up to 66% of cases no resumption of growth can be identified. Imbedding a metallic marker in the metaphysis allows early identification of this occurrence. Treat such patients as if they had an unresectable physeal bar.

J. Patients with an unresectable bar are faced with progressive shortening, potential joint distortion, and in the case of eccentrically located or peripheral bars, progressive angular deformity. In very young patients with substantial growth remaining, repeated osteotomies may be performed. Quite frequently progressive joint distortion will occur. When this occurs, complete the epiphysiodesis to prevent progressive deformity or repeated surgeries. Completion of the epiphysiodesis will lead to progressive limb length inequality because of unchecked normal growth in the opposite limb. This can be treated by epiphysiodesis of the opposite limb, lengthening of the affected limb, or combinations. See p 298.

PATIENT AT RISK FOR PARTIAL PHYSEAL ARREST

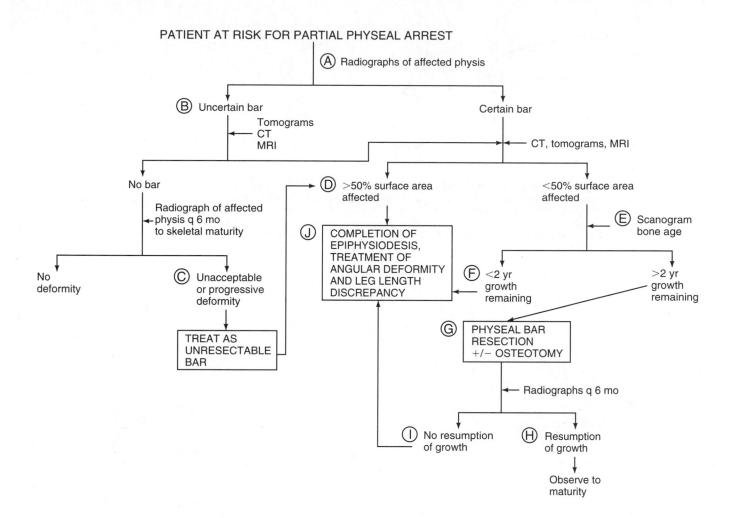

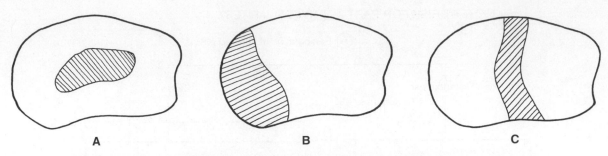

A   B   C

Figure 1 Classification of partial physeal arrest. **A,** Central arrests are characterized by bony bridge within the substance of the physis. The bridge is surrounded by relatively healthy physis. **B,** Peripheral bridges are characterized by an eccentric location of the arrest, in contact with the perimeter of the physis. **C,** Linear arrests are a variation of central arrests characterized by a through-and-through bridge, with healthy physis on either side. These typically occur after type IV fractures of the medial malleolus.

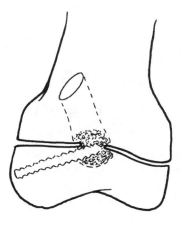

Figure 2 Resection of a central physeal bar is accomplished by access through a metaphyseal window, as illustrated in this case, or metaphyseal osteotomy. The bony bridge is removed, and the cavity created across the physis is filled with interpositional material to prevent re-formation of the bony bridge. If methylmethacrylate is used, it should be anchored to the epiphyseal side of the physis with a pin embedded in the epiphysis so that with resumption of growth the inert material remains with the epiphysis.

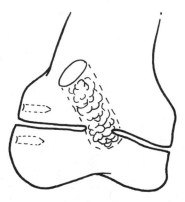

Figure 3 Fat may be used to pack the cavity. Metallic marks should be embedded in the metaphyseal and epiphyseal bone to monitor growth subsequent to the procedure.

References

Bright RW. Operative correction of partial epiphyseal plate closure by osseous-bridge resection and silicone-rubber implant: An experimental study in dogs. J Bone Joint Surg [Am] 1974; 56:655.

Canadell J, de Pablos J. Breaking bony bridges by physeal distraction: A new approach. Int Orthop 1985; 9:223.

Kasser JR. Physeal bar resections after growth arrest about the knee. Clin Orthop 1990; 255:68.

Langenskiöld A. An operation for partial closure of an epiphysial plate in children, and its experimental basis. J Bone Joint Surg [Br] 1975; 57:325.

Langenskiöld A. Surgical treatment of partial closure of the growth plate. J Pediatr Orthop 1981; 1:3.

Letts RM. Management of Pediatric Fractures. New York: Churchill Livingstone, 1994.

Ogden JA. Current concepts review: The evaluation and treatment of partial physeal arrest. J Bone Joint Surg [Am] 1987; 69:1297.

Osterman K. Operative elimination of partial premature epiphyseal closure: An experimental study. Acta Orthop Scand (Suppl) 1972; 147:1.

Peterson HA. Review: Partial growth plate arrest and its treatment. J Pediatr Orthop 1984; 4:246.

Williamson RV, Staheli LT. Partial physeal growth arrest: Treatment by bridge resection and fat interposition. J Pediatr Orthop 1990; 10:769.

HAND SURGERY

DISTAL INTERPHALANGEAL JOINT INJURIES

A. Avulsion of the insertion of either the flexor or extensor tendon may occur with or without a bony fragment. Specific tendon function should be assessed and radiographs examined for the presence of a fragment, either dorsally at the distal interphalangeal (DIP) joint or volarly in the flexor sheath.

B. Zone I extensor injuries are those distal to the central slip insertion onto the middle phalanx.

C. Extension splinting of the DIP joint should leave the proximal interphalangeal joint free for motion. In closed tendon avulsions, splinting is slowly weaned after 6 to 8 weeks, but resumed if extensor lag develops. Night splinting may be beneficial for several months to prevent recurrence of deformity (Fig. 1).

D. An extension splint is used to protect longitudinal K-wiring of the DIP joint. Following K-wire removal at 6 weeks, night splinting should be continued for an additional 2 months.

E. Open reduction and internal fixation (ORIF) with K-wires or pull-out suture are required for displaced fragments comprising >50% of the dorsal articular surface of the distal phalanx to prevent subluxation and restore articular congruity (Fig. 2).

F. In comminuted fractures, early range of motion (ROM) may allow articular fragments to contour about the middle phalanx head to restore some degree of joint surface. The development of painful post-traumatic arthritis is best treated with arthrodesis.

G. Late treatment of mallet deformities is often unrewarding because of extensor shortening and adhesions, which limit normal extensor gliding and joint motion.

H. For chronic mallet deformity with DIP subluxation, ORIF of the fracture fragment or excision with reinsertion of the extensor tendon into bone via a pull-out suture may be tried. If unsuccessful, or in the presence of arthritis, arthrodesis is recommended.

I. Dislocations of the DIP joint are often open injuries. Following debridement and reduction, the integrity of the long flexor and extensor tendons and collateral ligaments should be ascertained. Unstable or open injuries are pinned with a longitudinal K-wire, whereas closed stable injuries may merely require splinting.

J. Infrequently, closed reduction fails due, most commonly, to interposition of the proximally disrupted volar plate, as well as flexor tendon or bony fragments.

DIP INJURY

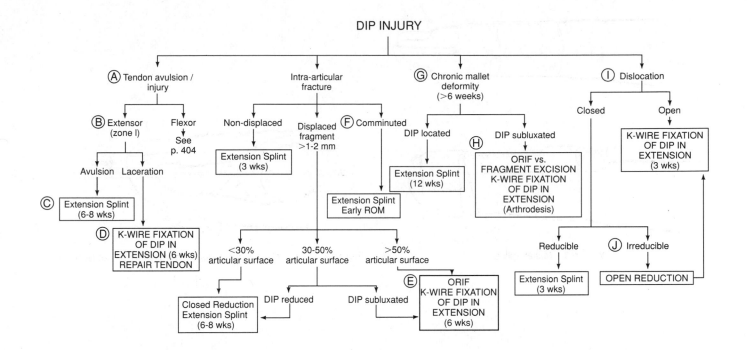

(A) Tendon avulsion / injury

(B) Extensor (zone I)

Flexor
See
p. 404

Avulsion

Laceration

(C) Extension Splint (6-8 wks)

(D) K-WIRE FIXATION OF DIP IN EXTENSION (6 wks) REPAIR TENDON

Intra-articular fracture

Non-displaced

Extension Splint (3 wks)

Displaced fragment >1-2 mm

(F) Comminuted

Extension Splint Early ROM

<30% articular surface

30-50% articular surface

>50% articular surface

Closed Reduction Extension Splint (6-8 wks)

DIP reduced

DIP subluxated

(E) ORIF K-WIRE FIXATION OF DIP IN EXTENSION (6 wks)

(G) Chronic mallet deformity (>6 weeks)

DIP located

DIP subluxated

Extension Splint (12 wks)

(H) ORIF vs. FRAGMENT EXCISION K-WIRE FIXATION OF DIP IN EXTENSION (Arthrodesis)

(I) Dislocation

Closed

Open

K-WIRE FIXATION OF DIP IN EXTENSION (3 wks)

Reducible

(J) Irreducible

Extension Splint (3 wks)

OPEN REDUCTION

353

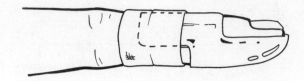

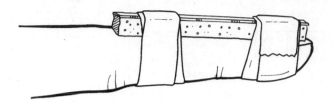

Figure 1 Mallet splint.

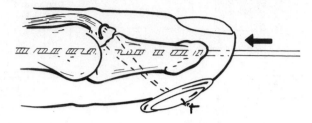

Figure 2 Terminal extensor avulsion repair with pull-out technique.

References

ASSH. Regional Review Courses in Hand Surgery: 1994. Aurora, CO: American Society for Surgery of the Hand, 1994.

Dray GJ, Eaton RG. Dislocations & ligament injuries in the digits. In: Green DP, ed. Operative Hand Surgery. 3rd ed. New York: Churchill-Livingstone, 1993: 767.

Stern P. Fractures of the metacarpals and phalanges. In: Green DP, ed. Operative Hand Surgery. 3rd ed. New York: Churchill-Livingstone, 1993: 695.

Thayer DT. Small joint injuries: DIP injuries. Hand Clin 1988; 4(1):1.

PROXIMAL INTERPHALANGEAL JOINT FRACTURES

A. Radiographic evaluation should include posteroanterior (PA), true lateral, and oblique views of the joint. Occasionally, anteroposterior (AP) and lateral tomograms are helpful in providing additional information regarding fracture displacement and degree of comminution. Articular injuries require anatomic reduction, with stable fixation allowing early range of motion (ROM).

B. Condylar fractures generally result from axial load injury. Type I fractures are nondisplaced and stable, Type II are unicondylar and unstable, and Type III are bicondylar or comminuted.

C. Nonoperative treatment (splinting only) of Type I fractures requires close radiographic follow-up to prevent malunion resulting from interval fracture displacement. Otherwise, stabilization may be obtained with percutaneous pinning (or a screw) under fluoroscopic control. Articular step-off should generally be 1 mm or less.

D. Unicondylar fractures that cannot be closed-reduced with traction, manual pressure, or use of a towel clamp through the skin are approached dorsally between the central slip and lateral band. Anatomic reduction is followed by fixation with pins or screws (Fig. 1).

In bicondylar fractures, the condyles are first attached to each other, and then secured to the shaft fragment with pins, screws, or a plate (mini-condylar). When possible, lateral placement of the plate avoids contact with the extensor mechanism and may lessen adhesion formation. However, these injuries are often associated with some degree of extensor lag, flexion contracture, and/or chronic swelling.

E. Impaction fractures of the base of the middle phalanx have been likened to pilon fractures of the distal tibia. Both result from axial loading and are characterized by articular comminution and lack of subchondral support. Operative intervention may be worthwhile if the articular surface can be reconstructed and fixed with wires and/or screws. The subchondral defect is then packed with cancellous graft to support the articular surface, much as in tibial plateau fractures.

F. Comminuted fractures may benefit from distraction for 3 to 6 weeks via distal skeletal traction through the middle phalanx or a hinged external fixator with early ROM to "mold" articular joint surfaces. The less than optimal results that may ensue are reflective of the severe nature of the initial injury.

PIP FRACTURE

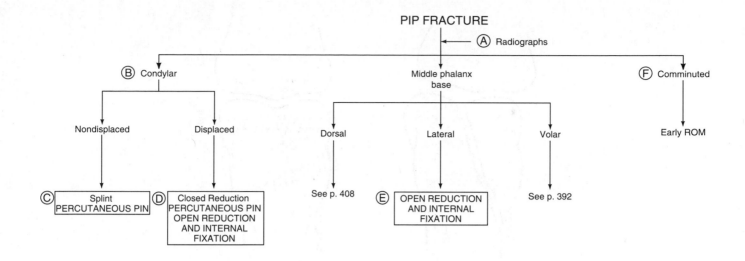

See p. 408

See p. 392

357

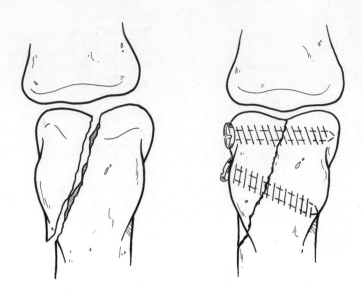

Figure 1   Open reduction and internal fixation of a unicondylar fracture of proximal interphalangeal joint.

References

Agee JM. Unstable fracture dislocations of the proximal inter-phalangeal joint of the fingers: A preliminary report of a new treatment technique. J Hand Surg 1978; 3:386.

ASSH. Regional Review Courses in Hand Surgery: 1994. Aurora, Colorado: American Society for Surgery of the Hand, 1994.

Buchler U, Fisher T. Use of a minicondylar plate for metacarpal and phalangeal periarticular injuries. Clin Orthop 1987; 214:53.

Ford D, El-Hadidi S, PG L, Burke F. Fractures of the phalanges: Results of internal fixation using 1.5 mm and 2 mm AO screws. J Hand Surg 1987; 12B:28.

Kuczynski K. The proximal interphalangeal joint: Anatomy and causes of stiffness of the fingers. J Bone Joint Surg 1968; 50B:656.

London P. Sprains and fractures involving the interphalangeal joints. Hand 1971; 3:155.

Margles SW. Intra-articular fractures of the metacarpophalangeal and proximal interphalangeal joints. Hand Clin 1988; 4(1):67.

McCue FC, Honner R, Johnson MC, Geick JH. Athletic injuries of the proximal interphalangeal joint requiring surgical treatment. J Bone Joint Surg 1970; 52A:937.

Schenck R. Dynamic traction and early passive movement for fractures of the proximal interphalangeal joint. J Hand Surg 1986; 11A:850.

Stern P. Fractures of the metacarpals & phalanges. In: Green DP, ed. Operative Hand Surgery. 3rd ed. New York: Churchill Livingstone, 1993; 718.

PROXIMAL INTERPHALANGEAL JOINT DISLOCATIONS

A. Radiographic evaluation includes posteroanterior (PA), true lateral, and oblique radiographs of the proximal interphalangeal (PIP) joint. The type and length of immobilization following injury is based on functional stability, as determined during active range of motion (ROM) and passive stress testing. Long-term joint swelling and stiffness are not uncommon.

B. Acute dorsal PIP dislocations result from hyperextension and longitudinal compression forces (Fig. 1):

- *Type I (hyperextension)*—joint surfaces are in contact, with avulsion of the distal volar plate insertion onto the base of the middle phalanx, with longitudinal splitting of the collateral ligament.
- *Type II (dorsal dislocation)*—as in Type I, with dorsal dislocation of the middle phalanx on the proximal phalanx (bayonet).
- *Type III (proximal dislocation)*—fracture of the volar base of the middle phalanx.

Stable injuries are Types I and II, and Type III with less than 40% articular involvement, as a portion of the collateral ligament remains attached to the middle phalanx. Type III injuries with fractures comprising greater than 40% of the articular surface are unstable, as the bulk of the collateral ligament remains attached to the fracture fragment. In such cases, if stability and joint congruity are obtained with moderate (approximately 75°) flexion, closed treatment is indicated.

C. An initial period of immobilization for 1 to 2 weeks is followed by controlled ROM exercises, avoiding potential re-dislocation in extension. Close radiographic follow-up is required to ensure continued joint reduction early in treatment.

D. Reducible injuries will demonstrate articular congruity in flexion without dorsal joint space widening (V-sign). Active flexion exercises are performed in a dorsal blocking splint following initial immobilization with close radiographic follow-up.

Irreducible injuries require open reduction and internal fixation (ORIF) of the fracture fragment or excision of small fragments and advancement of the volar plate into a volar trough at the base of the middle phalanx (volar plate arthroplasty) (Fig. 2). If severely comminuted, early motion in traction (skeletal or dynamic external fixator) may be tried.

E. Lateral PIP dislocations usually occur in extension, with the radial collateral ligament injured six times more frequently than the ulnar. Associated injuries may involve the volar plate, extensor mechanism, or bone.

F. Volar PIP dislocations are rare and result from axial loading and rotation with the PIP in flexion. The condyle may buttonhole between the central slip and lateral band, preventing closed reduction. Flexion of the metacarpophalangeal and PIP joints relaxes the lateral band, thereby facilitating reduction with gentle traction.

G. Uncommonly, open reduction is required and performed through a mid-axial incision on the side of suspected ligament injury. Interposed tissue (usually lateral band) is removed with repair of collateral ligament and lateral band as needed.

PIP DISLOCATION

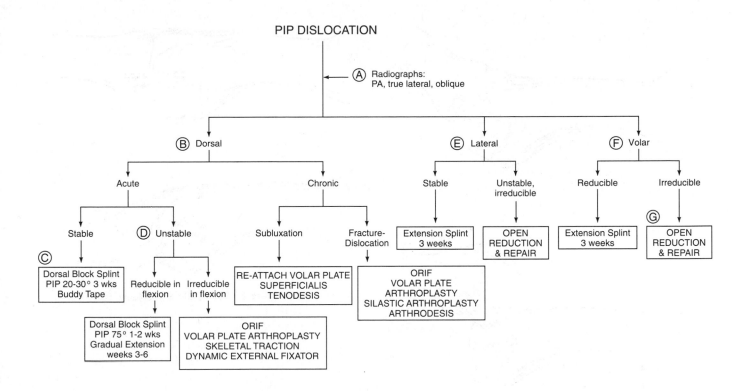

(A) Radiographs:
PA, true lateral, oblique

(B) Dorsal

- Acute
  - Stable
    - (C)
    - Dorsal Block Splint PIP 20-30° 3 wks Buddy Tape
  - (D) Unstable
    - Reducible in flexion
      - Dorsal Block Splint PIP 75° 1-2 wks Gradual Extension weeks 3-6
    - Irreducible in flexion
      - ORIF VOLAR PLATE ARTHROPLASTY SKELETAL TRACTION DYNAMIC EXTERNAL FIXATOR
- Chronic
  - Subluxation
    - RE-ATTACH VOLAR PLATE SUPERFICIALIS TENODESIS
  - Fracture-Dislocation
    - ORIF VOLAR PLATE ARTHROPLASTY SILASTIC ARTHROPLASTY ARTHRODESIS

(E) Lateral

- Stable
  - Extension Splint 3 weeks
- Unstable, irreducible
  - OPEN REDUCTION & REPAIR

(F) Volar

- Reducible
  - Extension Splint 3 weeks
- Irreducible
  - (G)
  - OPEN REDUCTION & REPAIR

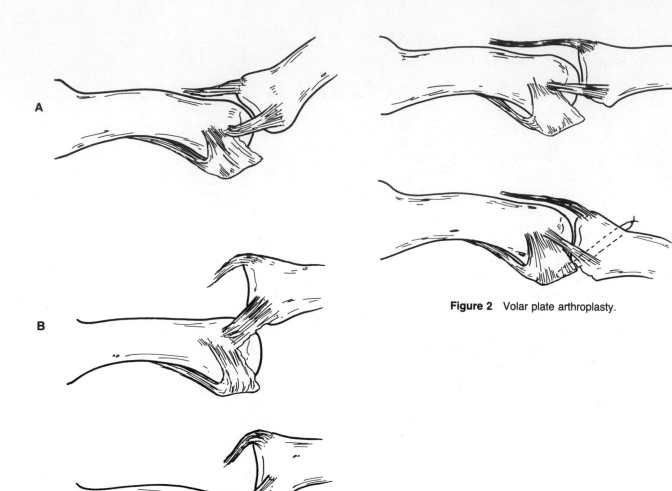

Figure 2 Volar plate arthroplasty.

Figure 1 Dorsal PIP dislocation. **A,** Type I (hyperextension). **B,** Type II (dorsal dislocation). **C,** Type III (fracture−dislocation).

References

Agee JM. Unstable fracture dislocations of the proximal interphalangeal joint of the fingers: A preliminary report of a new treatment technique. J Hand Surg 1978; 3:386.

ASSH. Regional Review Courses in Hand Surgery: 1994. Aurora, Colorado: American Society for Surgery of the Hand, 1994.

Bowers WH. The proximal interphalangeal joint volar plate: II—A clinical study of hyperextension injury. J Hand Surg 1981; 6:77.

Dray GJ, Eaton RG. Dislocations & ligament injuries in the digits. In: Green DP, ed. Operative Hand Surgery. 3rd ed. New York: Churchill-Livingstone, 1993: 767.

Eaton RG, Malerich NM. Volar plate arthroplasty for the proximal interphalangeal joint: A ten year review. J Hand Surg 1980; 5:260.

Kuczynski K. The proximal interphalangeal joint: Anatomy and causes of stiffness of the fingers. J Bone Joint Surg 1968; 50B:656.

Lubahn JD. Dorsal fracture dislocations of the proximal interphalangeal joint. Hand Clin 1988; 4:15.

McCue FC, Honner R, Johnson MC, Geick JH. Athletic injuries of the proximal interphalangeal joint requiring surgical treatment. J Bone Joint Surg 1970; 52A:937.

McElfresh EC, Dobyns JH, O'Brien ET. Management of fracture-dislocation of the proximal interphalangeal joints by extension-block splinting. J Bone Joint Surg 1972; 54A:1705.

Spinner M, Choi BY. Anterior dislocations of the proximal interphalangeal joint: A cause of rupture of the central slip of the extensor mechanism. J Bone Joint Surg 1970; 52A:1329.

Stern P, Lee A. Open dorsal dislocations of the proximal interphalangeal joint. J Hand Surg 1985; 10A:364.

Wilson RL, Liechty BL. Volar dislocation of the proximal interphalangeal joint. Hand Clin 1986; 2:329.

FINGER CARPOMETACARPAL INJURIES

A. Complex ligamentous support and bony stability confer minimal motion to the index and long carpometacarpal (CMC) joints, while the small CMC allows approximately 30° of motion in the sagittal plane. The stable index and long metacarpal bases interdigitate with the trapezoid and capitate. Soft tissue support is conferred by dorsal, volar, and interosseous ligaments with additional stability provided by wrist flexor and extensor insertions.

   Subtle injuries may be missed on radiographs due to bony overlap, particularly on the lateral view. Additional information is obtained from a 30° semipronated lateral view, which projects a true lateral of the small CMC joint. Attention must be directed at each individual articulation to avoid occult injuries, with plain tomography helpful in this regard.

B. Sprains result from palmar flexion and torsional forces, with local tenderness, swelling, and pain and/or instability on stress testing. The small CMC joint is most often injured.

C. Adequate CMC immobilization usually requires a short arm cast that includes adjacent metacarpophalangeal (MP) joints in moderate flexion, leaving the IP joints free. With early healing, a short arm cast well-molded in the palm may be utilized in order to prevent MP stiffness. Long-term symptoms are uncommon.

D. Chronic CMC pain is relatively uncommon and may sometimes respond to interval immobilization with a splint or cast. Long-standing symptoms resulting from instability and/or degenerative arthritis are more definitively managed with arthrodesis using crossed K-wires, staples, or screws.

E. CMC fracture-dislocations result from direct or longitudinal forces and more commonly involve the dorso-ulnar border of the hand. Multiple fracture-dislocations are usually the result of major trauma and/or crush injury with associated soft tissue injury. Displacement is usually dorsal.

F. Fixation of large intra-articular fragments with K-wires and/or small screws may be worthwhile to reduce post-traumatic arthritis. Joint reduction should be held by pinning the involved metacarpal to the carpus and/or adjacent metacarpal for 6 weeks. In the small finger, the extensor carpi ulnaris (ECU) may cause re-displacement of dorsal CMC dislocations unless the metacarpal is pinned to the carpus following closed reduction (Fig. 1).

   Open reduction and internal fixation (ORIF) may be required if interposed soft tissue prevents closed reduction or if anatomic fracture reduction cannot be obtained with traction. Loss of motion at the ulnar CMC joints may result in diminished grip strength.

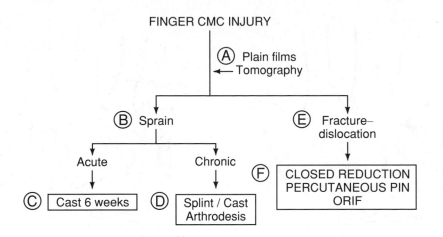

FINGER CMC INJURY

Ⓐ Plain films
← Tomography

Ⓑ Sprain

Ⓔ Fracture–
dislocation

Acute

Chronic

Ⓒ Cast 6 weeks

Ⓓ Splint / Cast
Arthrodesis

Ⓕ CLOSED REDUCTION
PERCUTANEOUS PIN
ORIF

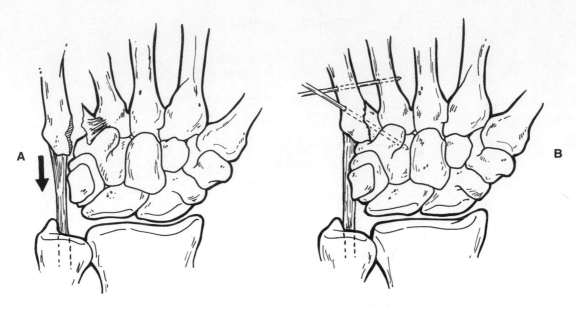

Figure 1 Small metacarpal-hamate fracture-dislocation ("reverse" Bennett's). **A,** Proximal pull by ECU. **B,** Closed reduction, percutaneous pinning.

References

ASSH. Regional Review Courses in Hand Surgery: 1994. Aurora, Colorado: American Society for Surgery of the Hand, 1994.

Bora F, Didizian N. The treatment of injuries to the carpometacarpal joint of the little finger. J Bone Joint Surg 1974; 56A:1459.

Dray GJ, Eaton RG. Dislocations & ligament injuries in the digits. In: Green DP, ed. Operative Hand Surgery. 3rd ed. New York: Churchill-Livingstone, 1993: 779.

Hartwig R, Louis D. Multiple carpometacarpal dislocations. A review of four cases. J Bone Joint Surg 1979; 61A:906.

Henderson J, Arafa M. Carpometacarpal dislocation: An easily missed diagnosis. J Bone Joint Surg 1987; 69B:212.

Rawles JJ. Dislocations and fracture-dislocations at the carpometacarpal joints of the fingers. Hand Clin 1988; 4:103.

Stern P. Fractures of the metacarpals & phalanges. In: Green DP, ed. Operative Hand Surgery. 3rd ed. New York: Churchill-Livingstone, 1993: 712.

PHALANGEAL FRACTURES

A. Radiographic evaluation of phalangeal fractures should include posteroanterior (PA), true lateral, and oblique views for each digit. Additional radiographic views are rarely necessary.

B. Extra-articular fractures of the distal phalanx often result from axial impact or crush injuries and usually do not require reduction. Extension splinting, including the distal interphalangeal (DIP) joint only, is useful for comfort and protection for 3 to 6 weeks.

   The nail plate should be removed when nail bed laceration is suspected, especially for subungual hematomas comprising 50% or greater of the nail plate. Fractures of the distal phalanx with associated nail bed injury are essentially open and require irrigation and debridement. Nail bed lacerations are carefully repaired with fine absorbable suture under loop magnification, and the cleansed nail or nonadherent gauze is placed under the nail fold to prevent adhesion of the underlying nail bed.

C. Physeal injuries of the distal phalanx are often open and are usually Salter I fractures. Following debridement, open reduction is performed with longitudinal pinning of the fracture across the DIP joint. Nonphyseal fractures may sometimes be stabilized without crossing the DIP joint.

D. Fracture deformity of the middle phalanx is governed by the pull of the terminal extensor and FDS tendons. Fractures distal to the FDS insertion display apex volar angulation, whereas those proximal to the FDS insertion have apex dorsal angulation. Proximal phalangeal fractures display apex volar angulation as the interossei flex the proximal fragment and the central slip extends the distal fragment (Fig. 1). Rotation must be carefully assessed, and is best accomplished by viewing the orientation of the fingernails in composite flexion. The fingertips should form a gentle cascade with-

out significant overlap and point toward the scaphoid. Most fractures should be mobilized within 3 weeks to avoid tendon adhesion and joint contracture, though splinting should be continued between exercise until healing is complete (approximately 6 weeks).

E. Nondisplaced and impacted fractures have some degree of intrinsic stability, allowing early protected mobilization with buddy-taping, after a short (<3 weeks) period of immobilization in a safe-position short-arm cast or splint (wrist dorsiflexed, metacarpophalangeal joints flexed, interphalangeal joints extended).

F. Percutaneous pinning of unstable fractures with crossed or longitudinal (canal filling Ender's-type) K-wires (Fig. 2), if stable, allows early range of motion (ROM) and avoids the soft tissue destruction of open treatment, both of which tend to result in improved ROM by minimizing the potential for adhesion formation. Care must be taken to avoid tethering the extensor mechanism when inserting the K-wires, which are subsequently removed upon evidence of early healing (3 to 6 weeks).

G. Internal fixation may include use of K-wires, interosseous wiring, screws, and/or plates (Figs. 3 and 4). When possible, plate application laterally instead of dorsally avoids the problem of excessive bulk underneath the extensor mechanism. Ideally, internal fixation should achieve rigidity sufficient to allow early active ROM, thereby minimizing potential stiffness that results from postoperative adhesions. Bone defects may require bone grafting.

H. Severely comminuted fractures require maintenance of length through the use of traction, longitudinal (Ender's-type) K-wires, external fixation, or a spanning plate (with or without bone graft).

PHALANGEAL FRACTURE

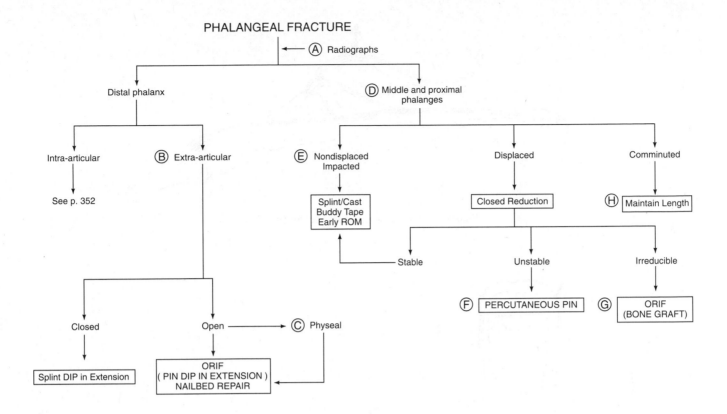

See p. 352

369

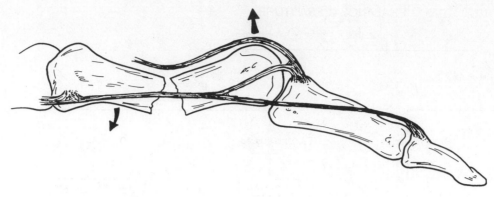

Figure 1   Proximal phalangeal fracture deformity.

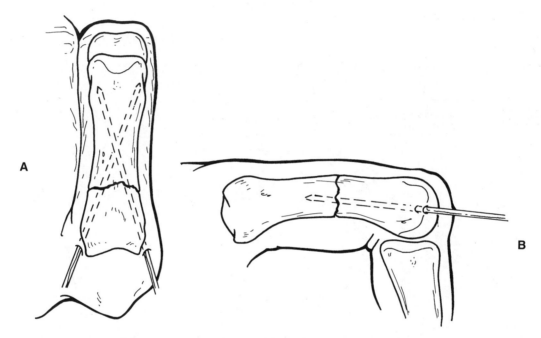

Figure 2   Percutaneous pinning. **A,** Antegrade. **B,** Retrograde.

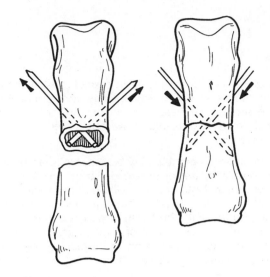

Figure 3 Open reduction, cross-pinning "inside-out" method.

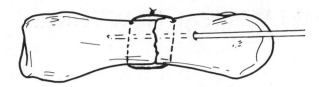

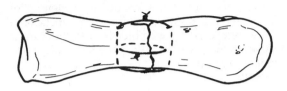

Figure 4 Interosseous wiring with and without cross pinning.

References

ASSH. Regional Review Courses in Hand Surgery: 1994. Aurora, Colorado: American Society for Surgery of the Hand, 1994.

Belsky MR, Eaton RG, Lane LB. Closed reduction and internal fixation of proximal phalangeal fractures. J Hand Surg 1984; 9A:725.

Crawford GP. Screw fixation for certain fractures of the phalanges and metacarpals. J Bone Joint Surg 1976; 58A:487.

Freeland A, Jabaley M, Hughes J. Stable fixation of the hand and wrist. New York: Springer-Verlag, 1986.

Green DP, Anderson JR. Closed reduction and percutaneous pin fixation of fractured phalanges. J Bone Joint Surg 1973; 55A:1651.

Hastings H. Unstable metacarpal and phalangeal fracture treatment with screws and plates. Clin Orthop 1987; 214:37.

Lister G. Intraosseous wiring of the digital skeleton. J Hand Surg 1978; 3:427.

Stern P. Fractures of the metacarpals & phalanges. In: Green DP, ed. Operative Hand Surgery. 3rd ed. New York: Churchill-Livingstone, 1993: 726.

Woods GL. Troublesome shaft fractures of the proximal phalanx: Early treatment to avoid late problems at the metacarpophalangeal and proximal phalangeal joints. Hand Clinics 1988; 4:75-85.

METACARPAL FRACTURES

A. Most metacarpal fractures involve the neck or shaft. Metacarpal head fractures are rare and may be associated with ligamentous avulsion. Complete subcapital fractures may result in avascular necrosis. Injuries to the physis may produce growth arrest with shortening, but rarely cause functional problems. Collateral ligament avulsion fractures off the metacarpal head are best seen radiographically with the Brewerton view (anteroposterior [AP] of the hand with metacarpophalangeal [MP] joints flexed 45° and fingers on the cassette).

B. Metacarpal neck fractures usually result from axial loading, as in a direct blow, and demonstrate apex dorsal angulation with volar comminution. Dorsal wounds are often indicative of puncture from human teeth and require exploration with I & D (irrigation and debridement) to prevent infection. Compensatory carpometacarpal (CMC) joint motion allows greater malreduction in the sagittal plane for the ring and small than for the index and long fingers.

C. Most metacarpal neck fractures can be easily treated nonoperatively with a safe position splint. The relative indications for closed reduction and percutaneous pinning include apex dorsal angulation >15° in the index and long metacarpals or > 40° in the ring and small metacarpals, the latter due to greater compensatory CMC motion. Open reduction and internal fixation (ORIF) may be required when a closed reduction cannot be obtained (Fig. 1).

D. Safe position splinting immobilizes the MP joints in flexion in order to place the collateral ligaments on stretch and thereby minimize their contracture. The interphalangeal (IP) joints are placed in extension, as contracture in this position is more easily treated than in flexion.

E. Malunion in flexion results in cosmetic loss of the dorsal "knuckle" with attendant palmar prominence of the metacarpal head. The latter may be associated with pain and resultant weakness with attempted power grip.

F. Percutaneous pinning may be accomplished by retrograde placement of intramedullary K-wires from the metacarpal head fossae (collateral ligament origins) with care taken to avoid tethering of the dorsal extensor. Pinning with the MP in flexion aids in fracture reduction and assessment of rotation and aids postoperative extensor excursion by displacing the sagittal hood distally (Figs. 2 and 3).

G. Transverse metacarpal shaft fractures usually result from axial loading, whereas oblique or spiral fractures result from rotational forces transmitted through the finger. Angulation is usually apex dorsal due to the volar forces exerted on the distal fragment by the interossei. The more proximal the fracture, the less angulation can be tolerated. Shortening is limited by the inter-volar plate ligament.

H. Angulatory malunion is tolerated less in shaft fractures than in fractures at the neck because, for every degree of angulation proximally, the resultant arc of displacement distally increases as the distance between the fracture site and MP joint increases.

I. ORIF may include use of lag screws alone for long oblique and spiral fractures at least twice the diameter of the shaft in length, plates, interosseous wiring, and/or K-wires (Figs. 4 to 6). The goal is to provide stability sufficient to allow immediate range of motion to minimize postoperative adhesions.

METACARPAL FRACTURE

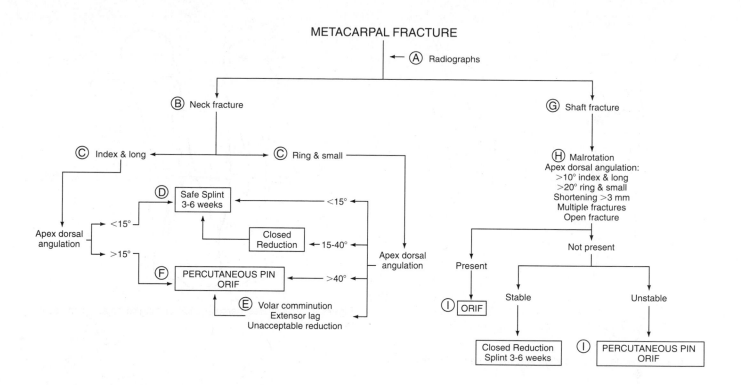

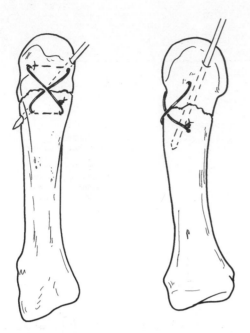

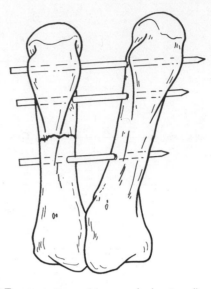

Figure 3 Transverse percutaneous pinning to adjacent metacarpal.

Figure 1 Oblique pinning and dorsal tension band of neck fracture.

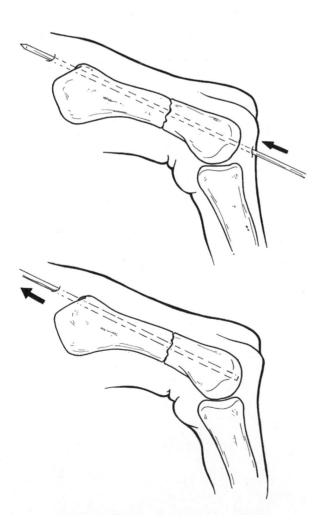

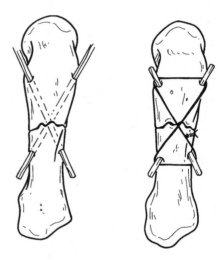

Figure 4 Cross pinning with dorsal tension band.

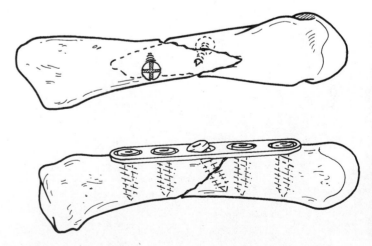

Figure 2 Retrograde percutaneous pinning.

Figure 5 Screw or plate fixation of oblique or spiral fractures.

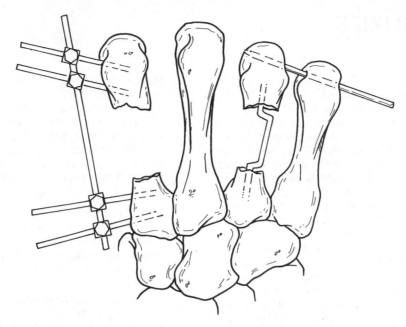

Figure 6 External fixation, intramedullary wire spacer, and pinning to adjacent metacarpal to maintain length in cases of bone loss.

References

ASSH. Regional Review Courses in Hand Surgery: 1994. Aurora, CO: American Society for Surgery of the Hand, 1994.

Barton N. Fractures of the hand. J Bone Joint Surg 1984; 66B:159.

Buchler U, Fischer T. Use of a mini-condylar plate for metacarpal and phalangeal periarticular injuries. Clin Orthop 1987; 214:53.

Burkhalter W. Hand fractures. Instructional Course Lectures 1990; 34:249.

Crawford GP. Screw fixation for certain fractures of the phalanges and metacarpals. J Bone Joint Surg 1976; 58A:487.

Edwards GJ, O'Brien E, Heckman M. Retrograde cross-pinning of transverse metacarpal and phalangeal fractures. Hand 1982; 14:141.

Freeland A, Jabaley M, Hughes J. Stable fixation of the hand and wrist. New York: Springer-Verlag, 1986.

Hastings H. Unstable metacarpal and phalangeal fracture treatment with screws and plates. Clin Orthop 1987; 214:37.

Hastings HI, Carroll CI. Treatment of closed articular fractures of the metacarpophalangeal and proximal interphalangeal joints. Hand Clin 1988; 4:503.

Heim U, Pfeiffer K. Small fragment set manual. In Internal Fixation of Small Fractures. 2nd ed. New York: Springer-Verlag, 1982.

Lane C. Detecting occult fractures of the metacarpal head: The Brewerton view. J Hand Surg 1977; 2:131.

Light T, Ogden J. Metacarpal epiphyseal fractures. J Hand Surg 1987; 12A:460.

Lister G. Intraosseous wiring of the digital skeleton. J Hand Surg 1978; 3:427.

Margles S. Intra-articular fractures of the metacarpophalangeal and proximal interphalangeal joints. Hand Clin 1988; 4:67.

McElfresh EC, Dobyns JH. Intra-articular metacarpal head fractures. J Hand Surg 1983; 8:383.

Melone CJ. Rigid fixation of phalangeal and metacarpal fractures. Orthop Clin North Am 1986; 17:421.

Stern PJ. Fractures of the metacarpals & phalanges. In: Green DP, ed. Operative Hand Surgery. 3rd ed. New York: Churchill-Livingstone, 1993: 695.

Viegas S, Tencer A, Woodard P, Williams C. Functional bracing of fractures of the second through fifth metacarpals. J Hand Surg 1987; 12A:139.

CARPAL INJURIES

A. Radiographic evaluation of the carpus may be accomplished with a wrist series, which includes a neutral posteroanterior (PA) (shoulder abducted 90°, elbow flexed 90°, forearm rotation neutral, wrist flexion/extension and deviation neutral) and neutral lateral (shoulder abducted 0°, elbow flexed 90°, forearm rotation neutral, wrist flexion/extension and deviation neutral). The series is completed with pronated PA views of the wrist in radial and ulnar deviation, along with an anteroposterior (AP) grip or clenched fist view.

Carpal dislocations are classified according to the relative alignment of the radius, lunate, and capitate. Perilunate injuries describe dislocation of the carpus about the lunate, such that the radius and lunate maintain their colinear alignment. With lunate dislocation, the lunate is volar to the carpus while the radius and capitate maintain their colinear alignment. Figures 1 and 2 illustrate the volar and dorsal carpal ligaments.

B. Trans-scaphoid perilunate dislocation results from dorsiflexion injury, with ulnar deviation and intercarpal supination. Energy dissipation across the carpus results in ligamentous disruption, fracture of the radial styloid, and/or carpal fracture (e.g., *trans*-scaphoid, *trans*-triquetral). Suboptimal results are often obtained with closed reduction alone without supplemental fixation due to the development of late carpal subluxation and consequent instability as well as post-traumatic arthritis resulting from malalignment. Postoperatively, the wrist is generally immobilized in a thumb spica cast for approximately 3 months.

C. Lunate dislocation may be thought of as the final stage of progressive perilunar instability, with energy dissipation resulting in ligamentous disruption about the lunate, which dislocates volarly as the carpus collapses into a stable configuration. In this instance, focal compression of median nerve by the lunate and associated soft tissue swelling may result in acute carpal tunnel syndrome requiring immediate carpal tunnel release.

In the absence of sensory findings, an attempt at closed reduction of the lunate at the time of injury may prevent subsequent development of median nerve compression. Interestingly, avascular necrosis of the lunate is uncommon. Postoperatively, the wrist is generally immobilized in a thumb spica cast for approximately 3 months.

D. Acute scapho-lunate (S-L) dissociation involves disruption of the intrinsic S-L ligament and is demonstrated by widening of the S-L interval on PA radio-graphs (compared to the contralateral side). Provocative testing includes axial loading, to induce a diastasis, with an AP clenched fist radiograph. Arthrography, magnetic resonance imaging, and arthroscopy may aid in the diagnosis. Operative results appear better following recent injury; stiffness, persistent instability, and late arthritis are potentially complicating factors. Postoperatively, the wrist is generally immobilized in a thumb spica cast for approximately 3 months.

E. The etiology of Kienböck's disease is unknown but thought to be related to antecedent trauma, with microfracture perhaps disrupting the vascular supply to the lunate. The following staging system may be used (see Fig. 3):
- *Stage 0:* Normal x-ray; abnormal bone scan or MRI
- *Stage I:* Linear or compression fracture
- *Stage II:* Increased bony density
- *Stage III:* Collapse
- *Stage IV:* Arthritis

Treatment is controversial, with procedures directed at diminishing force transmission through the lunate early in the disease process to allow revascularization without collapse (Stages I, II, and sometimes III). This may include carpal unloading using an external fixator with slight distraction, or joint leveling techniques, such as radial shortening or ulnar lengthening (Fig. 4). Other approaches are directed at restoring a collapsed lunate with bone graft and/or direct revascularization (Stage III). Late treatment for arthritis consists of salvage by proximal row carpectomy or arthrodesis (Stage IV).

F. The classification of carpal instabilities remains controversial. Common patterns involve malalignment of the scaphoid with respect to the lunate on lateral radiograph (Fig. 5). Dorsal intercalary segmental instability (DISI) describes a dorsiflexed lunate, with the scaphoid rotated into flexion, and is indicative of chronic S-L instability (rotary subluxation of the scaphoid). Alternatively, volar intercalary segmental instability (VISI) describes a flexed lunate and is indicative of chronic luno-triquetral (L-T) instability.

Symptoms of carpal instability include pain, weakness, and a palpable and/or audible pop that may be reproduced with certain maneuvers by the patient. Attempted ligamentous reconstruction is often unrewarding, and the long-term results of limited arthrodesis are as yet unknown.

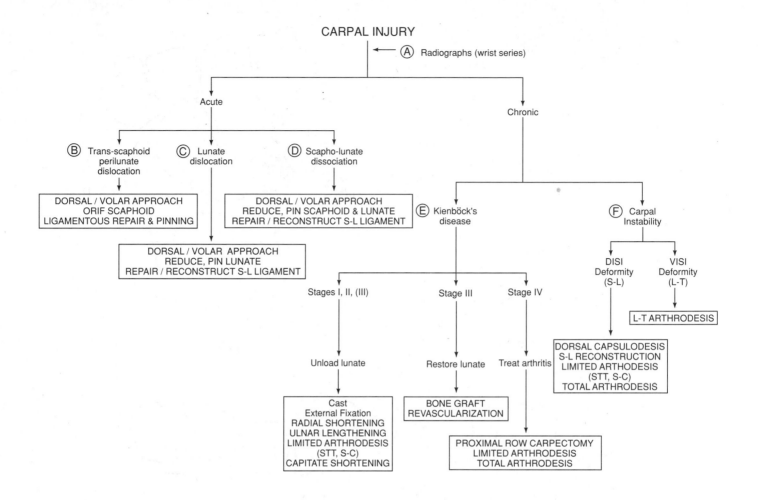

CARPAL INJURY

Ⓐ Radiographs (wrist series)

Acute

Chronic

Ⓑ Trans-scaphoid perilunate dislocation

Ⓒ Lunate dislocation

Ⓓ Scapho-lunate dissociation

DORSAL / VOLAR APPROACH
ORIF SCAPHOID
LIGAMENTOUS REPAIR & PINNING

DORSAL / VOLAR APPROACH
REDUCE, PIN SCAPHOID & LUNATE
REPAIR / RECONSTRUCT S-L LIGAMENT

Ⓔ Kienböck's disease

Ⓕ Carpal Instability

DORSAL / VOLAR APPROACH
REDUCE, PIN LUNATE
REPAIR / RECONSTRUCT S-L LIGAMENT

DISI Deformity (S-L)

VISI Deformity (L-T)

Stages I, II, (III)

Stage III

Stage IV

L-T ARTHRODESIS

DORSAL CAPSULODESIS
S-L RECONSTRUCTION
LIMITED ARTHODESIS
(STT, S-C)
TOTAL ARTHRODESIS

Unload lunate

Restore lunate

Treat arthritis

Cast
External Fixation
RADIAL SHORTENING
ULNAR LENGTHENING
LIMITED ARTHRODESIS
(STT, S-C)
CAPITATE SHORTENING

BONE GRAFT
REVASCULARIZATION

PROXIMAL ROW CARPECTOMY
LIMITED ARTHRODESIS
TOTAL ARTHRODESIS

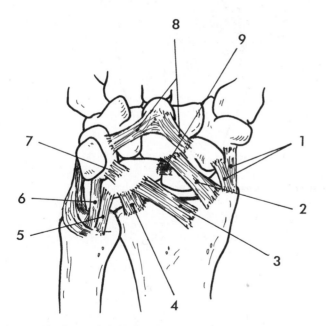

Figure 1   Volar carpal ligaments: (1) radial collateral ligament, (2) radio-scapho-capitate ligament, (3) long radio-lunate ligament, (4) short radio-lunate ligament, (5) ulno-lunate ligament, (6) ulno-triquetral ligament, (7) luno-triquetral ligament, (8) V-deltoid ligaments, (9) scapho-lunate ligament.

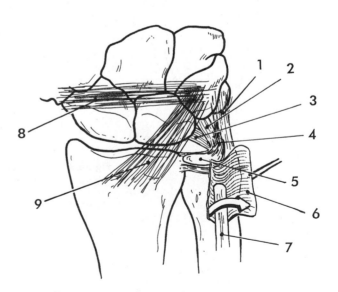

Figure 2   Dorsal carpal ligaments and TFCC: (1) ulnar collateral ligament, (2) ulno-triquetral ligament, (3) ulno-lunate ligament, (4) ulno-carpal meniscus homologue, (5) triangular cartilage (articular disc), (6) extensor carpi ulnaris sheath, (7) extensor carpi ulnaris, (8) dorsal intercarpal ligament, (9) dorsal radiocarpal (radiotriquetral) ligament.

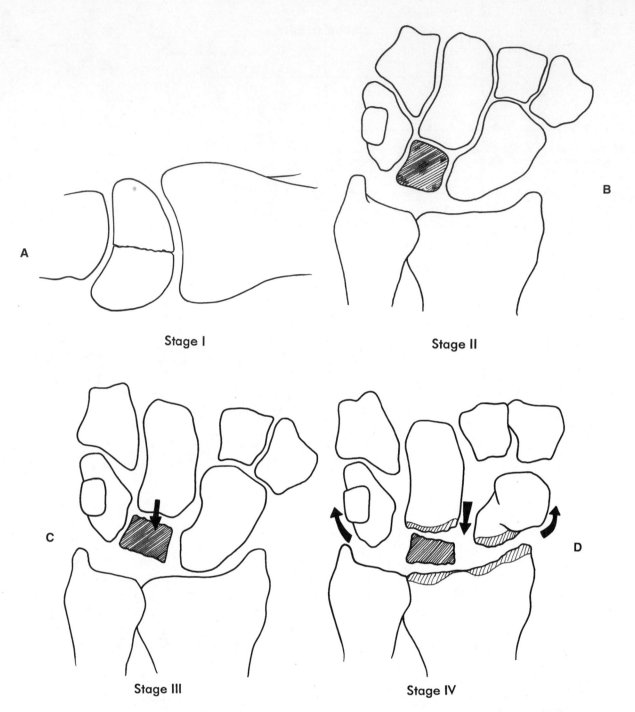

Stage I

Stage II

Stage III

Stage IV

Figure 3 Classification of Kienböck's disease.

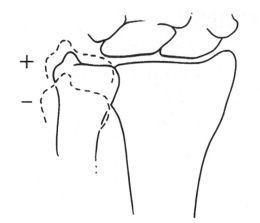

Figure 4 Ulnar variance.

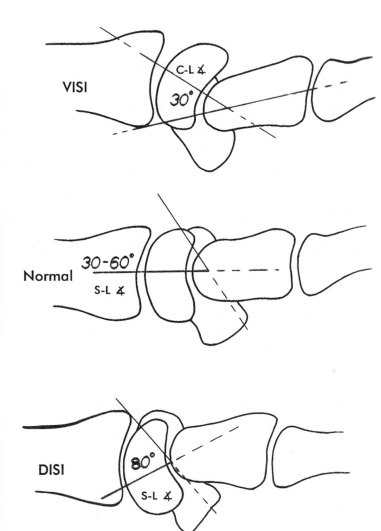

Figure 5 Carpal instability patterns.

References

Amadio P, Taleisnik J. Fractures of the carpal bones. In: Green DP, ed. Operative Hand Surgery. 3rd ed. New York: Churchill Livingstone, 1993: 799.

ASSH. Regional Review Courses in Hand Surgery: 1994. Aurora, Colorado: American Society for Surgery of the Hand, 1994.

Beckenbaugh RD, Shives TC, Dobyns JH, Linscheid RL. Kienbock's disease: The natural history of Kienbock's disease and consideration of lunate fractures. Clin Orthop 1980; 149:98.

Blatt G. Capsulodesis in reconstructive hand surgery: Dorsal capsulodesis for the unstable scaphoid and volar capsulodesis following excision of the distal ulna. Hand Clin 1987; 3:81.

Crosby EB, Linscheid RL, Dobyns JH. Scaphotrapezial trapezoidal arthrosis. J Hand Surg 1978; 3:223.

Dobyns JH, Linscheid RL, Chao EYS, et al. Traumatic instability of the wrist. AAOS Instructional Course Lectures 1975; 24:182.

Gelberman RH, Salamon PB, Jurst JM, Posch JL. Ulnar variance with Kienbock's disease. J Bone Joint Surg 1975; 57A:674.

Green DP. Carpal dislocations and instabilities. In: Green DP, ed. Operative Hand Surgery. 3rd ed. New York: Churchill-Livingstone, 1993: 861.

Kleinman WB. Management of chronic rotary subluxation of the scaphoid by scapho-trapezio-trapezoid arthrodesis: Rationale for the technique, post-operative changes in biomechanics and results. Hand Clin 1987; 3:113.

Kleinman WB, Steichen JB, Strickland JW. Management of chronic rotary subluxation of the scaphoid by scapho-trapezio-trapezoid arthrodesis. J Hand Surg 1982; 7:125.

Lichtman DM, Schneider JR, Swafford AR, Mack GR. Ulnar midcarpal instability: Clinical and laboratory analysis. J Hand Surg 1981; 6:515.

Linscheid RL, Dobyns JH, Beaubout JW, Bryan RS. Traumatic instability of the wrist: Diagnosis, classification and pathomechanics. J Bone Joint Surg 1972; 54A:1612.

Mayfield JK, Johnson RP, Kilcoyne RF. Carpal dislocations: Pathomechanics and progressive perilunar instability. J Hand Surg 1980; 5:226.

Palmer AK, Dobyns JH, Linshceid RL. Management of post-traumatic instability of the wrist secondary to ligament rupture. J Hand Surg 1978; 3:507.

Rayhack JM, Linscheid RL, Dobyns JH, et al. Posttraumatic ulnar translation of the carpus. J Hand Surg 1987; 12A:529.

Taleisnik J. Wrist: anatomy, function and injury. AAOS Instructional Course Lectures 1978; 27:61.

Taleisnik J. Post-traumatic carpal instability. Clin Orthop 1980; 149:73.

Watson HK, Goodman ML, Johnson TR. Limited wrist arthrodesis: Part II: Intercarpal radiocarpal combinations. J Hand Surg 1981; 6:223.

Watson HK, Hempton RD. Limited wrist arthrodesis: Part I—The triscaphoid joint. J Hand Surg 1980; 5:320.

THUMB CARPOMETACARPAL INJURIES

A. Thumb carpometacarpal (CMC) injury results from axial forces on a flexed metacarpal. Radiographs should include hyperpronated anteroposterior (AP) and true lateral views. Stability is afforded by the strong volar ligament and, to a lesser degree, the interlocking bony contours of the saddle-shaped joint.

B. Pure dislocation of the thumb CMC joint is rare and usually results in dorsal and radial displacement of the metacarpal. Reduction is generally obtained by axial traction and may be maintained by pinning the joint for 3 to 6 weeks.

C. Impediments to closed reduction include interposed capsule or small bone fragments. Careful radiographic scrutiny is necessary to ensure adequate reduction.

D. Fracture-dislocation injuries include Bennett's (volar ulnar metacarpal base) and Rolando (T or Y intra-articular metacarpal base) fractures with resultant proximal, dorsal, and radial migration of the metacarpal. Treatment objectives include anatomic restoration of the joint surface and restoration of joint stability. Nondisplaced fractures may be closely monitored in a short arm thumb spica cast.

E. When the Bennett's fracture fragment comprises <15% of the articular surface, closed reduction by axial traction and direct digital pressure with percutaneous K-wire stabilization of the CMC joint may be employed (Fig. 1).

F. For large Bennett's fracture fragments comprising >25% of the articular surface or in cases of failed closed reduction, open reduction through a volar approach with fixation using lag screws or K-wires is used. Rigid internal fixation may permit early range of motion. Otherwise, short arm thumb spica cast immobilization is continued for approximately 6 weeks.

Simple (two-part) Rolando fractures are managed by restoration of the articular surface and stabilization with a plate (Fig. 2). Bone grafting may be required if metaphyseal compaction exists. More comminuted fractures may require external fixation to restore length, with or without adjunctive limited internal fixation.

Malunion may result in CMC subluxation and arthritis. Occasionally, subluxation may be corrected by first metacarpal osteotomy, while soft tissue arthroplasty may be employed for cases of isolated CMC arthritis. Persistent subluxation with arthritis is best treated with CMC arthrodesis.

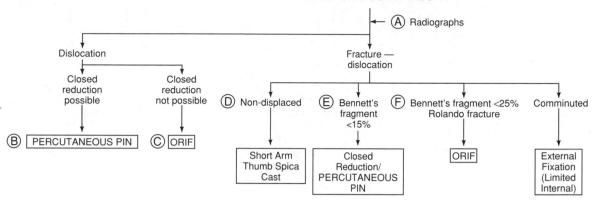

THUMB CMC JOINT INJURY

Ⓐ Radiographs

Dislocation

Fracture — dislocation

Closed reduction possible

Closed reduction not possible

Ⓓ Non-displaced

Ⓔ Bennett's fragment <15%

Ⓕ Bennett's fragment <25% Rolando fracture

Comminuted

Ⓑ PERCUTANEOUS PIN

Ⓒ ORIF

Short Arm Thumb Spica Cast

Closed Reduction/ PERCUTANEOUS PIN

ORIF

External Fixation (Limited Internal)

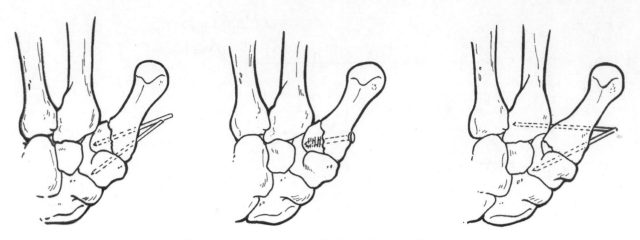

Figure 1 Pinning or screw fixation of Bennett's fracture.

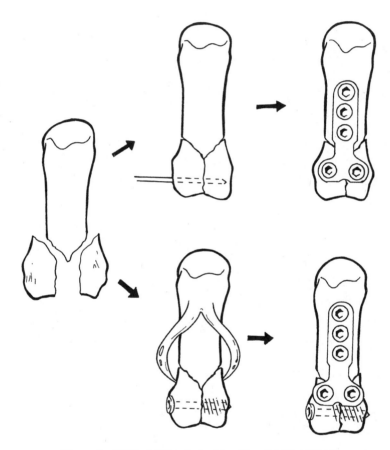

Figure 2 ORIF of Rolando fracture (T or Y intra-articular).

References

ASSH. Regional Review Courses in Hand Surgery: 1994. Aurora, Colorado: American Society for Surgery of the Hand, 1994.

Breen T, Gelberman R, Jupiter J. Intra-articular fractures of the basilar joint of the thumb. Hand Clin 1988; 4:491.

Chen V. Dislocation of the carpometacarpal joint of the thumb. J Hand Surg 1987; 12B:246.

Cooney W, Lucca M, Linscheid R. The kinesiology of the thumb trapeziometacarpal joint. J Bone Joint Surg 1981; 63A:1371.

Dray GJ, Eaton RG. Dislocations & ligament injuries in the digits. In: Green DP, ed. Operative Hand Surgery. 3rd ed. New York: Churchill Livingstone, 1993: 787.

Eaton RG, Lane LB, Littler JW, Keyser JJ. Ligament reconstruction for the painful thumb carpometacarpal joint: A long-term assessment. J Hand Surg 1984; 9A:692.

Foster R, Hastings HI. Treatment of Bennett, Rolando, and vertical intra-articular trapezial fractures. Clin Orthop 1987; 214:121.

Freeland A, Jabaley M, Hughes J. Stable fixation of the hand and wrist. New York: Springer-Verlag, 1986.

O'Brien ET. Fractures of the metacarpals & phalanges. In: Green DP, ed. Operative Hand Surgery. 2nd ed. New York: Churchill Livingstone, 1988: 765.

Pagalidis T, Kuczyinski K, Lamb D. Ligamentous stability of the base of the thumb. Hand 1981; 13:29.

Pellegrini VJ. Fractures at the base of the thumb. Hand Clin 1988; 4:87.

Ruedi T, Burri C, Pfeiffer K. Stable internal fixation of fractures of the hand. J Trauma 1971; 11:381.

Segmuller G. Surgical Stabilization of the Skeleton of the Hand. Baltimore: Williams & Wilkins, 1977.

SCAPHOID FRACTURES

The scaphoid articulates with five bones, is predominantly covered by articular cartilage, and is the most frequently fractured carpal bone (Fig. 1). Blood supply to the proximal pole may be tenuous, with approximately one third of scaphoids having one or no vascular foramina proximal to the scaphoid waist (mid-portion) (Fig. 2). As a result, proximal fractures require longer periods of immobilization for union, with avascular necrosis of the proximal pole seen in 30% of mid-third fractures and almost 100% of proximal pole fractures.

The radial artery sends a branch to the dorsal ridge, supplying 80% of the scaphoid, including the proximal pole, as well as a volar branch to the distal tuberosity, supplying 20% of the bone. Thus, the volar approach is less likely to interfere with proximal pole vascularity, while the dorsal approach may be required for (Herbert) screw placement in a proximal pole fracture.

A. Scaphoid fractures are often missed on radiographs. Radiographs should include a pronated view of the wrist in ulnar deviation, to extend the scaphoid and place its long axis in profile. Snuff box tenderness, despite negative radiographs, demands immobilization and follow-up radiographs at 1 week, at which time resorption at the fracture site may more clearly demonstrate a fracture. Long-arm casting appears to improve the union rate, though elbow immobilization should not exceed 6 weeks to avoid permanent elbow flexion contracture.

B. Immediate, stable open reduction and internal fixation (ORIF) of acute fractures may allow early, protected range of motion and possibly avoid late stiffness, though not yet clinically demonstrated to yield union rates superior to immobilization. Reduction should be within 1 mm with screw fixation using a Herbert or countersunk cancellous screw.

C. Management of the chronic, painless scaphoid non-union with observation versus ORIF is controversial.

Treatment of painful non-unions is influenced by patient age, occupation/demands, fracture location, proximal pole avascular necrosis, and the number of previous operations.

D. Non-union without collapse requires debridement of the fracture site, with cancellous bone graft and immobilization with a compression screw (e.g., Herbert, AO) or K-wires if screw purchase is unobtainable due to small fragment size. Alternatively, Russe cortico-cancellous inlay grafts may be used as a source of bone graft and to stabilize the fracture, with or without additional K-wires, if needed (Fig. 3).

E. Collapse of the scaphoid results in a "hump-back" deformity, which may be corrected with the use of a volar cortico-cancellous iliac crest wedge graft (Fig. 4), as in an opening wedge osteotomy, and screw (if possible) or K-wire fixation.

F. Localized radio-scaphoid arthritis with a stable fibrous scaphoid non-union and impingement at the radial styloid tip in an elderly, inactive patient may sometimes respond to limited radial styloidectomy. Care must be taken to avoid excessive resection as the origins of the important radio-carpal ligaments may be disrupted.

G. In the face of significant arthritis involving the scaphoid fossa of the radius, or in the multiply-operated patient, salvage-type procedures are indicated. After excision of the proximal scaphoid, the wrist may operate through the lunate fossa with the lunate, as occurs following fusion of the lunate-capitate-triquetrum-hamate, or with the capitate, as in proximal row carpectomy. In severe disease, total wrist arthrodesis is indicated.

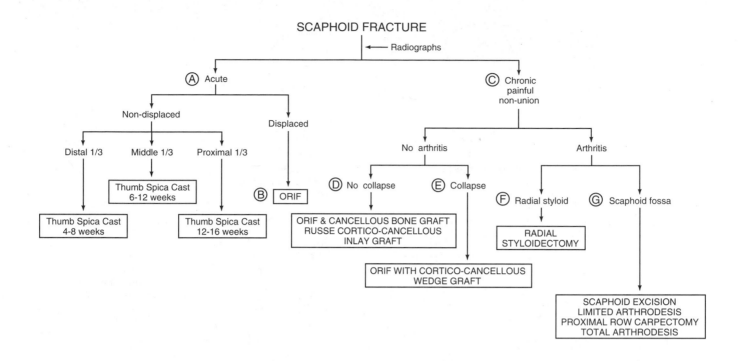

References

Adams BD, Blair WF, Reagan DS, et al. Technical factors related to Herbert screw fixation. J Hand Surg 1988; 13A:893.

ASSH. Regional Review Courses in Hand Surgery: 1994. Aurora, Colorado: American Society for Surgery of the Hand, 1994.

Burgess RC. The effect of a simulated scaphoid malunion on wrist motion. J Hand Surg 1987; 12A:774.

Cooney WP, Dobyns JH, Linscheid RL. Nonunion of the scaphoid: Analysis of the results from bone grafting. J Hand Surg 1980; 5:343.

Cooney WP, Linscheid RL, Dobyns JH. Scaphoid nonunion: Role of anterior interpositional bone grafts. J Hand Surg 1988; 13A:635.

Herbert TJ. Management of the fractured scaphoid using a new bone screw. J Bone Joint Surg 1984; 66B:114.

Mack GR, Lichtman DM. Scaphoid non-union. In: Lichtman DM, ed. The Wrist and Its Disorders. Philadelphia: W.B. Saunders, 1988: 293.

Monsivais JJ, Nitz PA, Scully TJ. The role of carpal instability in scaphoid nonunion: Casual or causal? Hand Surg 1986; 11B:201.

Nakamura R, Hori M, Horii E, et al. Reduction of the scaphoid fracture with DISI alignment. J Hand Surg 1987; 12A:1000.

Obletz BE, Halbstein BM. Nonunion of fractures of the carpal navicular. Journal Bone Joint Surg 1938; 20:424.

Osterman AL, Bora FW, Maiting E. Herbert screw fixation for scaphoid nonunion. Proc Am Soc Surg Hand 1988; 43:4.

Russe O. Fracture of the carpal navicular: Diagnosis, non-operative treatment and operative treatment. J Bone Joint Surg 1960; 42A:759.

Taleisnik J. Fractures of the carpal bones. In: Green DP, ed. Operative Hand Surgery. 2nd ed. New York: Churchill Livingstone, 1988: 813.

Taleisnik J, Kelly PJ. The extraosseous and intraosseous blood supply of the scaphoid bone. J Bone Joint Surg 1966; 48A:1125.

Vender MI, Watson HK, Wiener BD, et al. Degenerative change in symptomatic scaphoid nonunion. J Hand Surg 1987; 12A:514.

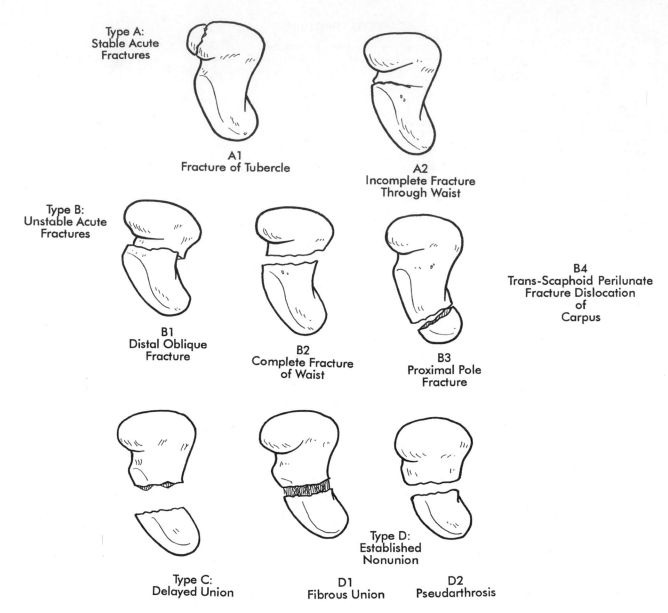

Figure 1 Scaphoid fracture classification.

Type A:
Stable Acute
Fractures

A1
Fracture of Tubercle

A2
Incomplete Fracture
Through Waist

Type B:
Unstable Acute
Fractures

B1
Distal Oblique
Fracture

B2
Complete Fracture
of Waist

B3
Proximal Pole
Fracture

B4
Trans-Scaphoid Perilunate
Fracture Dislocation
of
Carpus

Type C:
Delayed Union

Type D:
Established
Nonunion

D1
Fibrous Union

D2
Pseudarthrosis

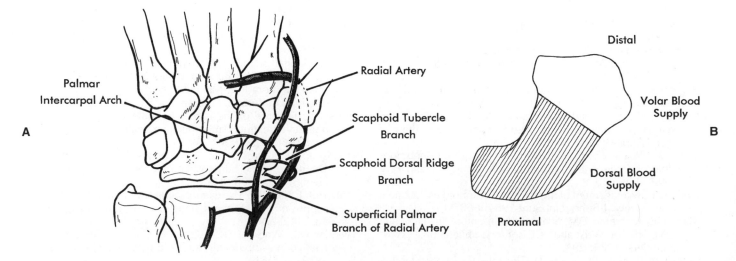

A

Palmar
Intercarpal Arch

Radial Artery

Scaphoid Tubercle
Branch

Scaphoid Dorsal Ridge
Branch

Superficial Palmar
Branch of Radial Artery

Distal

Volar Blood
Supply

Dorsal Blood
Supply

Proximal

B

Figure 2 Scaphoid blood supply.

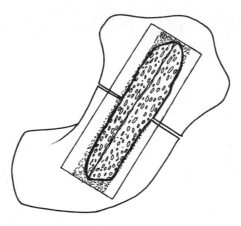

Figure 3 Russe cortico-cancellous volar inlay bone graft.

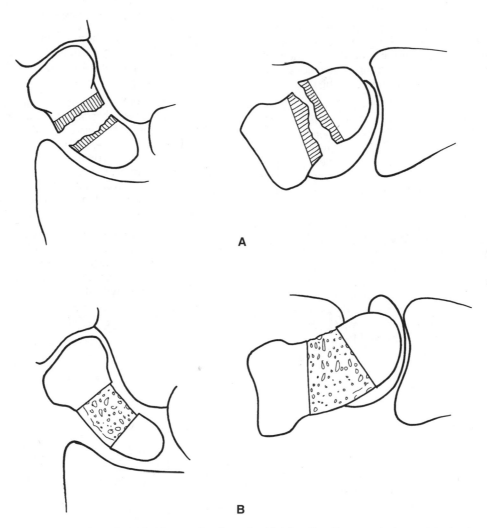

A

B

Figure 4 Correction of scaphoid non-union "humpback" deformity with compression-resistant volar cortico-cancellous bone graft.

THUMB METACARPOPHALANGEAL JOINT INJURIES

A. Injuries to the ulnar collateral ligament (UCL) of the thumb metacarpophalangeal (MP) joint result from forced radial abduction and occur five to eight times more frequently than radial collateral ligament injury. Associated injuries may involve the volar plate, dorsal capsule, adductor insertion, and fracture of the proximal phalanx. Instability is defined as joint opening of >30° compared to the contralateral thumb on stress testing under adequate anesthesia. Radial deviation force should be applied to the MP joint in full extension and in slight flexion, as the latter removes volar plate contribution to stability.

B. The Stener lesion involves interposition of the adductor aponeurosis between the distally avulsed collateral ligament and its insertion onto the base of the proximal phalanx, thereby preventing direct contact between bone and ligament required for healing (Figs. 1 and 2).

C. Avulsion fractures displaced >5 mm are less likely to heal with restoration of sufficient ligament tension to provide adequate stability. Large fracture fragments comprising >15% of the articular surface require anatomic reduction and fixation to avoid joint incongruity with resultant development of post-traumatic arthritis.

D. Repair of ligament avulsion from its insertion (or origin) may be accomplished with "pull-out" sutures tied over a button on the radial surface of the thumb or over the proximal phalanx itself. Alternatively, a bone anchor may be employed. Mid-substance tears are less common and may be sutured directly, though results may be less than satisfactory in such instances. The repair should be protected by MP joint pinning in ulnar deviation and slight flexion.

E. Results of reconstructive procedures for chronic MP UCL laxity are unpredictable, with arthrodesis constituting a reliable and functional solution, especially in patients with minimal contralateral MP range of motion. Less predictable options include tendon transfer (e.g., adductor advancement) or ligament reconstruction with tendon graft (palmaris longus).

F. Radial collateral ligament injuries result from forced adduction or rotation with the MP joint in flexion with no comparable Stener lesion. Treatment is similar to UCL injuries, though chronic disability is often less, as the joint remains stable in pinch.

G. Dorsal MP dislocations result from hyperextension injury and, while not usually associated with collateral ligament injury, must be assessed for stability following reduction.

H. Closed reduction is best accomplished under median and radial wrist block with distal pressure applied to dorsal base of the proximal phalanx. Interposition of volar plate, sesamoids, or flexor pollicis longus may prevent closed reduction. Flexion and adduction of the metacarpal will relax the thenar muscles, which may be slung around the metacarpal head, while flexion of the wrist and interphalangeal joint will relax the flexor pollicis longus.

I. Open reduction may be performed dorsally or volarly, though the latter allows for surgical repair of the volar plate in the rare instance of distal detachment from the base of the proximal phalanx. In such cases, the sesamoids remain with the metacarpal.

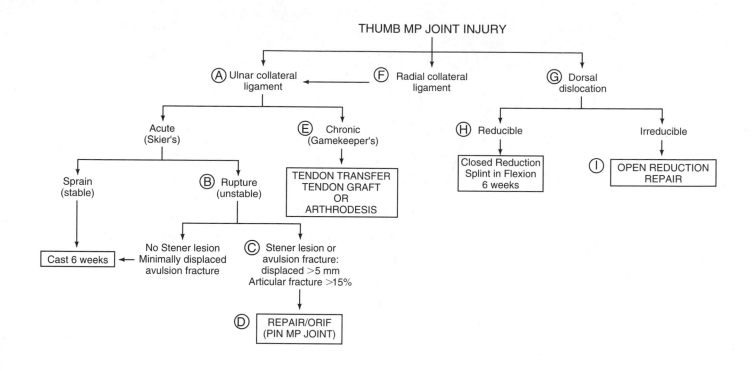

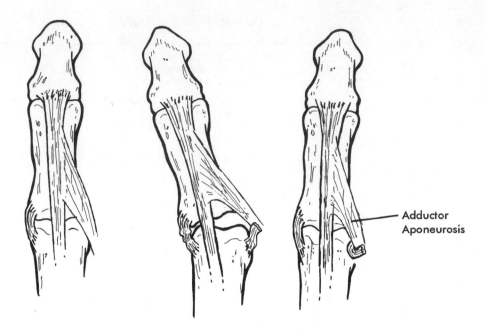

Figure 1 Stener lesion.

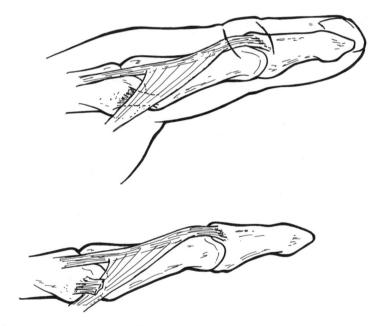

Figure 2 Stener lesion.

References

ASSH. Regional Review Courses in Hand Surgery: 1994. Aurora, Colorado: American Society for Surgery of the Hand, 1994.

Dray GJ, Eaton RG. Dislocations & ligament injuries in the digits. In: Green DP, ed. Operative Hand Surgery. 3rd ed. New York: Churchill-Livingstone, 1993: 781.

Miller RJ. Dislocations and fracture dislocations of the metacarpophalangeal joint of the thumb. Hand Clin 1988; 4:45.

O'Brien ET. Fractures of the metacarpals & phalanges. In: Green DP, ed. Operative Hand Surgery. 2nd ed. New York: Churchill-Livingstone, 1988: 763.

Smith RJ. Post-traumatic instability of the metacarpophalangeal joint of the thumb. J Bone Joint Surg 1977; 59A:14.

Stener B. Displacement of the ruptured ulnar collateral ligament of the metacarpophalangeal joint of the thumb. J Bone Joint Surg 1962; 44B:869.

FINGER METACARPOPHALANGEAL JOINT INJURIES

A. Dorsal dislocations of the metacarpophalangeal (MP) joint of the finger result from hyperextension injury and are most common in the index and small fingers. The volar plate ruptures at its origin proximally and may become interposed in the joint (complex injury), thereby preventing relocation. Traction further increases the tension on the intrinsic and flexor tendons, which surround the metacarpal head like a noose, sometimes making closed reduction difficult. Volar MP finger dislocations are rare and may be accompanied by interposition of dorsal capsule or volar plate.

B. Closed reduction is facilitated by flexion at the wrist to relax the flexor tendons. Excessive traction, which tightens the noose about the metacarpal head, is avoided. Rather, gentle volar and distal pressure on the dorsal base of the proximal phalanx is applied to slide it over the metacarpal head.

C. Open reduction for complex, irreducible dislocations (Fig. 1) is accomplished by division of the A1 pulley through a palmar approach. The tension on one side of the noose about the metacarpal head is thereby diminished, allowing the volar plate and metacarpal head to fall back into place. Formal repair of the volar plate is not necessary, and the MP joint is initially immobilized in a safe position splint (Figs. 2 and 3) and subsequently protected in a dorsal blocking splint for a total of 4 to 6 weeks.

D. Lateral MP dislocations involve collateral ligament injury.

E. Fracture-dislocations require open reduction and restoration of articular congruity. There is often an impaction injury to the articular surface of the metacarpal head or proximal phalangeal base, which necessitates elevation. Fixation may involve use of K-wires, screws/plates, absorbable pins, and even suture. Reconstructive options for substantial cartilage and bone loss or in cases of post-traumatic arthritis are limited and include, most reliably, arthrodesis, in addition to soft tissue arthroplasty, Silastic arthroplasty, osteochondral graft, and joint transfer.

F. Complications include injury to neurovascular structures during the surgical approach, as the bundle may be draped over the metacarpal head in a very subcutaneous position. Post-traumatic arthritis may ensue following multiple and vigorous reduction attempts or from initial chondral injury. Stiffness results from associated soft tissue injury, late reduction, and prolonged immobilization.

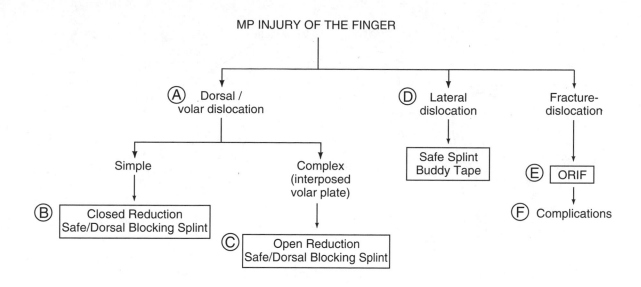

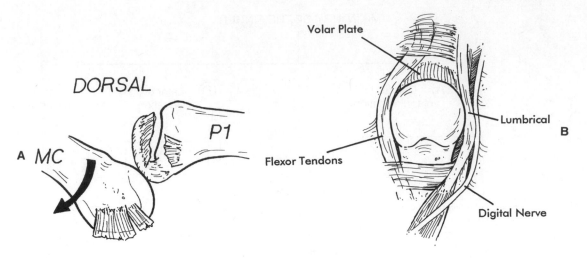

Figure 1 Irreducible dorsal MP dislocation with interposed volar plate. **A,** Lateral view. **B,** Palmar view.

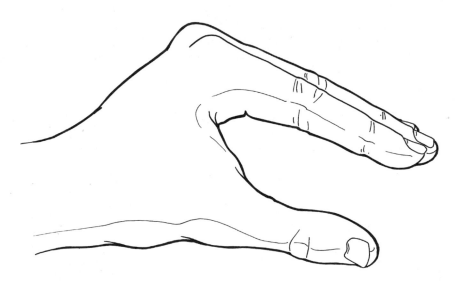

Figure 2 Safe position splinting (intrinsic plus).

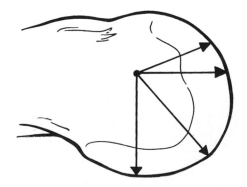

Figure 3 CAM effect of metacarpal head (collateral ligaments taut in flexion, lax in extension).

References

ASSH. Regional Review Courses in Hand Surgery: 1994. Aurora, CO: American Society for Surgery of the Hand, 1994.

Becton JL, Christian JD, Goodwin HN, Jackson JG. A simplified technique for treating the complex dislocation of the index metacarpophalangeal joint. J Bone Joint Surg 1975; 57A:698.

Dray GJ, Eaton RG. Dislocations & ligament injuries in the digits. In: Green DP, ed. Operative Hand Surgery. 3rd ed. New York: Churchill Livingstone, 1993: 767.

Hastings H, Carroll C. Treatment of closed articular fractures of the metacarpophalangeal and proximal interphalangeal joints. Hand Clin 1988; 4:503.

Hubbard LF. Metacarpophalangeal dislocations. Hand Clin 1988; 4:39.

Kaplan EB. Dorsal dislocation of the metacarpophalangeal joint of the index finger. J Bone Joint Surg 1957; 39A:1081.

Margles SW. Intra-articular fractures of the metacarpophalangeal and proximal interphalangeal joints. Hand Clin 1988; 4:67.

Stern PJ. Fractures of the metacarpals and phalanges. In: Green DP, ed. Operative Hand Surgery. 3rd ed. New York: Churchill Livingstone, 1993: 695.

Wilson RL, Liechty BL. Volar dislocation of the proximal interphalangeal joint. Hand Clin 1986; 2:329.

DISTAL RADIUS FRACTURES

A. The rationale for the operative treatment of distal radius fractures is based on the improved clinical results seen with restoration of normal anatomy. Radiographs in traction following closed reduction are helpful in determining the severity of injury and potential for instability. Poor results have been associated with residual dorsal tilt >20° (normal, 11−12° of volar tilt), radial inclination <10° (normal, 22−23°), articular incongruity >2 mm, and radial translation >2 mm. Concomitant injury to the distal radioulnar joint, carpal ligaments, and TFCC (triangular fibrocartilaginous complex) should not be overlooked, with a goal towards their anatomic restoration as well.

B. Initial immobilization is best accomplished with a sugar tong splint because of its additional rotational control and tolerance for post-injury edema. Large, potentially unstable fracture fragments, such as the radial styloid, may be optimally stabilized with a percutaneous K-wire to ensure reduction. Radiographic follow-up within 1 week allows for detection of subsequent fracture displacement and assessment of fracture immobilization by the splint as well as digital range of motion (ROM) and edema control.

   Treatment may be continued in the sugar tong splint after tightening with tape or switched to a short arm cast if strict rotational control is not necessary. In any event, elbow immobilization should not generally exceed 3 weeks to avoid the development of an elbow contracture.

   Fracture healing is usually sufficient to allow use of a removable volar wrist splint and gentle active ROM exercises at 4 to 6 weeks dependent on the appearance of fracture consolidation on x-ray and a nontender fracture site on palpation.

C. Unstable injuries are often the result of cortical comminution (dorsal with Colles', volar in Smith's), requiring external or internal support to prevent collapse (Fig. 1). Impact forces at the time of injury may sufficiently compress trabecular bone, especially in older individuals with osteopenia, to require iliac crest bone grafting of the metaphyseal defect created upon restoration of original length.

D. Many brands of external fixators are available with two fixation pins usually placed in the mid-distal radius and two in the index metacarpal. Fracture reduction may be obtained by using longitudinal traction with finger traps and 10 to 15 lbs of weight. Fluoroscopic evaluation allows for assessment of reduction parameters, and subsequent manipulative adjustments may be necessary prior to fixator placement. Care must be taken to avoid over-distraction of the carpus by the fixator, which may lead to impairment of digital ROM and possible neurapraxia.

   Close follow-up is needed to ensure proper edema control and adequate digital ROM, and to guard against pin tract infection. The fixator may be removed in 6 to 8 weeks dependent on fracture healing and degree of comminution. Hinged fixators have not been shown to provide results superior to traditional fixators.

E. Assessment of intra-articular injury is done by careful evaluation of plain films, including those obtained in traction after reduction. Conventional biplanar tomography often provides important additional information, as may CT reconstruction (at additional cost).

F. An acceptable reduction should fall within the parameters outlined in A for restoration of normal distal radial anatomy.

G. After satisfactory closed reduction, large fragment articular shear fractures without comminution (Barton—dorsal/volar lip, Chauffeur's—radial styloid; see Fig. 1) may be immobilized in a cast, with percutaneous fixation for additional stability.

H. Comminuted intra-articular fractures, including die-punch lesions (depressed lunate fossa fragment(s) resulting from axial loading by the lunate; Figs. 1 and 2), require accurate restoration of the articular surface via closed or open methods, with external fixation to unload the joint surface to prevent collapse (Fig. 3). Metaphyseal defects, more common with elderly, osteopenic bone, are filled with iliac crest bone graft.

I. Complications following distal radius fractures include malunion and post-traumatic arthritis resulting from such or from chondral damage at the time of injury. Median nerve damage may result from direct trauma by sharp fracture fragments or stretching at the time of injury and from compression due to local swelling. Indications for exploration and decompression include initial complete lack of function despite fracture reduction, progressive palsy, and deterioration following closed reduction.

   Additional complications include digital stiffness, tendon rupture, development of reflex sympathetic dystrophy, and even Volkman's ischemic contracture. Close follow-up with attention to rehabilitation is essential to help avert many of these problems.

DISTAL RADIUS FRACTURE

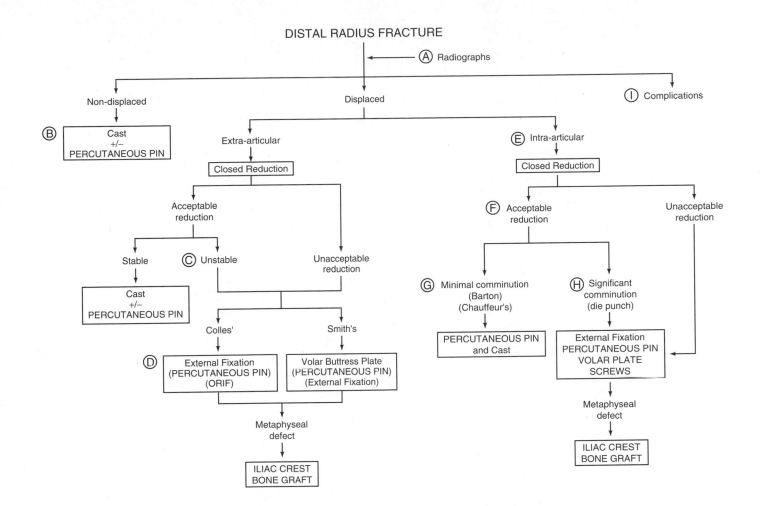

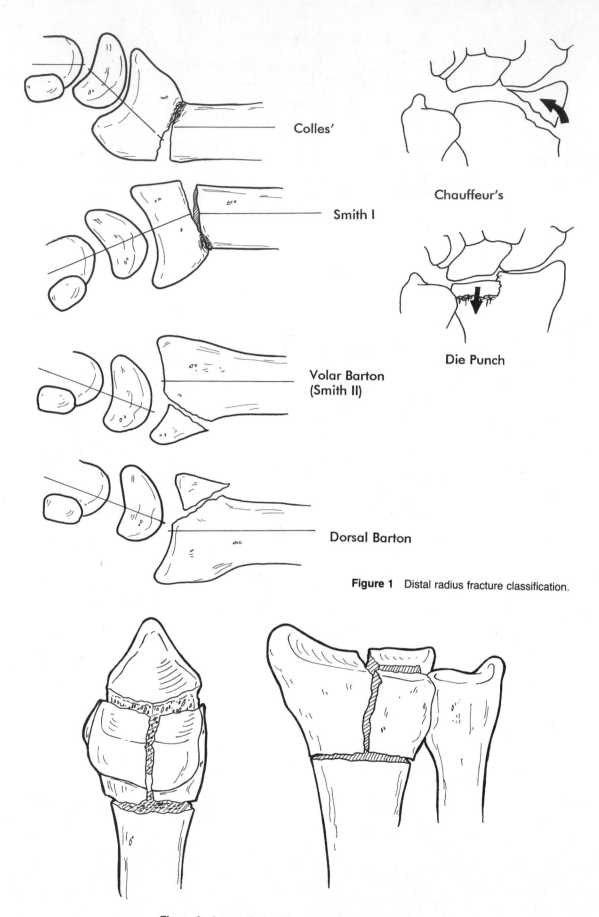

Colles'

Smith I

Chauffeur's

Die Punch

Volar Barton
(Smith II)

Dorsal Barton

Figure 1 Distal radius fracture classification.

Figure 2 Intra-articular "die-punch" fracture (Melone).

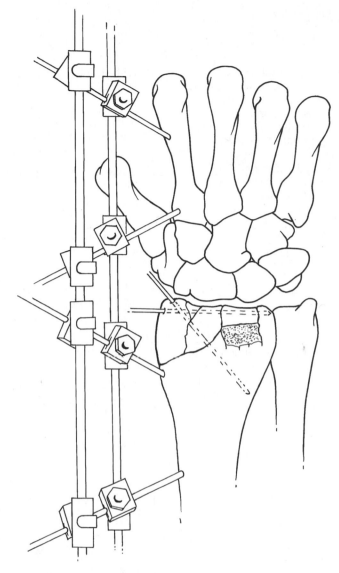

Figure 3 External fixation, percutaneous pinning of an intra-articular fracture.

References

ASSH. Regional Review Courses in Hand Surgery: 1994. Aurora, Colorado: American Society for Surgery of the Hand, 1994.

Bradway JK, Amadio PC, Cooney WP. Open reduction and internal fixation of displaced, comminuted intra-articular fractures of the distal end of the radius. J Bone Joint Surg 1989; 71A:839.

Fernandez DL. Correction of post-traumatic wrist deformity in adults by osteotomy, bone-grafting, and internal fixation. J Bone Joint Surg 1982; 64A:1164.

Fernandez DL. Radial osteotomy and Bowers' arthroplasty for malunited fractures of the distal end of the radius. J Bone Joint Surg 1988; 70A:1538.

Jupiter JB. Current concepts review: Fractures of the distal end of the radius. J Bone Joint Surg 1991; 73A:461.

Knirk JL, Jupiter JB. Intra-articular fractures of the distal end of the radius in adults. J Bone Joint Surg 1986; 68A:647.

Melone CP. Open treatment for displaced articular fractures of the distal radius. Clin Orthop 1986; 202:103.

Melone CP. Unstable fractures of the distal radius. In: Lichtman DM, ed. The Wrist and Its Disorders. 2nd ed. Philadelphia: W.B. Saunders, 1988: 160.

Palmer AK. Fractures of the distal radius. In: Green DP, ed. Operative Hand Surgery. 2nd ed. New York: Churchill Livingstone, 1993: 929.

Short WH, Palmer AK, Werner FW, et al. A biomechanical study of distal radial fractures. J Hand Surg 1987; 12A:529.

Szabo RM, Weber SC. Comminuted intraarticular fractures of the distal radius. Clin Orthop 1988; 230:39.

Villar RN, Marsh D, Rushton N, et al. Three years after Colles' fracture: A prospective review. J Bone Joint Surg 1987; 69B:635.

Weber SC, Szabo RM. Severely comminuted distal radial fracture as an unsolved problem: Complications associated with external fixation and pins and plaster techniques. J Hand Surg 1986; 11A:157.

FINGERTIP INJURIES

The fingertip (that portion of the digit distal to the flexor and extensor insertions) is the most commonly injured part of the hand. The volar pulp is highly innervated and contains fibroseptae, which anchor the volar skin to the distal phalanx. The nail provides support for the volar pulp, protects the distal tuft, and plays an important role in sensibility and fine manipulation (Fig. 1).

The nail plate should be removed when nail bed laceration is suspected, especially for subungual hematomas comprising ≥50% of the nail plate. Fractures of the distal phalanx with associated nail bed injury are essentially open and require incision and drainage. Nail bed lacerations are carefully repaired with fine absorbable suture under loupe magnification, and the cleansed nail or nonadherent gauze is placed under the nail fold to prevent adhesion of the underlying nail bed.

Fingertip injuries have been anatomically classified by Allen (Fig. 2): I, pulp only; II, pulp and nail bed; III, pulp, nail bed, and bone distal to the lunula; and IV, lunula to flexor/extensor insertion. Management of these injuries, however, depends also on the obliquity of tissue loss. Treatment should be directed at maintaining maximal length while providing sensation and satisfactory cosmetic appearance, maintaining joint motion, and avoiding painful neuromas.

A. Composite, nonvascularized grafts may survive in sharp, distal amputations, especially in children. Split-thickness skin grafting in adults reduces defect size with shrinkage, but does not offer the wound stability of a full-thickness graft.

B. V-Y flaps provide sensible skin, with volar (Atasoy) flaps (Fig. 3) applicable for transverse or dorsal oblique injury and double lateral (Kutler) flaps (Fig. 4) for volar oblique injury.

C. Volar advancement flaps (Fig. 5) are indicated for thumb injury, but may be associated with interphalangeal flexion contracture.

D. Cross finger flaps (Fig. 6) offer coverage for larger defects, but may result in joint stiffness and involve surgery on normal digits.

E. Thenar flaps (Fig. 7) offer more subcutaneous tissue, but are primarily indicated for children, due to the potential for joint stiffness.

F. Primary closure with shortening should include careful proximal neurectomies to avoid neuroma formation, with shortening sufficient to provide tension-free closure.

G. Replantation is not generally considered for distal fingertip amputations due to potential problems with small vessel size, inadequate venous outflow, unpredictable sensory return, prolonged recovery, and additional expense.

References

Allen MJ. Conservative management of fingertip injuries in adults. The Hand 1980; 12:257.

ASSH. Regional Review Courses in Hand Surgery: 1994. Aurora, Colorado: American Society for Surgery of the Hand, 1994.

Atasoy E, Iokimidis E, Kasdan ML, et al. Reconstruction of the amputated fingertip with a triangular volar flap: A new surgical procedure. J Bone Joint Surg 1970; 52A(5):921.

Beasley RW. Local flaps for surgery of the hand. Orthop Clin North Am 1970; 1:219.

Browne EZ. Skin grafts. In: Green DP, ed. Operative Hand Surgery. 3rd ed. New York: Churchill Livingstone, 1993: 1711.

Fisher RH. The Kutler method of repair of finger-tip amputations. J Bone Joint Surg 1967; 49A:317.

Idler RS, Strickland JW. Management of soft tissue injuries to the fingertip. Orthop Rev 1982; XI(10):25.

Kutler W. A new method for fingertip amputation. JAMA 1947; 133:29.

Lister G. Local flaps to the hand. Hand Clin 1985; 1(4):621.

Lister G. Skin flaps. In: Green DP, ed. Operative Hand Surgery. 3rd ed. New York: Churchill Livingstone, 1993: 1741.

Louis DS. Amputations. In: Green DP, ed. Operative Hand Surgery. 3rd ed. New York: Churchill Livingstone, 1993: 53.

Macht SD, Watson HK. The Moberg advancement flap for digital reconstruction. J Hand Surg 1980; 5:372.

McGregor IA, Morgan G. Axial random pattern flaps. Br J Plast Surg 1973; 26:202.

Melone CP, Beasley RW, Carstens JH. The thenar flap—an analysis of its use in 150 cases. J Hand Surg 1982; 7:291.

Posner MA, Smith RJ. The advancement pedicle flap for thumb injuries. J Bone Joint Surg 1971; 53A:1618.

Shepard GH. Management of acute nailbed avulsions. Hand Clin 1990; 6(1):39.

Van Beek AL, Kassan AL, Adson MH, Dole V. Management of acute fingernail injuries. Hand Clin 1990; 6(1):23.

Zook EG, Brown R. The perionychium. In: Green DP, ed. Operative Hand Surgery. 3rd ed. New York: Churchill-Livingstone, 1993: 1283.

FINGERTIP INJURY

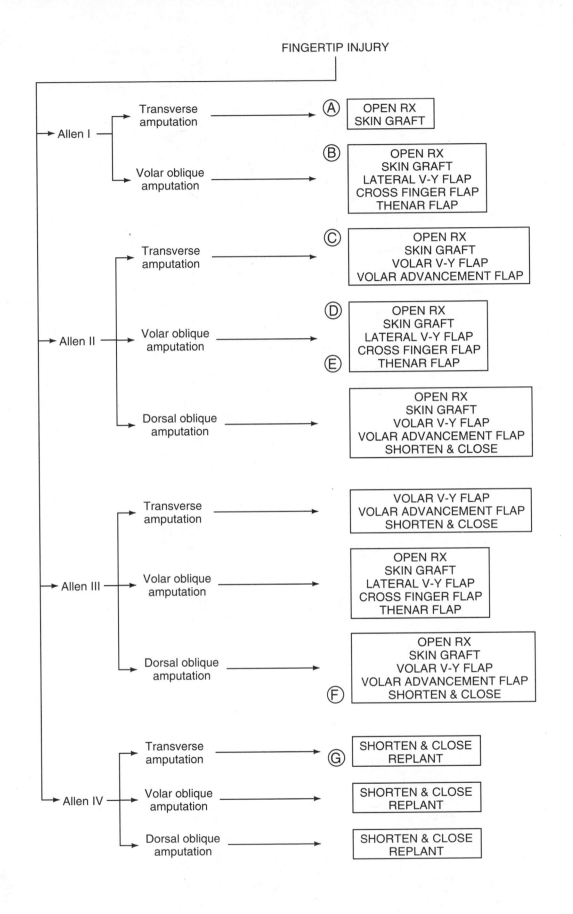

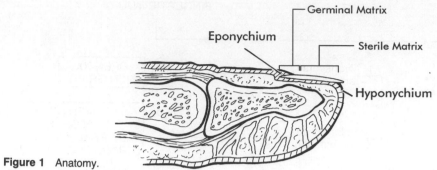

Figure 1 Anatomy.

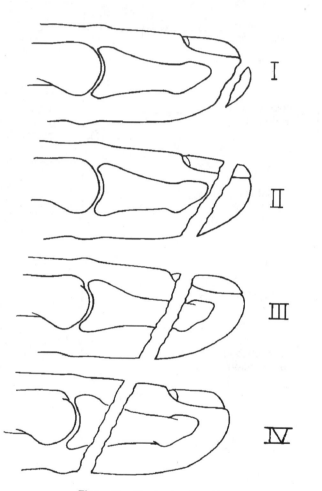

Figure 2 Allen's classification.

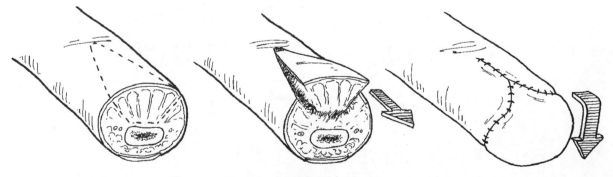

Figure 3 Volar V-Y flap (Atasoy).

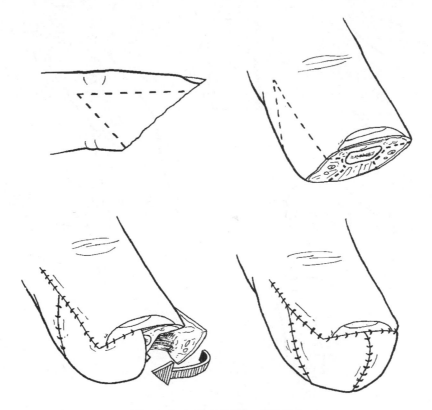

Figure 4 Lateral V-Y flaps (Kutler).

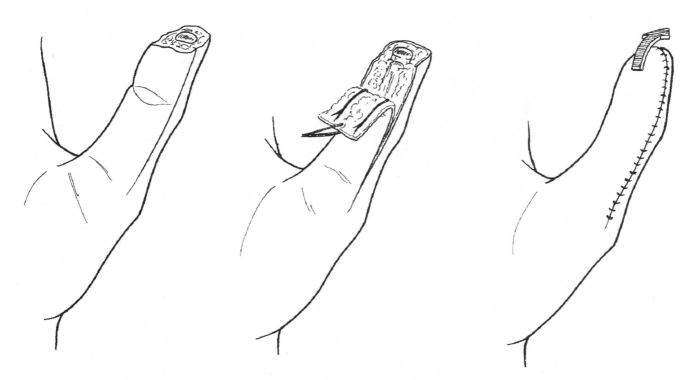

Figure 5 Volar advancement flap (Moberg).

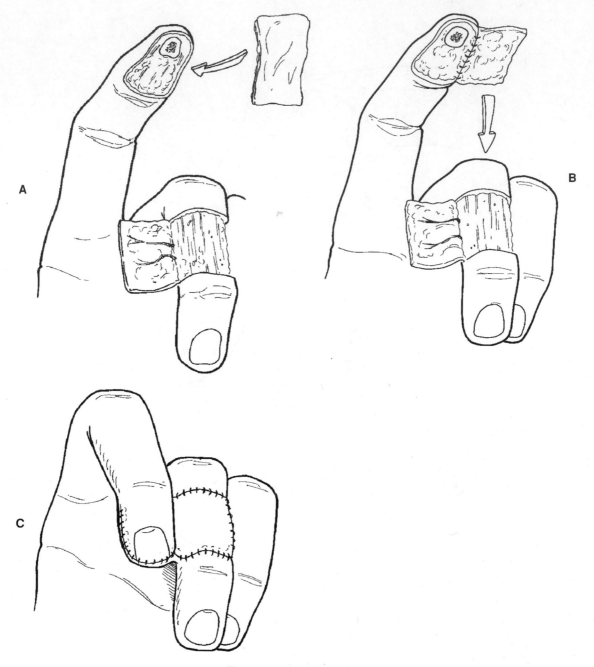

Figure 6 Cross-finger flap.

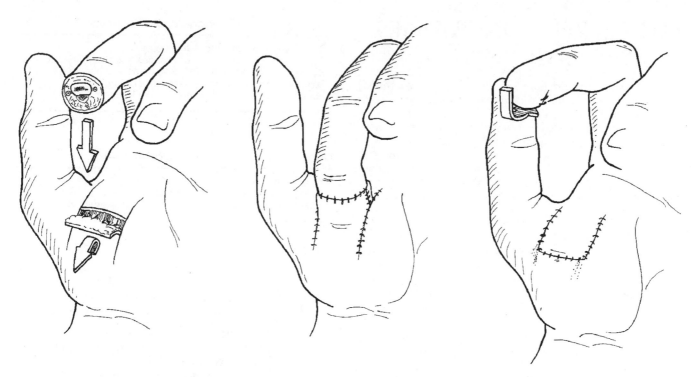

Figure 7 Thenar flap.

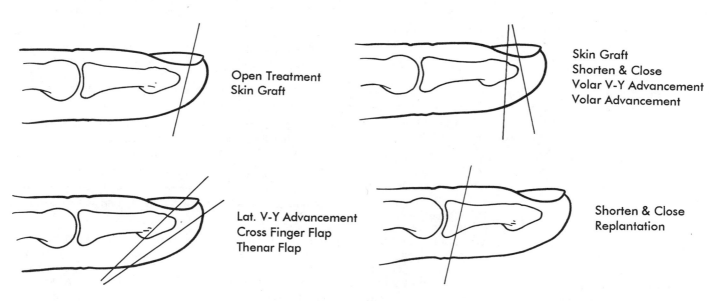

Open Treatment
Skin Graft

Skin Graft
Shorten & Close
Volar V-Y Advancement
Volar Advancement

Lat. V-Y Advancement
Cross Finger Flap
Thenar Flap

Shorten & Close
Replantation

Figure 8 Treatment.

FLEXOR TENDON INJURIES

A. Thorough examination of the traumatized hand should include testing of every flexor tendon. Each flexor digitorum profundus (FDP) and flexor pollicis longus (FPL) is tested by isolated distal interphalangeal (DIP) flexion against resistance. Flexor digitorum superficialis (FDS) function is ascertained by holding the other digits in full extension while resisting active proximal interphalangeal (PIP) flexion of the digit in question (quadriga effect). Note that some small fingers have a normally nonfunctional FDS, while many index fingers have independent FDP tendons. A "floppy" DIP joint indicates flexion via the FDS alone.

Pain with resistance may indicate a partial tendon injury. Additional indirect tests include an extensor posture of the affected digit at rest, lack of normal tenodesis effect with wrist range of motion (ROM), and lack of flexion with manual compression of proximal muscle bellies in the forearm.

Flexor tendon injuries in the fingers and thumb are classified according to anatomic zones (Tables 1 and 2 and Figs. 1 and 2).

B. While repair of acute tendon injuries in "tidy" wounds may be performed electively up to 3 weeks after injury, repair should probably be accomplished within the first days following injury, if possible, as delay allows for retraction of the proximal tendon and adhesion formation. Atraumatic technique must be practiced.

C. Insertion of a distal FDP laceration or avulsion is best accomplished via a pull-out suture technique with a dorsal nail button. Advancement should be limited to 1 cm to prevent loss of flexor/extensor balance.

D. Zone II is referred to as "no-man's land," as injuries here occur in the narrow space provided by the fibro-osseous theca, with a high potential for subsequent adhesion formation. Concomitant FDS and FDP repair provides superior results, with potential for preservation of the vincular blood supply (Fig. 3) and independent PIP flexion, provision for a smooth gliding bed for the FDP, and possible reduction in PIP hyperextension. Bruner or mid-lateral incisions are recommended. Sheath repair may facilitate tendon gliding, but has not been shown to conclusively affect clinical results.

TABLE 1   Flexor Tendon Zones of Fingers

Zone I—FDS insertion to FDP insertion
Zone II—A1 (entrance to fibro-osseous theca) to FDS insertion
Zone III—distal edge of transverse carpal ligament to A1
Zone IV—underneath transverse carpal ligament
Zone V—proximal to transverse carpal ligament

TABLE 2   Flexor Tendon Zones of Thumb

Zone I—A2 to FPL insertion
Zone II—A1 to A2 (fibro-osseous theca)
Zone III—radial edge of transverse carpal ligament to A1

Early ROM protocols (e.g., Duran and Kleinert) are directed toward reducing adhesion formation joints through protected motion in dorsal splints: wrist, 20° flexion; MP, 50° flexion; IP, full extension.

E. Zone IV injuries occur under the transverse carpal ligament, which should be closed via Z-lengthening in order to prevent volar bow-stringing of the flexor tendons with the wrist in a flexed position in the splint.

F. In chronic injuries, direct repair is often impossible due to loss of tendon substance and myostatic contracture.

G. Primary tendon grafting may be considered when soft tissues are relatively intact, including pulleys and the potential for postoperative scarring minimal, provided passive ROM is preserved. Otherwise, staged reconstruction should be considered.

H. Tendon grafting is secured proximally out of the fibro-osseous theca with a tendon weave and inserted distally into the distal phalanx with a pull-out technique.

I. The position of DIP tenodesis is usually slight (~15°) flexion. Crossed K-wires may be used for arthrodesis in neutral to slight flexion or a Herbert screw used in full extension.

J. Most commonly, the palmaris longus is used for tendon graft (ipsilateral, if available). Other potential sources include the plantaris or toe extensor tendon. Satisfactory results can be achieved provided the prerequisites of tissue equilibrium and good passive ROM are obtained first.

FLEXOR TENDON INJURY

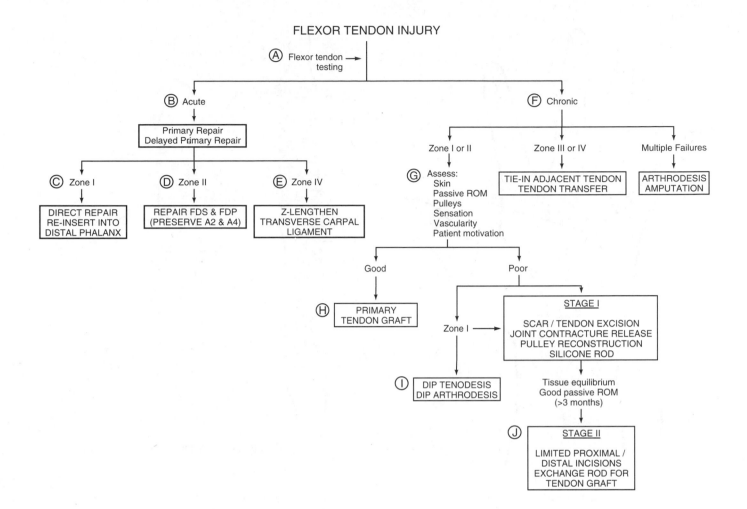

(A) Flexor tendon → testing

(B) Acute

Primary Repair
Delayed Primary Repair

(C) Zone I

DIRECT REPAIR
RE-INSERT INTO
DISTAL PHALANX

(D) Zone II

REPAIR FDS & FDP
(PRESERVE A2 & A4)

(E) Zone IV

Z-LENGTHEN
TRANSVERSE CARPAL
LIGAMENT

(F) Chronic

Zone I or II

(G) Assess:
Skin
Passive ROM
Pulleys
Sensation
Vascularity
Patient motivation

Zone III or IV

TIE-IN ADJACENT TENDON
TENDON TRANSFER

Multiple Failures

ARTHRODESIS
AMPUTATION

Good

(H) PRIMARY
TENDON GRAFT

Poor

Zone I →

(I) DIP TENODESIS
DIP ARTHRODESIS

STAGE I

SCAR / TENDON EXCISION
JOINT CONTRACTURE RELEASE
PULLEY RECONSTRUCTION
SILICONE ROD

Tissue equilibrium
Good passive ROM
(>3 months)

(J) STAGE II

LIMITED PROXIMAL /
DISTAL INCISIONS
EXCHANGE ROD FOR
TENDON GRAFT

407

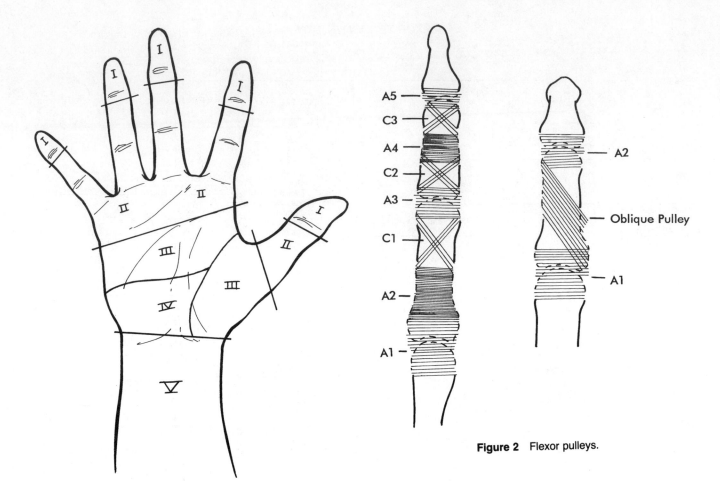

Figure 1   Flexor tendon zones.

Figure 2   Flexor pulleys.

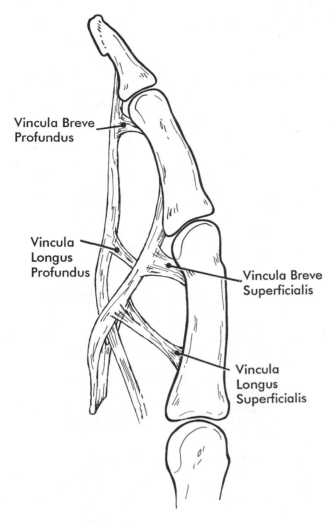

Vincula Breve Profundus

Vincula Longus Profundus

Vincula Breve Superficialis

Vincula Longus Superficialis

Figure 3   Vincular blood supply.

References

Amadio PC, Wood MB, Cooney WP, Bogard SD. Staged flexor tendon reconstruction in the fingers and hand. J Hand Surg 1988; 12:559.

ASSH. Regional Review Courses in Hand Surgery: 1994. Aurora, CO: American Society for Surgery of the Hand, 1994.

Boyes JH, Stark HH. Flexor tendon grafts in the fingers and thumb: a study of factors influencing results in 1000 cases. J Bone Joint Surg 1971; 53A:1332.

Chow JA, Thomes LJ, Dovell S, et al. Controlled motion rehabilitation after flexor tendon repair and grafting. A multicentre study. J Bone Joint Surg 1988; 70B:591.

Doyle JR. Anatomy of the finger flexor tendon sheath and pulley system. J Hand Surg 1988; 13A:473.

Doyle JR, Blythe WF. Anatomy of the flexor tendon sheath and pulleys of the thumb. J Hand Surg 1977; 2:149.

Duran R, Houser RG. Controlled passive motion following flexor tendon repair in zones 2 and 3. In: AAOS Symposium on Tendon Surgery in the Hand. St. Louis: C.V. Mosby, 1975.

Hunter JM, Salisbury RE. Flexor tendon reconstruction in severely damaged hands: a two-stage procedure using a silicone-dacron reinforced gliding prosthesis prior to tendon grafting. J Bone Joint Surg 1967; 53A:829.

Ketchum LD. Primary tendon healing: a review. J Hand Surg 1977; 2:428.

Kleinert HE, Kutz JE, Ashbell TS, et al. Primary repair of lacerated flexor tendons in "no man's land". J Bone Joint Surg 1967; 49:577.

LaSalle WB, Strickland JW. An evaluation of digital performance following two-stage flexor tendon reconstruction. J Hand Surg 1982; 7:411.

Leddy JP. Flexor tendons—Acute injuries. In: Green DP, ed. Operative Hand Surgery. 3rd ed. New York: Churchill-Livingstone, 1993: 1823.

Lister GD, Kleinert HE, Kutz JE, Atasoy E. Primary flexor tendon repair followed by immediate controlled mobilization. J Hand Surg 1977; 2:441.

Manske PR. Flexor tendon healing. J Hand Surg 1988; 13B:237.

Savage R. The influence of wrist position on the minimum force required for active movement of the interphalangeal joints. J Hand Surg 1988; 13B:262.

Schneider LH, Hunter JM. Flexor tendons—Late reconstruction. In: Green DP, ed. Operative Hand Surgery. 3rd ed. New York: Churchill Livingstone, 1993: 1853.

Stark HH, Zemel NP, Boyes JH, et al. Flexor tendon graft through intact superficialis tendon. J Hand Surg 1977; 2:456.

Strickland JW. Management of flexor tendon injuries. Orthop Clin North Am 1983; 14:827.

Strickland JW, Glogovac SV. Digital function following flexor tendon repair in zone II: A comparison of immobilization and controlled passive motion techniques. J Hand Surg 1980; 5:537.

Urbaniak JR, Cahill JD, Mortensen RA. Tendon suturing methods: Analysis of tensile strengths. In: AAOS Symposium on Tendon Surgery in the Hand. St. Louis: C.V. Mosby, 1975.

Verdan C. Half a century of flexor tendon repair: Current status and changing philosophies. J Bone Joint Surg 1972; 54A:472.

EXTENSOR MECHANISM INJURIES

A. Zone I injuries occur between the central tendon insertion onto the middle phalanx and the terminal extensor insertion onto the distal phalanx (Figs. 1 to 3). The treatment of these injuries is covered in the chapter on distal interphalangeal (DIP) injuries (pp 352-355).

B. Zone II extensor injuries occur between the transverse portion of the metacarpophalangeal (MP) extensor hood and the central tendon insertion onto the middle phalanx. Closed injuries result from forced flexion of the proximal interphalangeal (PIP) joint with avulsion of the central slip insertion. Volar migration of the lateral bands produces the characteristic boutonniere deformity of flexion at the PIP joint and extension at the DIP joint (Figs. 4 and 5).

C. Suture repair of the central slip should be protected with temporary pinning of the PIP in extension for approximately 6 weeks. During that time, active DIP flexion exercises ensure adequate mobilization and dorsal positioning of the lateral bands.

D. Open treatment of closed injuries is indicated when there is proximal displacement of an avulsion fracture >2 to 3 mm or when the fracture fragment comprises a substantial portion of the joint surface (e.g., 20% to 30%) with resultant articular incongruity.

E. Fixation of avulsion fractures is often difficult and usually involves use of small K-wires, mini-fragment screw, or tension band technique. Following fixation, the PIP joint should be pinned in extension to protect the central slip insertion.

F. Chronic boutonniere deformity (Fig. 4) associated with PIP joint contracture must first be treated with mobilization of the PIP joint into extension, via serial casting or dynamic splinting, while maintaining free DIP motion. Operative release, in addition to extensor reconstruction, may be indicated when passive PIP extension cannot be obtained, though often with suboptimal results.

G. Many techniques are available for reconstruction of the chronic boutonniere deformity. The most simple involves transection of the terminal extensor at the proximal middle phalangeal level. This allows for proximal sliding of the lateral bands with restoration of tension at the central slip. The oblique retinacular ligament is responsible for DIP extension.

Alternatively, distally transected lateral bands may be sutured dorsally to reinforce the central slip insertion if significant scarring is present. If central slip substance is missing, a free tendon graft may be used or the ulnar lateral band transferred dorsally to the central slip insertion. Finally, an elongated central slip may be shortened and reapproximated primarily, with or without V-Y advancement.

H. Zone III extensor injuries are those involving the sagittal bands and transverse portion of the extensor hood at the MP joint. Lack of IP extension indicates additional involvement of the intrinsic tendons on either side of the hand. In chronic cases with attrition of the sagittal band (e.g., rheumatoid arthritis), the extensor tendon subluxates into the inter-metacarpal valley. The patient cannot "obtain" active MP extension, but can "maintain" MP extension once the joint is passively placed there, due to relocation of the tendon dorsally over the MP joint.

I. Postoperative splinting should maintain the wrist at +20° and MP at 15° for 8 weeks while allowing active PIP and DIP range of motion (ROM). All joints are allowed active ROM at 4 weeks and passive ROM at 6 weeks.

J. Zone IV extensor injuries occur proximal to the MP joint. With attempted extension, the MP remains flexed, while the IP joints extend. Repairs underneath the dorsal retinaculum may require partial compartmental release to allow unobstructed tendon passage. Total release may result in bowstringing. Alternatives to primary repair include side-to-side repair with an adjacent extensor or tendon transfer using EIP or EDQ.

EXTENSOR MECHANISM INJURY

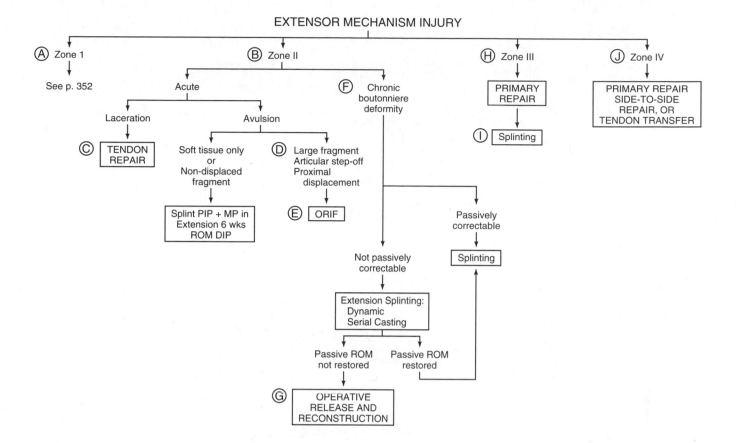

Ⓐ Zone 1

See p. 352

Ⓑ Zone II

Acute

Laceration

Ⓒ TENDON REPAIR

Avulsion

Soft tissue only
or
Non-displaced
fragment

Splint PIP + MP in
Extension 6 wks
ROM DIP

Ⓓ Large fragment
Articular step-off
Proximal
displacement

Ⓔ ORIF

Ⓕ Chronic
boutonniere
deformity

Not passively
correctable

Extension Splinting:
Dynamic
Serial Casting

Passive ROM
not restored

Passive ROM
restored

Ⓖ OPERATIVE
RELEASE AND
RECONSTRUCTION

Passively
correctable

Splinting

Ⓗ Zone III

PRIMARY
REPAIR

Ⓘ Splinting

Ⓙ Zone IV

PRIMARY REPAIR
SIDE-TO-SIDE
REPAIR, OR
TENDON TRANSFER

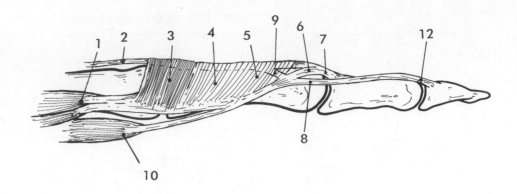

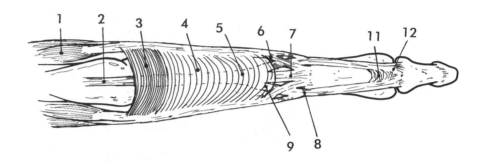

Figure 1 Extensor anatomy: (1) interosseous muscle, (2) common extensor tendon, (3) sagittal band, (4) transverse fibers, interosseous hood, (5) oblique fibers, interosseous hood, (6) medial interosseous band, (7) central slip, common extensor, (8) lateral conjoined tendon, (9) lateral slip, common extensor, (10) lumbrical muscle, (11) triangular ligament, (12) terminal extensor.

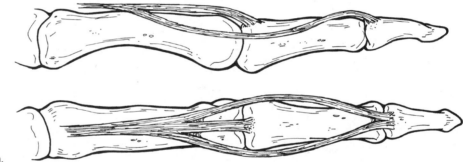

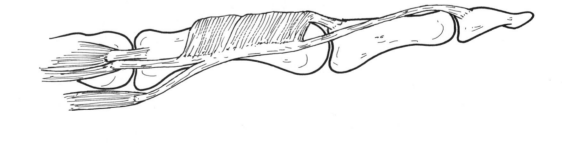

Figure 2 Extrinsic contribution.

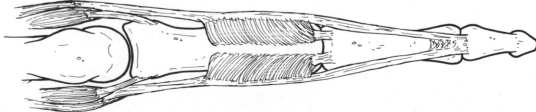

Figure 3 Intrinsic contribution.

412

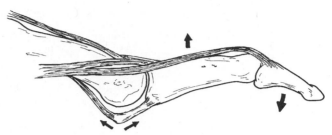

Figure 5 Swan-neck deformity.

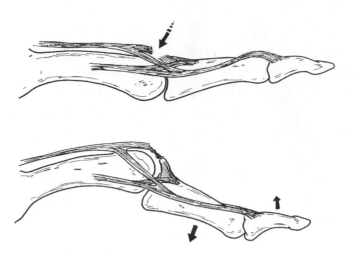

Figure 4 Boutonniere deformity.

References

ASSH. Regional Review Courses in Hand Surgery: 1994. Aurora, CO: American Society for Surgery of the Hand, 1994.

Bowers WH, Hurst LC. Chronic mallet finger: The use of Fowlers central slip release. J Hand Surg 1978; 3:373.

Burton RI. Extensor tendons—Late reconstruction. In: Green DP, ed. Operative Hand Surgery. 3rd ed. New York: Churchill Livingstone, 1993: 1955.

Curtis RM, Reid RL, Provost JM. A staged technique for repair of the traumatic boutonniere deformity. J Hand Surg 1983; 8:167.

Dolphin JA. Extensor tenotomy for chronic Boutonniere deformity of the finger. Report of two cases. J Bone Joint Surg 1965; 47A:161.

Doyle JR. Extensor tendons—Acute injuries. In: Green DP, ed. Operative Hand Surgery. 3rd ed. New York: Churchill Livingstone, 1993: 1925.

Elliott RA. Injuries to the extensor mechanism of the hand. Orthop Clin North Am 1970; 1:335.

Froehlich JA, Akelman E, Herndon JH. Extensor tendon injuries at the proximal interphalangeal joint. Hand Clin 1988; 4:25.

Harris C, Rutledge GL. The functional anatomy of the extensor mechanism of the finger. J Bone Joint Surg 1972; 54A:713.

Kaplan EB. Anatomy, injuries and treatment of extensor apparatus of the hand and digits. Clin Orthop 1959; 13:24.

Littler JW. The finger extensor mechanism. Surg Clin North Am 1967; 47:415.

Littler JW, Eaton RG. Redistribution of forces in correction of boutonniere deformity. J Bone Joint Surg 1967; 49A:1267-1274.

Matev I. Transposition of the lateral slips of the aponeurosis in treatment of long standing "boutonniere deformity" of the fingers. J Plast Surg 1964; 17:281.

Nalebuff EA, Millender LH. Surgical treatment of the boutonniere deformity in rheumatoid arthritis. Orthop Clin North Am 1975; 6:753.

Nalebuff EA, Millender LH. Surgical treatment of the swan neck deformity in rheumatoid arthritis. Orthop Clin North Am 1975; 6:733.

Smith RJ. Balance and kinetics of the fingers under normal and pathological conditions. Clin Orthop 1974; 104:92.

Snow JW. Use of a retrograde tendon flap in repairing a severed extensor tendon in the PIP joint area. Plas Reconstr Surg 1973; 51:555-558.

Snow JW. A method for reconstruction of the central slip of the extensor tendon of a finger. Plast Reconstr Surg 1976; 57:455.

Souter WA. The boutonniere deformity: A review of 101 patients with division of the central slip of the extensor expansion of the fingers. J Bone Joint Surg 1967; 49B:710.

Stark HH, Boyes JH, Wilson JN. Mallet finger. J Bone Joint Surg 1962; 44A:1061.

Thompson JS, Littler JW, Upton J. The spiral oblique retinacular ligament (SORL). J Hand Surg 1978; 3:482.

Tubiana R, Valentin P. The anatomy of the extensor apparatus of the fingers. Surg Clin North Am 1964; 44:897.

Urbaniak JR, Hayes MG. Chronic boutonniere deformity: An anatomic reconstruction. J Hand Surg 1981; 6:379.

SPINE SURGERY

FRACTURES AND SUBLUXATIONS OF THE ATLAS

A. The patient presenting with neck trauma is first assessed for the ABCs of life support. There is a high correlation of injuries of the cervical spine (C-spine) with external evidence of head and scalp trauma; however, patients can have significant C-spine injury with no sign of direct cranial trauma. Associated sub-atlantal fractures of the spinal column occur in approximately 50% of atlas fractures. Most of these segmental fractures either involve the odontoid process or the pedicle of C1. The complete neurologic examination should include evaluation of all of the cranial nerves. Dysesthesias or altered sensation along the course of the greater occipital nerve may be a presenting complaint in patients with an atlas fracture.

B. The radiographic signs of atlantoaxial injuries are often subtle. The pre-vertebral soft tissue shadow on the lateral radiograph should be <5 mm wide at C2 and 5–10 mm wide in front of the ring of the atlas. The lateral C-spine view may show fractures of the posterior ring of the atlas. The open-mouth odontoid view is especially helpful in detecting subtle displacement of the lateral masses in relationship to the superior articulating facets of the axis. Patients with incomplete osseous closure of the ring of the atlas may present with widening of the lateral masses without evident fracture. Rotatory subluxations may be visualized on the open-mouth odontoid with asymmetry of the joint space or the wink sign being noted, which is overlap of the inferior facet of C1 over C2, giving the appearance of no C1-C2 joint on the affected side.

C. Computed tomographic (CT) scans are especially helpful in identifying and evaluating Jefferson (burst) fractures and atlantoaxial rotatory subluxations. It is critical that the CT slice through the upper C-spine be parallel with the ring of C1. Dynamic CT scans, in which two separate scans of the C1-C2 complex are obtained with the patient maximally rotated first to one side and then to the other side, will confirm atlantoaxial rotatory subluxation.

D. Dynamic radiographs, which include lateral flexion-extension radiographs and cine-radiography, may be necessary to diagnose either an acute transverse ligament rupture or chronic atlantoaxial instability after healing of an atlas fracture. The prerequisites for flexion-extension radiographs include: (1) a neurologically intact patient, (2) performance of all movements actively by the patient, (3) no altered state of consciousness (including intoxication), and (4) direct physician supervision of the radiographic study. If adequate flexion-extension views are unobtainable, the fracture must be managed as a potentially unstable lesion.

E. Isolated fractures of the posterior arch of the atlas are secondary to hyperextension with or without axial loading of the upper C-spine. With this injury there is approximately a 50% chance that some other cervical injury is also present. The fractures most often occur at the junction of the lateral mass and the posterior arches. Since there is no compromise to atlantoaxial stability, management in the cervical orthosis is recommended. The Jefferson (or burst) fracture may involve four fractures, two anterior and two posterior to the lateral masses. Due to the spreading of the lateral masses and the arch, neurologic compromise rarely occurs. Bilateral offset of the lateral masses in relationship to the superior articulate facets of C2 on the open-mouth odontoid view is diagnostic of a burst injury. Experimental work has shown that if the total offset bilaterally is >7 mm, a probable transverse ligament rupture is also present. The free fragment of the medial tubercle of the lateral mass evident on CT scan or open-mouth odontoid views signifies an avulsion injury to the transverse ligament rather than a mid-substance tear. If the transverse ligament is intact, the injury is stable and can be treated with a cervical orthosis.

F. Burst fractures (Fig. 1) associated with wide spreading of the lateral masses can be adequately treated with halo immobilization for 3 months. For widely displaced fractures, evidence suggests that preliminary traction for 6 to 8 weeks to achieve partial reduction of the lateral masses leads to a better clinical result as regards post-injury upper cervical pain. Because this treatment involves bed rest with traction for 6 to 8 weeks with its concomitant risks, the clinical efficacy of this treatment has yet to be proven. Most Jefferson fractures will reunite without any chronic atlantoaxial instability. Fractures with >7 mm displacement signifying rupture of the transverse ligament must be checked for chronic atlantoaxial instability after removal of the halo. This can be done with flexion-extension views at the time of halo removal and subsequently when the patient has regained range of motion (ROM), if the initial flexion-extension views are negative. If C1–2 instability is present, a CT scan is necessary to determine the status of the healing of the arch of C1. If the arch is healed, a posterior atlantoaxial arthrodesis is sufficient for spine stabilization. If, however, there is non-union of the posterior arch of the atlas, occipital to C2 fusion is necessary.

G. Lateral mass fractures can consist of a single fracture anterior and posterior to the lateral mass with minimal displacement, which is a stable injury and can be treated with cervical orthosis, or a displaced lateral mass fracture or a comminuted lateral mass fracture, which is best treated with halo immobilization.

H. Transverse ligament ruptures occur from direct blows to the occiput. If the distance between the anterior ring of C1 and the anterior cortex of the odontoid process

FRACTURE OR SUBLUXATION OF ATLAS

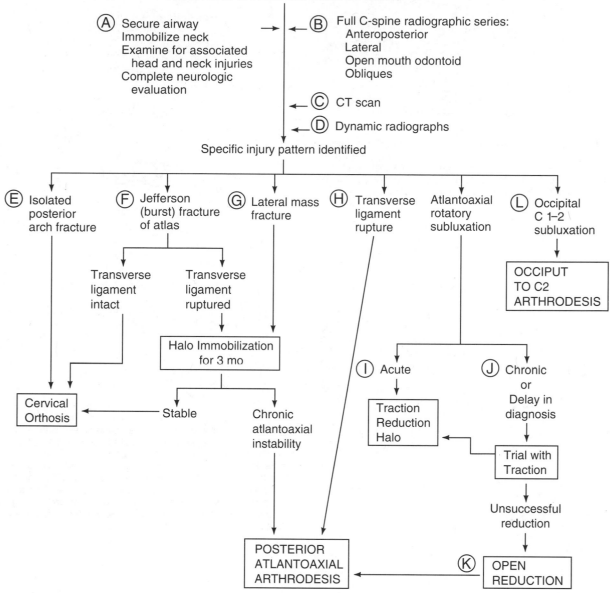

Ⓐ Secure airway
Immobilize neck
Examine for associated
   head and neck injuries
Complete neurologic
   evaluation

Ⓑ Full C-spine radiographic series:
   Anteroposterior
   Lateral
   Open mouth odontoid
   Obliques

Ⓒ CT scan

Ⓓ Dynamic radiographs

Specific injury pattern identified

Ⓔ Isolated posterior arch fracture

Ⓕ Jefferson (burst) fracture of atlas

Ⓖ Lateral mass fracture

Ⓗ Transverse ligament rupture

Atlantoaxial rotatory subluxation

Ⓛ Occipital C 1–2 subluxation

Transverse ligament intact

Transverse ligament ruptured

OCCIPUT TO C2 ARTHRODESIS

Halo Immobilization for 3 mo

Cervical Orthosis

Stable

Chronic atlantoaxial instability

Ⓘ Acute

Ⓙ Chronic or Delay in diagnosis

Traction Reduction Halo

Trial with Traction

Unsuccessful reduction

POSTERIOR ATLANTOAXIAL ARTHRODESIS

Ⓚ OPEN REDUCTION

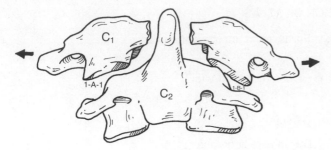

Figure 1 Jefferson's fracture with displacement of the lateral masses of C1. If total displacement (*A* + *B*) is >7 mm, the transverse ligament is also ruptured. The neural canal is expanded with this fracture so most patients are neurologically normal, but this is an unstable fracture and requires halo immobilization.

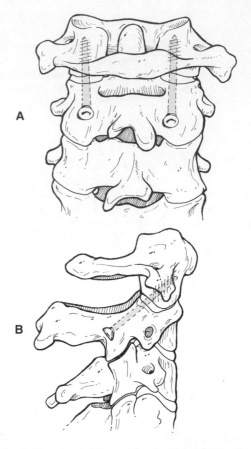

Figure 2   A, Technique of trans-articular screw fixation for a C1-2 arthrodesis. The AP view shows that the screws cross the C1-2 articulation but are medial to the foramen of the vertebral artery. **B,** On the lateral view, the screws begin at the midline of the C1-2 inferior facet and traverse the lamina and pedicle through the C1-2 joint. Before placement of the screws, the articular cartilage of the C1-2 joint is removed. After placement of the screws, corticocancellous bone grafts are secured in place across the lamina of C1 to C2 with either wire or heavy nonabsorbable suture.

on the lateral flexion radiograph is >5 mm in an otherwise normal spine, a transverse ligament rupture is present. If the distance is >9 to 10 mm, additional ruptures of the alar ligaments and apical ligaments of the odontoid process have been sustained. Spontaneous healing of a transverse ligament does not normally occur; therefore routine posterior atlantoaxial fusion is indicated.

I. Patients with acute traumatic atlantoaxial rotatory subluxation present with pain, torticollis, and decreased ROM. The diagnosis may be made on open-mouth odontoid views but is confirmed with the dynamic CT scans. If the symptoms are of short duration, reduction can be readily achieved by head halter or skull traction and maintained in a halo vest. Although the halo does not rigidly block flexion-extension loads in the sagittal plane or axial loads to the upper C-spine, it does adequately control rotational forces.

J. Chronic atlantoaxial rotatory subluxation is often due to a delay in diagnosis. It should be initially treated with a trial of skull traction and attempt at reduction. If reduction is achieved, the patient should be held in a halo for approximately 3 to 6 months. If reduction cannot be achieved or if there are neurologic signs, reduction and posterior atlantoaxial fusion should be performed. Fusion should also be performed on patients with recurrent atlantoaxial rotatory subluxation after an initially successful reduction with traction, which is not maintained.

K. The surgical construct for a posterior atlantoaxial arthrodesis should be chosen based on the degree of mechanical instability of the C1–2 complex. Simple midline Gallie fusions suffice for most cases, but interlaminar fusion using trapezoidal blocks or autogenous bone graft may be required in greater degrees of instability. Transarticular screw fixation as described by Magerl should be considered for patients with greater degrees of instability. This technique, however, requires the ability to completely reduce the C1–2 joint and familiarity with the anatomy of the atlantoaxial joint and the technique of screw placement (Fig. 2). The Magerl technique has the advantage of not requiring a halo while the fusion is consolidating. Approximately 50% of normal cervical rotation is lost after C1–2 arthrodesis in adults.

L. Occipital C1–2 subluxations or dislocations are extremely rare and generally fatal. Diagnosis may be difficult, and the use of Powers ratio based on a lateral radiograph centered at C1–2 may be helpful in making the diagnosis. Powers ratio is the distance between the basion and the C1 posterior arch, divided by the distance between the opisthion and the C1 anterior arch. The normal value for the Powers ratio is 1.0. If the diagnosis is made, these patients are best treated by occipital-cervical fusion.

References

Botte MJ, Byrne TP, Garfin SR. Application of the halo device for immobilization of the cervical spine utilizing and increasing torque pressure. J Bone Joint Surg 1987; 69A:750.

Fielding W, Hawkins R. Atlantoaxial rotatory fixation. J Bone Joint Surg 1977; 59A:37.

Fielding W, VanCochran G, Lansing J, Hohl M. Tears of the transverse ligament of the atlas. J Bone Joint Surg 1974; 56A:1683.

Fowler JL, Sandhu A, Fraser RD. A review of fractures of the atlas vertebra. J Spinal Disord 1990; 3:19.

Griswold D, Albright J, Schiffman E, et al. Atlantoaxial fusion for instability. J Bone Joint Surg 1978; 60A:285.

Jeanneret B, Magerl F. Primary fusion C1/2 in odontoid fractures: Indications, technique, and results of transarticular screw fixation. J Spinal Disorders 1992;5:464.

Koch R, Nickel V. The halo vest: An evaluation of motion and forces across the neck. Spine 1978; 3:103.

Levine A, Edwards C. Treatment of injuries in the C1–2 complex. Orthop Clin North Am 1986; 17:31.

Levine AM, Edwards CC. Traumatic lesions of the occipito-atlantoaxial complex. Clin Orthop 1989; 239:53.

Powers B, Miller MD, Kramer RS, et al. Traumatic anterior atlanto-occipital dislocation. Neurosurgery 1979; 4:12.

Schlicke L, Callahan R. A rational approach to burst fractures of the atlas. Clin Orthop 1981; 154:18.

Segla L, Grimm J, Stauffer S. Non-union of fractures of the atlas. J Bone Joint Surg 1987; 69A:1423.

Spence K, Decker S, Sell K. Bursting atlantal fracture associated with rupture of the transverse ligament. J Bone Joint Surg 1970; 52A:543.

White AA IIII, Panjabi MM. Clinical biomechanics of the spine, ed. 2. Philadelphia, J.B. Lippincott.

FRACTURES OF THE AXIS

A. A lateral radiograph of the upper cervical spine (C-spine) should be obtained in all trauma patients who complain of neck pain, have evidence of head, fascial or neck trauma, or have altered consciousness. A lateral C-spine radiograph will pick up approximately 85% of injuries to the C-spine and should be adequate to assess alignment from the skull to the T1 vertebral body.

B. If a C-spine injury is suspected, obtain a full C-spine series, including anteroposterior (AP), oblique, and open-mouth odontoid views, all of which can be obtained without moving the patient. Nondiagnostic radiographs can be supplemented with either computed tomography (CT), with sagittal and coronal reconstructions of the axis, or polytomography. These studies are not necessary if the plain films are diagnostic and nonsurgical care is planned.

C. CT, with sagittal and coronal reconstructions, visualizes most fractures of the axis well. The addition of a magnetic resonance imaging (MRI) scan is helpful in patients with evidence of neurologic injury or in those patients where no bony fracture is visualized, but ligamentous injury is suspected.

D. Polytomography may still play a role in the evaluation of type II odontoid fractures and lateral facet fractures, where the injury is primarily in the horizontal plane.

E. Isolated fractures to the lamina or vertebral body are uncommon. In particularly those patients presenting with anterior avulsion fractures to the C-spine, associated injuries should be sought. If these minor injuries are not associated with upper C-spine instability, they can be easily managed by mobilization using an intermediate class of orthosis (e.g., Philadelphia collar with thoracic extension, SOMI brace or four-poster brace).

F. The Anderson/D'Alonzo classification (Fig. 1) of odontoid process fractures is useful in evaluating the prognosis for fracture union with nonoperative treatment. Type II fractures through the body or base of the odontoid have a reported prevalence of non-union of 5–64%. Type III fractures, which extend into the cancellous bone of the axis, have an excellent prognosis with adequate reduction and external immobilization.

G. Type I fractures of the odontoid are thought to represent an avulsion injury of the tip of the dens by the alar ligament. This injury is very rare, and since it is located above the transverse ligament, there is no associated atlantoaxial instability. In most cases, a soft cervical collar can be used for symptomatic relief. Type II odontoid process fractures may be displaced anteriorly or posteriorly. There is greater potential for neurologic injury with posterior displacement. Fracture reduction and halo immobilization is the preferred treatment for patients who have no risk factors

for non-union (risk factors are age >40 years, fractures with primarily posterior translation, and displacement >5 mm). Consider primary posterior atlantoaxial arthrodesis for patients with one or more of these risk factors.

H. Various surgical constructs for C1–2 arthrodesis have been recommended for odontoid process fractures. The Gallie midline fusion is preferred for anteriorly displaced odontoid fractures in which the posterior wiring can be used as a modified tension band fixation. The Brooks interlaminar fusion is preferred for posteriorly displaced fractures in which rigid fixation is necessary, but posterior displacement of the ring should be avoided. Prior to any posterior arthrodesis, the integrity of the C1 posterior arch must be verified radiographically. For those patients who have reducible but highly unstable type II fractures of the odontoid, or those who have contraindications to halo immobilization, consider transarticular screw fixation of the atlantoaxial articulation. The preferred postoperative immobilization depends upon the stability offered by the surgical construct. Either cervical orthotic or halo immobilization may be indicated.

I. For patients with reducible type II odontoid fractures in whom maintenance of the atlantoaxial motion is preferred or halo immobilization is not possible, consider anterior screw fixation of the odontoid process.

J. Type III odontoid process fractures may be displaced or undisplaced. After closed reduction in traction or in a halo, under x-ray control, union can be expected in >90% of cases with simple halo cast or vest immobilization for 3 months.

K. Isolated facet fractures of the axis are extremely uncommon. When present, if instability is noted, treatment is reduction and halo cast or vest immobilization for 3 months.

L. Bilateral pedicle fractures of the axis (hangman's fracture, traumatic spondylolisthesis of the axis) are most commonly due to hyperextension and axial load forces to the upper C-spine (Fig. 2). Variable degrees of C2–3 interspace disruption and/or tearing of the posterior atlantoaxial membrane may be present. Interruption of the posterior longitudinal ligament allows significant horizontal translation of the cervicocranium on C3, resulting in neurologic damage. Pedicle fractures are, therefore, classified according to the extent of soft tissue disruption.

M. Type I pedicle fractures have minimal disruption of the anterior or posterior longitudinal ligaments and the C2–3 disc. There is usually <2 to 3 mm of displacement of the fracture site or translation of the body of C2 on C3. Integrity of the soft tissues can be confirmed by flexion-extension radiographs. Absolute prerequisites for obtaining flexion-extension radiographs include: (1) absence of any demonstrable neurologic deficit, (2) absence of an altered state of conscious-

NECK TRAUMA

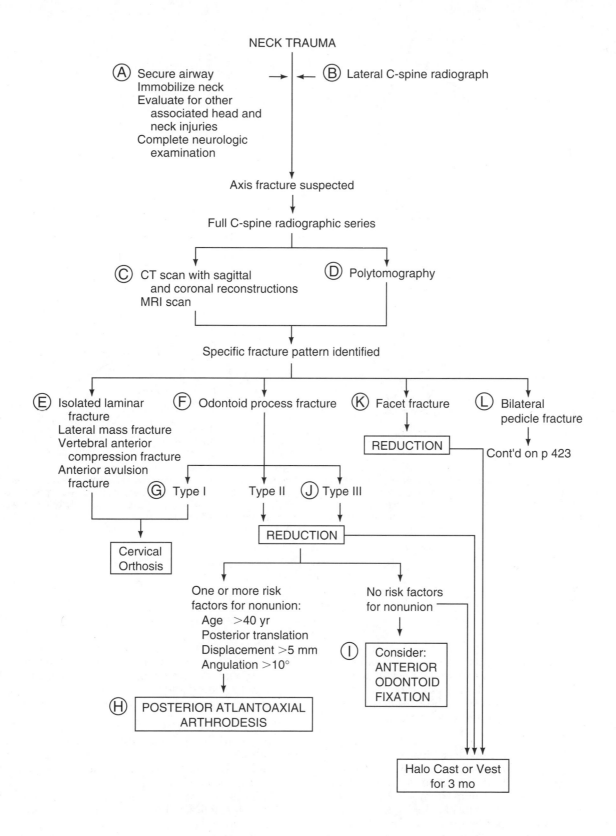

Ⓐ Secure airway
Immobilize neck
Evaluate for other
  associated head and
  neck injuries
Complete neurologic
  examination

Ⓑ Lateral C-spine radiograph

Axis fracture suspected

Full C-spine radiographic series

Ⓒ CT scan with sagittal
and coronal reconstructions
MRI scan

Ⓓ Polytomography

Specific fracture pattern identified

Ⓔ Isolated laminar
fracture
Lateral mass fracture
Vertebral anterior
  compression fracture
Anterior avulsion
  fracture

Ⓕ Odontoid process fracture

Ⓚ Facet fracture

Ⓛ Bilateral
pedicle fracture

REDUCTION

Cont'd on p 423

Ⓖ Type I   Type II   Ⓙ Type III

Cervical
Orthosis

REDUCTION

One or more risk
factors for nonunion:
  Age >40 yr
  Posterior translation
  Displacement >5 mm
  Angulation >10°

No risk factors
for nonunion

Ⓘ Consider:
ANTERIOR
ODONTOID
FIXATION

Ⓗ POSTERIOR ATLANTOAXIAL
ARTHRODESIS

Halo Cast or Vest
for 3 mo

421

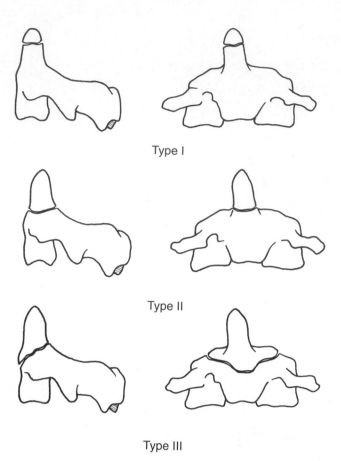

Type I

Type II

Type III

Figure 1 Fractures of the odontoid are classified into three types, depending on the line of the fracture through the odontoid. Type I fractures are stable. The treatment of type II and type III fractures depends on the age of the patient and the degree and direction of displacement.

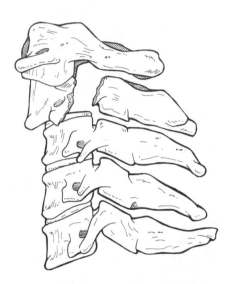

Figure 2 A traumatic spondylolisthesis of the axis (hangman's fracture) is a fracture through the pars interarticularis/pedicle of C2, which allows for anterior subluxation of the body of C2. These are rarely associated with neurologic dysfunction.

ness including intoxication, and (3) ability of the patient to actively flex and extend the neck without assistance. If adequate flexion-extension views are unattainable, the fracture must be considered potentially unstable. Stable injuries can be managed by an intermediate cervical orthosis.

N. Type II fractures are grossly unstable and are managed by careful closed reduction, using skull tong traction. Use no more than 20 lb of traction, to avoid distraction of the cervico-cranium from the rest of the C-spine. Halo cast immobilization for 3 months is necessary to achieve either union of the pedicle fracture or spontaneous fusion between the bodies of C2 and C3. Patients should have a radiograph in the halo, in both supine and upright positions, to document that the halo is preventing significant translation of the fracture. In those patients in whom significant loss of reduction is noted, 2–3 weeks of traction in bed followed by halo immobilization should be performed.

Some loss of position of the reduction can be expected if rigid immobilization of the upper C-spine in the halo is not achieved. Nonunions of type II pedicle fractures should be treated with anterior C2–3 fusion.

O. Type II-A fractures are felt to be related to a force vector primarily in flexion. They generally present with less displacement but more angulation than type II injuries. The degree of displacement in angulation increases when traction is applied, in contrast to type II injuries, which reduce in light traction. Therefore, type II-A injuries should be treated with reduction in the halo under x-ray control, and halo cast or vest immobilization for 3 months. Again, obtain both supine and upright x-ray films prior to discharge. Differentiation between type II and type II-A fractures can be difficult. Generally the type II-A fracture line is more horizontal in orientation, but many times only the fracture's response to traction permits differentiation.

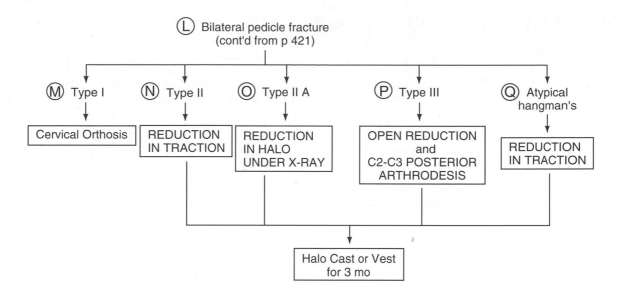

P. The type III pedicle fracture is felt to represent a pure flexion injury and involves complete soft tissue disruption between the bodies of C2 and C3 and an associated unilateral or bilateral facet dislocation. The posterior arch of C2 represents a free fragment; therefore closed reduction of such facet injuries is impossible and open reduction is mandatory. After open reduction of the C2 posterior elements with fusion posteriorly of C2-C3, the pedicle fracture can be treated by closed reduction and halo immobilization or incorporation of the C1 vertebrae into the posterior arthrodesis.

Q. Atypical bilateral pedicle fractures exit through the junction of the vertebral body with the pedicle, and on at least one side, the pedicle is still in continuity with the posterior cortex of the vertebral body. Therefore, with translation the spinal cord may be compressed between the posterior ring of C1 and the aspect of the posterior vertebral body of C2, which is attached to the pedicle. When these fractures are displaced, there is a higher incidence of neurologic injury than with the typical type II bilateral pedicle fracture. If neurologic deficit is noted, MRI of the upper C-spine should be obtained for evaluation of the cervical cord. These fractures can typically be treated with reduction and immobilization in a halo vest or a cast. However, great care must be taken to confirm stability in the halo, prior to immobilization of the patient, due to the higher risk of neurologic injury with displacement.

References

Anderson L, D'Alonzo R. Fracture of the odontoid process of the axis. J Bone Joint Surg 1974; 56A:1663.

Bohler J. Anterior stabilization for acute fractures and nonunions of the dens. J Bone Joint Surg 1982; 64A:18.

Brooks A, Jenkins E. Atlantoaxial arthrodesis by the wedge compression method. J Bone Joint Surg 1978; 60A:279.

Bucholz R. Unstable hangman's fractures. Clin Orthop 1981; 154:119.

Clark CR, White AA III. Fractures of the dens: A multi-center study. J Bone Joint Surg 1985; 67A:1340.

Dunn M, Seljeskoy E. Experience in the management of odontoid process injuries: An analysis of 128 cases. Neurosurgery 1986; 18:306.

Etter C, Coscia M, Jaberg H, et al. Direct anterior fixation of dens fractures with a cannulated screw system. Spine 1991; 16(Suppl 3):525.

Fielding W, Hawkins R, Ratzan S. Spine fusion for atlantoaxial instability. J Bone Joint Surg 1976; 58A:400.

Francis W, Fielding W, Hawkins R, Hensinger R. Traumatic spondylolisthesis of the axis. J Bone Joint Surg 1981; 63B:313.

Hadley M, Browner C, Sonntag V. Axis fractures: A comprehensive review of management and treatment in 107 cases. Neurosurgery 1985; 17:281.

Hanssen A, Cabanela M. Fractures of the dens in adult patients. J Trauma 1987; 27:928.

Jeanneret B, Magerl F. Primary fusion C1/2 in odontoid fractures: Indications, technique, and results of transarticular screw fixation. J Spinal Disorders 1992; 5:464.

Johnson R, Hart D, et al. Cervical orthoses: A study comparing their effectiveness in restricting cervical motion in normal subjects. J Bone Joint Surg 1977; 59A:332.

Levine A, Edwards C. Treatment of injuries in the C1−2 complex. Orthop Clin North Am 1986; 12:31.

Schatzker J, Rorabeck C, Waddell J. Fractures of the dens (odontoid process): An analysis of 37 cases. J Bone Joint Surg 1971; 53B:392.

Southwick W. Management of fractures of the dens. J Bone Joint Surg 1980; 62A:482.

Starr JK, Eismont FJ. Atypical hangman's fractures. Spine 1993; 18:1954.

LOWER CERVICAL SPINE INJURIES

A. Patients with suspected lower cervical spine (C-spine) injuries are transported in either a Philadelphia halo orthosis or Philadelphia collar with the sand bags and the head taped to a spinal board. Upon arrival in the emergency room, all poly-trauma patients with altered states of consciousness and all patients with pain, point tenderness, or other associated head and neck injuries warrant the diagnosis of possible C-spine fracture or dislocation. Adherence to the ABCs of trauma management and evaluation for other associated injuries are mandatory. Obtain a complete history, physical and neurologic examination. Specific questioning about transient paralysis of paresthesias and documentation of any neurologic loss are imperative. Obtain a cross-table lateral view of the C-spine, giving special attention to evidence of soft tissue swelling or malalignment. The entire C-spine, from the occiput to T1, must be adequately visualized on the lateral radiograph. This often necessitates a swimmer's view of the cervical-thoracic junction. For patients who present with an incomplete neurologic deficit within the first 8 hours, high-dose methylprednisolone is beneficial.

B. If the emergency cross-table lateral radiograph is abnormal or equivocal, obtain a full C-spine series, including anteroposterior, oblique, and open-mouth odontoid views. Computed tomography (CT) scans and occasionally polytomography assist in detecting fractures of the pedicle, lamina, and facet joints. Further radiographic studies may be necessitated by the injury pattern identified.

C. Minor C-spine fractures generally are treated symptomatically. Spinous process fractures (e.g., the clay shoveler's fracture, a fracture of the tip of the spinous process of C7), can be caused by extension injuries to the neck or direct muscle pull on the spinous process. Treat with short-term immobilization for comfort and then gradual mobilization as symptoms subside. Transverse process fractures also generally are muscular avulsion fractures and can be treated symptomatically. In evaluation of laminar fractures, associated fractures of the facet must be ruled out, as these fractures often are unstable. The teardrop avulsion fracture, an extension injury, must be differentiated from the teardrop fracture, which is a flexion-rotation-axial compression injury and is unstable.

D. Flexion injuries to the C-spine consist of variable injury to the posterior ligaments and facet joint capsule. Patients who show >11° of intervertebral angulation or >3.5 mm of subluxation on the initial radiograph have an unstable posterior ligamentous injury and are treated with posterior cervical arthrodesis.

E. For patients who present with <11° of angulation but possible flexion injury to the C-spine, obtain dynamic radiographs. Prerequisites for flexion-extension views of the C-spine include: (1) a neurologically intact patient, (2) performance of all movements actively by the patient, (3) no altered state of consciousness (including intoxication), and (4) direct physician supervision of the radiographic study. If <11° of angulation is noted on the flexion-extension view, treat with a cervical orthosis and obtain repeat flexion-extension views in 10 days to 2 weeks. If >11° of angulation is noted, the patient should undergo posterior cervical arthrodesis.

F. Flexion-rotation injuries consist of the unilateral jumped facet (25% subluxation on lateral x-ray). Closed reduction of unilateral jumped facets should be attempted initially. This consists of placing the patient in cervical traction with progressive increase in weight (increments of 5 lbs) under radiographic control. Reduction of unilateral jumped facets not uncommonly requires at least some mild rotatory manipulation. Sequential neurologic examinations are performed with each addition of weight. Generally only 50% of these dislocations can be reduced. If the unilateral jumped facet is reduced with traction, evaluate for the presence of a facet fracture.

G. It is extremely difficult to hold the patient with unilateral facet fracture in a reduced position with a halo vest. If any neurologic deficit is present, the patient should definitely be treated with posterior cervical arthrodesis, incorporating a control of rotatory instability. This entails posterior spinous wiring with oblique wiring, triple-wire technique (Fig. 1), or, more recently, posterior cervical plating. Patients with facet fracture and no neurologic deficit may be treated with a halo vest, depending on the patient's wishes. With this form of treatment there generally is some residual subluxation even after healing of the facet fracture.

H. When a unilateral jumped facet is reduced in traction and no facet fracture is noted, treat with a halo vest for 3 months and assess stability after removal of the halo.

I. For irreducible unilateral or bilateral jumped facets, obtain an MRI prior to surgical open reduction. There is some controversy as to whether irreducible unilateral jumped facets require surgical intervention. For patients who have a neurologic deficit, I think that reduction and stabilization are imperative. Even without neurologic deficit, patients who are left unreduced do not do as well clinically as those who are operatively reduced and fused. If MRI shows no anterior spinal cord compression from soft disc, posterior cervical arthrodesis can be performed. The arthrodesis must incorporate rotational control (see G). Standard interspinous wiring is inadequate.

J. The patient with unreducible unilateral or bilateral jumped facets and anterior spinal cord compression should undergo anterior cervical discectomy with placement of interbody graft to remove the compressing disc material before undergoing posterior cervical arthrodesis as previously described.

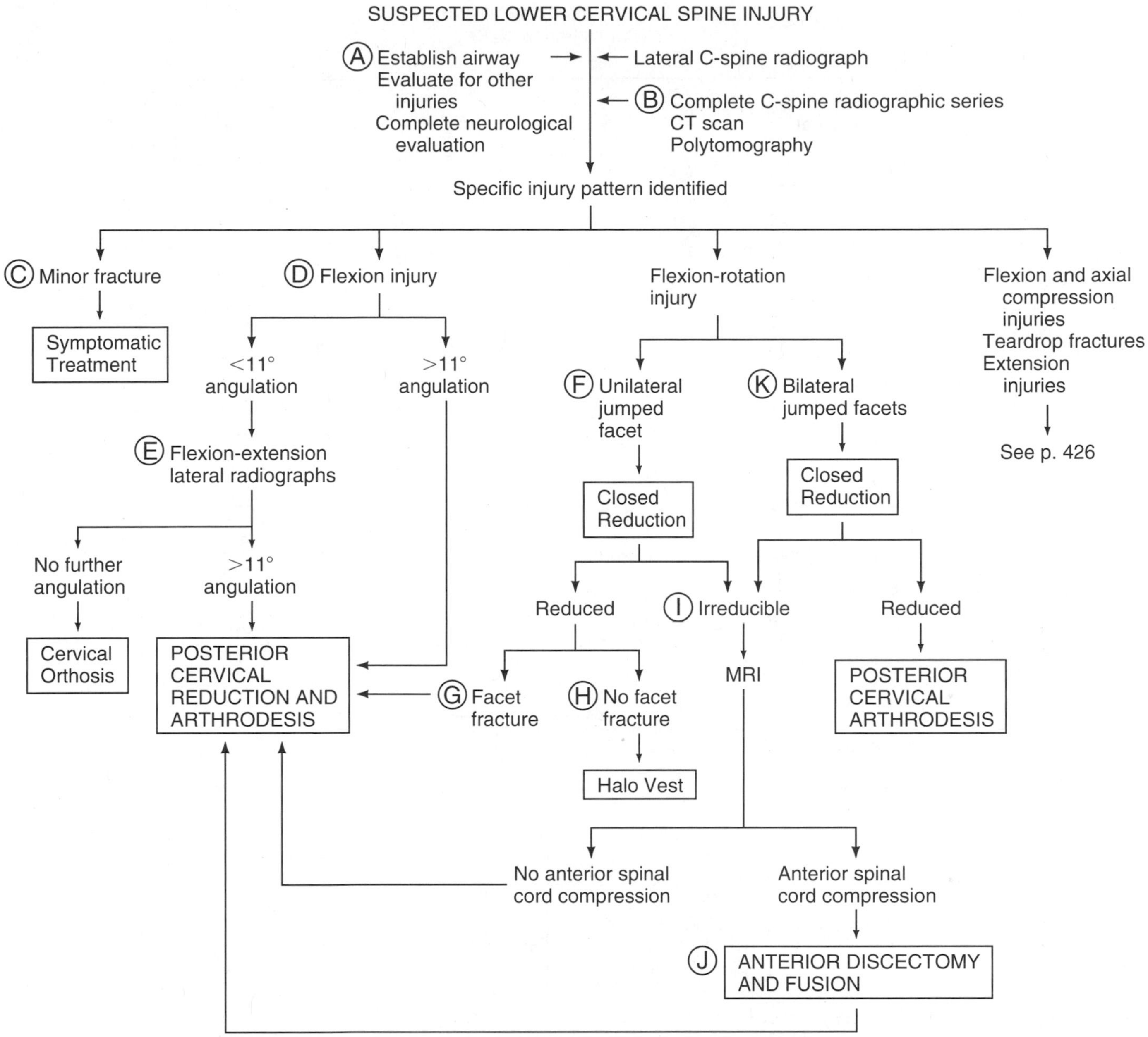

K. Place patients with bilateral jumped facets (Fig. 2) in cervical traction with sequentially added weights under radiographic control. It is imperative that the patient have normal mental status. If the patient's mental status is altered, obtain magnetic resonance imaging (MRI) of the C-spine before closed reduction. If the patient is neurologically intact and reducible with traction, perform posterior cervical arthrodesis. For the patient who presents with neurologic deficit and bilateral jumped facets, there is some controversy as to whether MRI should be performed prior to reduction. Historically the standard has been closed reduction with traction with sequential neurologic examination.

L. Flexion and axial compression injuries consist of compression fractures and burst fractures.

M. Anterior compression fractures that involve <25% of the anterior aspect of the body can be safely treated with a cervical orthosis for 8–12 weeks. For compression fractures >25%, and especially those >50%, it is imperative that posterior elements be evaluated to rule out disruption and instability of the posterior elements. If the posterior elements are felt to be intact, these compression injuries can also be treated with a cervical orthosis.

N. Compression fractures in which the posterior elements are disrupted have a very high rate of progressive flexion deformity with risk of neurologic injury. They should be treated with posterior cervical arthrodesis. They generally do not require anterior strut grafting, since the posterior cortex of the cervical vertebrae is intact.

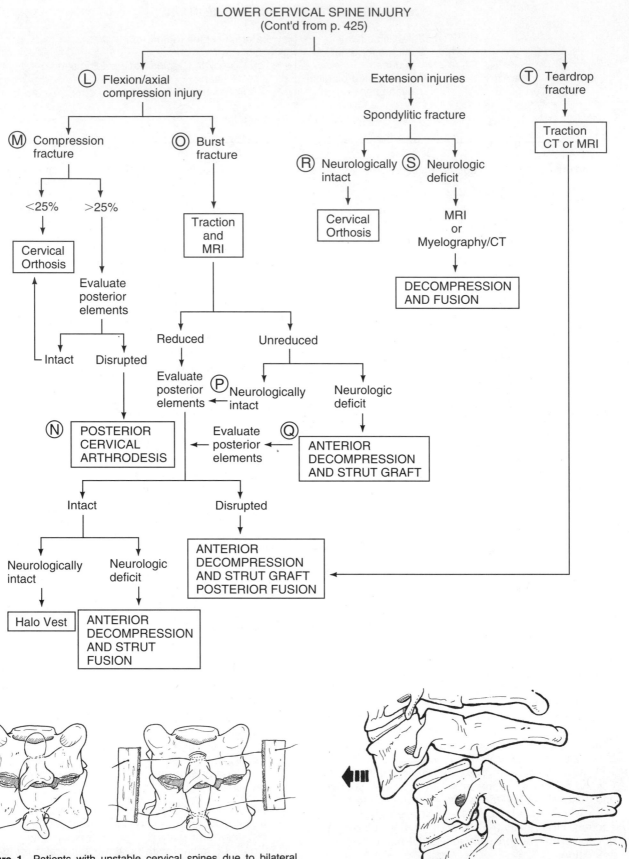

LOWER CERVICAL SPINE INJURY
(Cont'd from p. 425)

Ⓛ Flexion/axial compression injury

Extension injuries

Ⓣ Teardrop fracture

Spondylitic fracture

Traction CT or MRI

Ⓜ Compression fracture

Ⓞ Burst fracture

Ⓡ Neurologically intact

Ⓢ Neurologic deficit

<25%   >25%

Cervical Orthosis

Traction and MRI

Cervical Orthosis

MRI or Myelography/CT

Evaluate posterior elements

DECOMPRESSION AND FUSION

Intact   Disrupted

Reduced   Unreduced

Evaluate posterior elements

Ⓟ Neurologically intact

Neurologic deficit

Ⓝ POSTERIOR CERVICAL ARTHRODESIS

Evaluate posterior elements

Ⓠ ANTERIOR DECOMPRESSION AND STRUT GRAFT

Intact   Disrupted

Neurologically intact

Neurologic deficit

ANTERIOR DECOMPRESSION AND STRUT GRAFT POSTERIOR FUSION

Halo Vest

ANTERIOR DECOMPRESSION AND STRUT FUSION

Figure 1 Patients with unstable cervical spines due to bilateral perched, jumped, or fractured facet joints need to be stabilized with a posterior fusion. The gold standard is a posterior spinous process wiring. The triple wire modification as designed by Bohlman, which incorporates iliac structural grafts, as shown here, provides rotation as well as flexion stability.

Figure 2 With bilateral facet dislocations the cephalad vertebrae are translated approximately 50% or more on the caudal vertebrae. This condition needs to be corrected surgically.

O. Place the patient with a C-spine burst fracture in cervical traction. Then, obtain either MRI or CT scan with intrathecal contrast to evaluate whether the vertebral body fragments have been reduced. If there is no residual compression on the neural elements, then evaluate the posterior elements. If they are disrupted, the patient should undergo anterior decompression and strut graft with associated posterior stabilization and fusion. If the posterior elements are intact and the patient is neurologically impaired, perform anterior decompression and strut fusion, followed by placement in a halo vest. If the patient is neurologically intact, treat with a halo vest.

P. Patients with residual bone fragments in the neural canal should undergo anterior decompression and strut grafting. For those who are neurologically intact, this can be done as a delayed procedure, with anterior strut grafting alone performed if the posterior elements are intact and anterior-posterior fusion performed if posterior elements also are disrupted. Patients can undergo anterior plating after strut grafting, but these fusions should be augmented with a cervical orthosis or halo if the posterior elements are disrupted.

Q. Patients who are neurologically impaired and have residual fragments in the canal unreduced by traction should undergo immediate anterior decompression and strut grafting. If their posterior elements are also disrupted, undertake associated posterior fusion. Even patients with complete neurologic injury may gain nerve root recovery from decompression of residual bony compression of the spinal cord.

R. Extension injuries to the C-spine are generally most relevant in the patient with underlying spondylosis. If the patient with underlying cervical spondylosis presents with a hyperextension injury and evidence of instability, treatment depends on neurologic status. If the patient is neurologically intact, recognition of the instability is very important to prevent delayed neurologic loss. These patients generally are treated with a cervical orthosis for 6–8 weeks; most will self-stabilize.

S. For the patient with a spondylitic fracture and central cord syndrome, obtain MRI or a post-myelo-CT to evaluate neurologic compression. If compression is noted, the patient should undergo decompression of the area of injury with associated surgical stabilization and fusion.

T. In a teardrop fracture the anterior inferior wedge of the vertebral body is fractured off. It is associated with a sagittal split through the middle of the vertebral body on CT scan and associated disruption of the posterior elements. This is an extremely unstable fracture. When recognized, the patient should be placed in cervical traction. Obtain MRI or a post-myelo-CT. If there are residual bone and/or disc fragments in the canal, perform anterior decompression and strut grafting followed by posterior stabilization fusion. If there are no residual bony fragments in the canal and the patient is neurologically intact, treat with posterior stabilization and fusion.

References

Aebi M, Mohler J, Zäch GA, et al. Indication, surgical techniques, and results of 100 surgically treated fractures and fracture-dislocations of the cervical spine. Clin Orthop 1986; 203:244.

Allen BL Jr., Ferguson RL, Lehman TR, O'Brien RP. A mechanistic classification of closed, indirect fractures and dislocations of the lower cervical spine. Spine 1982; 7:1.

Benzel EC, Larson SJ. Recovery of nerve root function after complete quadriplegia from cervical spine fractures. Neurosurgery 1986; 19:809.

Bohlman HH. Acute fractures and dislocations of the cervical spine: An analysis of 300 hospitalized patients and review of the literature. J Bone Joint Surg 1979; 61A:1119.

Bohlman HH. Late anterior decompression and fusion for spinal cord injuries: Review of 100 cases with long-term results. Orthop Trans 1980; 4:42.

Bracken MD, Separd MJ, Collins WF, et al. A randomized controlled trial of methylprednisolone or naloxone in the treatment of acute spinal cord injury: Results of the Second National Acute Spinal Cord Injury Study. N Engl J Med 1990; 332:14405.

McAfee PC, Bohlman HH, Wilson WL. The triple wire fixation technique for stabilization of acute fracture-dislocations: A biomechanical analysis. Orthop Trans 1985; 9:142.

Ripa DR, Kowall MG, Meyer PR Jr., et al. Series of ninety-two traumatic cervical spine injuries stabilized with anterior ASIF plate fusion technique. Spine 1991; 16:546.

Robertson PA, Ryan MD. Neurologic deterioration after reduction of cervical subluxation: mechanical compression by disc tissue. J Bone Joint Surg 1992; 74B:224.

Rorabeck CH, Rock MG, Hawkins RS, et al. Unilateral facet dislocation of the cervical spine: An analysis of the results of 26 patients. Spine 1987; 12:23.

Templeton PA, Young JW, Miruisse SE, Buddemeyer EU. The value of retropharyngeal soft tissue measurements in trauma of the adult cervical spine: Cervical spine soft tissue measurements. Skeletal Radiol 1981; 16:98.

THORACOLUMBAR FRACTURES

A. Patients with thoracolumbar (TL) fractures are transported on a rigid spine board. Upon arrival to the emergency room, the patient should have a complete evaluation, including observation of the skin of the back as this could be pertinent as far as timing of any particular procedures. There also should be a complete neurologic examination. Hypotension may be related to neurologic injury as well as other associated injuries.

B. Patients with altered states of consciousness or other associated injuries should have a lateral cervical-spine radiograph and anteroposterior (AP) and lateral views of the TL spine as there is a prevalence of approximately 15%–20% of multi-level fractures of the spine. If an area of injury is suspected, further study with either computed tomography (CT) or polytomography may be of benefit. Once an unstable fracture is identified, transfer the patient to a roto-kinetic bed to prevent skin breakdown and augment pulmonary function.

C. Treatment of anterior compression fractures of the TL spine depends on the degree of angulation, the percent of compression of the anterior aspect of the body, and the presence of contiguous fractures. Patients with minimal compression (<20%) can generally be treated with ambulation and avoidance of flexion and lifting after the acute period of possible ileus has passed. All patients who sustain TL fractures should be evaluated for the development of possible ileus. Those with >20° of compression but <40° of anterior compression and <20° of coronal angulation generally are treated by placement in a hyperextension cast or thoracolumbosacral orthosis (TLSO). Patients with >40° of anterior compression, >20° of coronal angulation, or contiguous fractures whose percent compression and angulation added together is greater than the above, are treated with posterior instrumentation and fusion. A trial of hyperextension casting may be acceptable if the patient can be monitored very closely for worsening kyphotic position in the brace.

D. Burst fractures are fractures of both the anterior and posterior cortex of the vertebral body. When a possible burst fracture is identified, obtain further diagnostic evaluation with CT. Magnetic resonance imaging also may be helpful in evaluation of the patient with neurologic deficit. It is generally felt that these patients do better with surgical intervention. Patients with <30% canal compromise are treated with posterior instrumentation and fusion. There will be some clearing of the neural canal with distraction and reduction of the normal alignment of the spine by posterior instrumentation; this is generally adequate for patients with <30% canal compromise.

E. For patients with >50% canal compromise, some surgeons feel that anterior decompression with strut grafting and either anterior or subsequent posterior instrumentation and fusion is needed. The route of decompression is controversial. Transpedicular decompression of the neural canal with associated posterior stabilization and fusion is an acceptable alternative to anterior decompression. For patients with 30%–50% canal compromise, treatment depends on the particular location and character of the fracture and preference of the treating surgeon and patient. Burst fractures with associated laminar fracture can have neural elements trapped within the laminae; this must be considered during the approach.

F. Treatment of burst fractures in patients without neurologic deficit depends on the particular fracture pattern. Patients with <30% to 40% canal compromise and <20° kyphosis can be treated with hyperextension cast or TLSO. Patients with >40% canal compromise and ≥20° kyphosis or >50% loss of body height are generally thought to do better with posterior instrumentation, reduction, and fusion.

G. Flexion distraction injuries, often called seat-belt fractures or Chance fractures, are flexion injuries with the fulcrum of flexion placed anterior to the spine. The degree of instability depends on whether the anterior longitudinal ligament is intact. If it is intact, as it generally is, treatment depends on the location of the horizontal fracture line. If the fracture line goes through bone, treat the patient with reduction and placement in hyperextension cast or TLSO. If disruption is through the ligaments or disc space, posterior compressive instrumentation and fusion is the treatment of choice.

H. Fracture-dislocations constitute disruption of all three columns of the spine and require stabilization. Generally reduction is best obtained by approaching the fracture posteriorly. The type of instrumentation used should allow for placement of multiple sites of fixation to anatomically align the spine and then fuse across the area of fracture. Care should be taken so that no distraction is produced across the area of fracture. If there is significant loss of bone anteriorly, or compromise of the neural canal anteriorly after posterior reduction, instrumentation and fusion, then a staged anterior decompression and fusion with strut grafting may be necessary.

I. Isolated fractures of the spinous process or transverse process are generally stable and can be treated symptomatically. If the spinous process fracture is associated with a hyperextension injury, treatment depends on associated ligamentous disruptions. Treatment of facet fractures depends on whether a single facet or both facets are involved. Single facet fractures are generally stable; treat symptomatically. Evaluate bilateral facet fractures for the competency of the anterior and posterior longitudinal ligaments. If there is associated disruption of the anterior or middle column, the fracture is unstable and requires either bracing or surgical stabilization.

THORACOLUMBAR FRACTURE

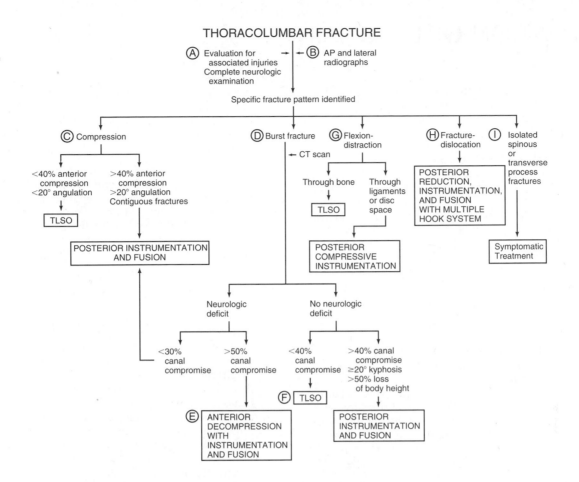

References

Aebi M, Etter C, Kehl T, et al. The internal skeletal fixation system: A new treatment of thoracolumbar fractures and other disorders. Clin Orthop 1988; 227:30.

An HS, Vaccano A, Cotler JM, et al. Low lumbar burst fractures: Comparison among body cast, Harrington rod, Luque rod and Steffe plate. Spine 1991; 61:5440.

Anderson PA, Aenlay MB, Rivara FP, et al. Flexion distraction and chance injuries to the thoracolumbar spine. J Orthop Trauma 1991; 5:153.

Bradford D, McBride G. Surgical management of thoracolumbar spine fractures with incomplete neurologic deficits. Clin Orthop 1987; 218:201.

Cammisa FP, Eismont FJ, Green BA. Dural laceration occurring with burst fractures and associated laminar fractures. J Bone Joint Surg 1989; 71:1044.

Dall B, Stauffer ES. Neurologic injury and recovery patterns in burst fractures at the T12, L1 or L2 motion segment. Clin Orthop 1988; 233:171.

Denis F, Armstrong G, Searls F, et al. Acute thoracolumbar burst fractures in the absence of neurologic deficit: A comparison between operative and non-operative treatment. Clin Orthop 1984; 189:142.

Gertzbein S. Scoliosis research society: Multi-center spine fracture study. Spine 1992; 17:528.

Gertzbein SD, Court-Brown CM. Flexion distraction injuries of the lumbar spine: Mechanisms of injury and classification. Clin Orthop 1988; 277:52.

Gertzbein SD, Court-Brown CM, Jacobs RR, et al. Decompression and circumferential stabilization of unstable spinal fractures. Spine 1988; 13:892.

Hanley E, Eskay M. Thoracic spine fractures. Orthopaedics 1989; 12:689.

Jones RF, Snowdon E, Coan J, et al. Bracing or thoracic and lumbar spine fractures. Paraplegia 1987; 25:386.

Kaneda K, Abami K, Fujiya M. Burst fractures with neurologic deficits of the thoracolumbar-lumbar spine. Results of anterior decompression and stabilization with anterior instrumentation. Spine 1984; 9:788.

McAfee PC. Biomechanical approach to instrumentation of thoracolumbar spine: A review article. Adv Orthop Surg 1985; 313.

Sasson A, Mores G. Complete fracture dislocation of the thoracic spine with neurologic deficit. Spine 1987; 12:67.

Tensor AF, Ferguson RL, Allen BL Jr. A biomechanical study of thoracolumbar spinal fractures with bone in the canal: Part II. The effect of flexion angulation, distraction, and shortening of motion segment. Spine 1985; 10:586.

Weinstein NJ, Collato P, Lehman TR. Thoracolumbar burst fractures treated conservatively: A long-term follow-up. Spine 1988; 13:33.

Willen J, Lindahl S, Instam L, et al. Unstable thoracolumbar fractures: A study by CT and conventional roentgenology of the reduction effect of Harrington instrumentation. Spine 1984; 9:214.

EVALUATION OF BACK PAIN

A. The current history of the pain syndrome should include questions regarding the four W's:
   • *When did it start?*
   • *Where is it now?*
   • *Where does it go?*
   • *What makes it better/worse?*
   The Quebec Classification is very useful in classifying disorders of the lumbar spine based on patient symptoms, duration, and work status. This pain is classified according to: pain without radiation; pain with radiation to the proximal part of the extremity; pain with radiation to the distal part of the extremity; pain with radiation to the limb with neurologic signs. Determine whether the major complaint is back pain or radiating extremity pain and record the relative contribution of each to the total symptom complaint. Use of a pain drawing (Fig. 1) is helpful for the initial evaluation and follow-up examinations.

B. When eliciting specifics of the past history, determine the frequency and character of other pain episodes as well as the nature and results of previous treatments. Probe for other medical problems as well as current medications and any allergies. When prior surgical intervention has occurred, ascertain whether there were clear indications for the surgery, the specifics of the intervention (operative reports, etc.), and the near and long-term results of the surgery relative to the preoperative complaints.

C. The physical examination should be consistent, patient to patient, and should be accomplished in a thorough but expeditious manner. Proceed logically with the patient first standing, then walking, and then bending. Have the patient sit over the end of the examination table for reflex and muscle strength testing. This is followed by the patient lying first supine and then side-to-side. The examination ends with the patient lying prone. In this way, patient movements on and off the table are minimized.

D. Watch the patient walk on the heels (L5 root integrity) and on the toes (S1 root integrity). Ask the patient to elevate the body weight against gravity on either leg (S1 root integrity). Look for any list of the trunk.

E. Common areas of local tenderness are at the lumbosacral junction and over the low lumbar paraspinal muscle masses. Tenderness over the sacroiliac joints and in the sciatic notch near the greater trochanter is not infrequent. The patient should be comfortably positioned to accurately palpate the tender structures: forward flexed over the examination table; side and prone lying.

F. Forward flexion and backward extension should be recorded with any limitation or trunk shift. Evaluate the symmetry of range of motion (ROM) in the major articulations of the lower extremities.

G. Sciatic stress testing can be performed with the patient (1) standing by means of a kick maneuver; (2) flexing forward over the examination table with the feet flat on the floor; (3) in the seated position; or (4) supine, to perform the classic straight leg raising test.

H. Deep tendon reflexes should be symmetrical. Knee jerk reflects L4 root integrity. Ankle jerk reflects S1 root integrity. Dorsiflexion strength of the great toe reflects L5 root integrity. Check sensation on the anteromedial pretibial area proximally (L4), on the dorsum of the foot between the great and second toes (L5), and on the lateral border of the foot (S1).

I. Standard imaging studies for back pain include plain/bending films, computed tomography (CT) scan, magnetic resonance imaging (MRI), bone/SPECT scan, myelogram, and discogram. Acute back pain without neurologic deficit can be treated initially without imaging studies. Informational yield from plain film radiographs is generally limited except to rule out spondylolisthesis. CT scan is superior to MRI for bone definition. MRI is valuable to assess soft tissue anatomy. Bone scan is indicated for suspected infectious or neoplastic lesions and occasionally to rule out inflammatory conditions such as osteoid osteoma. SPECT bone scan can provide axial views for improved uptake differentiation. Myelography is less commonly used with availability of high quality MRI but still is valuable if the diagnosis is uncertain and for intraspinal tumors. Discography remains somewhat controversial; however, in selected cases it can be the only test to identify discogenic pain.

J. Laboratory evaluation includes, but is not limited to, complete blood count/urinalysis, chemistry profile, sedimentation rate, rheumatoid factor, HLA-B27, and selected other tests. Routine or arthritic survey tests are not standard but are utilized when the history, examination, or patient response to the initial treatment regimen suggests a need for further investigation. If the patient presents with flank pain, especially with inguinal radiation, be certain to have the urine analyzed for blood and for crystals. Since viral neuropathy can masquerade as radiculopathy, consider a zoster level laboratory test to rule out herpes zoster in those cases with any cutaneous eruption in the affected limb.

K. Electromyograms and nerve conduction velocities are generally utilized in the evaluation of the more chronic conditions. Such testing can be quite useful in the demonstration of radiculopathies as distinguished from peripheral neuropathies. In addition, electrodiagnostics can be helpful in distinguishing situations of neurogenic claudication (spinal stenosis).

L. A working clinical diagnosis should classify the syndrome of symptom complaints. Be cautious about making a specific patho-anatomic diagnosis unless there is clear objective documentation.

BACK PAIN

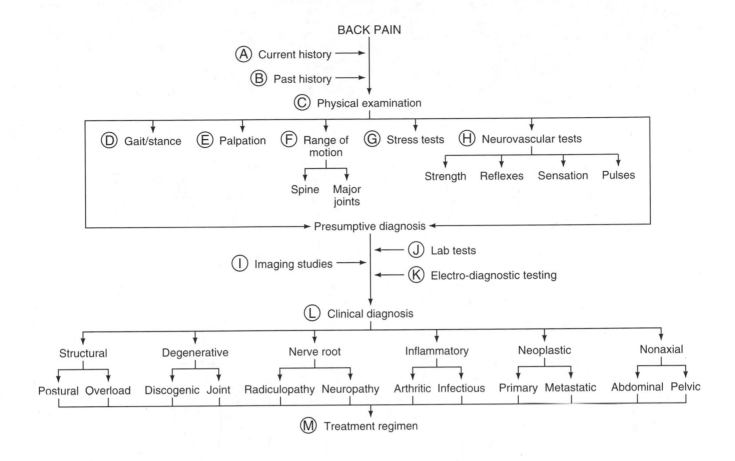

Ⓐ Current history ⟶

Ⓑ Past history ⟶

Ⓒ Physical examination

Ⓓ Gait/stance Ⓔ Palpation Ⓕ Range of motion Ⓖ Stress tests Ⓗ Neurovascular tests

Spine Major joints

Strength Reflexes Sensation Pulses

Presumptive diagnosis

Ⓘ Imaging studies ⟶ ⟵ Ⓙ Lab tests

⟵ Ⓚ Electro-diagnostic testing

Ⓛ Clinical diagnosis

Structural Degenerative Nerve root Inflammatory Neoplastic Nonaxial

Postural Overload Discogenic Joint Radiculopathy Neuropathy Arthritic Infectious Primary Metastatic Abdominal Pelvic

Ⓜ Treatment regimen

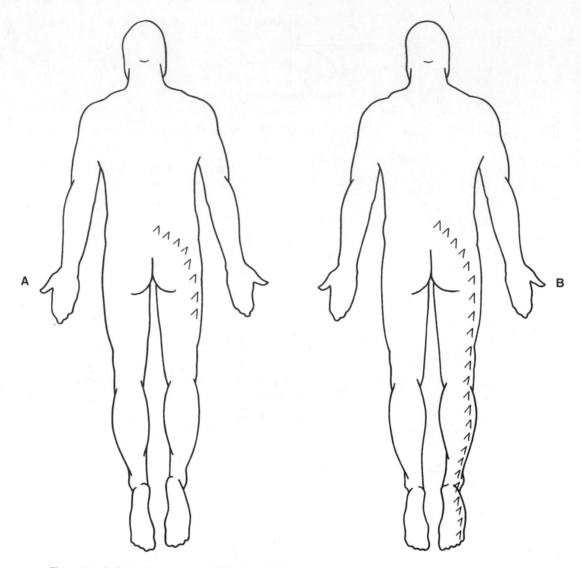

Figure 1 **A,** Pain drawing compatible with soft tissue strain or posterior element pain. **B,** Pain drawing characteristic of lumbar S1 radiculopathy.

M. The natural history of back pain is that most patients will recover within 4 weeks. For those who do not respond, further, more detailed investigation is warranted with appropriate diagnostic modification and specific treatment. However, if a cauda equina syndrome is suspected (bowel/bladder dysfunction; perineal sensory deficit) the clinician must complete the evaluation swiftly and initiate treatment promptly. Similarly, unremitting pain, despite an appropriate treatment regimen, should alert the physician to perform diagnostic studies to establish a patho-anatomic cause leading to specific intervention.

References

Aprill C. Diagnostic disc injection. In: Frymoyer JW, ed: The Adult Spine: Principles and Practice. New York: Raven Press, 1991; 403.

Bell G. Lumbar spine. Orthopaedic Knowledge Update 4. Am Acad Orthop Surg 1993; 491.

Deyo R. Conservative therapy for low back pain: Distinguishing useful from useless therapy. JAMA. 1983; 250:1057.

Deyo R, Diehl A. Lumbar spine films in primary care: Current use and effects of selective ordering criteria. J Gen Intern Med 1986; 1:20.

Hadler N. A critical appraisal of the fibrositis concept. Am J Med 1986; 81(Suppl 3A):26.

Kostuik J, et al: Cauda Equina syndrome and lumbar disc herniation. J Bone Joint Surg 1986; 68:386.

Liang M, Komaroff A. Roentgenograms in primary care patients with acute low back pain: A cost-effectiveness analysis. Arch Intern Med 1982; 142:1108.

Mooney V. Differential diagnosis of low back disorders. In: Frymoyer JW, ed: The Adult Spine: Principles and Practice. New York: Raven Press, 1991; 1551.

Mooney V, Robertson J. The facet syndrome. Clin Orthop 1976; 115:149.

Nachemson A. Advances in low back pain. Clin Orthop 1985; 200:266.

Saal J, et al: The Pseudoradicular syndrome: Lower extremity peripheral nerve entrapment masquerading as lumbar radiculopathy. Spine 1988; 13:926.

Spitzer W, et al. Scientific approach to the assessment and management of activity related spinal disorders: A monograph for clinicians. Report of the Quebec Task Force on Spinal Disorders. Spine 1987;12:1.

Weinstein J. The pain of discography. Spine 1988; 13:1344.

MANAGEMENT OF ACUTE LOW BACK PAIN

A. Most patients with acute low back pain experience resolution of their symptoms within 3 to 4 weeks; generally, only about 10% of cases have pain that persists beyond 2 months. Unrelieved pain with persistent or progressive neurologic deficit after 2 to 3 weeks of intensive conservative therapy should be thoroughly investigated by appropriate studies followed by surgical intervention if a specific patho-anatomic diagnosis can be established.

B. Cauda equina syndrome is relatively rare, being reported in approximately 1% to 3% of patients with confirmed disc herniations. Features include: rapid progression of neurologic symptoms and signs; bilateral leg pain; caudal sensory deficit; bladder overflow incontinence or retention; loss of rectal sphincter tone with or without fecal incontinence. The usual pathology in acute cauda equina syndrome is a large central disc herniation with extrusion. When this syndrome presents, one must proceed rapidly with appropriate imaging studies and emergent decompression of the neurologic elements.

C. Prolonged bed rest should be avoided. Patients may be up for bathroom functions and for meals. Sitting, especially in low or soft chairs should be avoided. Two to 3 days of modified bed rest seems to be as effective as 7 days. Extended bed rest can have deleterious side effects including muscle atrophy, generalized deconditioning, and bone mineral loss.

D. If there are no contraindications, nonsteroidal anti-inflammatory drugs (NSAIDs) are generally effective both for their anti-inflammatory and analgesic actions. Time-limited use of oral muscle relaxants, analgesics, and tricyclic antidepressants can also be helpful in the management of acute back pain. Selective injection techniques can be utilized effectively in the presence of acute radiculopathies.

E. Passive modalities may be used for short periods as analgesic supplements but should be followed by the initiation of early therapeutic exercises guided by an appropriately trained professional. Avoid long-term patient dependence on passive modalities.

F. Although commonly used, there is little objective evidence of efficacy for corsets and braces. Restriction of lumbar motion is counter-productive to the principle of early active motion in the repair of injured collagen tissue. However, there may be some rationale for the use of orthotic devices in selective postoperative situations and as temporary protective "reminders" in the worker population.

G. In multiple clinical trials, only "auto-traction" has been shown to be of any benefit. Manipulation in various forms has a long history of use and can be helpful in the management of acute low back pain without neurologic deficit.

H. Active/assistive exercises should be guided by a trained health care professional. An individualized program requires careful assessment and initiation of specific exercises depending on the particular clinical situation. Generally, range of motion or stretching exercises precede muscle strengthening techniques, which are followed thereafter by low impact aerobic activity. In the presence of a radiculopathy, the McKenzie extension regimen can be helpful to centralize the pain pattern and to diminish the extremity radiation. The flexion regimen of Williams is useful in mechanical low back syndromes without a major radicular component.

I. In the absence of uncontrolled pain or progressive neurologic deficit, reassessment may be delayed for 3 to 4 weeks since most patients will be significantly improved within this time frame. If symptoms persist, a more detailed investigation is warranted to establish a specific patho-anatomic diagnosis. However, the studies selected should be guided by the working clinical diagnosis.

J. The great majority of patients with acute low back pain respond to well-managed programs of conservative care. Less than 10% of such patients require surgical intervention.

K. Health care providers can make a major impact on the incidence and severity of low back pain by meaningful programs of patient education that emphasize such variables as: prevention, fitness and strength, life style habits, ergonomics, and stress management.

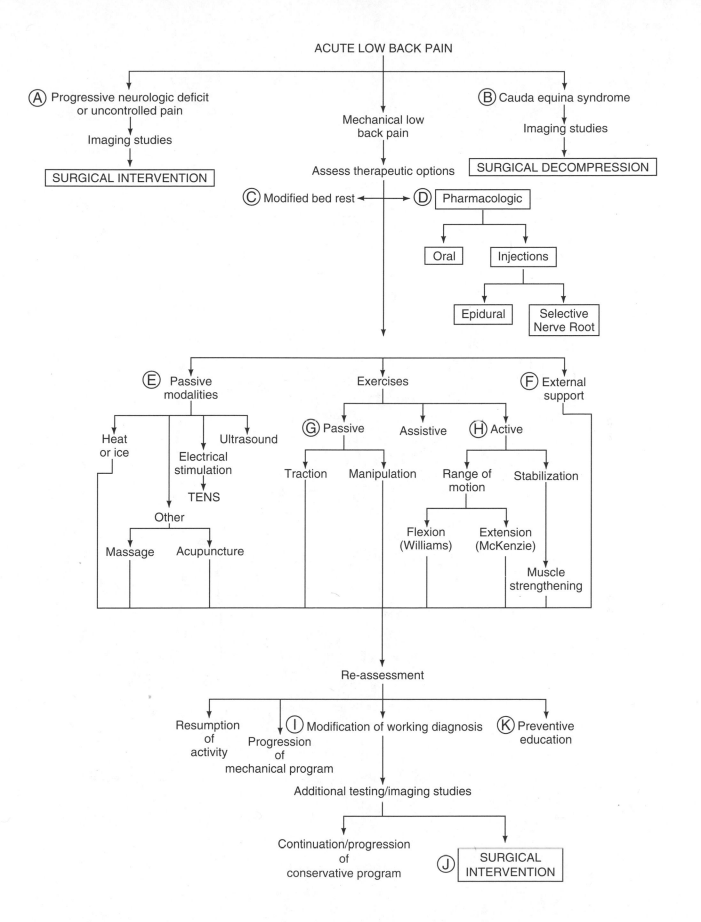

ACUTE LOW BACK PAIN

(A) Progressive neurologic deficit
or uncontrolled pain

Imaging studies

SURGICAL INTERVENTION

Mechanical low
back pain

Assess therapeutic options

(B) Cauda equina syndrome

Imaging studies

SURGICAL DECOMPRESSION

(C) Modified bed rest ←→ (D) Pharmacologic

Oral   Injections

Epidural   Selective
Nerve Root

(E) Passive
modalities

Exercises

(F) External
support

Heat
or ice

Ultrasound

Electrical
stimulation

TENS

Other

Massage   Acupuncture

(G) Passive   Assistive   (H) Active

Traction   Manipulation   Range of
motion   Stabilization

Flexion
(Williams)   Extension
(McKenzie)

Muscle
strengthening

Re-assessment

Resumption
of
activity

(I) Modification of working diagnosis

Progression
of
mechanical program

(K) Preventive
education

Additional testing/imaging studies

Continuation/progression
of
conservative program

(J) SURGICAL
INTERVENTION

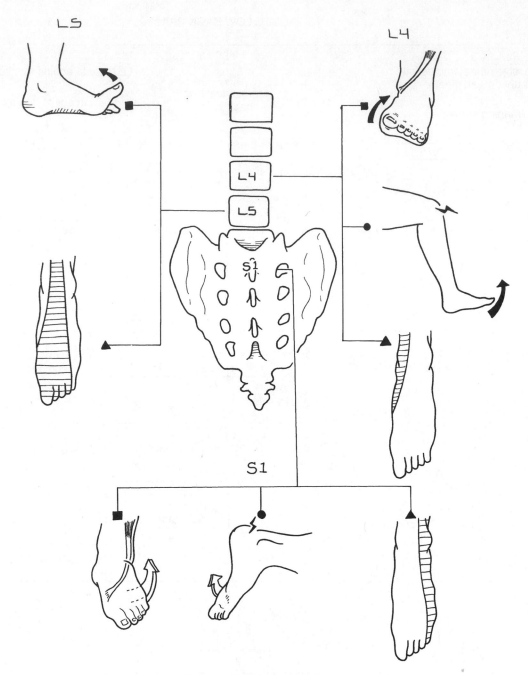

Figure 1 L4-S1 nerve root signs.

References

Alcoff J, et al. Controlled trial of imipramine for chronic low back pain. J Fam Pract 1982; 14:841.

Amlie E, et al. Treatment of acute low back pain with piroxicam: Results of a double-blind placebo-controlled trial. Spine 1987; 12:473.

Andersson G, et al. The intensity of work recovery in low back pain. Spine 1983; 8:880.

Bell G. Lumbar spine. Orthopaedic Knowledge Update 4. Am Acad Orthop Surg 1993; 491.

Bogduk N. Back pain: Zygapophysial blocks and epidural steroids. In: Cousins MJ, Bridenbaugh PO, eds: Neural Blockade in Clinical Anesthesia and Management of Pain. Philadelphia: Lippincott, 1988; 935.

Boyles W, et al: Management of acute musculo-skeletal conditions: Thoracolumbar strain or sprain. A double-blind evaluation comparing the efficacy and safety of carisoprodol with diazepam. Todays Therapeutic Trends. 1983; 1(1):1.

Deyo R. Nonoperative treatment of low back disorders: Differentiating useful from useless therapy. In: Frymoyer JW, ed: The Adult Spine: Principles and Practice. New York: Raven Press, 1991; 1567.

Deyo R, et al. How many days of bed rest for acute low back pain? A randomized clinical trial. N Engl J Med 1986; 315:1064.

Deyo R, Bass J. Lifestyle and low back pain: The influence of smoking and obesity. Spine 1989; 14:501.

Deyo R, Tsui-Wu Y. Descriptive epidemiology of low back pain and its related medical care in the United States. Spine 1987; 12:264.

Dillane J, et al. Acute back syndrome: A study from general practice. Br Med J 1966; 2:82.

DiMaggio A, Mooney V. The McKenzie program: Exercise effective against back pain. J Musculoskel Med 1987; December: 63.

Donelson R, McKenzie R. Mechanical assessment and treatment of spinal pain. In: Frymoyer JW, ed: The Adult Spine: Principles and Practice. New York: Raven Press, 1991; 1627.

Frymoyer J. Back pain and sciatica. N Engl J Med 1988; 318:291.

Haldeman S, Phillips R. Spinal manipulative therapy in the management of low back pain. In: Frymoyer JW, ed. The Adult Spine: Principles and Practice. New York: Raven Press, 1991; 1581.

Kostuik J, et al. Cauda equina syndrome and lumbar disc herniation. J Bone Joint Surg 1986; 68:386.

Krolner B, Toft B. Vertebral bone loss: An unheeded side effect of therapeutic bed rest. Clin Sci 1983; 64:437.

Larsson V, et al. Auto-traction for treatment of lumbago-sciatica: A multicentre controlled investigation. Acta Orthop Scan 1980; 51:791.

Mooney V. Differential diagnosis of low back disorders. In: Frymoyer JW ed: The Adult Spine: Principles and Practice. New York: Raven Press, 1991; 1551.

Nordin M, et al. The prevention and treatment of low back disorders. In: Frymoyer JW, ed: The Adult Spine: Principles and Practice. New York: Raven Press, 1991; 1641.

Nutter P. Aerobic exercise in the treatment and prevention of low back pain. State Art Rev Occup Med 1988; 3:137.

Quebec Task Force on Spinal Disorders. Scientific approach to the assessment and management of activity-related spinal disorders. Spine 1987; 12:S1.

Saal J, et al. The natural history of lumbar intervertebral disk extrusions treated nonoperatively. Spine 1990; 15:683.

Witt P. The physical therapist approach. In: Frymoyer JW, ed: The Adult Spine: Principles and Practice. New York: Raven Press, 1991; 1619.

MANAGEMENT OF CHRONIC LOW BACK PAIN

A. Refer to A and B of the chapter on Evaluation of Back Pain (p 430). It is important to critically review the nature of prior episodes and previous therapies. Establish whether the earlier treatments resulted in improvements or whether the pain seemed to subside despite the treatment regimen. Particularly in the case of prior surgery, ascertain if the surgical intervention helped the back pain, the leg pain, or both. Distinguish whether the current presenting residual problem is primarily back or leg pain and whether the leg pain is of a radicular nature. Patient-generated pain drawings are very useful for the initial evaluation and for follow-up recording. Refer to the Quebec Classification regarding disorders of the lumbar spine.

B. Review prior studies and accompanying reports. In establishing a working clinical diagnosis, try to define a viable pain generator if possible. Supplement earlier studies by additional testing as indicated to expand diagnostic probabilities. However, if previous treatment regimens were incomplete, a comprehensive program of conservative care is indicated before proceeding with invasive/provocative imaging studies.

C. Electrodiagnostic studies, including electromyography (EMG) and nerve conduction velocity measurements, can be helpful in the chronic situation, particularly in the differentiation of radiculopathy versus peripheral neuropathy. In addition, dynamic EMG studies before and after exercise can, at times, demonstrate changes that are compatible with neurogenic claudication in spinal stenosis.

D. Nonsteroidal anti-inflammatory medications are used if there is no medical contraindication. These are the mainstay of treatment in chronic cases and are supplemented by medications such as tricyclic antidepressants when indicated. Muscle relaxants are rarely indicated except as sleeping aids. Narcotics should be avoided in chronic cases except for exceptional situations such as in the postoperative patient or in the presence of recognized neoplasms.

E. In an attempt to distinguish a pain generator, selective injection techniques, guided by radiographic control, can be of both diagnostic and therapeutic benefit. Selective nerve roots can be individually injected as well as the facets and sacroiliac joints. Epidural steroids, either through the lumbar or caudal routes, can modify radicular symptoms.

F. The various passive modalities outlined in the chapter on Management of Acute Low Back Pain (p 434) may be utilized for short periods and as a prelude to structured therapeutic exercise programs. However, these passive modalities are often used indiscriminately for extended periods, resulting in patient dependence. On the other hand, selective relaxation techniques such as biofeedback can be well incorporated into a program for chronic back pain management since many patients with back pain have unresolved multiple stressful situations in their daily lives.

G. A structured, guided program of therapeutic exercise remains the basic mode of treatment for chronic low back pain when urgent surgery is not indicated (Figs. 1 to 4). Even for patients with a well-defined pathoanatomic lesion and with static neurologic deficit, programs of well-managed exercise are an important component of an intensive conservative regimen. These exercises should be modified according to the particular clinical presentation and should be supervised by a therapist specifically trained to evaluate and treat such patients. Generally, there is a progression of the routine from range of motion (ROM) exercises, through muscle strengthening, to low impact cardiovascular training.

H. Patients with chronic low back pain, particularly those who have been out of work for 4 to 6 months, tend to develop generalized deconditioning with significant ROM and strength deficits. In this population, quantitative functional evaluation by a variety of techniques can provide a baseline of information and direct a focused therapeutic exercise program to treat the deconditioned syndrome. Such techniques include, but are not limited to: inclinometer measurements for ROM, isokinetic trunk flexion/extension, torso rotation, and lift task determinations; upper and lower extremity bicycle ergometry; and progressive isoinertial lifting.

I. Patient education is a critical component of the therapy regimen. It should emphasize prevention; fitness, strength, and endurance; lifestyle habits; ergonomics; and stress management.

J. Reassessment should take place after 3 to 4 weeks of a structured program. As long as the patient is not *objectively* worse, the conservative program should continue even if there has been little improvement in the patient's self report of pain. Rather, the clinician should be guided by functional parameters of improvement and should deemphasize, as much as possible, the pain report as a measure of success.

K. The progressive exercise regimen is designed to maximize ROM and to stress stabilization techniques by means of muscle strengthening, coordination, and endurance. These principles have been well developed in the field of Sports Medicine and are equally appropriate for the treatment of soft tissue injuries in the low back. Cardiovascular fitness training through low impact aerobics seems beneficial in preventing recurrences for the chronic low back pain patient.

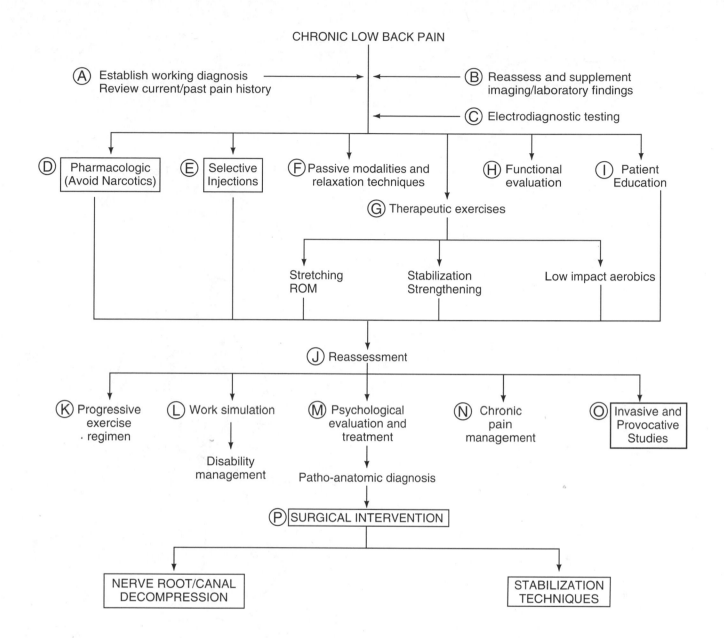

CHRONIC LOW BACK PAIN

(A) Establish working diagnosis
Review current/past pain history

(B) Reassess and supplement
imaging/laboratory findings

(C) Electrodiagnostic testing

(D) Pharmacologic
(Avoid Narcotics)

(E) Selective
Injections

(F) Passive modalities and
relaxation techniques

(H) Functional
evaluation

(I) Patient
Education

(G) Therapeutic exercises

Stretching
ROM

Stabilization
Strengthening

Low impact aerobics

(J) Reassessment

(K) Progressive
exercise
regimen

(L) Work simulation

(M) Psychological
evaluation and
treatment

(N) Chronic
pain
management

(O) Invasive and
Provocative
Studies

Disability
management

Patho-anatomic diagnosis

(P) SURGICAL INTERVENTION

NERVE ROOT/CANAL
DECOMPRESSION

STABILIZATION
TECHNIQUES

L. Work simulation/hardening is an important component of treatment for the chronic low back pain patient in the Workers' Compensation population. It is combined with ergonomic modifications as needed to assist the worker in establishing a return to the job environment. As such, work simulation is one component of the much more complex field of disability management for these patients.

M. Many patients with chronic low back pain have varying degrees of clinical depression that significantly aggravates their perception of pain and concomitant suffering. Somatization, sleep disturbances, substance abuse, and antisocial behavior are other aspects of the chronic pain syndrome that must be addressed by appropriate psychologic testing and treatment. In the more severely impaired patients, psycho-pharmaceutical intervention is indicated with the assistance of a psychiatrist.

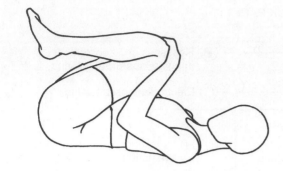

Figure 1 Flexion regimen.

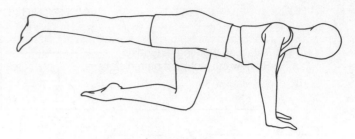

Figure 3 Stabilization techniques.

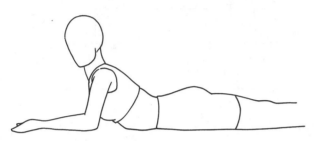

Figure 2 Extension regimen.

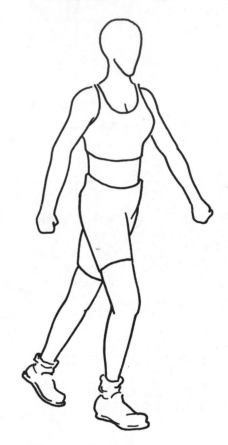

Figure 4 Aerobic fitness routine.

N. Chronic pain management with referral to a specialty clinic for intervention occasionally is required for intractable cases such as chronic canal scarring, reflex sympathetic dystrophy, recognized cancer, metabolic neuropathy, and substance abuse. Such a referral source is also helpful for selective injection techniques and when clinicians choose to refer their patients.

O. Invasive and provocative studies should be considered when 3 to 4 months of a well-managed, aggressive, conservative program has failed or when there has been documented, objective deterioration in the clinical presentation. As noted above, the patient's self report of pain alone should be viewed with caution in making this determination unless the clinician has developed a sufficient level of confidence in the particular patient. Under such circumstances, invasive and provocative testing can be viewed as preoperative maneuvers to establish, if possible, a specific pathoanatomic diagnosis prior to surgery. In this regard, computed tomographic (CT) myelography is an appro-

priate test; it is also often helpful in the evaluation of spinal stenosis cases. The CT discogram should be utilized when all other modes of investigation have failed to identify a specific pain generator, when the patient is considered to be reliable, and when the clinical diagnosis of internal disc disruption seems to be accurate. Despite these precautions, one must be cautious in the potential overinterpretation of discogram results, and one should have a high level of confidence in the experience of the discographer.

P. The details of surgical intervention for chronic low back pain are beyond the scope of this brief presentation. Nevertheless, the goal of surgery is adequate decompression of the neurologic elements and/or the treatment of a primary discogenic pain source. In addition, appropriate stabilization techniques in the form of arthrodesis with or without internal fixation devices should be undertaken when there is a defined clinical pattern of instability. See the references for further information.

References

Amlie E, et al. Treatment of acute low back pain with piroxicam: Results of a double-blind placebo-controlled trial. Spine 1987; 12:473.

Alcoff J, et al. Controlled trial of imipramine for chronic low back pain. J Fam Pract 1982; 14:841.

Aprill C. Diagnostic disc injection. In: Frymoyer JW, ed: The Adult Spine: Principles and Practice. New York: Raven Press, 1991; 403.

Berry H, Hutchinson D. Tizanidine and ibuprofen in acute low back pain: Results of a double-blind multicenter study in general practice. J Int Med Res 1988; 16:83.

Bogduk N. Back pain: Zygaphophysial blocks and epidural steroids. In: Cousins MJ, Bridenbaugh PO, eds: Neural Blockade in Clinical Anaesthesia and Pain Management. Philadelphia: Lippincott. 1988; 935.

Deyo R, et al. A controlled trial of transcutaneous electronic nerve stimulation (TENS) and exercise for chronic low back pain. N Engl J Med. 1990; 322:1627.

Deyo R, Bass J. Lifestyle and low back pain: The influence of smoking and obesity. Spine 1989; 14:501.

Donelson R, McKenzie R. Mechanical assessment and treatment of spinal pain. In: Frymoyer JW, ed: The Adult Spine: Principles and Practice. New York: Raven Press, 1991; 1627.

Garfin S, et al. Laminectomy: A review of the Pennsylvania hospital experience. J Spine Dis 1988; 1:116.

Gatchel R. Psycho-social assessment and disability management in the rehabilitation of painful spinal disorders. In: Mayer TG, Mooney V, Gatchel RJ: Contemporary Conservative Care for Painful Spinal Disorders. Philadelphia: Lea & Febiger. 1991; 441.

Herkowitz H, Kurz L. Degenerative lumbar spondylolisthesis with spinal stenosis: A prospective study comparing decompression with decompression and intertransverse process arthrodesis. J Bone Joint Surg 1991; 73:802.

Mayer T, et al. A prospective two-year study of functional restoration in industrial low back injury: An objective assessment procedure. JAMA 1987; 258:1763.

Mooney V. Differential diagnosis of low back disorders. In: Frymoyer JW, ed: The Adult Spine: Principles and Practice. New York: Raven Press, 1991; 1551.

Mooney V, Robertson J. The facet syndrome. Clin Orthop 1976; 115:149.

Nordin M, et al. The prevention and treatment of low back disorders. In: Frymoyer JW, ed: The Adult Spine: Principles and Practice. New York: Raven Press, 1991; 1641.

Nouwen A. EMG Biofeedback used to reduce standing levels of paraspinal muscle tension in chronic low back pain. Pain 1983; 17:353.

Nutter P. Aerobic exercise in the treatment and prevention of low back pain. State Art Rev Occup Med 1988; 3:137.

Polatin P. Psychoactive medications as adjuncts in functional restoration. In: Mayer TG, Mooney V, Gatchel RJ: Contemporary Conservative Care for Painful Spinal Disorders. Philadelphia: Lea & Febiger. 1991; 465.

Saal J, et al. The natural history of lumbar intervertebral disk extrusions treated nonoperatively. Spine 1990; 15:683.

Saal J, et al. The pseudoradicular syndrome: Lower extremity peripheral nerve entrapment masquerading as lumbar radiculopathy. Spine 1988; 13:926.

Spitzer W, et al. Scientific approach to the assessment and management of activity related spinal disorders: A monograph for clinicians. Report of the Quebec Task Force on Spinal Disorders. Spine 1987; 12:S1.

Waddell G. A new clinical model for the treatment of low back pain. Spine 1987; 12:632.

Waddell G. Non-organic physical signs in low back pain. Spine 1980; 5:117.

Weinstein J, et al. The pain of discography. Spine 1988; 13:1344.

West J, et al. Results of spinal arthrodeses with pedicle screw-plate fixation. J Bone Joint Surg 1991; 73:1179.

Wiskeski R, Rothmam R. Microdiscectomy techniques. Semin Spine Surg 1989; 1:54.

CERVICAL SPONDYLOSIS

A. Patients with cervical spondylosis present with symptoms ranging from localized neck pain to severe progressive myelopathy. History and physical examination are important to determine whether the onset of symptoms was acute or gradual and long term. It is important to understand the factors that aggravate the pain, including positional changes of the head and neck. The patient's perception of loss of neurologic function is also important. Plain radiographs generally are of little benefit in delineating the cause of neck and arm pain, and either magnetic resonance image (MRI) or myelography with post-contrast computed tomography (CT) scan are required to better delineate possible areas of neural compression.

B. Acute neck pain can arise from trauma, as in whiplash type injuries, or simply from unusual positioning of the neck during sleep or physical activity. Acute neck pain always is treated conservatively, with short-term immobilization, bed rest for 2–3 days, traction, nonsteroidal anti-inflammatory drugs (NSAIDs), and short-term use of muscle relaxants. Also, physical therapy with McKenzie-type exercises and electrical stimulation may be helpful. Judicious use of regional blocks can be helpful for subacute pain.

C. Patients who have evidence of multi-level spondylosis, whose primary complaint is neck pain with no neurologic loss, are treated with conservative means. Most of these patients' symptoms can be controlled without surgery. Patients who do not have multi-level disease may be candidates for further diagnostic evaluation.

D. When neck pain has been present for <1 year, conservative management is the treatment of choice. Patients who have had symptoms for >1 year and have isolated spondylosis may be candidates for discography. If discography produces exact concordant pain reproduction, anterior cervical fusion has approximately a 60%–70% success rate. If exact concordant pain is not reproduced, the patient should be managed by nonoperative means.

E. Patients who present with neck and arm pain classically fall into one of two diagnostic categories: (1) soft disc herniation or (2) spondylitic bone spurs (hard disc). This delineation often can be made on MRI or CT myelography.

F. Patients with soft disc herniation and progressive neurologic deficit should undergo surgical discectomy. The approach taken depends on the position and size of the herniation. If it is large and causes any spinal cord compression, or if it is peri-centrally placed, the patient will do best with an anterior cervical discectomy and interbody fusion (Fig. 1). Patients who have a lateral disc herniation or migration of a soft fragment into the foramen are treated by posterior microforaminotomy and removal of the fragment (Fig. 2). For those with a stable neurologic deficit or no deficit, conservative management consisting of NSAIDs, a trial of cervical traction, cervical McKenzie-type exercises, isometric cervical strengthening, progressive mobilization of the cervical spine, and judicious use of regional blocks may be of benefit. Short periods of immobilization of the neck may also be of benefit, but care must be taken not to allow the paracervical musculature to weaken due to prolonged brace wear. If symptoms do not resolve with conservative management, and if there is a clear lesion that correlates with the symptoms, the patient should undergo surgical discectomy. In the lumbar spine, the results of surgery start to fall off after 12 weeks, but there is no clear demarcation as to the length of time that conservative treatment should be undertaken for cervical disc herniations. In general, conservative management is continued as long as the symptoms and neurologic signs continue to improve. Patients who undergo surgery with associated fusion need immobilization while the graft is healing.

G. Spondylitic spurs can be off the disc space, classically off the area of the uncovertebral joint, but also they can be off the facet joint, causing nerve root impingement. Patients with neck and arm pain and neurologic deficit from spondylitic spur are less likely to improve with conservative management.

H. Surgical decompression is recommended for a patient with a neurologic deficit secondary to a spondylitic spur, if there is a clear correlation between the pathology and the symptoms. If the spondylitic spur is off the anterior disc space, it is approached anteriorly (Fig. 3). If it is off the facet joint, it is approached posteriorly with a microdecompression. For patients with no neurologic deficit but with neck and arm pain, a trial of conservative management should be undertaken. Patients also may get some symptomatic relief from cortisone injections. When there are multiple levels of spondylosis, and the precise level that is causing the symptoms is unclear, selective nerve root blocks or electromyelography may help in delineating the precise etiology and location of the symptoms. There are intradural connections between nerve rootlets that can effect the patient's clinical presentation. Patients may present with more than one root level radiculopathy from a single disc herniation. Again, if there is no resolution of symptoms with conservative management, surgical decompression should be considered.

I. Cervical spondylosis at its most advanced stages consists of spondylitic spurs or large central disc herniations that cause spinal cord compression and dysfunction.

CERVICAL SPONDYLOSIS

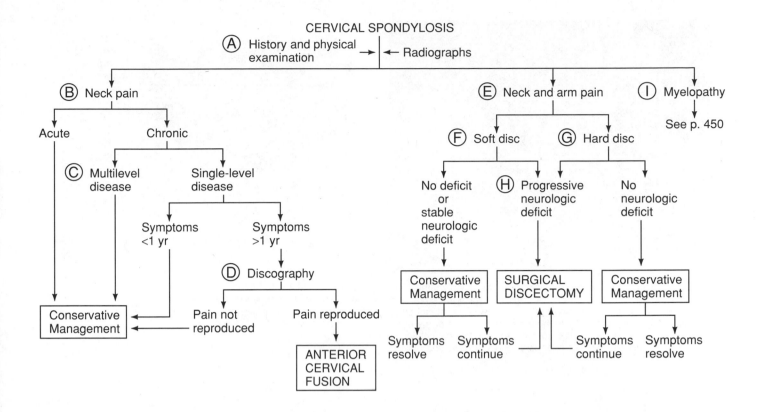

See p. 450

443

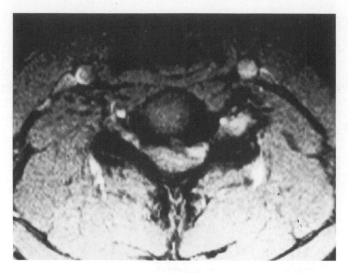

Figure 1 Young man with a left-sided cervical radiculopathy. This axial MRI image shows a large disk fragment which is central and to the left, causing compression of the left side of the spinal cord, and also disk fragments out into the foramen. Because of the large size of this disk and the spinal cord compression, this patient would best be approached by an anterior cervical discectomy and fusion.

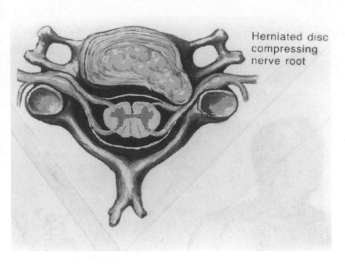

Figure 2 Lateral foraminal herniation in the cervical spine. Because the actual herniation is lateral to the spinal cord, this could be approached safely by a posterior foraminal decompression and discectomy with anticipated good results.

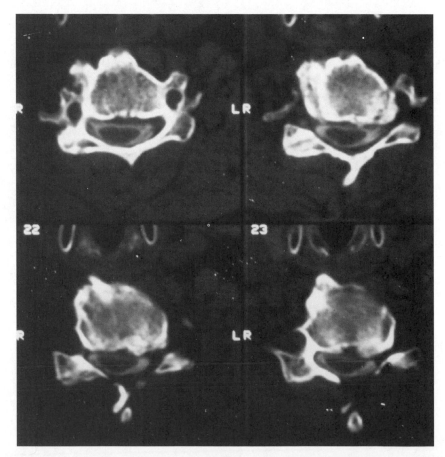

Figure 3 In this man who presented with symptoms of myelo-radiculopathy there is a large osteophytic bar across the anterior disk space with associated foraminal stenosis. This patient would best be approached by an anterior decompression, either a vertebrectomy or a wide discectomy.

References

Boden SD, Weisel SW. Conservative treatment for cervical disk disease. Semin Spine Surg 1989; 1:229.

Clement DH, O'Leary PF. Anterior cervical discectomy and fusion. Spine 1990; 15:1023.

Gore DR, Sepic SB, Gardner GM, et al. Neck pain: A long-term follow-up of 205 patients. Spine 1987; 12:1.

Gush MR, Wolf SL. Applications of transcutaneous electrical nerve stimulation in the management of patients with pain. Phys Ther 1985; 65:314.

Herkowitz HN, Kurz LT, Overholt DP. Surgical management of cervical soft disc herniation: A comparison between anterior and posterior approach. Spine 1990; 15:1026.

Johnson RM, Hart DL, et al. Cervical orthosis: A study in normal subjects comparing their effectiveness in restricting cervical motion. J Bone Joint Surg 1977; 59A:323.

Macnab I. Cervical spondylosis. Clin Orthop 1975; 109:69.

Manzo JM, Simmons EH, Kallen F. Intradural connections between adjacent cervical spinal roots. Spine 1987; 12:964.

Murphy MJ, Lieponis JV. Nonoperative treatment of cervical spine pain. The Cervical Spine. Philadelphia, J.B. Lippincott, 1989; 670.

Spurling RB, Segerberg LH. Lateral intervertebral disc lesions in the lower cervical region. JAMA 1953; 151:354.

Whitecloud TS III, Seago RA. Cervical discogenic syndrome: Results of operative intervention in patients with positive discography. Spine 1987; 12:313.

RHEUMATOID ARTHRITIS OF THE CERVICAL SPINE

A. Rheumatoid arthritis (RA) is a systemic autoimmune disease that classically involves multiple joints in the body. Typically approximately 60%–80% of patients with rheumatoid disease show some radiographic involvement of the cervical spine (C-spine). The severity of changes in the C-spine correlates with the severity of the peripheral disease; cervical subluxation is more likely in patients with peripheral peri-articular erosions. When evaluating the patient with RA, remember that they have a high incidence of abnormalities of other organ systems, and the evaluation should be comprehensive. Evaluate pulmonary or renal involvement so that proper medical treatment can be instituted prior to consideration of surgical intervention. Most patients with RA are taking anti-arthritic medications, ranging from the non-steroidal antiinflammatory drugs to various chemotherapeutic agents, most commonly methotrexate, and also corticosteroids. The use of corticosteroids mandates that the patient be covered with augmented corticosteroids during surgery.

Prior to undergoing surgical procedure, patients with RA should undergo evaluation of the C-spine to rule out instability. Classically that instability will fall into one of three patterns: basilar invagination, C1–2 instability, and subaxial subluxation (Fig. 1).

B. Basilar invagination consists of upward migration of the odontoid process towards the foramen magnum and may involve actual compression of the upper cervical cord and brain stem. Evaluation for basilar invagination on plain x-ray films can be difficult. Classically if the odontoid process is below Chamberlain's line (a line drawn from the anterior rim of the posterior foramen magnum to the hard palate), basilar invagination does not exist. Ranawat and associates have developed a measurement for evaluation of basilar invagination, which consists of drawing a line along the coronal axis of C1, connecting the center of the anterior arch of C1 with the center of the posterior arch of C1. A second line starts at the center of the sclerotic rim of C2 (the pedicles) and extends superiorly along the mid axis of the odontoid until it intercepts the first line. A measurement of <13 mm is considered abnormal. Similarly if the body of the axis is immediately behind the arch of the atlas on the lateral radiograph, this can be a useful sign of vertical instability.

C. When there is no evidence of significant basilar invagination, observation is the treatment of choice. For patients who have migration of the odontoid consistent with basilar invagination, a magnetic resonance image (MRI) can be useful. Distortion of the spinal cord on MRI correlates with signs of myelopathy, as does a brain stem cervico-medullary angle <135° (normal is 135–175°) on MRI. Cord compression on MRI also correlates with clinical signs of myelopathy (Fig. 2). When there is no evidence of cord compression, observation is the treatment of choice.

D. Patients who have cord compression on MRI but no clinical evidence of myelopathy are best treated by posterior occiput to C2 fusion. Cervical arthrodesis can be very beneficial in patients who do not have severe myelopathy. Therefore, fusion is indicated in patients who are at high risk for developing myelopathy. Patients who are clinically myelopathic and have evidence of basilar invagination can go directly forward with a posterior occiput to C2 fusion (Fig. 3). If the myelopathy resolves after this fusion they can be clinically observed for subaxial subluxation, which is more likely to occur after cervical-occipital fusion. As an alternative, patients with basilar invagination and clinical myelopathy can be placed in traction, and very slowly, over 1 to 2 weeks, can have careful reduction of their basilar invagination, followed by posterior occiput to C2 fusion. If the myelopathy does not resolve after fusion, these patients should be considered for anterior odontoid resection.

E. C1–2 instability (Fig. 4) also commonly occurs in patients with RA. One study found that rheumatoid atlantoaxial instability was present in 1 of 30 patients with any evidence of rheumatoid disease, 1 of 15 patients with clinical disease, and 1 of 5 patients hospitalized for rheumatoid disease. For patients who have documented instability on flexion-extension radiographs that is <5 mm and who are not clinically myelopathic, observation is the treatment of choice. Space available for the cord (i.e., a posterior atlanto-odontoid interval ≤13 mm) is a very important criterion for determining risk for myelopathy. Also, the severity of paralysis rather than its duration is the important factor in predicting the prognosis for neural recovery following surgery. Patients operated on with less severe myelopathy do better than those with severe myelopathy. For patients who have 5 to 10 mm of instability, the treatment depends on the presence or absence of neurologic involvement.

F. The most frequent symptom of C1–2 subluxation is pain localized to the upper neck or radiating to the occiput, forehead, or eyes. There may be paresthesias in the occipital area if the second cervical nerve root is compressed. With advancing spinal cord or medullary compression, these patients may complain of weakness of the arms or legs, paresthesias, vertigo, gait abnormalities, and poor coordination of the hands. In the later stages there may be involvement of the bowel and bladder. With involvement of the vertebral artery, the patients may have nystagmus or bulbar signs as well as episodic loss of consciousness. Often it is difficult to ascertain the evidence of my-

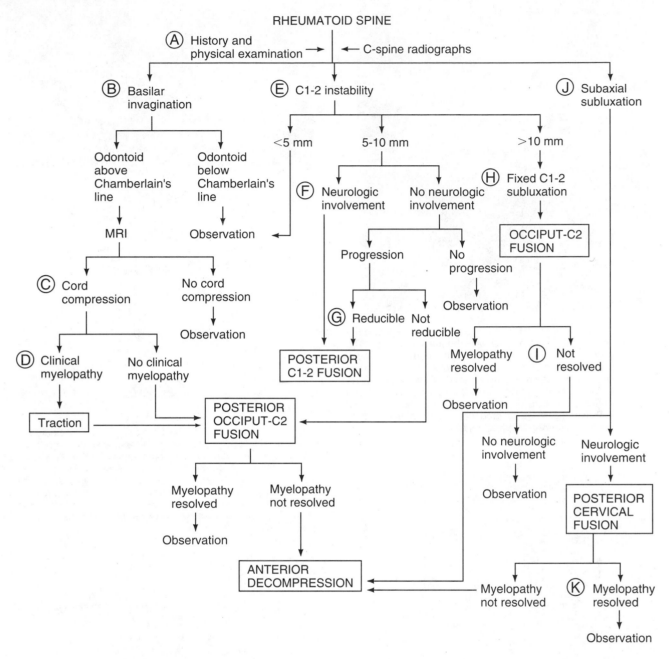

RHEUMATOID SPINE

(A) History and physical examination → ← C-spine radiographs

(B) Basilar invagination

(E) C1-2 instability

(J) Subaxial subluxation

Odontoid above Chamberlain's line → MRI

Odontoid below Chamberlain's line → Observation

<5 mm

5-10 mm

>10 mm

(H) Fixed C1-2 subluxation

(F) Neurologic involvement

No neurologic involvement

OCCIPUT-C2 FUSION

(C) Cord compression

No cord compression → Observation

Progression

No progression → Observation

(G) Reducible   Not reducible

Myelopathy resolved

(I) Not resolved

(D) Clinical myelopathy

No clinical myelopathy

POSTERIOR C1-2 FUSION

Observation

Traction →

POSTERIOR OCCIPUT-C2 FUSION ←

No neurologic involvement → Observation

Neurologic involvement

Myelopathy resolved → Observation

Myelopathy not resolved

POSTERIOR CERVICAL FUSION

ANTERIOR DECOMPRESSION ←

Myelopathy not resolved

(K) Myelopathy resolved → Observation

elopathy in these patients due to the severe involvement of their peripheral joints. For patients who have evidence of neurologic involvement with 5 to 10 mm of instability, a posterior C1–2 fusion is the treatment of choice (Fig. 5). Those who do not have neurologic involvement should have careful follow-up for progression of disease. Progression occurs in a variable number of patients. For those with documented progression, the treatment depends on the reducibility of the C1–2 subluxation and the possible need to decompress the spinal cord.

G. Patients who have documented progression of C1–2 instability and a reducible C1–2 articulation should have a posterior C1–2 fusion. If the subluxation is fixed or not reducible, consider a posterior occiput to C2 fusion with laminectomy of C1, due to the difficulty of getting a solid fusion to C1 in this situation.

H. Patients with >10 mm of subluxation are at high risk for development of myelopathy. If the subluxation is reducible, they should have a posterior C1–2 fusion. If the subluxation is fixed, they should have removal of the lamina of C1 posteriorly and an occiput to C2 fusion. If the myelopathy resolves with the posterior fusion, observation for further progression of subaxial instability is undertaken.

I. Patients whose myelopathy does not resolve and who have a fixed subluxation of C1 on C2 should undergo an anterior resection of the odontoid process. This can be carried out through a transoral approach and has a good success rate. After a posterior fusion is obtained, it is not necessary to place a graft anteriorly; therefore the risk of infection with odontoid resection without the need for anterior fusion is reduced.

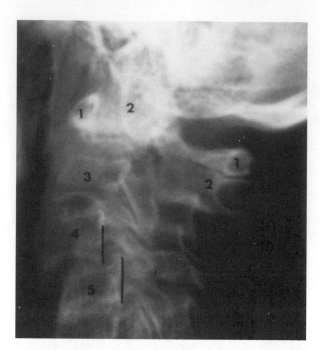

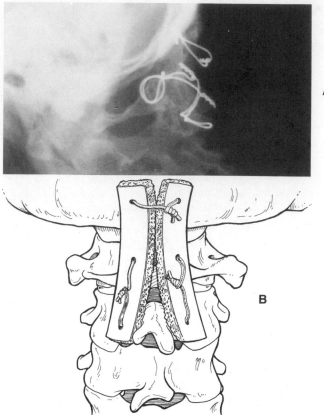

Figure 1 Lateral x-ray of a 54-year-old female who shows all three of the instability patterns associated with rheumatoid arthritis. The anterior ring of C1 has subluxed inferiorly on the body of C2, allowing for superior migration of the odontoid process into the foramen magnum. This constitutes basilar invagination. There also is some subluxation of C1 anteriorly in relation to the odontoid process and evidence of subaxial subluxation at the C4–5 level. The patient with this dramatic abnormality would probably require a pan-occiput-cervical fusion incorporating all the areas of instability.

Figure 3 The treatment for basilar invagination is occiput to cervical fusion. Classically this is done with wiring of bone grafts to the occiput and upper cervical vertebrae as depicted in **A**, showing a solid occiput to C2 fusion. **B**, The wires securing the grafts to the occiput are passed between the tables of the occiput. A sublaminar wire is passed under the lamina of C1 and connected to a wire that is passed through the spinous process of C2 to secure the grafts in position over the laminae, which have been previously cleaned of all soft tissue.

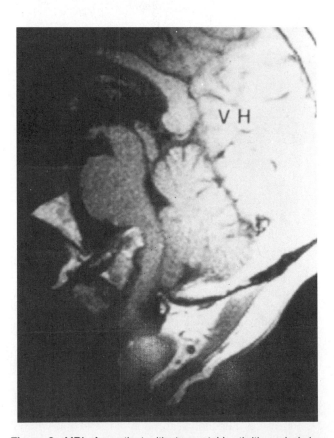

Figure 2 MRI of a patient with rheumatoid arthritis and obvious basilar invagination. The odontoid process has migrated superiorly through the foramen magnum, causing significant compression on the brain stem and decreasing the angle of the brain stem to <135°.

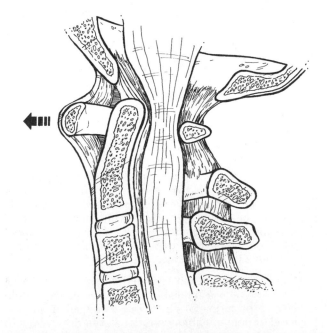

Figure 4 The articulation between the transverse ligament and the odontoid process is a synovial joint. With rheumatoid involvement of this articulation the transverse ligament becomes incompetent and this allows for anterior subluxation of C1 on C2.

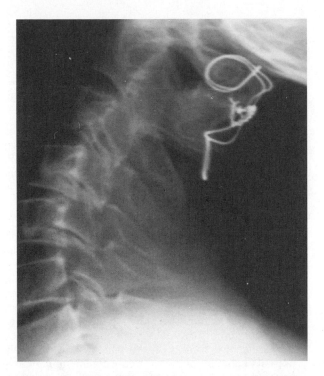

Figure 5 C1–2 Instability secondary to rheumatoid disease, treated with a C1 to C2 fusion using a modified Gallie technique with a sublaminar wire at C1 and a spinous processes wire at C2, wiring rectangular corticocancellous grafts down across the lamina. A solid arthrodesis has been achieved.

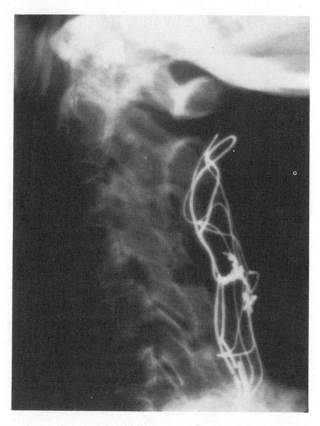

Figure 6 Lateral radiograph of a 52-year-old female with rheumatoid arthritis who had multi-level subaxial subluxations treated by a long posterior cervical fusion from C2 to C7. There is some residual subluxation at C4–5. In patients with subaxial subluxation and kyphotic deformity, all levels of the instability and deformity need to be incorporated into the fusion.

J. Patients with subaxial subluxation may have symptoms that range from neck pain to radicular arm pain to obvious myelopathy. The subaxial subluxation may occur at multiple levels. If there is no evidence of neurologic involvement, observation is the treatment of choice. If neurologic involvement is noted, the patient should undergo a posterior cervical fusion (Fig. 6). Posterior cervical fusion is recommended over anterior cervical fusion, because there are significant risks and complications with anterior fusion. When a solid posterior fusion is obtained and the myelopathy resolves, observation for subsequent levels of instability should be undertaken.

K. If myelopathy does not resolve, anterior decompression can be performed as a second procedure with good results.

References

Breedveld FC, Algra PR, Vielvoye CJ, Cats A. Magnetic resonance imaging in the evaluation of patients with rheumatoid arthritis and subluxations of the cervical spine. Arthritis Rheum 1987; 30:624.

Bundschuh CV, Modic MT, Kearny F, et al. Rheumatoid arthritis of the cervical spine: Surface coil MR imaging. Am J Neuro Rad 1988; 9:565.

Clark CR, Goetz DD, Menezes AH. Arthrodesis of the cervical spine in rheumatoid arthritis. J Bone Joint Surg 1989; 71A:381.

Crockard HA, Pozo JL, Ransford AO, et al. Transoral decompression and posterior fusion for rheumatoid atlanto-axial subluxation. J Bone Joint Surg 1986; 68B:350.

Delamarter RB, Dodge L, Bohlman HH, Gambetti PL. Orthopaedic transactions 1988; 12:54.

Dodge LD, Bohlman HH, Rechtine GR. Paralysis secondary to rheumatoid arthritis: Pathogenesis secondary to rheumatoid arthritis. Orthop Trans 11:473.

Fielding JW, Cochran G van B, Lawsing JF 3rd, Hohl M. Tears of the transverse ligament of the atlas: A clinical and biomechanical study. J Bone Joint Surg 1974; 55A:1683.

Heywood AWB, Learmonth ID, Thomas M. Cervical spine instability in rheumatoid arthritis. J Bone Joint Surg 1988; 70B:702.

Lipson SJ. Cervical myelopathy and posterior atlanto-axial subluxation in patients with rheumatoid arthritis. J Bone Joint Surg 1985; 67A:593.

Meijers KAE, Van Beusekom GT, Luyendik W, Dukjfjes F. Dislocation of the cervical spine with cord compression in rheumatoid arthritis. J Bone Joint Surg 1974; 56B:668.

Pellicci PM, Ranawat CS, Tsairs P, Bryan WJ. A prospective study of the progression of rheumatoid arthritis of the cervical spine. J Bone Joint Surg 1981; 63A:342.

Rana NA. Natural history of atlanto-axial subluxation in rheumatoid arthritis. Spine 1989; 14:1054.

Ranawat CS, O'Leary P, Pellicci P, et al. Cervical spine fusion in rheumatoid arthritis. J Bone Joint Surg 1979; 61A:1003.

Sharp J, Purser DW. Spontaneous atlanto-axial dislocation in ankylosing spondylitis and rheumatoid arthritis. Am Rheum Dis 1961; 20:47.

Weitheim SB, Bohlman HH. Occipito-cervical fusion: Indications, technique, and long-term results in thirteen patients. J Bone Joint Surg 1987; 69A:833.

Winfield J, Cooke D, Brook AS, Corbett M. A prospective study of the radiological changes in the cervical spine in early rheumatoid arthritis. Am Rheum Dis 42:613.

CERVICAL MYELOPATHY

A. Cervical myelopathy occurs in acute and chronic forms. For patients with acute myelopathy, it is important to ascertain in the history and physical examination whether they are at high risk for development of epidural hematomas, such as patients with ankylosing spondylitis or on anticoagulant therapy. Patients at high risk for disc space infection, such as those on immunosuppression, include patients with diabetes and patients with underlying diseases that affect the immune system. Also, any history of primary neoplasm needs to be obtained.

B. Treat the patient with acute myelopathy expeditiously. If there is no contraindication, begin corticosteroids. The exact regimen of cortisone use in this instance has not been clearly defined. Order a diagnostic work-up consisting of myelography with post-contrast computed tomography (CT) scan, magnetic resonance imaging (MRI), or both, depending on the particular lesion involved.

C. Depending on the patient's history and other predisposing factors, there may be a high index of suspicion for a specific lesion, such as a disc space infection in patients who are at high risk for infection. In that setting, technetium bone scan and/or gallium scan may also be of benefit.

D. Patients with an acute herniated disc with evidence of myelopathy should undergo anterior cervical discectomy and fusion.

E. For those patients with evidence of an epidural hematoma, first delineate the extent of the hematoma, define its cause, and correct any reversible bleeding abnormalities. Then decompress the area of hematoma. This is classically done by a laminectomy. For patients with an epidural abscess and acute myelopathy, delineate the extent of the abscess. If the patient has an underlying susceptibility to infection, this should be defined and the patient placed on appropriate antibiotics; then surgical decompression of the involved area of epidural abscess is undertaken. Again, this is classically done by a laminectomy. If, however, there is associated bony destruction anteriorly, the patient will require anterior debridement and stabilization, because in this setting laminectomy alone is associated with an increased incidence of neurologic loss.

F. Diagnosis of a disc space infection requires a high degree of clinical suspicion as patients may present with vague neck pain without any obvious fever or elevation of white blood cell count. Patients at high risk for infection who present with neck pain of unclear etiology, or especially neck pain that is worsened at night, are evaluated to rule out disc space infection. Technetium bone scan and gallium scan combination is better than technetium bone scan alone, and MRI is the most sensitive study for delineation of disc space infection. A patient with cervical myelopathy due to disc space infection should undergo anterior debridement down to normal viable tissue and then an autograft strut fusion and antibiotic therapy.

G. After debridement and anterior strut fusion, if there is any involvement of the posterior elements or evidence of instability there, fusion is augmented with a halo vest or cast to maintain proper spinal alignment. In the setting of spinal infection, instrumentation acutely is not recommended.

H. Acute cervical myelopathy can be caused by primary or metastatic tumors. Metastatic tumors are much more common than primary tumors. Primary tumors that can present with acute myelopathy include osteoblastoma, chordoma, eosinophilic granuloma, giant cell tumor, aneurysmal bone cyst, and isolated plasmacytoma. The treatment depends on the tumor type. For patients with acute myelopathy secondary to metastatic tumor, treatment depends on the presence of significant deformity. If the patient is in relatively normal alignment, a tumor is causing the neural compression, and the tumor is radiosensitive, radiation and bracing is the treatment of choice. When the spinal compression is caused by progressive collapse and deformity of the spinal column as well as tumor cells, the treatment of choice is surgical debridement and decompression as well as fusion. The type of fusion performed depends on the tumor type and the presumed longevity of the patient. If survival is anticipated to be longer than 6 months to a year, the construct should include a bone graft that will allow for fusion and long-term stabilization. If only very short-term survival is likely, methylmethacrylate can allow for immediate mobilization.

I. The most common form of chronic cervical myelopathy is secondary to spondylosis. Patients with chronic spinal cord dysfunction classically are >50 years of age; have varying symptoms of unsteadiness of gait, weakness, and atrophy of the upper extremities with loss of dexterity of the hands; and motor abnormalities tend to predominate over sensory abnormalities. They may have varying degrees of spasticity; hyperreflexia and long tract signs, such as extensor plantar responses tend to be late findings. The clinical course is marked by spontaneous exacerbations and remissions. The remissions do not constitute resolution of the myelopathic symptoms, but simply stabilization at a plateaued level of neurologic dysfunction.

J. For patients with a mild myelopathy that is stable and not progressive, consider observation. However, it should be noted that the degree of success with surgery for myelopathy is affected by the severity of the myelopathy and by the timing of the surgery in relationship to neural progression. Patients with more severe myelopathy, or those who are operated on while their myelopathy is actively progressing, do not have as good a prognosis for surgical intervention.

CERVICAL MYELOPATHY

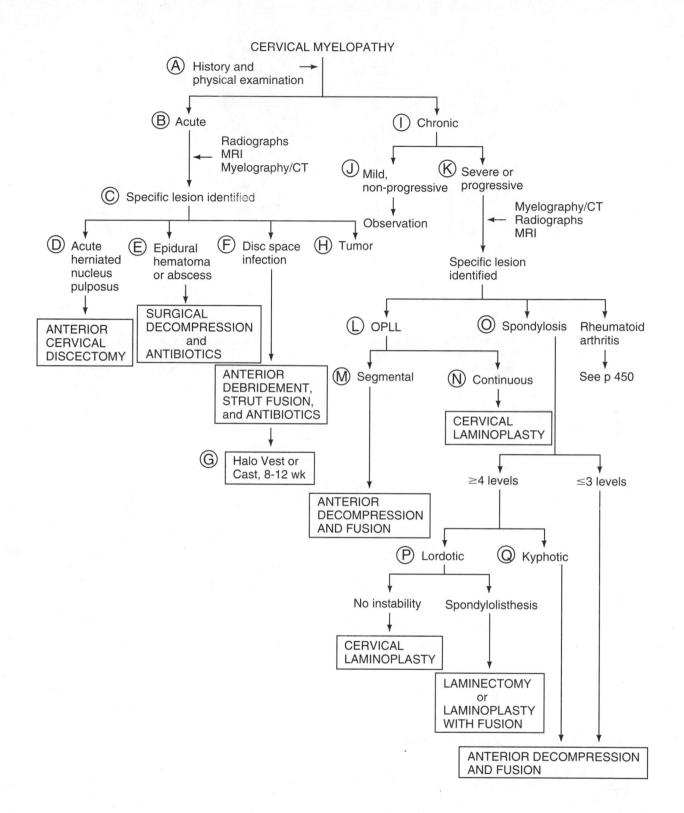

(A) History and physical examination

(B) Acute

Radiographs
MRI
Myelography/CT

(C) Specific lesion identified

(D) Acute herniated nucleus pulposus

(E) Epidural hematoma or abscess

(F) Disc space infection

(H) Tumor

ANTERIOR CERVICAL DISCECTOMY

SURGICAL DECOMPRESSION and ANTIBIOTICS

ANTERIOR DEBRIDEMENT, STRUT FUSION, and ANTIBIOTICS

(G) Halo Vest or Cast, 8-12 wk

(I) Chronic

(J) Mild, non-progressive

Observation

(K) Severe or progressive

Myelography/CT
Radiographs
MRI

Specific lesion identified

(L) OPLL

(O) Spondylosis

Rheumatoid arthritis

See p 450

(M) Segmental

(N) Continuous

CERVICAL LAMINOPLASTY

ANTERIOR DECOMPRESSION AND FUSION

≥4 levels

≤3 levels

(P) Lordotic

(Q) Kyphotic

No instability

Spondylolisthesis

CERVICAL LAMINOPLASTY

LAMINECTOMY or LAMINOPLASTY WITH FUSION

ANTERIOR DECOMPRESSION AND FUSION

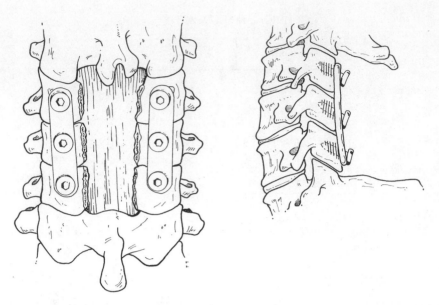

Figure 1 For patients who require laminectomy, lateral mass plates allow for rigid fixation with a high rate of successful fusion.

K. Patients with severe myelopathy or evidence of progression from a previous time are evaluated for the specific cause and location of the spinal cord compression with the thought of undergoing surgical decompression. In the cervical spine, the diagnostic tool of choice is myelography followed by post-contrast CT scan. MRI can be useful, however, in delineating intrinsic abnormalities within the substance of the spinal cord itself.

L. Patients with ossification of the posterior longitudinal ligament (OPLL) most commonly are of Asian or Middle Eastern descent. However, patients of any race or ethnic background can have OPLL.

M. Patients with segmental OPLL are generally best approached by an anterior decompression, removal of the ossified area, and fusion over the involved disc spaces.

N. Because the continuous form of OPLL tends to involve multiple levels, these patients are generally best approached by a cervical laminoplasty. Some evidence suggests that patients clinically do better with laminoplasty than with laminectomy, although this is controversial. Also, there may be less progression of the OPLL after laminoplasty than after laminectomy.

O. In cervical spondylitic myelopathy the surgical approach depends on the number of levels involved and the patient's anatomic alignment.

P. Patients who have involvement of four levels or more, are in a neutral or lordotic posture, and have no evidence of clinical instability can be treated with either laminectomy or laminoplasty. Evidence suggests that these patients have a better prognosis with laminoplasty. Because the spinal cord compression, even in patients with a normal lordosis, is typically anterior, the spinal cord may not move away from the anterior osteophytes with a posterior decompression, and the patient may have to undergo a secondary anterior decompression. Typically anterior decompression is safer and needs to be done over fewer disc levels if performed after posterior decompression. Patients who have evidence of instability, such as spondylolisthesis, but who are in a lordotic posture, should undergo a laminectomy and/or laminoplasty with associated interfacet fusion (Fig. 1).

Q. Patients with a kyphotic posture or who present with three disc levels or less of spinal cord compression should undergo an anterior decompression and fusion.

References

Bernard TN Jr., Whitecloud TS. Cervical spondylotic myeloradiculopathy: Anterior decompression and stabilization with autogenous fibular strut graft. Clin Orthop 1987; 221:149.

Bracken MD, Separd MJ, Collins WF, et al. A randomized controlled trial of methyl prednisolone or naloxone in the treatment of acute spinal cord injury: Results of the second national acute spinal cord injury study. N Engl J Med 1990; 332:1405.

Cervical Spinal Research Society. Cervical spondylotic myelopathy. Spine 1988; 13:828.

Epstein JA, Epstein NE. The surgical management of cervical spinal stenosis, spondylosis, and myeloradiculopathy by means of the posterior approach: The cervical spine, 2nd ed. Philadelphia, J.B. Lippincott, 1989; 625.

Herkowitz HN. A comparison of anterior cervical fusion, cervical laminectomy and cervical laminoplasty for the surgical management of multiple level spondylotic radiculopathy. Spine 1988; 13:774.

Hirabayaski K, Satoni K. Operative procedure and results of expansive open door laminoplasty. Spine 1988; 13:870.

Hukada S, Mochizuki T, Ogata M, et al. Operations for cervical spondylotic myelopathy: A comparison of the results of anterior and posterior procedures. J Bone Joint Surg 1985; 67B:609.

McAfee PC, Regan JJ, Bohlman HH. Cervical cord compression from ossification of the posterior longitudinal ligament in non-Orientals. J Bone Joint Surg 1987; 69B:569.

Nakano N, Nakano T, Nakano K. Comparison of the results of laminectomy and open door laminoplasty for cervical spondylotic myeloradiculopathy and OPLL. Spine 1988; 13:792.

Okada K, Shirasaki N, Hayashi H, et al. Treatment of cervical spondylitic myelopathy by enlargement of the spinal canal anteriorly, followed by arthrodesis. J Bone Joint Surg 1991; 73A:352.

White AA, Panjabi MM. Biomechanical considerations in the surgical management of cervical spondylotic myelopathy. Spine 1988; 13:856.

Yonenobu K, Fuji T, Ono K, et al. Choice of surgical treatment for multi-segmental cervical spondylotic myelopathy. Spine 1985; 10:710.

Zdeblick TA, Bohlman HH. Cervical kyphosis and myelopathy: Treatment by anterior corpectomy and strut grafting. J Bone Joint Surg 1989; 71A:170.

SPONDYLOLISTHESIS

A. Spondylolisthesis in the adult, with the exception of traumatic and pathologic spondylolistheses, typically presents with a long history of back pain that may be punctuated with waxing and waning symptoms. It is unusual for spondylolisthesis in the adult to present with acute neurologic loss. A more common scenario is the onset of intermittent radicular or neurogenic claudicatory-type symptoms that slowly become a more prominent part of the history. The physical findings vary depending on the degree of slippage and the acuteness of symptoms. It is important to remember that the spondylolisthesis may not be the cause of an adult patient's back pain. The incidence of disc degeneration is increased compared to the control population in patients over the age of 25, and this may be the cause of the patient's pain, not the listhesis itself.

B. Traumatic spondylolisthesis is caused most typically by a fall from a height. The fractures generally are not simply through the pars interarticularis, as is seen in isthmic spondylolisthesis, but may include the facets, the pedicles, and/or the pars interarticularis. The traumatic spondylolisthesis must be watched carefully for progressive slippage. For the patient with a traumatic spondylolisthesis of grade I or less, an attempt at allowing the fractures to heal by bracing should be the initial mode of treatment employed. If the listhesis is at the L5-S1 level, the thoracolumbosacral orthosis (TLSO) should incorporate one thigh into the brace. Maintain careful follow-up. If there is any evidence of progressive slippage in the brace, the patient should have surgical stabilization of the listhetic level. If the pedicles are intact, that can be a single level fusion with pedicle instrumentation. If the pedicles are not intact, perform a two-level fusion with fusion to the adjacent superior level. For patients with a grade II or greater listhesis of traumatic origin, perform direct surgical stabilization. Remember that sometimes it is difficult to delineate an acute fracture from a long-standing spondylolitic defect. Generally a bone scan is hot in an acute fracture but positive in only a small percentage of patients with a chronic listhesis. Also, on computed tomography (CT) scan an acute fracture often can be delineated by the absence of heavy sclerotic bone.

C. Degenerative spondylolisthesis is based on the advancement of the degenerative cascade with disc degeneration and facet degeneration over time, presenting with incompetence of the facet joint and anterior listhesis of the proximal on the distal vertebra. This most commonly occurs at the L4-5 level (Fig. 1) and to a lesser degree at L3-4 and L5-S1. It is felt that L5-S1 is protected because of the strong iliolumbar and lumbosacral ligaments. Typically these patients present with a long history of episodic back pain.

D. Degenerative spondylolisthesis may present with progressive neurogenic claudication that initially may be predominantly L5 nerve root related to impingement from the large osteophytes at the L4-5 facet. However, all nerve levels from the listhesis down may be involved, and patients may present with cauda equina syndrome. When there are symptoms of neurogenic claudication, perform the physical examination first with the patient at rest and then after exercise to the point of having symptoms. Typically the neurologic examination is normal with the patient at rest, and there may be some neurologic loss with exercise. As with spinal stenosis in general, consider a differential diagnosis of vascular claudication or peripheral neuropathy. If spinal stenosis is suspected, obtain a magnetic resonance imaging (MRI) or a myelogram and post-myelogram-CT to delineate the degree and exact levels of spinal stenosis present. For patients who present with a fixed neurologic deficit or symptoms of neurogenic claudication that are severely limiting function, consider surgical decompression and fusion. There is some controversy as to whether the fusion is needed, but Herkowitz and Kurz showed in a prospective study that patients with degenerative spondylolisthesis did better post-surgery when a concomitant fusion was performed.

E. Patients who have no neurologic symptoms but simply midline back pain with no other discernible cause are treated by non-operative means. Conservative management includes patient education, an exercise program, and perhaps intermittent bracing. The exercise program should emphasize posture and correct body mechanics as well as minimizing twisting and rotational motions. It should consist of a flexion regimen of abdominal strengthening, either isometric or isotonic, pelvic tilt, knee-to-chest exercises, and a low impact aerobic conditioning program. Bracing may be necessary on an intermittent basis to control the patient's symptoms. Other conservative modalities that can be tried are short periods of bed rest, symptomatic medications (predominantly nonsteroidal anti-inflammatories), traction, epidural injections, and facet joint infiltration for short-term relief of an acute exacerbation of symptoms. For patients with symptomatic spondylolysis or minimal spondylolisthesis unresponsive to conservative care, consider surgical repair of the defect.

F. When a patient continues to have severe back pain unresponsive to conservative management, undertake further evaluation. If the adjacent discs are normal and are painless on discography, consider surgical decompression and fusion of the old listhetic level. For patients who have multiple levels of disc degeneration, surgery does not tend to be beneficial, except to treat pain of neurologic origin.

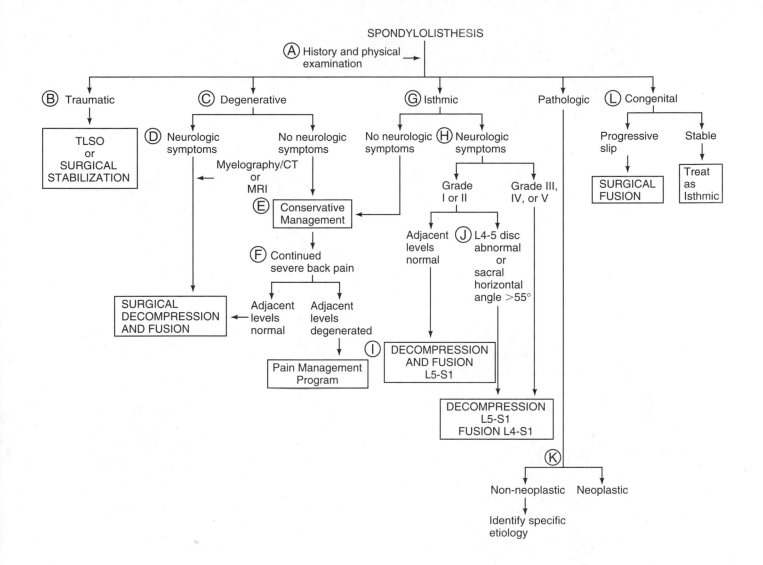

G. Isthmic spondylolisthesis (Fig. 2) occurs in two varieties: sub-type A, a lytic pars defect, and sub-type B, an elongation of the pars interarticularis. They are felt to be variations of the same etiology, a stress fracture of the pars interarticularis. The elongation occurs with repetitive stress fractures and healing over time. Again, in the adult with no neurologic symptoms, one cannot assume that the listhetic level is the etiology of the patient's pain. Evaluate the adjacent discs before considering surgical options. Most patients with simply midline back pain can be controlled by conservative means.

H. In patients with isthmic spondylolisthesis, the typical neurologic symptoms tend to be evidence of L5 radiculopathy related to the fibrocartilaginous mass at the side of the pars defect. Neurologic loss can also be attributed to a disc herniation at the adjacent levels, stretching of the nerve with the listhesis, far lateral syndrome where the nerve is caught between the transverse process of L5 and the sacral ala, or other causes of peripheral neuritis (diabetes).

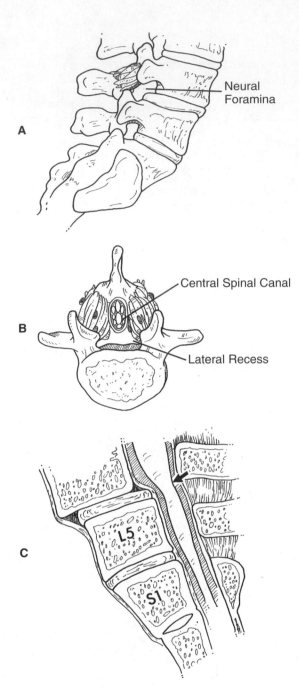

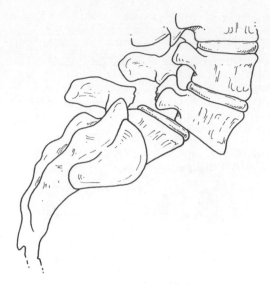

Figure 2 Isthmic spondylolisthesis. Bilateral defects in the pars interarticularis allow for anterior translation of L5 on S1 with resultant narrowing of the neuroforamina at L5–S1. This can occur at L4–5 or L3–4 as well but is much less common.

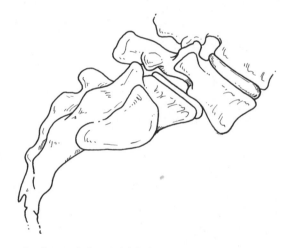

Figure 3 Congenital spondylolisthesis due to inadequate development of the L5–S1 facet complexes. Anterior listhesis of L5 allows the lamina to translate with the vertebral body of L5, causing severe spinal stenosis and cauda equina compression.

Figure 1 Degenerative spondylolisthesis most commonly occurs at the L4–5 level. **A,** Degeneration of the facet leads to facet hypertrophy, which in turn may lead to the facet becoming incompetent and allowing anterior translation. **B,** The hypertrophy of the inferior facet of the vertebrae above leads to central canal stenosis. The superior facet hypertrophy leads to narrowing of the lateral recess and neural foramina. **C,** With anterior listhesis the dural sac is narrow, causing pressure on the cauda equina.

I. For the patient with evidence of neurologic loss related to the listhesis itself, consider decompression and fusion. Patients who present with a grade I or grade II spondylolisthesis in which the other adjacent discs are normal can be treated by decompression of the L5 nerve roots and fusion simply of the L5—S1 interspace. There is some controversy as to whether decompression is absolutely necessary. In the adolescent, fusion alone seems to be adequate even in the presence of a neurologic deficit. However, in the adult, the tendency is to do a surgical decompression of the involved nerve roots.

J. Patients with a grade I or grade II spondylolisthesis in which the L4—5 disc is abnormal and the L3—4 disc is normal should be treated with a decompression of the L5—S1 interspace and fusion from L4 to S1. This is also the treatment of choice for patients who have a high sacral horizontal angle (>55°). For patients who have abnormal discs at L3—4 and L4—5, decompression and fusion of the L5—S1 interspace alone should be performed. Those who present with a grade III, grade IV, or grade V (spondyloptosis) spondylolisthesis are treated with decompression and fusion from L4 to S1. There is no one accepted technique for obtaining fusion in these patients. Successful methods include posterior in situ fusion alone, posterior lateral fusion with associated interbody fusion of L5—S1 via a fibular graft inserted from posterior, anterior fusion with associated posterior fusion, and multiple different types of instrumentation. For the patient with spondyloptosis, consideration may need to be given to complete spondylectomy of L5 and reduction of L4 onto the sacrum. In the adult, it is not recommended that the L5 vertebrae be reduced due to the high rate of neurologic injury.

K. Pathologic fractures consist of a defect in the posterior arch because of abnormalities of the bone itself, either underlying metabolic bone disease or neoplasia. For patients with spondylolisthesis due to metabolic bone disease, the specific etiology should be identified and the underlying problem treated, with the spondylolisthesis monitored for progression. The listhesis itself may stabilize with treatment of the underlying bone disease. If the pathologic fracture is due to neoplasia, treatment depends on tumor type, its sensitivity to radiation, neurologic involvement, and life expectancy of the patient.

L. Congenital spondylolisthesis consists of structural anomalies of the lumbosacral junction resulting in inadequate mechanical support to prevent forward slippage of L5 on S1 (Fig. 3). In the adolescent, congenital spondylolisthesis may present as a neurologic emergency because, unlike isthmic spondylolisthesis, the posterior lamina goes with the slipping vertebra of L5. Therefore, when congenital spondylolisthesis is identified in childhood, a single level fusion of L5—S1 should be performed. In patients who present as adults, the typical picture is generally more like that of isthmic spondylolisthesis. If there is no evidence of progressive slippage or neurologic deficit, conservative treatment can be entertained. Patients with evidence of progressive slippage or neurologic symptoms are treated with decompression and fusion.

References

Bradford DS, Iza J. Repair of the defect in spondylolysis or minimal degrees of spondylolisthesis by segmental wire fixation and bone grafting. Spine 1985; 10:673.

Farfan HF. The pathological anatomy of degenerative spondylolisthesis: A cadaver study. Spine 1980; 5:412.

Gaines RW. Treatment of spondyloptosis by two stage L5 vertebrectomy and reduction of L4 onto the S1. Spine 1985; 10:680.

Grobler LS, Wiltse LC. Classification, non-operative, and operative treatment of spondylolisthesis. The Adult Spine: Principles and Practice. New York: Raven Press, 1991; 1655.

Hanley EN Jr. Decompression and distraction-derotation arthrodesis for degenerative spondylolisthesis. Spine 1986; 11:269.

Herkowitz HN, Kurz LT. Degenerative lumbar spondylolisthesis with spinal stenosis: A prospective study comparing decompression with decompression and intertransverse process arthrodesis. J Bone Joint Surg 1991; 73A:802.

Lowe J, Schachner E, Hirschberg E, et al. Significance of bone scintigraphy in symptomatic spondylolysis. Spine 1984; 9:653.

Macnab I. Spondylolisthesis with an intact neural arch: The so-called pseudo-spondylolisthesis. J Bone Joint Surg 1950; 32:325.

Macnab I. Back ache. 2nd ed., Baltimore: Williams & Wilkins, 84.

Pennell RG, Maurer AH, Bonakdarpour A. Stress injuries of the pars interarticularis: Radiologic classification and indications for scintigraphy. Am J Radiol 1985; 145:763.

Rosenberg NJ. Degenerative spondylolisthesis: Predisposing factors. J Bone Joint Surg 1975; 57:467.

Smith MD, Bohlman HH. Spondylolisthesis treated by a single-stage operation combining decompression with in-situ posterolateral and anterior fusion. J Bone Joint Surg 1990; 72:415.

Weinstein JN, Walsh TR, Spratt KF, et al. Lumbar discography: A controlled prospective study of normal volunteers to determine the false positive rate. Presented at the annual meeting of the American Academy of Orthopedic Surgeons, New Orleans, 1990.

Wiltse LL, Newman PH, Macnab I. Classification of spondyloptosis and spondylolisthesis. Clin Orthop 1976; 117:23.

Wiltse LL, Rothman LG. Spondylolisthesis: Classification, diagnosis, and natural history. Semin Spine Surg 1989; 1(2):78.

Wiltse LL, Widell EH Jr, Jackson DW. Fatigue fracture: The basic lesion in isthmic spondylolisthesis. J Bone Joint Surg 1975; 51:17.

Wiltse LL, Winter RB. Terminology and measurement of spondylolisthesis. J Bone Joint Surg 1983; 65:768.

SPINAL INFECTIONS

A. Spinal infections are rare, constituting only 2%–4% of all cases of osteomyelitis. Often patients with vertebral osteomyelitis have few systemic symptoms, such as fever or sepsis, and may have normal white blood cell counts, and therefore delay in diagnosis is not uncommon. A high index of suspicion is necessary to accurately diagnose spinal infections in the early stages. Carefully question the patient about risk factors for spinal infection, including diabetes, alcoholism, drug addiction, or a compromised immune system, as in steroid use for rheumatoid arthritis or acquired immune deficiency syndrome. Ask the patient about travel to areas of endemic infection. For example, coccidioidomycosis is endemic in the southwestern United States. The history of other recent infections of other anatomic locations is also important. When spinal infection is suspected, the initial assessment needs to include laboratory studies, of which a complete blood cell count with differential, sedimentation rate, and C-reactive protein are important. The sedimentation rate and C-reactive protein will be valuable to follow as treatment begins. Obtain blood cultures from at least two separate sites of venipuncture. If the patient's tuberculin status is unknown, place a PPD along with appropriate controls. If granulomatous disease is considered, the patient should have an anteroposterior and lateral chest radiograph. Other radiographic studies that may be of benefit include a bone scan, gallium scan, and/or magnetic resonance imaging (MRI). A bone scan is highly sensitive in detecting lesions of osteomyelitis if they have been present >48 hours. It is less sensitive in picking up disc space infections, and the combined technetium bone scan and gallium scan have a higher sensitivity than technetium scanning alone for disc space infections. The most sensitive and specific test, however, is MRI, which also gives more detailed anatomic information on which to base treatment decisions.

B. Generally neurologic involvement occurs later in the course of spinal infection. Neurologic compromise can be caused by progressive spread of infected material into the epidural space or by collapse of the infected vertebrae with deformity or bone fragments causing neurologic involvement. Once blood cultures have been drawn and laboratory studies taken, the patient with suspected spinal infection and evidence of neurologic involvement is begun on a course of broad-spectrum antibiotics to cover the most likely causes of infection. Antibiotics are begun before definitive biopsy, because neurologic involvement requires expeditious treatment. If the symptoms, bone scan, or plain radiographs delineate a specific spinal location, obtain MRI or computed tomography (CT) scan. These studies are not mutually exclusive; MRI delineates the neural elements, the extent of infected material in and about the epidural space, and soft tissue abscesses associated with the lesion, while CT better delineates bony anatomy, which may be very helpful in planning the surgical approach. Often the radiographs suggest either pyogenic or granulomatous infection. Treatment decisions then are affected by the suspicion of granulomatous infection or by the absence or presence of deformity. A patient with suspected pyogenic infection or a deformity that will necessitate surgical intervention should go directly to surgical debridement and decompression of the neural elements. At the time of surgical decompression, specimens can be obtained for definitive pathology. Generally surgical debridement incorporates removal of all infected material at the apex of the deformity and the placement of anterior strut grafts. If the debridement allows for removal of most infected material down to viable tissue, bone grafts can be placed in the surgical site. If there is concern about the placement of nonvascularized bone grafts, then dependent upon the location of the lesion a vascularized rib can be placed as an anterior strut. Whether associated posterior instrumentation and fusion is required depends on the degree of deformity and stability of the lesion after strut grafting. In the setting of a pyogenic infection, posterior instrumentation and fusion is performed as a second-stage procedure. The duration of antibiotic therapy before posterior stabilization is adjusted to the individual patient's needs.

C. If granulomatous disease is suspected and no deformity is present, obtain a biopsy to confirm the pathology. If granulomatous disease is confirmed, adjust the patient's medical therapy appropriately. Also, place the patient in a spinal orthosis, which will significantly improve symptoms and may help with the neurologic involvement. If a deformity is present that would necessitate surgical intervention, the patient should proceed directly to surgical debridement and reconstruction. Again, debridement should allow for removal of most infected material down to viable tissue for placement of the bone grafts. In the setting of a purely granulomatous disease with no involvement of the posterior elements, surgical instrumentation may be done as a second stage on the same day as the debridement.

SUSPECTED SPINAL INFECTION

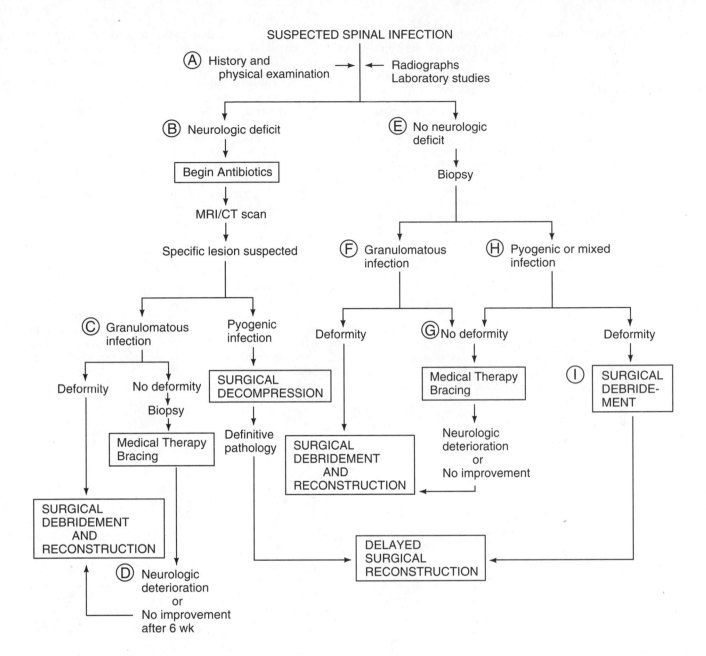

D. If at any point during medical therapy for a granulomatous infection the patient has neurologic deterioration, or if no improvement in neurologic status occurs after 6 weeks, surgical debridement, decompression, and reconstruction should be performed.

E. For the patient with no neurologic deficit, the initial work-up is the same. Once a specific location and lesion has been identified, biopsy is performed before initiation of antibiotic therapy. The biopsy is done under CT guidance or fluoroscopy to document proper placement of the biopsy needle.

F. When there is biopsy-proven granulomatous disease, further treatment depends on the presence of significant deformity. What constitutes significant deformity is somewhat controversial. As a rule, patients who have >50° of kyphosis from their normal alignment are at significant risk for progression of the deformity even with bracing. Medical treatment for >2 years is required for the anterior structures to heal sufficiently to support themselves. Therefore, surgical intervention is often the most expeditious mode of treatment. Surgery can be timed at an appropriate interval after initiation of antimicrobial therapy. For purely granulomatous disease, surgical debridement and reconstruction can generally proceed at the same time.

G. For patients without significant deformity and with documented granulomatous disease, the treatment of choice is medical therapy and bracing as needed.

H. For patients without neurologic involvement and with biopsy-proven pyogenic or mixed infections, treatment depends on the presence or absence of deformity. For those patients with no deformity, medical therapy with concomitant bracing is the treatment of choice. Medical therapy for pyogenic infection should consist of a minimum of 6 weeks of intravenous therapy and then 6 weeks to 6 months of oral therapy, depending upon the patient's clinical response. If at any point progressive deformity is noted or the patient fails to respond to medical therapy, consider surgical intervention.

I. For pyogenic infections with deformity, surgical debridement consists of anterior resection of all infected material and strut grafting. If posterior stabilization is necessary, it should be done as a delayed second-stage procedure after the patient has had appropriate medical therapy. The duration of antibiotic therapy before posterior stabilization is adjusted to the individual patient's needs. A patient who requires delayed posterior stabilization in the setting of spinal instability is placed in a roto-kinetic bed while awaiting definitive stabilization.

References

Abramovitz JN, Batson RA, Yablon JS. Vertebral osteomyelitis: The surgical management of neurologic complications. Spine 1986; 11:418.

Digby JM, Kersley JB. Pyogenic non-tuberculous spinal infection. J Bone Joint Surg [Br] 1979; 61:47.

Eismont FJ, Bohlman HH, Soni PL, et al. Pyogenic and fungal vertebral osteomyelitis with paralysis. J Bone Joint Surg 1983; 65A:19.

Eismont FJ, Wiesel SW, Brighton CT, et al. Antibiotic penetration into rabbit nucleus pulposus. Spine 1987; 12:254.

Emery SE, Chan DP, Woodward HR. Treatment of hematogenous pyogenic vertebral osteomyelitis with anterior debridement and primary bone grafting. Spine 1989; 14:284.

Guirguis AR. Pott's paraplegia. J Bone Joint Surg [Br] 1967; 49:658.

Hodgson AR, Skinsnes OK, Leong CY. The pathogenesis of Pott's paraplegia. J Bone Joint Surg 1967; 49:1147.

Hodgson AR, Stock FE. Anterior spine fusion for the treatment of tuberculosis of the spine. J Bone Joint Surg 1960; 42:295.

Shauffer RN. Pyogenic vertebral osteomyelitis. Orthop Clin North Am 1975; 6:1015.

Shitut RV, Goodpasture HC, Marsh HO. Diagnosing hematogenous vertebral pyogenic osteomyelitis. Comp Orthop March-April: 1987.

Szypryt EP, Hardy JG, Hinton CE, et al. A comparison between magnetic resonance imaging and scintigraphic bone imaging in the diagnosis of disc space infection in an animal model. Spine 1988; 13:1042.

Vincent KA, Benson DR, Voegeli TL. Factors in the diagnosis of adult pyogenic vertebral osteomyelitis. Orthop Trans 1988; 12:523.

Willis TA. Nutrient arteries of the vertebral bodies. J Bone Joint Surg 1949; 31:538.

SPINAL STENOSIS

A. The most common cause of spinal stenosis is degenerative change in the lumbar disc and facet joint complex. It typically affects men and women over the age of 60 and is more common with increasing age. The history and physical examination of patients with spinal stenosis differ significantly from those with unilateral lumbar disc herniation. Typically patients present with symptoms of neurogenic claudication, which is relieved by rest and classically also relieved by forward bending and recreated during lumbar extension. A thorough history is important for patients who present with these symptoms because spinal stenosis can also be caused by primary or metastatic tumors as well as certain metabolic disorders. The image study of choice for diagnosis of spinal stenosis has been myelography followed by contrast enhanced computed tomography (CT) scan. An anterior posterior diameter of <10 mm or a cross-sectional area of <100 mm^3 constitutes a diagnosis of spinal stenosis. More recently with the advent of magnetic resonance imaging (MRI), the need for myelography has diminished significantly. However, certain patients are still best evaluated by myelography and CT scan when MRI does not give a definitive explanation of the symptoms.

B. Congenital spinal stenosis is most commonly associated with achondroplasia or other forms of dwarfism. Patients who are otherwise normal, however, can have a neural canal that is congenitally narrow and predisposes them to symptoms of spinal stenosis with minimal degenerative changes or small disc herniations.

C. In congenital spinal stenosis, once neurogenic claudication is present, conservative treatment is relatively unsuccessful, and most patients do best with surgical decompression of the stenotic areas.

D. The most common forms of spinal stenosis are acquired, and the most common form of acquired spinal stenosis is that secondary to spondylosis. Spinal stenosis, however, can be caused by soft disc herniations if they are large enough, or by central disc herniations. They can also be caused by iatrogenic or metabolic disorders.

E. Classically soft disc herniations present with unilateral sciatica. However, central disc herniations can present with bilateral lower extremity symptoms without neurologic deficit typical of the symptoms of neurogenic claudication. For patients with symptoms it is important to rule out cauda equina syndrome, which consists of dysfunction of bowel and bladder, paresthesias in the perineal region, and bilateral lower extremity motor and sensory loss. For patients with evidence of a cauda equina syndrome, surgical decompression, carried out as expeditiously as possible, is the treatment of choice.

F. For patients with soft disc herniation and evidence of spinal stenosis, conservative management generally consists of nonsteroidal anti-inflammatory drugs (NSAIDs), physical therapy consisting of McKenzie-type exercises and spinal stabilization, and epidural steroid injections. These injections can be helpful in the short-term relief of symptoms, but their long-term benefit is uncertain. If neurologic symptoms fail to resolve with conservative management, the patient is a candidate for surgical decompression and discectomy.

G. Iatrogenic spinal stenosis commonly has two causes: (1) instability related to previous surgery, and (2) hypertrophic degenerative changes above an area of previous fusion. Typically in both instances, the treatment of choice is decompression accompanied by a concomitant posterolateral fusion. Some evidence suggests that in patients with clinical instability and those with spinal stenosis above previous fusion, instrumentation increases the success rate of spinal fusion.

H. Spondylosis is the most common form of acquired spinal stenosis. Typically patients present with evidence of neurogenic claudication. It is important to rule out peripheral vascular disease, which often resembles the symptoms of neurogenic claudication. Patients who have a fixed neurologic deficit should undergo surgical decompression, unless there are medical contraindications to surgical intervention.

I. There is still some controversy as to what constitutes instability. Classically there are two particular patterns of changes within the lumbar spine that most people agree constitute evidence of instability: (1) degenerative spondylolistheses where there is anterior or posterior subluxation of one vertebra on the adjacent vertebra, and (2) degenerative scoliosis in which progression of the curvature is documented. For patients with neurogenic claudication, fixed neurologic deficit, and no evidence of instability, decompression alone is the treatment of choice. For those with an associated instability pattern, posterolateral fusion should accompany surgical decompression. Again, evidence suggests that instrumentation increases the success rate of spinal fusion in spondylolistheses and degenerative scoliosis.

J. For patients with spondylosis and spinal stenosis who present with neurogenic claudication but no fixed neurologic deficit, consider a trial of conservative management. This typically consists of lumbar flexion type exercises, NSAIDs for a short time, and a slowly progressive low impact aerobic conditioning. Epidural steroids can be helpful in the short-term relief of symptoms. It is controversial, however, whether they have any significant long-term benefit. I feel they can be beneficial if used expeditiously and intermittently for patients who either are not candidates for surgical decompression or do not wish to undergo decompressive surgery.

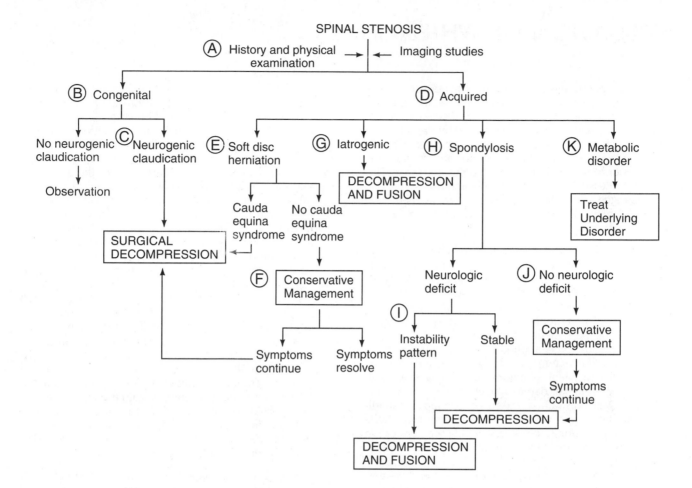

SPINAL STENOSIS

(A) History and physical → ← Imaging studies
examination

(B) Congenital

(D) Acquired

No neurogenic
claudication

(C) Neurogenic
claudication

(E) Soft disc
herniation

(G) Iatrogenic

(H) Spondylosis

(K) Metabolic
disorder

Observation

Cauda
equina
syndrome

No cauda
equina
syndrome

**DECOMPRESSION
AND FUSION**

**Treat
Underlying
Disorder**

**SURGICAL
DECOMPRESSION**

(F) **Conservative
Management**

Neurologic
deficit

(J) No neurologic
deficit

Symptoms
continue

Symptoms
resolve

(I) Instability
pattern

Stable

**Conservative
Management**

Symptoms
continue

DECOMPRESSION

**DECOMPRESSION
AND FUSION**

In the conservative management of patients with spinal stenosis, narcotic medication must be used with great caution. Most of these patients are elderly, and many elderly patients with spinal stenosis have signs of decompression that can be significantly exacerbated by narcotic medications. The risk of addiction and overmedication is also much greater in the elderly.

K. The two metabolic disorders that can lead to spinal stenosis are Paget's disease and acromegaly. Both constitute spinal stenosis by gradual enlargement of the bone, including the vertebral body, which narrows the spinal canal. Patients with Paget's disease can present with an acute neurologic crisis that requires emergent decompression. The treatment of choice for these metabolic disorders is the treatment of the underlying disorder; the spinal stenosis only requires treatment if the neurogenic claudication is unresponsive to medical therapy.

References

Cuckler JM, Bernini PA, Wiesel SW, et al. The use of epidural steroids in the treatment of lumbar radicular pain: A prospective, randomized, double-blind study. J Bone Joint Surg 1985; 65A:63.

Hall S, Bartleson JD, Onofino BM, et al. Lumbar spinal stenosis: Clinical features, diagnostic procedures and results of surgical treatment in 68 patients. Ann Intern Med 1985; 103:271.

Herkowitz HN, Kurz LT. Degenerative lumbar spondylolisthesis with spinal stenosis: A prospective study comparing decompression with decompression and intertransverse arthrodesis. J Bone Joint Surg 1991; 73A:802.

Katz JN, Lipson SJ, Larson MG, et al. The outcome of decompressive laminectomy for degenerative lumbar stenosis. J Bone Joint Surg 1991; 73A:809.

Kestwik JP, Harrington I, Alexander D, et al. Cauda equina syndrome and lumbar disc herniation. J Bone Joint Surg 1986; 68A:386.

Nasca RJ. Surgical management of lumbar spinal stenosis. Spine 1987; 12:809.

Rosen C, Kahanovitz N, Viola K, et al. A retrospective analysis of the efficacy of epidural steroid injections. Clin Orthop 1988; 228:270.

Sienkiewicz PJ, Flatley TJ. Post-operative spondylolisthesis. Clin Orthop 1987; 221:172.

Stokes IA, Frymoyer JW. Segmental motion and instability. Spine 1987; 12:688.

EVALUATION OF WHIPLASH

The initiating pathophysiologic event is hyperextension of the unrestrained neck as the torso is propelled forward secondary to a rear end impact. Forward and side motions of the cranium are restrained to some degree by the chest and the superior shoulder respectively. In the absence of a well made and correctly placed head restraint, the cranium hyperextends until the occiput strikes the thoracic area. This results in excessive stretching of the anterior soft tissue structures together with loading of the motion segments and posterior elements as well as large traction forces on the head-neck complex.

A. Ascertain the following information: When did the accident occur? What was the mechanism of injury? Was the person restrained? Was there loss of consciousness? What were the immediate/delayed symptoms? Most cases of whiplash result from an impact to the rear-end of a stationary vehicle. A disproportionate number of the patients are female. Try to determine the extent of force applied by inquiring about the amount of damage to the car; however, there can be significant physical symptoms and signs even with minimal vehicular damage. Determine whether the patient was a restrained passenger with lap and shoulder harnesses and whether the head rest stopped the cranium from going into excessive hyperextension. In addition, question the patient about any loss of consciousness or other potential cerebral symptoms such as being dazed. Similarly, explore whether there was any temporary loss of memory regarding the details of the incident. Ask about the onset of the symptoms and whether they were immediate or delayed.

B. It is important to explore whether the patient had prior cervical symptoms and/or treatments either secondary to a previous trauma or as the result of other causes. Determine the state of the patient's general health, current medications/allergies, and whether there has been time lost from work as a result of symptoms in the cervical spine. Pre-existing cervical discogenic degenerative disease may have an impact on the diagnosis and recovery potential of the patient.

C. Visualize the head and neck posture and look for persistent torticollis, which might indicate a unilateral facet problem. Carefully carry out a range of motion (ROM) examination of the cervical spine in all six planes: forward flexion, backward extension, right/left rotation, and right/left side bending. Record any asymmetrical restrictions and pain production. Also, examine the ROM of the major articulations of the upper extremities for symmetry or restrictions. Systematic palpation is important and should be carried out with the patient in both the erect and the supine positions. Elicit the presence or absence of tenderness in such areas as: posterior trapezius; sternocleidomastoid; superior/medial angle of the scapulae (scapulo-costal tenderness is quite common); spinous processes; paraspinal muscle mass over the facet joints; suboccipital area; brachial plexus in the supra-clavicular fossa; anterior cervical soft tissues; and the temporo-mandibular joints. Perform a neurologic examination including determination of the presence and symmetry of the biceps, triceps and brachio-radialis reflexes as well as muscular strength and sensation in the C5 through T1 nerve root distributions. Recognize that hyperextension trauma in the elderly can result in spinal cord damage particularly when there is preexisting cervical spondylosis. Headaches are a common associated symptom complaint with whiplash. Most such headaches are occipital and are often related to paraspinal muscular tension. However, persistent headaches and those associated with any other symptoms of cerebral concussion should alert the physician to the need for a more comprehensive neurologic examination and special cranial imaging studies. The presence of dysphagia must be evaluated thoroughly because of its prognostic significance. Look for symptoms and signs that might suggest vascular or sympathetic dysfunction implying a stretch injury to the cervical sympathetic chain (Barre syndrome). Finally, make a general assessment of the patient's emotional status, ability to cope with the trauma, and ability to comply with the treatment program. Recognize that a high percentage of such cases will become legal matters and that litigation seems to be more dependant on the severity of injury and particularly when headache persists.

D. Good quality radiographs should be obtained in all but relatively minor symptom complaint cases. These films should include: anteroposterior; odontoid views; right/left obliques; and lateral views in neutral as well as forward flexion and backward extension. In addition to evaluating these films for any bone/facet injury, the examiner should be sensitive to the prevertebral soft tissues for evidence of swelling or displacement. Bone injury can be evaluated more completely by computed tomography (CT) scan, often performed with contrast in the cervical spine. Magnetic resonance imaging (MRI) of the cervical spine is not an initial imaging study unless there is documented objective neurologic deficit; it is often utilized later in the evaluation process for those patients who fail to respond to treatment. If there are symptoms or signs of cerebral concussion, an MRI of the cranium is indicated. Cervical myelography with postmyelography CT scanning is also a later study in those cases where a surgical intervention is contemplated. For the less common situation of persistent suspected discogenic pain, cervical discography may be a definitive test to indicate the potential for disc excision and anterior cervical fusion.

E. Special testing is usually reserved for patients who do not respond to initial treatment protocols and for those with persistent symptoms. Electrodiagnostic examination includes electromyographic evaluation of the cervical innervated muscles (Fig. 1) and nerve conduction velocity studies of the major nerves in the upper extremities (Fig. 2). Electroencephalograms may be

WHIPLASH

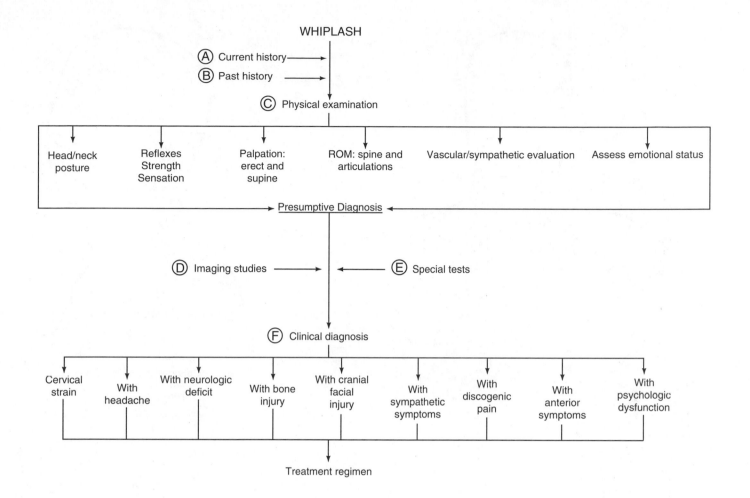

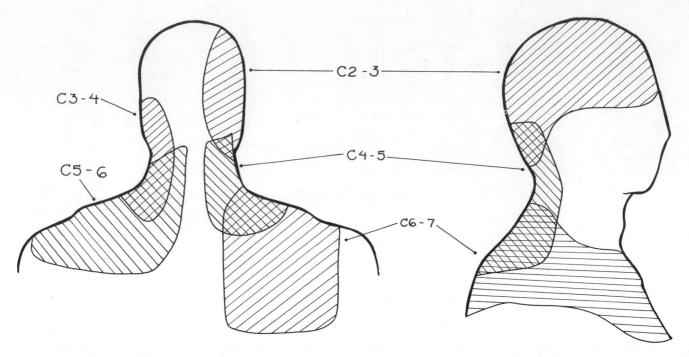

Figure 1 Patterns of referred cervical pain.

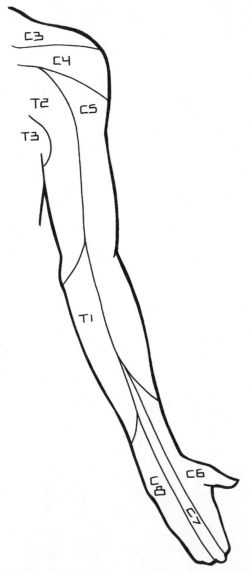

Figure 2 Dermatomal root distribution.

part of a more comprehensive neurologic evaluation for cases with postconcussion syndrome. Selective injection techniques include: cervical medial branch blocks and facet injections; selective nerve root injections; C1-C2 and greater occipital nerve blocks; C2-C3 and third occipital nerve blocks; cervical epidurals; and sympathetic blocks. Persistent psychophysiologic reactions and patterns of illness behavior can adversely affect recovery potential; such situations should be recognized and managed by appropriate referral for psychologic evaluation. Laboratory survey may be indicated for evaluation of otherwise unrecognized metabolic or rheumatic diathesis. Additional special investigations would include but not be limited to the following: vascular and sympathetic testing including ophthalmologic examination regarding diminished or absent corneal reflex; oral surgery examination for temporomandibular dysfunction; evaluation of esophageal integrity.

F. Establishing a clinical diagnosis based on the above principles is important even in the absence of a specific defined patho-anatomic pain generator. Most cases will respond to a treatment program based on the general diagnosis of cervical strain syndrome. However, as the symptom complex becomes more inclusive, it becomes important to extend the work-up to consider the other various possibilities listed.

References

Balla J. The late whiplash syndrome. Aust NZ J Surg 1980; 50:610.

Bland J. Disorders of the cervical spine. Philadelphia: WB Saunders. 1987; 224.

Bogduk N. Back pain. Zygapophysial blocks and epidural steroids. In: Cousins MJ, Bridenbaugh PO, eds: Neural Blockade in Clinical Anesthesia and Management of Pain. Philadelphia: JB Lippincott, 1988; 935.

Gay J, Abbott K. Common whiplash injuries of the neck. JAMA 1953; 152:1698.

Hohl M. Soft tissue injuries of the neck in automobile accidents. J Bone J Surg 1974; 56:1675.

Jackson R. The cervical syndrome. Springfield, IL: Charles C. Thomas, 1978.

Keefe F, et al. The psychology of chronic back pain. In: Frymoyer JW, ed: The Adult Spine: Principles and Practice. New York: Raven Press, 1991; 185.

LaRocca H. Cervical sprain syndrome: Diagnoses, treatment, and long-term outcome. In: Frymoyer JW, ed: The Adult Spine: Principles and Practice. New York: Raven Press, 1991; 1051.

Liu Y, et al. Subcortical EEG changes in rhesus monkeys following experimental hyperextension-hyperflexion (whiplash). Spine 1984; 9:329.

Miles K, et al. The incidence and prognostic significance of radiological abnormalities in soft tissue injuries to the cervical spine. Skeletal Radiol 1988; 17:493.

Norris S, Watt I. The prognosis of neck injuries resulting from rear-end vehicle collisions. J Bone J Surg 1983; 65:608.

Scher A. Hyperextension trauma in the elderly: An easily overlooked spinal injury. J Trauma 1983; 23:1066.

Severy D, et al. Controlled automobile rear-end collisions: An investigation of related engineering and medical phenomena. Can Serv Med J 1955; 11:727.

Stringer W, et al. Hyperextension injury of the cervical spine with esophageal perforation. J Neurosurg 1980; 53:541.

Weinberg S, Lapointe H. Cervical extension-flexion injury (whiplash) and internal derangement of the temporomandibular joint. J Oral Maxillo Fac Surg 1987; 45:653.

Winston K. Whiplash and its relationship to migraine. Headache 1987; 27:452.

MANAGEMENT OF WHIPLASH

A. Most patients with acute cervical strain syndrome experience resolution of their symptoms within 4 to 6 weeks. Unrelieved pain with persistent or progressive neurologic deficit after 2 to 3 weeks of intensive conservative therapy should be thoroughly investigated by appropriate studies, followed by surgical intervention if a specific patho-anatomic diagnosis can be established.

B. If bone stability is in question or if there is evidence of perched or locked facets, aggressive intervention is indicated. See pages 416-429.

C. Soft collar support or more formal orthotic devices are helpful in the acute phase. However, patients tend to become dependent on such devices with resultant aggravation of a deconditioned status. Wean patients away from such devices early in the treatment regimen unless there is a clear indication for their use based on objective patho-anatomic derangement. Instead, institute a program of therapeutic exercises, stressing guided range of motion (ROM), muscle strengthening, and low impact cardiovascular conditioning.

D. If there are no contraindications, nonsteroidal anti-inflammatory drugs are generally effective both for their anti-inflammatory and analgesic actions. Time-limited use of oral muscle relaxants, analgesics, and tricyclic antidepressants can also be helpful in the management of the acute condition. Selective injection techniques can be utilized effectively both for radiculopathies and for persistent facet related pain.

E. Preventive education should be included in any management program for whiplash. If the head rest of a car seat is not properly positioned, it can aggravate a hyperextension injury by acting as a fulcrum rather than a restraint. The head rest should be as close as possible to the posterior cranium.

F. Active/assistive exercises (Fig. 1) should be guided by a trained health care professional. An individualized treatment program requires careful assessment and the initiation of specific exercises depending on the particular clinical situation. Following the principles of Sports Medicine, ROM/stretching exercises precede muscle strengthening/stabilization techniques, which are followed thereafter by low impact aerobic activity.

G. Passive modalities include such treatments as: heat or ice; ultrasound; electrical stimulation and TENS; massage; and acupuncture. Passive exercises include traction and manipulation. These techniques may be used for short periods as analgesic supplements and as assistive methods for early active therapeutic exercises guided by an appropriately trained professional. Avoid permitting patients to become dependent on any passive technique of treatment.

H. When symptoms persist beyond a normal expected healing time, a thorough evaluation is indicated with appropriate studies selected according to the suspected clinical diagnosis to establish objective documentation of a patho-anatomic diagnosis. In such circumstances, surgical intervention may be the rational choice of treatment. Such surgery usually has as its goal the adequate decompression of the neurologic elements and/or the treatment of a primary discogenic pain source. Additionally, appropriate stabilization techniques in the form of arthrodesis with or without internal fixation devices should be undertaken in those cases where there is a defined clinical pattern of instability. In any event, surgery should rarely be contemplated before 6 to 9 months of appropriate, well-managed, conservative care in the absence of progressive neurologic deficit.

I. Many patients with chronic symptoms develop varying degrees of clinical depression, which significantly aggravates their perception of pain and concomitant suffering. Somatization, sleep disturbance, substance abuse, and anti-social behavior are other aspects of a chronically impaired patient. These issues must be addressed by appropriate psychologic testing and treatment. In the more severely involved patients, psycho-pharmaceutical intervention is indicated with the assistance of a psychiatrist.

J. Reassessment should take place after 3 to 4 weeks of a structured program. As long as the patient is not *objectively* worse, the conservative program should continue even if there has been little improvement in the patient's self report of pain. Rather, the clinician should be guided by functional parameters of improvement and should de-emphasize, as much as possible, the pain report as a measure of success. Most patients with acute cervical strain respond to well-managed programs of conservative care. A history of prior neck injury, pre-existing degenerative changes, and the persistence of headache seem to alter the prognosis for early recovery.

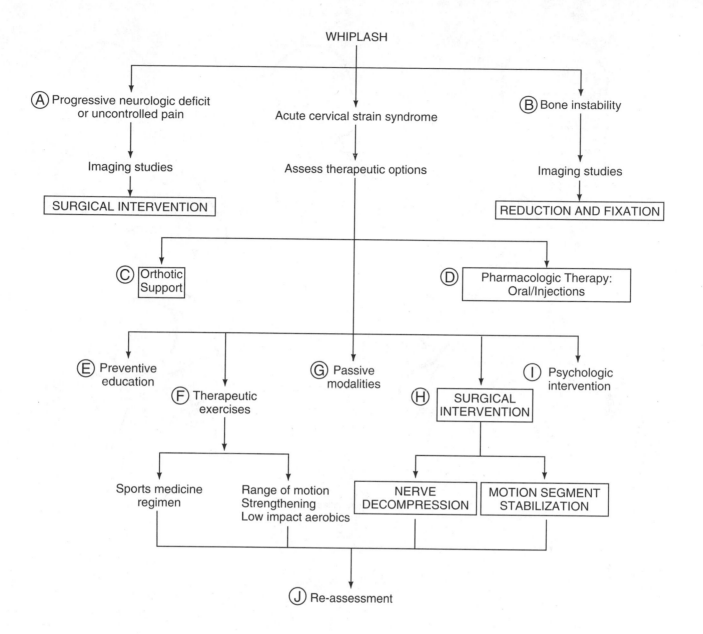

WHIPLASH

Ⓐ Progressive neurologic deficit
or uncontrolled pain

Acute cervical strain syndrome

Ⓑ Bone instability

Imaging studies

Assess therapeutic options

Imaging studies

SURGICAL INTERVENTION

REDUCTION AND FIXATION

Ⓒ Orthotic
Support

Ⓓ Pharmacologic Therapy:
Oral/Injections

Ⓔ Preventive
education

Ⓖ Passive
modalities

Ⓘ Psychologic
intervention

Ⓕ Therapeutic
exercises

Ⓗ SURGICAL
INTERVENTION

Sports medicine
regimen

Range of motion
Strengthening
Low impact aerobics

NERVE
DECOMPRESSION

MOTION SEGMENT
STABILIZATION

Ⓙ Re-assessment

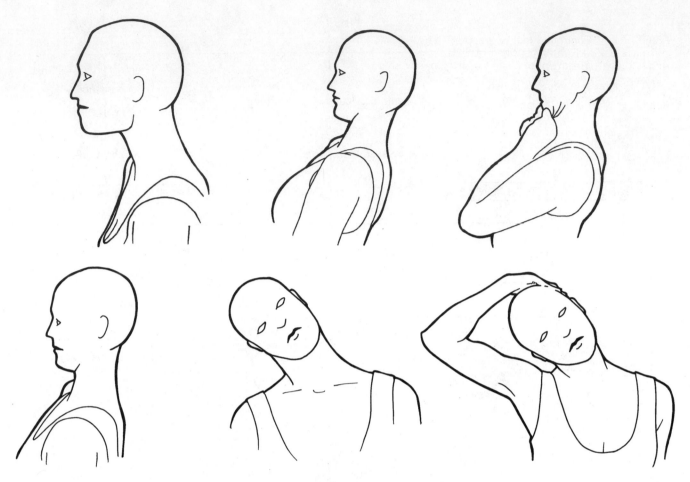

Figure 1 Therapeutic exercises for cervical syndrome.

References

Alcoff J, et al. Controlled trial of imipramine for chronic low back pain. J Fam Pract 1982; 14:841.

Amlie E, et al. Treatment of acute low back pain with piroxicam: Results of a double-blind placebo-controlled trial. Spine 1987; 12:473.

Bogduk N. Back pain. Zygapophysial blocks and epidural steroids. In: Cousins MJ, Bridenbaugh PO, eds: Neural Blockade in Clinical Anesthesia and Management of Pain. Philadelphia: Lippincott, 1988;935.

Bogduk N, Marsland A. The cervical zygapophyseal joints as source of neck pain. Spine 1988; 13:610.

Donelson R, McKenzie R. Mechanical assessment and treatment of spinal pain. In: Frymoyer JW, ed: The Adult Spine: Principles and Practice. New York: Raven Press, 1991;1627.

Ducker T. Cervical radiculopathies and myelopathies: Posterior approaches. In: Frymoyer JW, ed: The Adult Spine: Principles and Practice. New York: Raven Press, 1991;1187.

Gatchel R. Psychosocial assessment and disability management in the rehabilitation of painful spinal disorders. In: Mayer TG, Mooney V, Gatchel RJ: Contemporary Conservative Care for Painful Spinal Disorders. Philadelphia: Lea & Febiger. 1991;441.

Larocca H. Cervical sprain syndrome: Diagnoses, treatment, and long-term outcome. In: Frymoyer JW, ed: The Adult Spine: Principles and Practice. New York: Raven Press, 1991;1051.

Mealy K, et al. Early mobilization of acute whiplash injuries. Br Med J [Clin Res] 1986; 292:656.

Norris S, Watt I. The prognosis of neck injuries resulting from rear-end vehicle collisions. J Bone Joint Surg [Br] 1983; 65:608.

Olney D, Marsden A. The effect of head restraints and seat belts on the incidence of neck injury in car accidents. Injury. 1986; 17:365.

Polatin P. Psychoactive medications as adjuncts in functional restoration. In: Mayer TG, Mooney V, Gatchel RJ: Contemporary Conservative Care for Painful Spinal Disorders. Philadelphia: Lea & Febiger. 1991;465.

Whitecloud T. The anterior approach. In: Frymoyer JW, ed: The Adult Spine: Principles and Practice. New York: Raven Press, 1991;1165.

Whitecloud T, Kelley L. Anterior and posterior surgical approaches to the cervical spine. In: Frymoyer JW, ed: The Adult Spine: Principles and Practice. New York: Raven Press, 1991;987.

Winston K. Whiplash and its relationship to migraine. Headache 1987; 27:452.

Witt P. The physical therapist approach. In: Frymoyer JW, ed: The Adult Spine. Principles and Practice. New York: Raven Press, 1991;1619.

MANAGEMENT OF THORACIC PAIN

A. The differential diagnosis of thoracic pain includes both spinal and extraspinal etiologies. Early in the evaluation process, the clinician must ascertain the presence or absence of neurologic impairment and use this information as a baseline in subsequent examinations. Determine when the pain began and where it is currently; ascertain if the pain has any radicular component and what makes it better or worse. Specifically, ask if there is any night or rest pain and seek information regarding the presence of any sensory alterations, weakness/instability, or any bowel/bladder incontinence. Thoracic pain may be referred from both the cervical and the lumbar regions. Although pain is the most common complaint, the patient may present initially with neurologic signs of myelopathy including: incoordination of gait with lower extremity weakness and/or spasticity; altered sensation in the extremities and/or perineal area; bowel and/or bladder dysfunction. The pain pattern itself may be variable, but mostly the presenting complaint is of thoracic back pain with some pattern of referred discomfort. The quality of the pain has been described as dull, throbbing, aching, sharp, or burning with associated various levels of intensity. The types of radiation range from a local generalized spread of pain to more specific patterns of dermatomal distribution with occasional anterior spread through rather than around the chest. In the evaluation process, consider the anterior chest wall as a source of thoracic pain with the recognition of such conditions as Tietze's syndrome and rib-tip pain. Posterior element symptoms are not uncommon and include pain of facet origin as well as those syndromes related to the articulations between the rib head and the transverse process and/or vertebral body. Ascertain whether the pain is episodic or constant and whether or not it is relieved by recumbency. Night pain tends to suggest a neoplastic or infectious etiology.

B. Examination of the patient's gait and stance, including one-leg elevation of body weight, provides information regarding muscular strength and coordination. Palpation of the posterior thorax can be reasonably accurate with the patient flexed over the examination table and while resting on a pillow; in this position and with the feet flat on the floor, one can be generally sure regarding the absence of any significant lumbar sciatic tension. Palpation also includes the anterior and lateral chest wall, the abdomen, and flank regions. A range of motion examination should assess the cervical and lumbar spines as well as the major articulations of the upper and lower extremities in addition to careful palpation for areas of local tenderness. Careful neurovascular examination is critical in the diagnostic work-up; deep tendon reflexes, muscle strength, and sensory testing should be supplemented by a search for hallmarks of spasticity or ataxia. Recall that a thoracic or abdominal aneurysm is an uncommon but serious and potentially treatable cause of thoracic pain.

C. Good quality radiographs and/or a bone scan with SPECT imaging generally are satisfactory in the initial evaluation process. As magnetic resonance imaging (MRI) with or without gadolinium enhancement has become better defined in this area, it seems to be supplanting water soluble myelography with computed tomography scanning. However, the latter technique still is quite useful, particularly for intracanal neoplastic lesions and to differentiate bone spur formation as well as soft tissue or disc calcification. Thoracic discograms, although still somewhat controversial, do have a place in the evaluation process for patients with suspected thoracic discogenic pain in whom the symptoms are persistent and felt to be genuine, and in whom all other tests have failed to define an objective patho-anatomic pain generator.

D. Laboratory analysis includes but is not limited to: complete blood count, chemistry profile, urinalysis, sedimentation rate, rheumatoid factor, HLA-B27, Bence Jones protein, electrophoresis, and zoster levels. Specific evaluation may be needed for documentation of osteoporosis or osteomalacia including amino acid assays and bone biopsy for histomorphometry as well as bone density measurements. Selective injections can be quite helpful diagnostically and include such techniques as facet and/or costotransverse/costovertebral blocks as well as thoracic epidural injections. Electrodiagnostic evaluations can be of assistance in the differential diagnosis of cervical radiculopathies masquerading as thoracic pain. In addition, intercostal motor conduction time has been described for the diagnosis of nerve root compression. A vascular work-up should seek to rule out the presence of thoracic or lumbar aortic aneurysm as a cause of thoracic pain. Also, in the surgical treatment of thoracic problems, the uniqueness of the vascular supply to the spinal cord and the attendant critical vascular zones must be kept in mind. Although somewhat less common than in lumbar or cervical conditions, chronic thoracic pain complaints can be related to unresolved psychosocial issues that must be properly evaluated and managed if meaningful progress is to be made. Other diagnostic testing includes evaluation of persistent thoracic pain after thoracotomy.

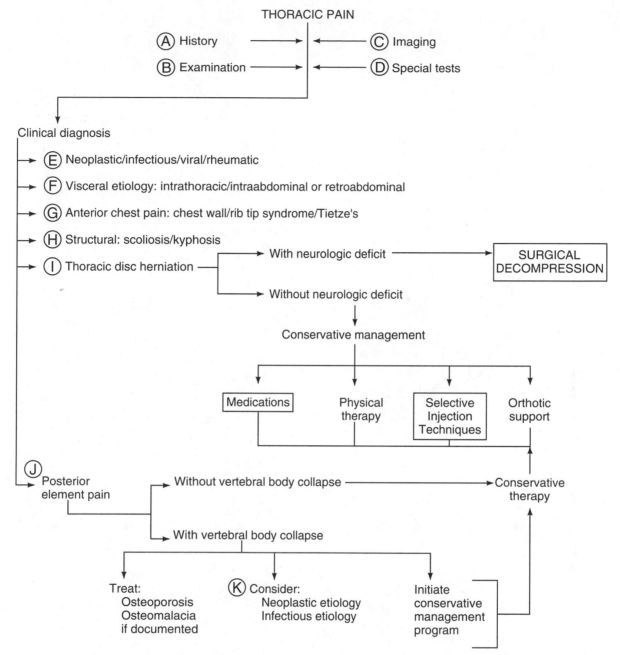

THORACIC PAIN

(A) History   →   ←   (C) Imaging

(B) Examination   →   ←   (D) Special tests

Clinical diagnosis

→ (E) Neoplastic/infectious/viral/rheumatic

→ (F) Visceral etiology: intrathoracic/intraabdominal or retroabdominal

→ (G) Anterior chest pain: chest wall/rib tip syndrome/Tietze's

→ (H) Structural: scoliosis/kyphosis

→ (I) Thoracic disc herniation — → With neurologic deficit — → **SURGICAL DECOMPRESSION**

     → Without neurologic deficit

     Conservative management

     | Medications | Physical therapy | Selective Injection Techniques | Orthotic support |

(J) Posterior element pain → Without vertebral body collapse — → Conservative therapy

     → With vertebral body collapse

Treat: Osteoporosis Osteomalacia if documented

(K) Consider: Neoplastic etiology Infectious etiology

Initiate conservative management program

E. The spine is a common area for metastatic disease processes particularly from primary sources in the lung, breast, thyroid, and kidneys. Intracanal neoplasms include both primary and metastatic extradural tumors as well as intradural/extramedullary and intramedullary neoplasms. Also, primary bone lesions, particularly round cell tumors such as myeloma, should be included in the differential diagnosis. Vertebral osteomyelitis and disc space infection must be considered as well. Both neoplastic and infectious lesions tend to have nonremitting pain that is not relieved by recumbency. These conditions can often be discriminated by good quality MRIs with gadolinium enhancement and by bone scans with SPECT imaging. A cutaneous eruption should alert the clinician to the possibility of herpes zoster, and zoster levels should be obtained; the pain of herpes zoster usually precedes the onset of the typical eruption. If morning stiffness is a characteristic of the presenting symptom complex, and particularly if there are other joint or soft tissue complaints, a laboratory rheumatic survey should be undertaken.

F. Visceral conditions that may masquerade as thoracic pain include intrathoracic cardiovascular, pulmonary or mediastinal lesions; intra-abdominal hepatic or gastrointestinal problems; and retroperitoneal lesions including renal or ureteral sources of pain.

G. Local injection techniques as well as laboratory surveys can assist in the differentiation of anterior chest wall syndromes such as costochondritis and rib-tip syndrome. In addition, musculo-fascial pain and polymyalgia rheumatica should be considered.

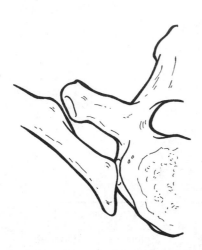

Figure 1 Costotransverse articulation.

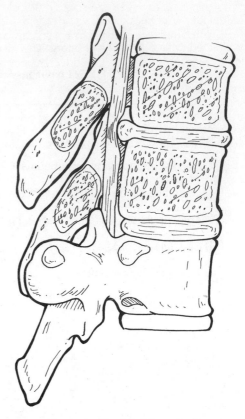

Figure 3 Herniated thoracic disc.

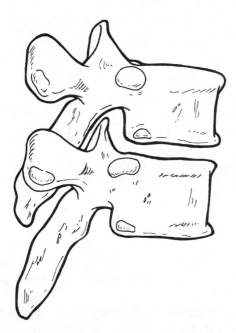

Figure 2 Costovertebral articulation.

H. Structural pain may be secondary to degenerative joint disease with diagnosis and treatment being successfully directed to facet and/or costotransverse or costovertebral osteoarthritis (Figs. 1 and 2). Superimposition of degenerative changes and hypertrophy of the zygapophyseal joints in combination with a scoliotic deformity may result in spinal stenosis. In addition, such cases may demonstrate: lateral recess stenosis; herniated discs, particularly at the inferior end of the curve; and spinal cord compressive myelopathy.

I. Most thoracic disc herniations are small and are located beneath the posterior longitudinal ligament (Fig. 3). Symptomatic herniations without neurologic signs are usually lateral or centrolateral. The overall incidence of clinically significant thoracic disc herniation has been estimated to be approximately one in one million people and between 0.2% and 1.8% of all disk operations. Although thoracic disc herniation has been reported in children and in association with Scheuermann's disease, most patients are adults in the fourth to sixth decades with the herniation usually involving the lower third of the thoracic spine. In the absence of neurologic deficit, a regimen of conservative care can be quite successful. Such a program could include the judicious administration of oral medications and selective injection techniques as well as the temporary use of an external orthotic support. The mainstay of conservative treatment should be individualized physical therapy with structured, graduated exercises supplemented by initial passive modalities supervised by a trained therapist. When surgery is indicated, the recommended treatment is anterior transthoracic disc excision with or without fusion.

J. Vertebral body wedge compression is common in osteoporosis and causes thoracic pain secondary to the fracture phenomenon. In the later stages, posterior element pain can persist and can be amenable to selective injection techniques. Adult vertebral body collapse, in the absence of documented osteoporosis or osteomalacia, may indicate metastatic or primary neoplasms. It has been estimated that more than half of patients who have metastatic disease have involvement of the spine, and neurologic deficits occur in 20% of these cases. However, in stable benign situations with posterior element pain a conservative management program as discussed in I above should be initiated. The reader is also referred to the conservative management discussion of chronic back pain, sections E-J, p. 438.

K. Neoplastic or infectious etiologies in the presence of neurologic deficit usually require surgical decompression. Radiation therapy and/or chemotherapy may be indicated in those tumors that are expected to respond to such treatments.

References

Aprill C. Diagnostic disc injection. In: Frymoyer JW, ed: The Adult Spine: Principles and Practice. New York: Raven Press, 1991;403.

Ashby E. Abdominal pain of spinal origin: Value of intercostal block. Ann Roy Col Surg Eng 1977; 59:242.

Bluestone R. Ankylosing spondylitis. In Arthritis and Allied Conditions. Philadelphia: Lea & Febiger. 1985;819.

Bogouk N. Back pain: Zygaphophysial blocks and epidural steroids. In: Cousins MJ, Bridenbaugh PO, eds: Neural Blockade in Clinical Anesthesia and Pain Management. Philadelphia: Lippincott, 1988;935.

Bohlman H, Zdeblick T. Anterior excision of herniated thoracic discs. J Bone Joint Surg 1988; 70:1038.

Bradford D, Garcia A. Neurological complications in Scheuermann's disease. J Bone Joint Surg 1969; 51:567.

Caldwell J, et al. Determinations of intercostal motor conduction time in diagnosis of severe root compression. Arch Phys Med Rehab 1968; 24:515.

Dommisse G. The blood supply of the spinal cord. J Bone Joint Surg [Br] 1974; 56:225.

Gatchel RJ. Psychosocial assessment and disability management in the rehabilitation of painful spinal disorders. In: Mayer TG, Mooney V, Gatchel RJ: Contemporary Conservative Care for Painful Spinal Disorders. Philadelphia: Lea & Febiger. 1991;441.

Griffiths H, Jones D. Pyogenic infection of the spine: A review of twenty-eight cases. J Bone Joint Surg [Br] 1971; 53:383.

Hawkins B, et al. Use of the B27 test in the diagnosis of ankylosing spondylitis. Arthritis Rheum 1981; 24:743.

Keefe F, et al. The psychology of chronic back pain. In: Frymoyer JW, ed: The Adult Spine: Principles and Practice. New York: Raven Press, 1991;185.

Kostuik J. Adult kyphosis and scoliosis. In: Frymoyer JW, ed: The Adult Spine: Principles and Practice. New York: Raven Press, 1991;1369.

MacCartee C, et al. Ruptured calcified thoracic disc in a child: Report of a case. J Bone Joint Surg [Am] 1972; 54:1272.

McBeath A, Keene J. The rib-tip syndrome. J Bone Joint Surg 1975; 57:795.

Nathan H, et al. The costovertebral joints. Anatomical clinical observations in arthritis. Arth Rheum 1964; 7:228.

Otani K, et al. The surgical treatment of thoracic and thoracolumbar disc lesions using the anterior approach. Spine 1977; 2:266.

Raney F. Costovertebral-costotransverse joint complex as the source of local or referred pain. J Bone Joint Surg 1966; 48:1451.

Rawlings M. Differential diagnosis of the painful chest. Geriatrics 1963; 18:139.

Ross J, et al. Thoracic disc herniation: MR imaging. Radiology 1987; 165:511.

Skubic J, Kostuik J. Thoracic pain syndromes and thoracic disc herniation. In: Frymoyer JW, ed: The Adult Spine. New York: Raven Press, 1991;1443.

Weinstein J. Differential diagnosis and surgical treatment of primary benign and malignant neoplasms. In: Frymoyer JW, ed: The Adult Spine: Principles and Practice. New York: Raven Press, 1991;829.

Weinstein JN. Spinal tumors. In: Weinstein JN, Wiesel SW: The Lumbar Spine. Philadelphia: WB Saunders. 1990;741.

Weinstein J. Thoracolumbar spine: Reconstruction. Orthopaedic Knowledge Update 4. American Academy of Orthopaedic Surgeons. 1993;475.

Weinstein J, et al. The pain of discography. Spine 1988; 13:1344.

Weinstein J, McLair R. Primary tumors of the spine. Spine 1987; 12:843.

SPORTS MEDICINE

RECURRENT ANTERIOR SHOULDER INSTABILITY

Recurrence is directly related to the patient's age. First-time dislocators in the 15- to 25-year-old age group have the highest risk, approximately 50%–70%. From anatomic studies, the glenohumeral ligamentous complex has been better defined. The importance of the inferior glenohumeral ligament as a static restraint to an anterior translation has been determined. Arthroscopic evaluation of first-time dislocators has given us anatomic information regarding the "essential lesion." Capsular and labral avulsions off of the anterior and inferior glenoid create the Bankart lesion. This lesion compromises the function of the inferior glenohumeral ligament. Persistent capsular incompetency or labral detachment leads to recurrent instability. Anterior recurrent instability can present with recurrent dislocations or subluxations of traumatic or atraumatic etiology.

A. Patients with a traumatic history can often give an accurate detail of the initial episode. A typical mechanism includes forced abduction and external rotation producing an anterior dislocation or subluxation. Spontaneous reduction may occur or a manipulative reduction by a physician or trainer may be necessary. Subsequently, patients may experience recurrent dislocations with the addition of trauma or arm positioning. Some describe a "dead-arm" during recurrent subluxations. Atraumatic recurrent instability is also seen. Patients typically have generalized ligamentous laxity and may be involved in activities that repetitively stress the capsular restraints. Occasionally, these patients may not appreciate that they have an unstable shoulder. Translation maneuvers, apprehension testing, and provocative testing can delineate the degree and direction of the instability. The overlap between impingement and instability must be kept in mind. Translation maneuvers are performed with the patient seated or supine. Contralateral comparison is essential in that there is a wide variability in patients' inherent laxity. First, "load" the humerus into the glenoid to center the joint. Then, apply posterior and anterior forces. An appreciation of the amount of translation is obtained by noting the humeral head relationship to the anterior or posterior glenoid rim. Elicit the "sulcus sign" by an inferiorly directed force on the adducted arm, noting the distance that the humeral head moves away from the undersurface of the acromion. Provocative testing is accomplished with the "crank test" or the "apprehension sign." By placing the arm in the abducted and externally rotated position, note recreation of the patient's symptoms or apprehension. Often, the patient will say, "If you go any further, it will come out."

B. True anteroposterior (AP) views of the glenohumeral joint, transcapular lateral and axillary lateral views define the direction of instability and any associated fractures. The presence of a Hill-Sachs lesion or an anterior inferior glenoid rim avulsion are diagnostic of anterior instability episodes. Computed tomography (CT), arthrograms, and fluoroscopy may give added information in confusing cases. CT arthrography can be used to delineate a labral avulsion from the anterior inferior glenoid. Fluoroscopy is most helpful in differentiating the direction of subluxation in patients with a difficult physical examination (i.e., a swimmer with a positive apprehension sign and significant posterior asymmetry on the load and shift test), which also recreates their symptoms. Again, recreation of the symptoms during the examination is key.

C. Conservative treatment consisting of rotator cuff strengthening and scapular stabilization benefits most atraumatic subluxators and some patients with traumatic recurrent instability. Those patients who voluntarily subluxate their shoulder should undergo counseling and are not operative candidates. Rehabilitation focuses on concentric and eccentric strengthening. Patients with posterior capsular tightness will benefit from a stretching program and internal rotation. Avoid programs that stress the anterior capsule (i.e., stretching in the abducted and externally rotated position).

D. Patients with recurrent disabling instability undergo arthroscopic or open exploration of the glenohumeral joint. If a Bankart lesion is present, perform a Bankart repair. If the pathologic lesion is capsular redundancy, perform a capsular tightening procedure.

E. Open repair of a Bankart lesion is the standard procedure for most cases. The goal is to create stability without loss of motion. Excessive anterior tightening can lead to osteoarthrosis due to limitation of external rotation. The use of screws or staples in repairs can lead to several complications including hardware loosening and joint penetration. Arthroscopic techniques have yet to equal the good results of open techniques.

F. If, at the time of arthroscopy or open exploration, no Bankart lesion is present, perform a capsular tightening procedure. This can be done by the horizontal capsular incision and a "cruciate repair" overlapping the anterior capsule. It can also be performed with a vertical incision in the capsule bringing the inferior limb superiorly, much like an inferior capsular shift procedure.

RECURRENT ANTERIOR SHOULDER INSTABILITY

(A) Clinical Evaluation ⟶   (B) Imaging

Maintenance ⟵ (C) Rehabilitation ⟶ Counseling for voluntary subluxation

(D) | ARTHROSCOPIC OR OPEN EVALUATION |

Bankart lesion   Capsular insufficiency

(E) | ARTHROSCOPIC OR OPEN BANKART REPAIR | (F) | OPEN CAPSULAR PLICATION |

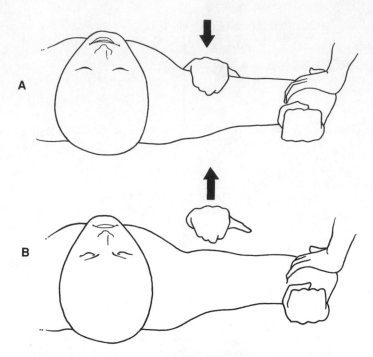

Figure 1 **A,** Relocation test. With the patient supine, a posteriorly directed force on the proximal humerus allows greater external rotation prior to a sensation of impending dislocation. **B,** Release test. With the sudden release of the posterior force, the patient becomes anxious.

References

Baker CL, Uribe JW, Whitman L. Arthroscopic evaluation of acute initial anterior shoulder dislocations. Am J Sports Med 1990; 181:25.

Hawkins RJ, Angelo RL. Glenohumeral osteoarthrosis: A late complication of Putti-Platt repair. J Bone Joint Surg 1990; 72A:1193.

Hovelius L: Anterior dislocation of the shoulder in teenagers and young adults: A five-year prognosis. J Bone Joint Surg 1987; 69A:393.

O'Brien SJ, Neves MC, Arnoczky SP, et al. The anatomy and histology of the inferior glenohumeral ligament complex of the shoulder. Am J Sports Med 1990; 18:449.

Rockwood CA Jr. Glenohumeral instability in the shoulder. In Matsen FA III, Rockwood CA Jr (eds). The shoulder. Philadelphia: WB Saunders Co, 1990.

Rockwood CA Jr, Burkhead WZ Jr, Brna J. Subluxation of the glenohumeral joint: A response to rehabilitative exercise in traumatic versus atraumatic instability. American Shoulder and Elbow Surgeons 2nd Open Meeting, New Orleans, 1986.

Rowe CR. Prognosis and dislocation of the shoulder. J Bone Joint Surg 1956; 38A:957.

Rowe CR. Recurrent transient anterior subluxation of the shoulder: The "dead-arm" syndrome. Clin Orthop 1987; 223:11.

Schwartz RE, O'Brien SJ, Warren RF, et al. Capsular restraints to anterior-posterior motion of the abducted shoulder: A biomechanical study. Orthop Trans 1988; 17:727.

Silliman JF, Hawkins RJ. Current concepts and recent advances in the athlete's shoulder. Clin Sports Med 1991; 10:693.

Zuckerman JD, Matsen FA III. Complications about the glenohumeral joint related to the use of screws and staples. J Bone Joint Surg 1984; 66A:175.

POSTERIOR SHOULDER INSTABILITY

Posterior instability of the shoulder continues to be a diagnostic dilemma. Most cases of posterior dislocation are misdiagnosed. Chronically locked or missed posterior dislocations still occur due to the difficulty in diagnosis. Recurrent posterior subluxation is being diagnosed more frequently, especially in athletes. Cadaveric studies have demonstrated the importance of the superior glenohumeral ligament and anterior capsular structures in posterior shoulder instability.

A. The mechanism and violence of the injury are important to note. Common etiologies of posterior dislocations include seizure disorders, major trauma, electric shock, and alcoholism. Typically, the arm is in a forward flexed, internally rotated position and adducted at the time of the injury. Less commonly, an anterior blow to the shoulder can produce posterior dislocation. Physical examination of an acute traumatic posterior dislocation reveals a prominent coracoid process, squaring of the anterior lateral acromion, fullness in the posterior deltoid, and an internal rotation deformity. These patients typically have a significant amount of pain. Patients with chronic locked dislocations show functional forward elevation and internal rotation. However, they are unable to externally rotate their arm at the side and may reveal a marked internal rotation deformity as much as 60°. These patients may also show a limitation of supination when the arm is held in a forward flexed position. Recurrent posterior subluxation is by far the most common form of posterior instability. Take care to differentiate these patients from those with multidirectional instability. Typically, there are four different subsets of patients with posterior subluxation: voluntary/habitual (emotionally disturbed); voluntary/not willful (muscular control); involuntary with positional changes; and involuntary/unintentional. These patients rarely remember a traumatic episode that began their shoulder problems. They typically give a history of their shoulder slipping out of socket, but "popping back in." Stress on the rotator cuff can create tendinitis, which also can obscure the diagnosis. Most of these patients cannot demonstrate their instability during examination. Some patients, however, can do so with arm position or selective muscular contraction. After subluxation, a typical clunk is palpated during the relocation. Also, symptomatic posterior translation with the load and shift test is helpful in determining a diagnosis.

B. Anteroposterior views (AP) in the plane of the glenohumeral joint, axillary lateral, and transcapular lateral views are necessary to determine the bony anatomy and joint position. Stress radiographs in the position of subluxation are helpful in determining the direction of instability. Fluoroscopy can also help to confirm the diagnosis of subluxation. In the rare case of a posterior dislocation, the axillary view is most helpful. This view gives an appreciation for the size of the humeral head defect and the changes on the glenoid rim. In the case of longstanding posterior dislocation, a computed tomography (CT) scan is sometimes necessary to determine the extent of head involvement and the status of the glenoid.

C. Patients with posterior subluxation typically present with pain; instability symptoms are secondary. Patients with subluxation do not progress to recurrent dislocations. The pathoanatomy differs from that of anterior instability in that typically no Bankart lesion is present. A redundancy of the posterior capsule and pouch contributes to posterior instability.

D. Habitual or willful voluntary dislocators do not do well with surgical treatment. These patients should be distinguished from those who, by arm position or muscular contraction, can demonstrate a subluxation episode. If any doubt exists, these patients should undergo psychiatric evaluation and placement in a rehabilitation program.

E. Involuntary or unintentional subluxators respond well to rotator cuff strengthening, scapular stabilization, and progressive shoulder girdle rehabilitation. Depending on the severity of the pain associated with the instability, these patients should progress from isometrics to isotonics and isokinematics when available. Return to activities is facilitated by activity specific rehabilitation.

F. If an adequate trial of rehabilitation fails, surgical stabilization is advised. These patients should undergo a detailed evaluation under anesthesia to substantiate that the instability is unidirectional and posterior. Arthroscopic evaluation is beneficial in athletes or if the evaluation is not conclusive. Typically these patients are treated with a posterior capsular plication or shift as an open procedure. They are casted postoperatively in neutral rotation, adduction, and slight shoulder extension.

G. Posterior dislocation is rare. Alcoholism, seizure disorders, electrocution, or violent trauma is the typical etiology.

H. Acute posterior dislocations are more difficult to reduce without anesthetics than anterior dislocations. After muscle spasm has been eliminated, gentle traction and anterior force on the head usually accomplish a reduction. If reduction is difficult, slight internal rotation and lateral traction on the proximal humerus may be necessary. These patients are then casted in neutral rotation and slight extension for 3 weeks. If closed reduction is unsuccessful, open reduction through an anterior approach is necessary.

I. Chronic posterior dislocation occurs when an acute locked dislocation is either missed by the original physician or no attention was sought. As the initial pain abates, these patients typically complain of functional

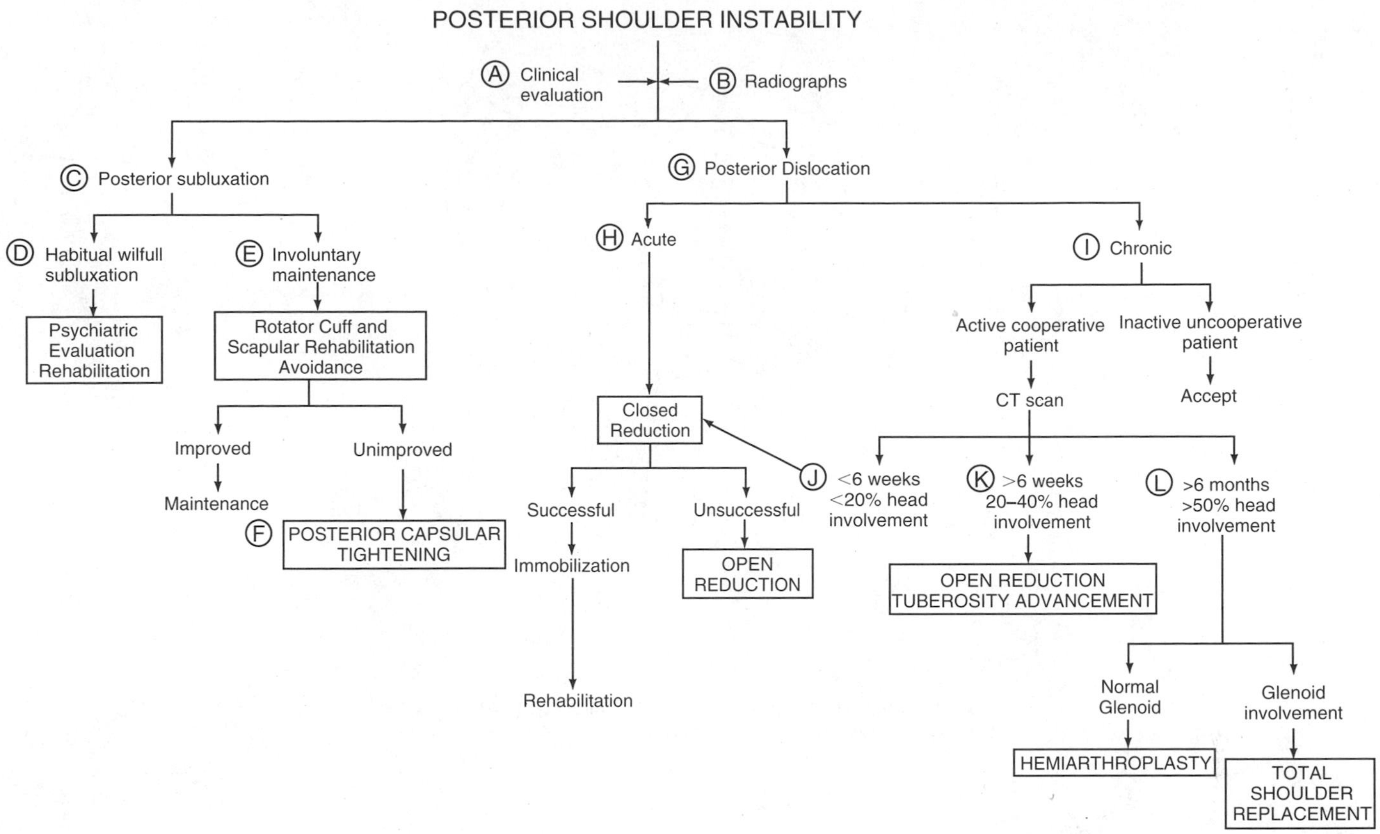

POSTERIOR SHOULDER INSTABILITY

(A) Clinical evaluation ——— (B) Radiographs

(C) Posterior subluxation

(D) Habitual wilfull subluxation

Psychiatric Evaluation Rehabilitation

(E) Involuntary maintenance

Rotator Cuff and Scapular Rehabilitation Avoidance

Improved

Maintenance

Unimproved

(F) POSTERIOR CAPSULAR TIGHTENING

(G) Posterior Dislocation

(H) Acute

Closed Reduction

Successful

Immobilization

Rehabilitation

Unsuccessful

OPEN REDUCTION

(I) Chronic

Active cooperative patient

CT scan

Inactive uncooperative patient

Accept

(J) <6 weeks <20% head involvement

(K) >6 weeks 20–40% head involvement

OPEN REDUCTION TUBEROSITY ADVANCEMENT

(L) >6 months >50% head involvement

Normal Glenoid

HEMIARTHROPLASTY

Glenoid involvement

TOTAL SHOULDER REPLACEMENT

483

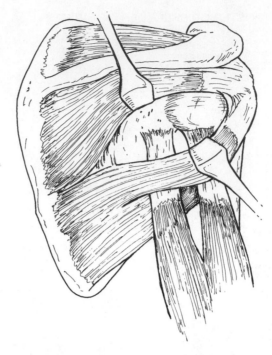

Figure 1 Repair of posterior shoulder instability. Interval is developed within the substance of the infraspinatus tendon.

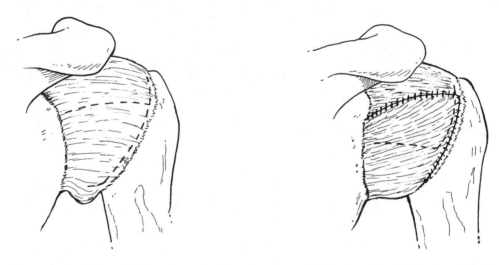

Figure 2 Capsular redundancy is resolved by advancing an inferior flap. Infraspinatus tenodesis is often needed to reinforce the capsule.

problems from loss of range of motion. In the inactive or uncooperative patient, the deformity can be accepted.

J. Active patients with chronic posterior dislocations and disability undergo operative reduction. Preoperative CT scan is used to evaluate the status of the humeral head and glenoid. If the dislocation is <6 weeks old and if <20% of the humeral head is involved, closed reduction is attempted.

K. If the dislocation is >6 weeks old and 20%–40% of the humeral head is involved, open reduction and tuberosity or subscapularis transfer into the defect is indicated. This is done through an anterior approach.

L. If the dislocation is of >6 months duration or if >50% of the humeral head is destroyed, hemiarthroplasty or total shoulder replacement is necessary depending on the status of the glenoid. The humeral component should be placed in less retroversion than a standard arthroplasty. If the dislocation is of <6 months duration, approximately 20° of retroversion is necessary. If the dislocation is of >6 months duration, the humeral components should be placed neutral version.

References

Colfield RH, Irving JF. Evaluation and classification of shoulder instability with special reference to examination under anesthesia. Clin Orthop 1987; 32.

Hawkins RJ. Recurrent posterior instability. J Bone Joint Surg 1984; 66A:169.

Hawkins RJ. Locked posterior dislocation of the shoulder. J Bone Joint Surg 1987; 69A:9.

Hawkins RJ, McCormack RG. Posterior shoulder instability. Orthopaedics 1988; 11:101.

Matsen FA III, Thomas SC, Rockwood CA Jr. Glenohumeral instability. In Rockwood CA Jr, Matsen FA III (eds). The shoulder. Philadelphia: WB Saunders Co, 1990.

Rowe CR, Pierce DS, Clark JG, et al. Voluntary dislocation of the shoulder: A preliminary report on a clinical electromyographic and psychiatric study of twenty-six patients. J Bone Joint Surg 1973; 55A:445.

Rowe CR, Zarins B. Chronic unreduced dislocations of the shoulder. J Bone Joint Surg 1982; 64A:494.

Schwartz E, Warren RF, O'Brien SJ, Fronek J. Posterior shoulder instability. Orthop Clin North Am 1987; 18(3):409.

MULTIDIRECTIONAL INSTABILITY OF THE SHOULDER

In 1962, Carter Rowe discussed atraumatic instability of the shoulder in more than one direction. Neer's classic article defined the syndrome of multidirectional instability as anteroposterior (AP) instability with a component of inferior instability. Neer's large series had an equal male/female ratio and approximately one-half the patients had a history of trauma. Altchek's series of athletes all had traumatic etiologies. Other etiologies described are repetitive minor injury and varying degrees of inherent ligamentous laxities such as mild forms of Ehlers-Danlos syndrome. This disorder is now recognized as being more common than originally appreciated. Many failed reconstructions for anterior or posterior unidirectional shoulder instability can be attributed to unrecognized multidirectional instability.

A. A traumatic event should not diminish suspicion for multidirectional instability. Many patients, however, present without specific injury history but might be exposed to multiple repeated trauma and stretching of the shoulder capsule. Pain symptoms in these patients are often vague. Fatigue and an inability to carry a heavy load with the arm at the side or overhead are common. These patients can also present with a pain pattern similar to rotator cuff impingement tendinitis, i.e., night pain, rest pain, and pain worsened by activities. They also can present with transitory numbness in the hand or arm. Many of these patients are athletes, in particular those who are involved in sports that place major stress on the shoulder capsule such as swimming and gymnastics.

B. In patients with multidirectional instability, the physical examination is the key to the diagnosis. Assessment of the skin for excess laxity and spreading of scars gives a general index for generalized tissue laxity. Examination of patellar mobility, hyperextensible elbows and metacarpophalangeal joints, and also excursion in the contralateral shoulder indicate the patient's inherent joint laxity. Compare anterior and posterior excursion to the contralateral side with the load and shift test. Elicit the sulcus sign by an inferiorly directed force on the adducted arm, noting the distance that the humeral head moves away from the acromion. Asymmetry in the sulcus sign or asymmetry of AP excursion in the contralateral shoulder is a diagnostic key. Inferior excursion of the humeral head is typically ≥2 cm in patients with significant inferior laxity. Recreation of the patient's symptoms at the time of this inferior excursion is pathognomonic. At times,

a differential injection with 1% lidocaine is helpful in determining the source of pain. Perform anterior and posterior apprehension tests to determine the component of the patient's instability and pain pattern coming from those directions. Inferior apprehension can also be tested by an inferiorly directed force on the abducted arm. Many of these patients are diagnosed in the operating room during preoperative examination under anesthesia for AP instability. At that time, a significant difference between the contralateral shoulder examination in both the inferior plane and the AP plane forms a diagnosis of multidirectional instability. This is particularly important in a heavily muscled patient or one who showed muscle guarding during an awake examination.

C. Standard AP, axillary lateral, and trans-scapular views give an appropriate evaluation for the bony anatomy of the shoulder. Stress radiographs in the erect patient with 25 lb in each hand can be used to substantiate inferior laxity.

D. Patients with inherent laxity of the capsular structures often depend on dynamic stabilization from the rotator cuff and scapula. Therefore, many of these patients respond relatively quickly to internal and external rotator strengthening exercises. Also, all parts of the deltoid should be strengthened with progressive resistance exercises. Isometric exercises appear to be particularly suited to these patients and can be limited to a range of neutral joint position. These patients are also trained to avoid situations that tend to irritate their shoulder. Nonsteroidal anti-inflammatory drugs (NSAIDs) can be used to treat symptoms of tendinitis.

E. The great majority of these patients respond to conservative treatment. Surgical treatment is indicated when pain and disability are unabated by conservative measures (Fig. 1). The procedure of choice is an inferior capsular shift. Postoperatively, patients are immobilized for 8–12 weeks depending on the inherent joint laxity and surgical findings. Many of these patients should be immobilized in a cast, maintaining the arm in neutral flexion and extension with approximately 10° of external rotation. Consider patients with significant resting sulcus and significant laxity in the superior cuff and capsule for superior capsular plication and coracohumeral ligament reconstruction.

MULTIDIRECTIONAL INSTABILITY OF THE SHOULDER

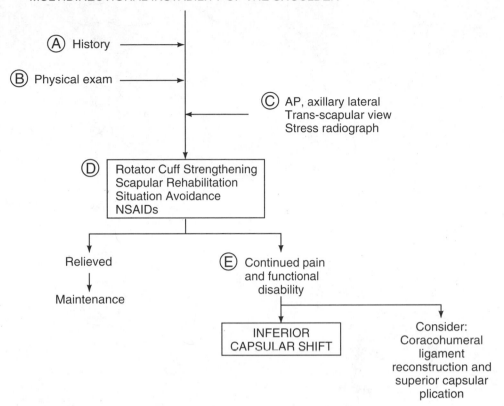

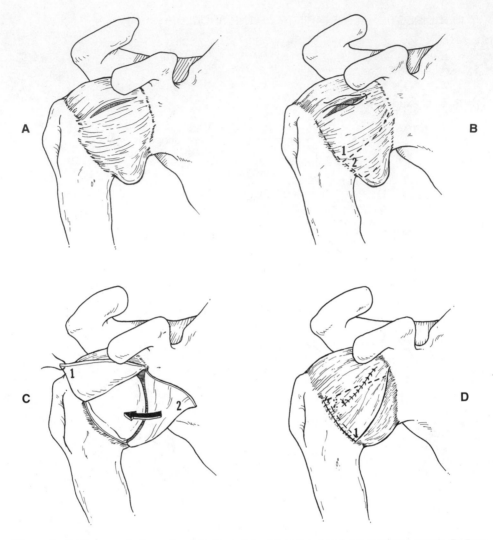

Figure 1 **A,** Common findings of a defective rotator interval and redundant inferior pouch. **B,** Rotator interval is closed. Redundancy is reduced by creating an inferior and superior flap. **C,** Medially based superior and inferior flaps are created. The inferior capsular flap is elevated posteriorly by externally rotating the arm. **D,** Inferior flap is advanced superior to eliminate the inferior punch.

References

Altchek DW, Warren RF, Skyhar MJ, Ortiz G. T-Plasty modification of the Bankhart procedure for multidirectional instability of the anterior and inferior types. J Bone Joint Surg 1991; 73A:105.

Jobe FW, Moynes DR, Brewster CE. Rehabilitation of shoulder joint instabilities. Orthop Clin North Am 1987; 18:473.

Matsen FA III, Thomas SE, Rockwood CA Jr. Anterior glenohumeral instability. In Rockwood CA Jr, Matsen FA III (eds). The shoulder. Philadelphia: WB Saunders, 1990.

Neer CS II, Foster CR. Inferior capsular shift or involuntary inferior and multidirectional instability of the shoulder: A preliminary report. J Bone Joint Surg 1980; 62A:897.

Neer CS II. Involuntary inferior multidirectional instability to the shoulder: Etiology, recognition and treatment. Instr Course Lect 1985; 34:232.

Neer CS II. Voluntary inferior and multidirectional instability of the shoulder: Etiology, recognition and treatment. In Neer CS II (ed). The shoulder. Philadelphia: WB Saunders, 1990.

Norris TR. Diagnostic techniques for shoulder instability. Instr Course Lect 1985; 34:239.

Rockwood CA Jr, Matsen FA III (eds). The shoulder. Philadelphia: WB Saunders, 1990.

Rowe CR. Acute and recurrent dislocations of the shoulder. J Bone Joint Surg 1962; 44A:998.

ACUTE ANTERIOR CRUCIATE LIGAMENT INJURY

The diagnosis of an acutely torn anterior cruciate ligament (ACL) is based on the circumstance of the injury as reported by the patient and the stability assessment during the physical examination. Many acute tears go undiagnosed due to the wide variety of presentations. Biomechanically, the three bands of the ACL are the primary restraint to anterior translation of the tibia with respect to the femur. Most commonly, the tear is interstitial and irreparable. Occasionally, in adolescents, the ligament is avulsed from its bony attachment and is amenable to primary repair.

A. In the general population, up to 70% of acute ACL injuries occur during sporting events. A decelerating, twisting, cutting, or jumping injury is associated with a pop or giving way episode. Severe swelling within 2–6 hours may occur. Functional instability occurs during running, cutting, and jumping activities. Subsequent swelling episodes are less severe. Because associated meniscal and articular injuries are common; locking, catching, and joint line pain can be present.

B. Examination of the uninjured knee is used as a baseline. Determine muscle tone, range of motion (ROM), and ligamentous stability. Examine the injured knee for swelling, joint line tenderness, effusion, ROM, and collateral ligament stability. Evaluate for posterior cruciate ligament (PCL) injury. Lachman's test of assessing the anterior translation of the tibia on the femur with the knee in 20°–30° of flexion is the most accurate diagnostic examination. Anterior drawer and pivot shift testing are also performed. Classification is based on the amount of translation with 0 being normal, 1+ less than 5 mm, 2+ between 5–10 mm, 3+ between 10–15 mm, and 4+ greater than 15 mm. It is also classified as single plane (i.e., anterior) or rotatory (i.e., anterolateral) if collateral ligaments are involved. Instrumented measurement with an arthrometer can be helpful in knees that are difficult to examine (i.e., extremely large knees).

C. Standing anteroposterior (AP) view, lateral, and patellar views are necessary to rule out bony injury in ACL deficient knees. The presence of a lateral capsular avulsion or Segond's sign is associated with ACL tear. Other intraarticular and periarticular fractures affect the treatment plan for these injuries. Magnetic resonance imaging (MRI) is sometimes indicated for planning purposes. This is particularly helpful when a decision to treat ligamentous tear conservatively necessitates evaluation of meniscal and chondral injuries.

D. No one algorithm fits all patients with ACL disruption. Many factors are unique to that individual and must be considered independently. The factors include: acuity; associated ligamentous, meniscal, or articular cartilage injury; age and activity level; degree of instability; and the patient's ability to modify activities. Activity level is the most important factor. If a patient's occupation or recreational activities require cutting, turning, pivoting, jumping, or other high risk activities, reconstruction is indicated. If they can modify their lifestyles, many patients do well with conservative treatment. NSAI, physical therapy, and ROM exercises are prescribed acutely. Crutch gait may be necessary for a short time. Optional bracing may assist patients in returning to low demand activity. Patients who are not candidates for reconstruction may require arthroscopy if mechanical symptoms develop. ACL stump debridement, meniscectomy, chondroplasty, and loose body excision may be required to improve function.

E. Skeletally mature patients with functional instability, an active lifestyle, and a desire for knee stability should undergo ACL reconstruction. The result of repair of intersubstance ACL tears is poor. The most reliable technique is using the autogenous central third bone patellar tendon bone graft intra-articularly. Other autogenous material include semitendinosus and gracilis tendons singularly or in combination. These grafts are best suited for acute reconstructions and can augment ligament repair. Patients should be operated on only when the inflammation and restricted ROM from the initial injury has resolved. Some studies demonstrate that early intervention increases the risk of postoperative arthrofibrosis.

F. Skeletally immature patients may present with avulsion fractures that can be repaired by primary ORIF or arthroscopically. Mid-substance tears in these patients can be treated conservatively or operatively. Conservative treatment includes activity modification, muscle rehabilitation and re-training, and bracing. In very young patients with significant growth potential, delaying an intra-articular procedure when possible is preferable. Do not use staples to fixate the graft. Hamstring grafts using the over the top method with limited notch plasty may be considered. Take care on the femoral side fixation not to violate the femoral growth plate. In patients approaching skeletal maturity, central third patellar tendon bone tendon bone graft is the most reliable procedure.

ACUTE ANTERIOR CRUCIATE LIGAMENT INJURY

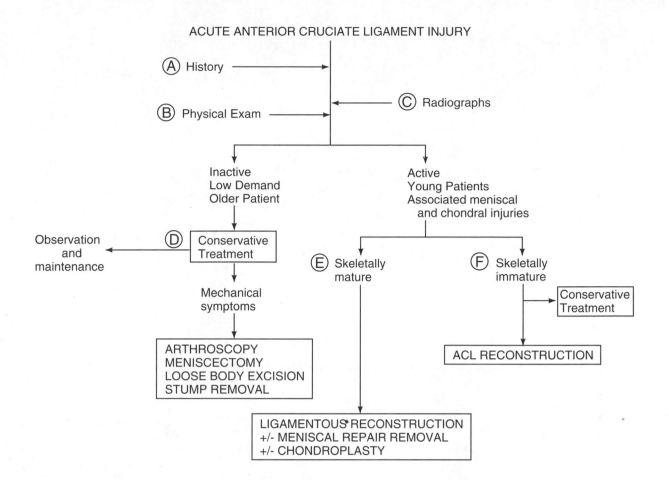

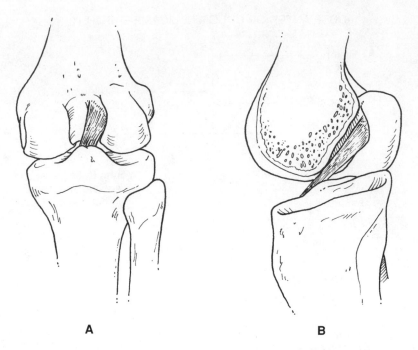

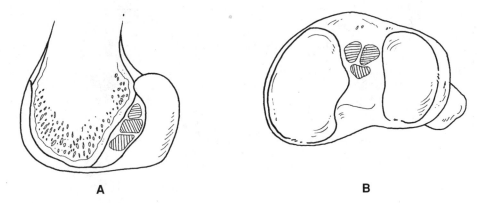

Figure 1 **A,** Anatomic femoral attachment of anterior cruciate ligament. **B,** Course of ligament through notch.

Figure 2 Attachment sites for anterior cruciate ligament. **A,** Femoral attachment. **B,** Tibial attachment.

References

Amiel D, Cleiner JB, Akeson WH. Natural history of anterior cruciate ligament autograft of patellar tendon origin. Am J Sports Med 1986; 14:449.

Cawley PW, France EP, Paulos LE. The current state of functional knee bracing research: A review of the literature. Am J Sports Med 1991; 19:226.

Clanton TO, DeLee JC, Sanders B, et al. Knee ligament injuries in children. J Bone Joint Surg 1979; 61A:1195.

Dandy DJ, Flanagan JP, Steenmeyer B. Arthroscopy in the management of the ruptured anterior cruciate ligament. Clin Orthop 1982; 1967:43.

Daniel DM, Stone ML, Sacks R, et al. Instrumented measurement of the anterior knee laxity in patients with acute anterior cruciate ligament disruption. Am J Sports Med 1985; 13:401.

DeHaven KE. Diagnosis of acute knee injuries with hemarthrosis. Am J Sports Med 1980; 8:9.

Lipscomb B, Anderson A. Tears of the anterior cruciate ligament in adolescents. J Bone Joint Surg 1986; 68A:19.

McCarroll JR, Rettig AC, Shelbourne KD. ACL injuries in the young athlete with open physes. Am J Sports Med 1988; 16:44.

Noyes FR, Bassett RW, Grood EF, Butler DL. Arthroscopy in acute traumatic hemarthrosis of the knee: Incidence of anterior cruciate tears and other injuries. J Bone Joint Surg 1980; 52A:687.

Sgaglione NA, Warren RF, Wickiewicz TL, et al. Primary repair with semitendinosus tendon augmentation of acute anterior cruciate ligament injuries. Am J Sports Med 1990; 18:64.

Shelbourne KD, Wilckens JH, Mollabashy A, DeCarlo M. Arthrofibrosis in acute anterior cruciate ligament reconstruction: The affect of timing of reconstruction and rehabilitation. Am J Sports Med 1991; 19:332.

Torg JS, Conrad W, Kalen V. Clinical diagnosis of anterior cruciate ligament instability in the athlete. Am J Sports Med 1976; 4:84.

Warner JP, Warren RF, Cooper DE. Management of acute anterior cruciate ligament injury. In: Instructional Course Lectures, American Academy of Orthopaedic Surgeons, Vol. 50, pp 219-232, Park Ridge, Ill., American Academy of Orthopaedic Surgeons, 1991.

Woods GW, Stanley RF Jr, Tullos HS. Lateral capsular sign: X-ray clue to significant knee instability. Am J Sports Med 1979; 7:27.

ACUTE POSTERIOR CRUCIATE LIGAMENT INJURY

A. Injuries to the posterior structures of the knee are less common than other soft-tissue injuries about the knee and are frequently missed at initial assessment. Mechanism of injury can often give the first clue. A direct blow anteriorly that hyperextends the knee (Fig. 1, A) obviously places the posterior capsule and cruciate at risk. This occurs in kicking sports such as soccer as well as in contact sports such as football. The other mechanism involves a direct blow anteriorly to a flexed knee—such as in a motorcyclist (Fig. 1, B). This drives the tibia posteriorly and often produces a pure posterior cruciate ligament (PCL) injury. On physical examination, bruising anteriorly, especially on the anteromedial aspect of the proximal tibia, should alert the clinician to the possibility of posterior soft tissue injury. Clinical tests for posterior instability have classically been the posterior sag and the posterior drawer. Daniel et al. and Shelbourne et al. have recently described adaptations of these tests that make interpretation easier. Determining posterolateral instability is clinically much more difficult. Hughston and Norwood described the classic test (Fig. 2), which has been refined by Loomer.

B. Radiographs have routinely only been helpful in determining bony avulsion of the PCL (Fig. 3, A). Recently, Jakob has used stress radiographs to document posterior translation, but the reproducibility of his results is uncertain. The MRI illustrates the posterior cruciate well in the standard cuts, allowing for documentation of pure PCL injuries (Fig. 3, B). Posterolateral corner injuries are less well documented by MRI.

C. Bony avulsions of the PCL tend to occur in younger patients and require reduction and fixation if displaced. Torisu demonstrated that fixation on delayed unions or nonunions is feasible but should probably be reserved for the symptomatic displaced large fragment in the high-demand athlete.

D. Controversy persists over the treatment of midsubstance tears of the PCL. Numerous outcome studies have shown good long-term results of nonoperative treatment of pure PCL injuries. All authors have agreed that associated ligamentous injuries may worsen the results. Other studies have suggested that patellofemoral and medial compartment arthritis are more frequent after PCL injuries and that early surgical reconstruction is advisable. Both Jakob and Parolie have suggested that posterior subluxation >15 mm that does not reduce with internal rotation may indicate more serious posterior disruption requiring surgical intervention.

E. Posterolateral instability may or may not have an associated PCL injury. The lateral corner injury usually involves the arcurate ligament, producing an increased posterolateral sag with external rotation of the tibia. Acute mild posterolateral rotatory instability (PLRI) may be treated with bracing in flexion to allow the posterior capsule to tighten down. Quadriceps rehabilitation following this is crucial and return to sport should occur only when the injured quadriceps are at least equal to the noninjured side when tested on a Cybex–equivalent. Chronic mild PLRI requires a change in the level of sport.

F. Moderate or severe acute PLRI requires surgical reconstruction. Differentiation between mild and moderate PLRI is examiner subjective but should center on the amount of posterolateral tibial rotation and sag. More commonly, PLRI presents as a chronic condition. Surgical decision making in this setting is more difficult as soft tissues have often stretched and reconstruction may have to be done in conjunction with an osteotomy. If the initial tear is discernible, an attempt can be made to repair it. Most often, scarring is such that the original pathology cannot be isolated. Advancement of the posterolateral complex (arcuate ligament, popliteus and fibular collateral ligament)—with or without a bone block—is recommended. Hughston reports superior objective results (90%) and less satisfactory subjective (60%) and functional (40%) results.

G. Examination of a knee suspected of having posterior instability requires full evaluation of all other major ligaments. All authors agree that combination major ligament injuries require surgical intervention.

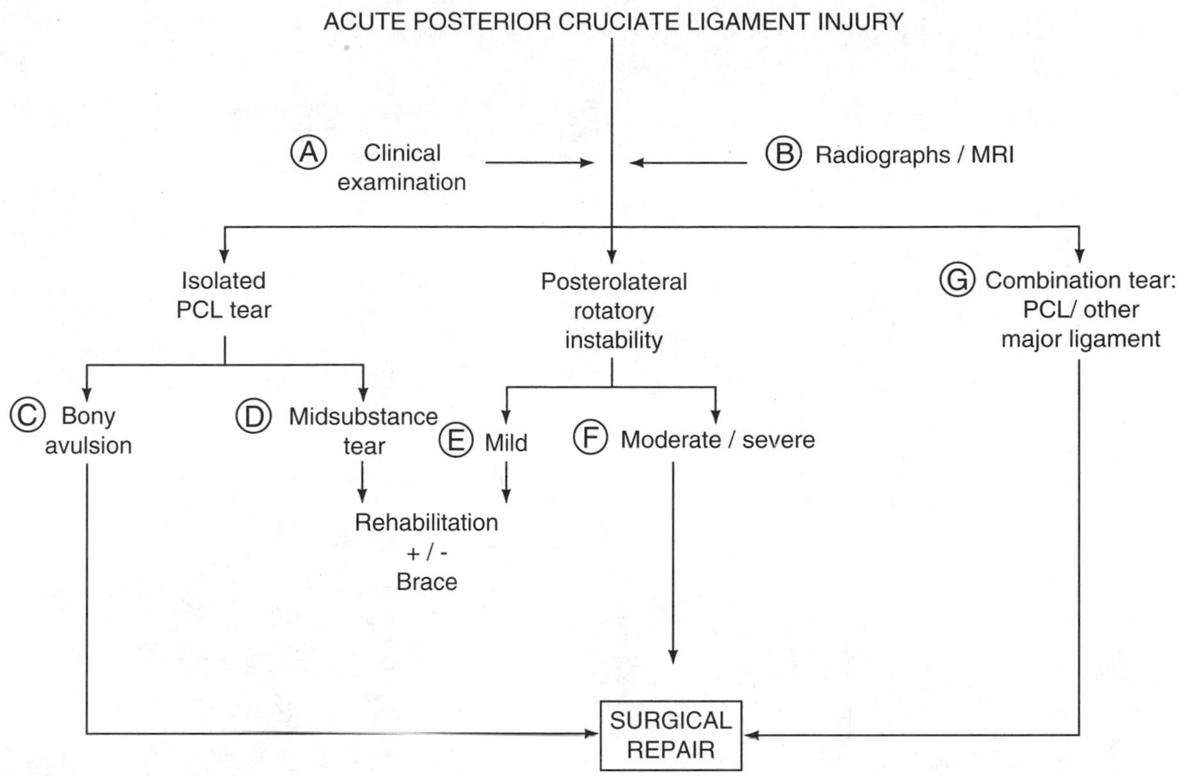

ACUTE POSTERIOR CRUCIATE LIGAMENT INJURY

(A) Clinical examination → ← (B) Radiographs / MRI

Isolated PCL tear

Posterolateral rotatory instability

(G) Combination tear: PCL/ other major ligament

(C) Bony avulsion

(D) Midsubstance tear

(E) Mild

(F) Moderate / severe

Rehabilitation + / - Brace

SURGICAL REPAIR

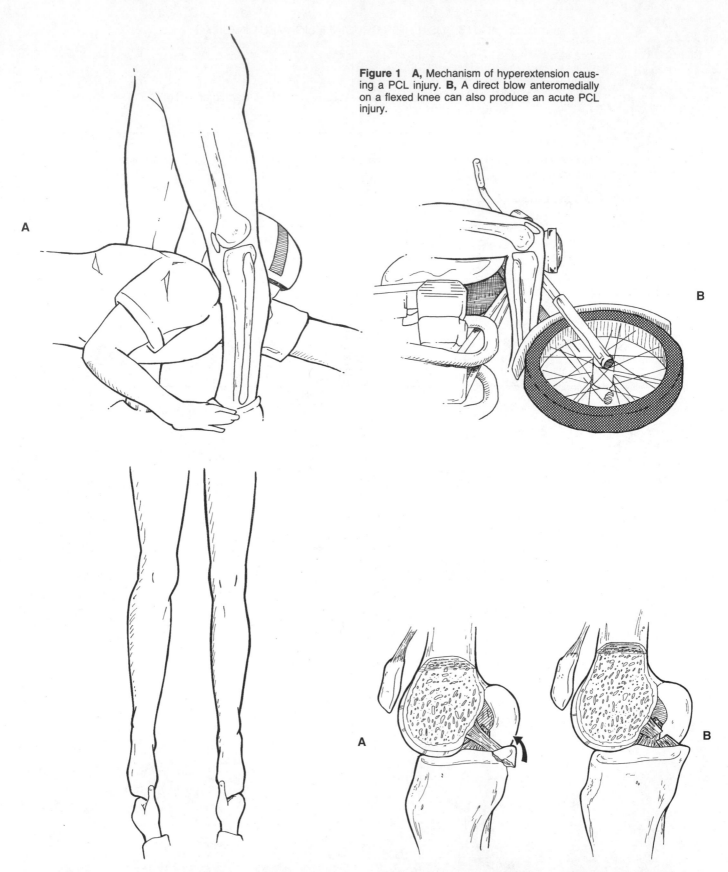

Figure 1 **A,** Mechanism of hyperextension causing a PCL injury. **B,** A direct blow anteromedially on a flexed knee can also produce an acute PCL injury.

Figure 2 Hughston's test for posterolateral instability. Both legs are extended with the examiner holding the great toe. If PLRI is present, the affected knee rotates externally and sags posterolaterally.

Figure 3 PCL injuries can be bony avulsions or mid-substance injuries. **A,** Displaced bony avulsion requires reduction and fixation. **B,** Midsubstance tears have normal radiographs.

References

Clancy WG, Shelbourne KD, Zoellner GB, et al. Treatment of knee joint instability secondary to rupture of the posterior cruciate ligament: Report of a new procedure. J Bone Joint Surg 1983; 65A:310.

Cross MJ, Powell JF: Longterm follow-up of posterior cruciate ligament rupture: A study of 116 cases. Am J Sports Med 1984; 12:292.

Daniel DM, Stone ML, Barnett P, Sachs R. Use of the quadriceps active test to diagnose posterior cruciate disruption and measure posterior laxity of the knee. J Bone Joint Surg 1988; 70A:386.

DeLee JC, Riley MB, Rockwood CA: Acute posterolateral rotatory instability of the knee. Am J Sports Med 1983; 11:199.

Fowler PJ, Messieh SS. Isolated posterior cruciate injuries in athletes. Am J Sports Med 1987; 15:553.

Hess H, Hubertz R. Soccer injuries in sports injuries: Mechanisms, prevention and treatment. In: Schneider RC, Kennedy JC, Plant ML, eds. Baltimore: Williams & Wilkins, 1985.

Hughston JC. Posterolateral rotatory instability. In: Hughston JC. Knee Ligaments: Injury and Repair. Philadelphia: Mosby-Year Book, 1993.

Hughston JC, Norwood LA. The posterolateral drawer test and external rotational recurvatum test for posterolateral rotatory instability of the knee. Clin Orthop 1980; 147:82.

Jakob RP. Acute posterior cruciate ligament tears—Diagnosis and management in knee surgery: Current practice. In: Aichroth PM, Cannon WD, eds. New York: Raven Press, 1992.

Kannus P, Bergfeld J, Jarvinen M, et al. Injuries to the posterior cruciate ligament of the knee. Sports Med 1991; 12:110.

Kennedy JC. The injured knee. In: Schneider RM, Kennedy JC, Plant ML, eds. Sports Injuries: Mechanisms, Prevention and Treatment. Baltimore: Williams & Wilkins, 1985.

Kennedy JC, Grainger RW. The posterior cruciate ligament. J Trauma 1967; 7:367.

Loomer RL. A test for knee posterolateral rotatory instability. Clin Orthop 1991; 264:235.

Parolie JM, Bergfeld JA. Longterm results of non-operative treatment of isolated posterior cruciate injuries in the athlete. Am J Sports Med 1986; 14:35.

Shelbourne KD, Benedict F, McCarrol JR, Rettig AC. Dynamic posterior shift test. An adjuvant in evaluation of posterior tibial subluxation. Am J Sports Med 1989; 17:275.

Torg JS, Barton TM, Pavlov H, Stine R. Natural history of the posterior cruciate ligament deficient knee. Clin Orthop 1983; 246:208.

Torisu T. Avulsion fracture of the tibial attachment of the posterior cruciate ligament: Indications and results of delayed repair. Clin Orthop 1973; 143:107.

ANTERIOR CRUCIATE LIGAMENT DEFICIENT KNEE

The true natural history of the anterior cruciate ligament (ACL) deficient knee is unknown. Many of these injuries go undiagnosed and unreported. Many studies have shown recurrent meniscal injury, degenerative arthrosis, and functional disability with untreated anterior instability. However, others have stated that disruption of the ACL does not necessarily lead to dysfunction. Still others report that operated knees were not improved compared with conservatively treated knees.

A. The patient typically can relate the original injury to the present symptoms. Twisting, decelerating, cutting, or jumping injury with a giving way episode or an associated pop and significant swelling are commonly described. Correlate recent symptoms of pain, swelling, and giving way with current level of activities. Note the frequency and total number of giving way episodes or swelling. Unfortunately, many of these patients have had previous surgery or even previous reconstructions that have failed. Examine for thigh atrophy, patellofemoral stability and crepitance, osteophytes and loose bodies, or mechanical symptoms from mensical disease. Anterior drawer and Lachman's testing are graded as in acute ACL injury (p 490). Record the status of the end point of the anterior translation—firm or soft. Pivot shift testing demonstrates anterolateral transitory motion similar to the described giving way episodes and may actually recreate the patient's complaints.

B. Radiography includes standard standing bilateral anteroposterior (AP) views, lateral views, notch and patellar views. Assess degenerative changes. Intracondylar eminence peaking, joint space narrowing, notch encroachment, and multi-compartmental degenerative joint disease (DJD) may be seen even in young patients with ACL deficiency.

C. Arthrometry, in experienced hands, gives an objective measure of translation. Side-to-side comparison is useful in understanding the degree of instability.

D. Skeletally immature patients who demonstrate functional instability and have failed conservative measures including bracing, are candidates for reconstruction. Autogenous semitendinosus graft, routed intra-articularly over the top of the femur, and extra-articular reconstructions (EAR) are performed to prevent violations of the femoral growth plate. Standard central bone-patellar tendon-bone (BTB) grafts with interference fixation, however, yield the most reliable and reproducible results.

E. Treat inactive, older patients, or patients with significant degenerative joint disease and no pivot or giving way episodes with activity modification and maintenance rehabilitation programs with functional bracing for low level activity. These patients occasionally require arthroscopy for meniscal or chondral lesions to improve function.

F. Active patients with functional instability benefit from ACL reconstruction. Autogenous patellar tendon or hamstring tendon grafts are most commonly performed for primary reconstructions. Careful placement, tensioning, and graft fixation are critical to the success of the procedure. Obtaining normal range of motion (ROM) postoperatively is essential. With interference fixation, immediate weight bearing and full ROM are permitted postoperatively. Early rehabilitation allows return to most sports and work-related activities within 4–6 months. Allograft reconstruction is usually reserved for salvage of previous failed autogenous reconstructions. Consider extra-articular backup with an IT bank tenodesis in allograft procedures for chronic ACL insufficiency. Excellent results can be obtained with allograft reconstructions. However, disease transmission, graft availability, and expense make it a salvage choice. The most reproducible and reliable surgery in the ACL-deficient knee is the central third BTB autograft.

References

Amiel D, Cleiner JB, Akeson WH. Natural history of anterior cruciate ligament autograft of patellar tendon origin. Am J Sports Med 1986; 14:449.

Daniel DM, Stone ML, Sacks R, et al. Instrumental measurement of the anterior knee laxity in patients with acute anterior cruciate ligament disruption. Am J Sports Med 1985; 13:401.

Fetto GF, Marshall JL. The natural history and diagnosis of the anterior cruciate ligament insufficiency. Clin Orthop 1980; 147:29.

Hawkins RJ, Misamore GW, Merit TR. Follow-up of the acute non-operated isolated anterior cruciate ligament tear. Am J Sports Med 1986; 14:205.

Indelicato PA, Linton RC, Huegel M. The results of fresh-frozen patellar tendon allografts for chronic ACL deficiency of the knee. Am J Sports Med 1992; 20:118.

McCarroll JR, Rettig AC, Shelbourne KD. ACL injuries in the young athlete with open physes. Am J Sports Med 1988; 16:44.

McDaniel WJ Jr, Dameron TB Jr. Untreated rupture of the anterior cruciate ligament: A follow-up study. J Bone Joint Surg 1980; 62A:696.

Noyes FR, Barber-Westin ST, Robert SC. Use of allografts for failed treatment of rupture of the anterior cruciate ligament. J Bone Joint Surg 1994; 76A:1019.

Noyes FR, Mooar PA, Mathews DS, Butler DL. The symptomatic anterior cruciate deficient knee: Part 1—The long-term functional disability in athletically active individuals. J Bone Joint Surg 1983; 65A:154.

Sandberg R, Balkfors B, Neilson B, Westlin N. Operative versus non-operative treatment of recent injuries to the ligaments of the knee: A prospective randomized study. J Bone Joint Surg 1987; 69A:1120.

Steiner ME, Brown C, Zarins B, et al. Measurement of anterior-posterior displacement of the knee: A comparison of the results with instrumented devices and with clinical examination. J Bone Joint Surg 1990; 72A:1307.

ANTERIOR CRUCIATE LIGAMENT DEFICIENT KNEE

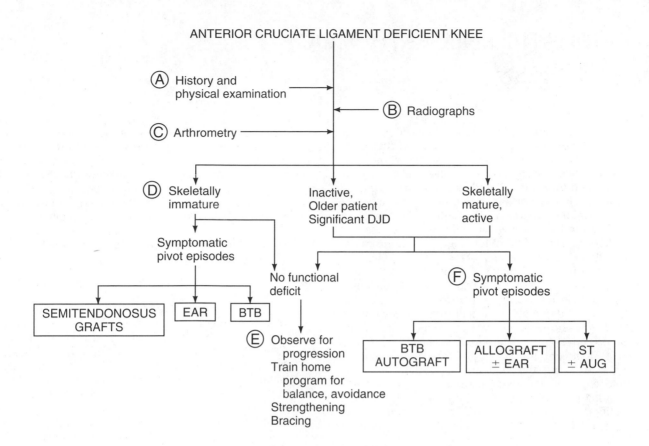

ATRAUMATIC KNEE PATHOLOGY
IN ATHLETES

A. Improper technique, overtraining and ill-fitting equipment are the more common causes of soft tissue inflammation about the knee in athletes. Poor warm-up programs often result in increased iliotibial band tightness; while overtraining produces stress fractures and tendonitis (Fig. 1). An accurate history of the athlete's recent training regimen should include details of warm-up and warm-down activities as well as changes in intensity or duration of training. Physical examination often pinpoints the area of inflammation. Iliotibial band syndrome is frequently symptomatic at the joint line just above Gerdy's tubercle. Stress fractures usually occur in the posteromedial aspect of the proximal tibia. Radiographs are usually normal. Bone scans are diagnostic for stress fractures, which usually occur posteriorly or posteromedially on the proximal tibia. Treatment consists of physical therapy modalities to decrease the inflammation while continuing protected strengthening. Workouts in the pool allow continued cardiorespiratory conditioning without loading the injured extremity. Orthotics and specialized coaching sessions may help prevent recurrence.

B. Patellofemoral symptoms are almost as frequent in athletes as in the general population. This anterior knee pain can be divided into two basic groups—that associated with obvious maltracking (subluxation or dislocation) and that without significant tracking pathology. The latter responds well to physical therapy that emphasizes vastus medialis strengthening—usually by cycling—and iliotibial band stretch. Braces are also used but their effectiveness is uncertain. Recent laboratory studies suggest that subtle maltracking may be the cause and that these changes may be reversible. Differential diagnosis of anterior knee pain should include osteochondritis dissecans of the patella, symptomatic plica, and reflex sympathetic dystrophy.

C. Instability of the patella in the femoral groove is usually lateral (Fig. 2). Most authors recommend conservative treatment initially for subluxation and the majority of dislocations. Hawkins identified several at-risk factors that may mandate early surgery in dislocations, including intra-articular loose bodies and severe ligamentous laxity with a family history of dislocations. A long-term follow-up study by a group in Sweden found poorer results in the operative cases. This suggests that demonstrated failure of an established physical therapy regimen is needed prior to surgical consideration. A number of procedures have been used with varying degrees of success. The underlying principle of the surgical procedures has been to realign the patellar tracking mechanism. Although lateral release is a component of most procedures, it is rarely successful as the sole procedure. Both proximal and distal realignment procedures have been advocated. At present, it would appear that distal realignment, such as with the Elmslie-Trillat procedure, is well tolerated in the adolescent population. However, adult patients seem to have better results with proximal realignment such as vastus medialis advancement.

D. Effusions, locking or catching and vague generalized knee discomfort, often with no history of trauma, are the usual modes of presentation of an unusual form of knee problem—diseases of the synovium. Connective tissue disorders such as rheumatoid arthritis and Reiter's disease do occur in athletes; once diagnosed, they are usually treated by established medical regimens. Presenting with the same symptoms and physical examination, but with no laboratory abnormalities are localized synovial diseases such as pigmented villonodular synovitis (PVNS) and synovial chondromatosis. Several radiologic studies have demonstrated the usefulness of magnetic resonance imaging (MRI) in establishing the diagnosis. Thickened synovium is easily visualized on the MRI. The variation in signal between the blood products of PVNS and the chondral bodies found in synovial chondromatosis allow for differential diagnosis on MRI. Treatment involves removal of both diseased and residual synovium as recurrence rates are high. Traditionally this has been done as an open synovectomy, but recent experiences suggest that lower recurrence rates and less morbidity may be possible with arthroscopic synovectomy.

E. Tumors occur not infrequently about the knee and not infrequently in athletes. The most common symptomatic benign tumor is an osteochondroma, which may arise either in the distal femur or the proximal tibia. Radiographs will demonstrate those on the distal femur, but a CT scan may be needed to visualize the more sessile lesions of the proximal tibia. Treatment depends on the persistence of symptoms. A number of malignant tumors may also present about the knee. Giant cell tumors (Fig. 3) often present as joint line or collateral ligament insertion pain. Symptoms such as night pain, pain at rest and gradually increasing pain warrant further work-up for diagnosis. Minimal or equivocal changes on radiographs can be substantiated with either bone scan or MRI. Treatment depends on pathology and should be carried out in concert with the oncology team.

ATRAUMATIC KNEE PATHOLOGY IN ATHLETES

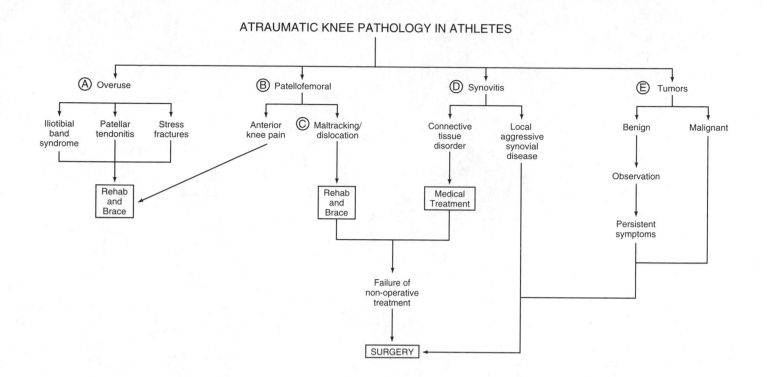

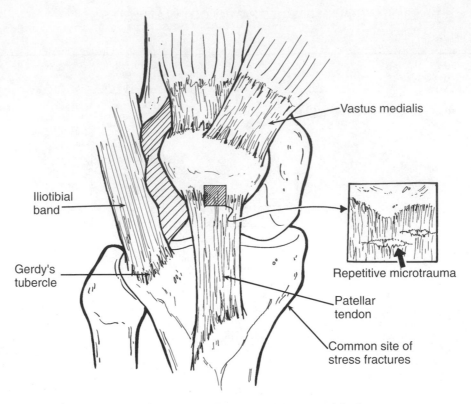

Figure 1 Common sites of overuse injuries around the knee.

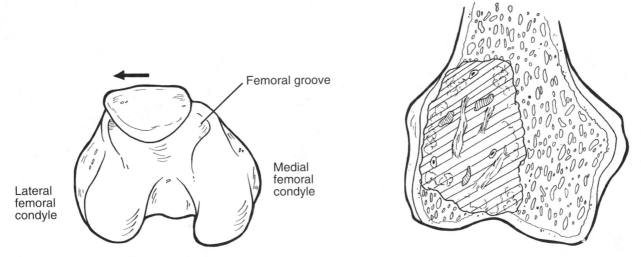

Figure 2 Lateral position of maltracking patella in femoral groove.

Figure 3 Giant cell tumor occupying most of the lateral femoral condyle.

References

Aalberg JR. Synovial hemangioma of the knee: A case report. Acta Orthop Scan 1990, 61:88.

Arnbjornsson A, Egund N, Rydling O, et al. The natural history of recurrent dislocation of the patella. J Bone Joint Surg 1992; 748:140.

Bessette GC, Hunter RE. The Maquet procedure: A retrospective review. Clin Orthop 1988; 232:159.

Brukner P, Khan K. Lateral, medial and posterior knee pain. In: Brukner P, Khan K, eds. Clinical Sports Medicine. Sydney: McGraw-Hill, 1993.

Campanacci M, Baldini N, Boriani S, Sudanese A. Giant cell tumor of the bone. J Bone Joint Surg 1987; 69A:106.

Coolican MR, Dandy DJ. Arthroscopic management of synovial chondromatosis of the knee. J Bone Joint Surg 1989; 71B:498.

Fisher RL. Conservative treatment of patellofemoral pain. Orthop Clin North Am 1986; 17:269.

Fulkerson JP, Shea KP. Disorders of patellofemoral alignment: Current concepts review. J Bone Joint Surg 1990; 72A:1424.

Gebhardt MD, Ready JE, Mankin HJ. Tumors about the knee in children. Clin Orthop 1990; 255:86.

Hawkins RJ, Bell RH, Arisette G. Acute patellar dislocations: The natural history. Am J Sports Med 1986; 14:117.

Johnson DP, Eastwood DM, Witherow PJ: Symptomatic synovial plica of the knee. J Bone Joint Surg 1993; 75A:1485.

Kransdorf MJ, Moser RP, Vinh TN, et al: Primary tumors of the patella. Skelet Radiol 1989; 18:365.

Lyu S-R, Wu J-J. Snapping syndrome caused by the semitendinosis tendon. J Bone Joint Surg 1989; 71A:303.

Mandebaum BR, Grant TT, Hartzman S, et al. The use of MRI to assist in diagnosis of pigmented villonodular synovitis of the knee joint. Clin Orthop 1988; 231:135.

Marcove RC, Arlen M, eds. In Atlas of Bone Pathology, Philadelphia: J.B. Lippincott, 1992.

Milgram C, Finestone A, Shlamkovitch N. Patellofemoral pain caused by overactivity. J Bone Joint Surg 1991; 73A:1041.

Moller BN, Moller-Larsen F, Frich LH. Chondromalacia induced by patellar subluxation in the rabbit. Acta Orthop Scand 1989; 60:188.

Musculo PL, Ayerza MA, Calabrese ME, Gruerberg M. The use of bone allograft for reconstruction after resection of giant-cell tumor close to the knee. J Bone Joint Surg 1993; 75A:1656.

Pfeiffer WH, Gross ML, Seeger LL. Osteochondritis dissecans of the patella. Clin Orthop 1991; 271:207.

Ray JM, Clancy WG, Leman RA. Semimembranous tendonitis: An overlooked cause of medial knee pain. Am J Sports Med 1988; 16:347.

Rukeras O. Brace with a lateral pad for patellar pain. Acta Orthop Scand 1990; 61:319.

Shipley M (ed). In A Colour Atlas of Rheumatology. 3rd ed. Ayresbury: Wolfe Publishing, Mosby—Year Book Europe Ltd, 1993.

Sojbjerg JO, Lauritzen J, Hvid I, Boe S. Arthroscopic determination of patellofemoral malalignment. Clin Orthop 1987; 215:243.

Sundarams M, McGuire MH, Fletcher J, et al. Magnetic resonance imaging of lesions of synovial origin. Skelet Radiol 1986; 15:110.

Thompson RC, Vener JJ, Griffiths HJ, et al. Scanning electron-microscopic and magnetic resonance imaging studies of injuries to the patellofemoral joint after acute transarticular load. J Bone Joint Surg 1993; 75A:704.

Tutjen R. Reflex sympathetic dystrophy of the knee. Clin Orthop 1986; 209:234.

Wootan JR, Cross MJ, Wood DG. Patellofemoral malalignment: A report of 68 cases treated by proximal and distal patellofemoral reconstruction. Injury 1990; 21:169.

Yates CK, Grana WA. Patellofemoral pain in children. Clin Orthop 1990; 255:36.

MENISCAL DERANGEMENT

The meniscus fibrocartilage serves to increase knee stability, joint congruency, improve nutrition and lubrication of the articular cartilage. The menisci bear 50%–70% of the load from the femur to the tibia and translate compression loads to hoop stress. The peripheral 2–3 mm has a demonstrable blood supply in the adult. This blood supply is more prevalent in the anterior and posterior horns and in children. The entire meniscus, however, is metabolically active. Patients with ligamentous instability are particularly prone to meniscal tears. Meniscectomy in these patients significantly increases the risk of osteoarthritis. Preadolescent patients do very poorly after a meniscectomy. The goal of treatment is to preserve as much meniscus as possible.

A. Patients with unstable tears complain of pain, catching, popping, or locking. Findings are more subtle with degenerative or stable tears. Examination for associated injury including anterior cruciate ligament (ACL), posterior cruciate ligament (PCL), or collateral ligamentous damage is indicated due to this high association of meniscal tears with ligamentous injury. Effusion, thigh wasting, and joint line tenderness are commonly seen. Compare range of motion (ROM) to the contralateral knee. Prone extension comparing heel height differences often reveals asymmetry and subtle extension deficits in knees with meniscal tears. Compression testing, such as McMurray's or Apley's maneuvers, may elicit pain during the examination.

B. Standing anteroposterior (AP), lateral, notch, and patellar views give an overall assessment of joint congruity and the presence or absence of joint space narrowing or degenerative joint disease (DJD). Magnetic resonance imaging (MRI) has replaced arthrography as the diagnostic ancillary procedure of choice. Only after failure of conservative treatment, and in the absence of a clear diagnosis from physical examination and history, should this study be used. Its accuracy is dependent on many factors. Grade I and II signals are intrameniscal and usually should be observed. Grade III signals have a high correlation with full-thickness meniscal tears. The capability to rule out a meniscal tear is limited by a high false-negative rate.

C. Patients complaining of joint line pain, catching, popping, or locking are first treated conservatively. In many patients the initial symptoms resolve without sequela. Ice, nonsteroidal anti-inflammatory drugs (NSAIDs), crutch gaiting, and ROM exercises along with activity modifications are indicated. If the symptoms resolve, the patient can return to normal activities. If symptoms continue and ROM is limited, arthroscopic evaluation is indicated.

D. Meniscal tears in the avascular zone (i.e., inner third) or complete irreparable tears are excised to a stable rim. Preservation of the posterior horns and as much stable rim as possible is the goal especially in ACL deficient knees.

E. Reparable tears are of traumatic origin in the vascular region of the meniscus (peripheral third) and >7 mm long. Patients with a reparable tear associated with an ACL tear have a 90% chance of healing the repair if the knee is stabilized. If the knee is not stabilized, up to 40% of the repairs fail. Using anatomic landmarks and careful approach, injury to the peroneal nerve laterally and saphenous nerve medially can be avoided.

F. Partial thickness tears and stable vertical or oblique tears <5 mm long can be left alone.

G. Patients with chronic symptoms of effusions or joint line tenderness with catching undergo a trial of activity modification, NSAIDs, rehabilitation, and impact modification with shoe inserts. If this fails, arthroscopic partial meniscectomy is indicated. Rarely, the meniscus is brittle and degenerated to the extent that total meniscectomy is necessary.

MENISCAL DERANGEMENT

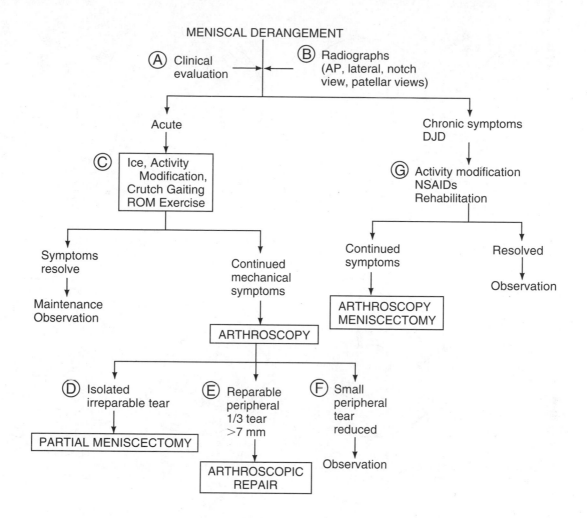

(A) Clinical evaluation   (B) Radiographs (AP, lateral, notch view, patellar views)

Acute

Chronic symptoms DJD

(C) Ice, Activity Modification, Crutch Gaiting ROM Exercise

(G) Activity modification NSAIDs Rehabilitation

Symptoms resolve

Continued mechanical symptoms

Continued symptoms

Resolved

Maintenance Observation

ARTHROSCOPY

ARTHROSCOPY MENISCECTOMY

Observation

(D) Isolated irreparable tear

(E) Reparable peripheral 1/3 tear >7 mm

(F) Small peripheral tear reduced

PARTIAL MENISCECTOMY

ARTHROSCOPIC REPAIR

Observation

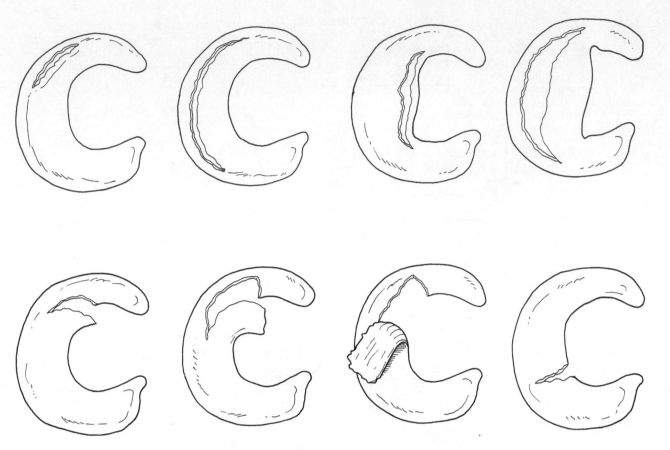

Figure 1 Meniscal cartilage tears present in a variety of anatomic patterns. The goal of treatment is to preserve as much stable tissue as possible

References

DeHaven JE. Decision making factors in treatment of meniscal lesions. Clin Orthop 1990; 252:49.

Fischer FP, Fox JM, Delpizzio W, et al. Accuracy of diagnosis of magnetic resonance imaging of the knee: Multi-center analysis of 1,014 patients. J Bone Joint Surg 1991; 73A:2.

Jackson GW, Jennings LD, Maywood RM, et al. Magnetic resonance imaging in the knee. Am J Sports Med 1988; 16:29.

Medlar RC, Mandiberg JA, Lyne DD. Meniscectomies in children: A report of long-term results. Am J Sports Med 1980; A:87.

Morgan Casscells SW. Arthroscopic meniscal repair: A safe approach to posterior horns. Arthroscopy 1986; 2:3.

Raunest J, Oberle A, Louhnert J, et al. The clinical value of magnetic resonance imaging in the evaluation of meniscal disorders. J Bone Joint Surg 1991; 73A:11.

Shoemaker SC, Markols L. The role of the meniscus in anterior posterior stability and loaded anterior cruciate deficient knee. J Bone Joint Surg 1986; 68A:71.

Warren RF. Meniscectomy in apparent anterior cruciate ligament deficient patient. Clin Orthop 1990; 252:563.

UNSTABLE ANKLE

A. Historically initial assessment of the unstable ankle included standard radiographs. The low yield on these examinations prompted the use of arthrograms and "tenograms"; but these were difficult to perform and also low yield for diagnosis. Several recent studies suggest that, at least for the soft tissue pathology, the most accurate radiologic examination may be the MRI.

B. One of the cardinal symptoms of an unstable ankle is giving way, particularly on uneven ground. "Going over" on the ankle is usually secondary to lateral ankle pathology such as collateral dysfunction or peroneal tendon dislocation or it may be due to hindfoot pathology such as tarsal coalition.

C. Lateral ligament injury about the ankle is extremely common. Injuries may involve one or more of the lateral ligaments. Lively debate continues over surgical versus nonsurgical treatment in the acute setting, but most authors prefer rehabilitation as the majority of patients do well. Nonoperative treatment includes physical therapy as well as specific exercises for proprioception. Anti-inflammatories may be beneficial. Some form of ankle support on return to sport is strongly recommended, especially in ankle-at-risk sports such as basketball. Studies show that bracing is a more consistent support than taping. Lateral ligament injuries that take >2 months to resolve may involve either an os fibulare or a syndesmosis injury. Occasionally a small avulsion fracture may occur at the tip of the fibula—a delayed or nonunion may produce persistent pain. The syndesmosis injury is more subtle (Fig. 1) but the patients frequently have pain when the fibula is compressed towards the tibia above the ankle. These do not always need surgical placement of a syndesmosis screw, but probably warrant slower progression of weight bearing.

D. Patients with persistent lateral ligament instability may require surgical repair. Numerous operations have been described and all have satisfactory results at long-term follow-up. Recent trends are towards using the injured ligament or neighboring nonessential tissue and preserving soft tissue structures that contribute to dynamics of the foot.

E. Peroneal tendon dislocation occurs after disruption of the superior peroneal retinaculum (SPR), which holds the tendons against the fibula (Fig. 2). The initial injury is similar to that for lateral ligament injuries and, as a result, the SPR injury often is missed initially. If appreciated initially, it can be treated nonoperatively. Most patients present with chronic symptoms requiring surgical reconstruction of the retinaculum.

F. Tarsal coalition of the hindfoot—commonly calcaneo-navicular or talo-calcaneal—may present with giving way as well as peroneal spasm. Although a congenital deformity, the commonest age of presentation is adolescence. Treatment varies widely, but most agree that signs of degenerative changes in adjacent joints of the foot preclude bar resection, leaving triple arthrodesis as the treatment of choice for the very symptomatic patient.

G. Recurrent locking is the second most common chronic ankle symptom. Although spasm in adjacent tendons may cause pseudolocking, the causes of classic locking are usually mechanical. Articular cartilage flaps or loose bodies (osteochondritis dissecans) and synovial hypertrophy secondary to an underlying disease process are the most common causes.

H. Osteochondritis dissecans of the talus has two different forms—medial and lateral. The lateral injury (Fig. 3, A) is usually post-traumatic and produces an anterolateral shallow wafer that is easily displaced. Unless undisplaced and asymptomatic, surgical treatment with debridement and drilling of the defect is recommended.

I. Medial osteochondritis of the talus (Fig. 3, B) is a true avascular necrosis. The lesion is posteromedial, has a deep crater and not infrequently occurs in adolescents. In the younger patient a lesion in-situ may heal with protected weight bearing. Displaced lesions or in situ lesions that do not heal with protection require either pinning or excision and drilling of the defect.

J. Symptomatic synovitis of the ankle can arise from either a generalized connective tissue disease such as rheumatoid arthritis or from a local synovial disease such as pigmented villonodular synovitis or synovial chondromatosis. The systemic diseases frequently respond to medical treatment while the localized synovial diseases require arthroscopic synovectomy. Failure of medical treatment is a good indication for arthroscopic synovectomy.

K. Sports that require extremes of ankle dorsiflexion or plantarflexion can lead to anterior or posterior impingement. Anterior impingement is usually secondary to spur formation on the anterior tibia and/or the neck of the talus. Posterior impingement, seen particularly in ballet dancers, is often caused by a large os trigonum. Most authors recommend aggressive rehabilitation and brace, with surgery reserved for failures of nonoperative treatment.

UNSTABLE ANKLE

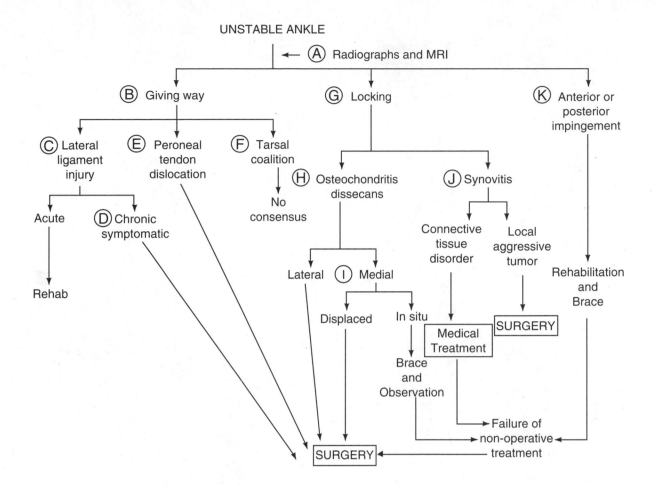

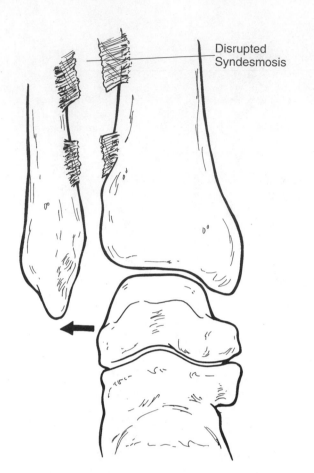

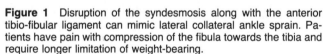

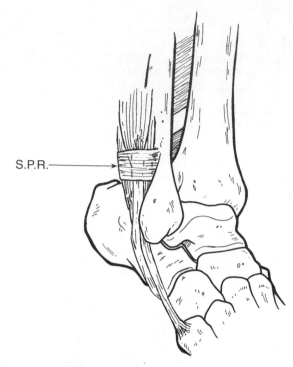

Figure 1 Disruption of the syndesmosis along with the anterior tibio-fibular ligament can mimic lateral collateral ankle sprain. Patients have pain with compression of the fibula towards the tibia and require longer limitation of weight-bearing.

Figure 2 Disruption of the superior peroneal retinaculum (SPR) can occur with inversion injuries and leads to instability of the peroneal tendons at the distal end of the fibula.

Figure 3 **A,** Lateral osteochondritis dissecans of the talus is usually anterior and follows an acute ankle injury. **B,** Medial osteochondritis is a true avascular necrosis and is usually posterior on the talus.

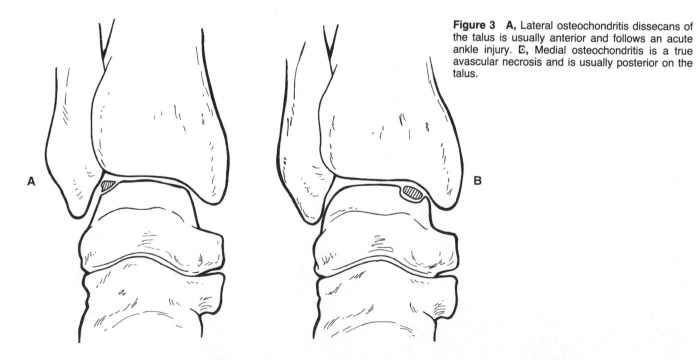

References

Berg EE. The symptomatic os subfibular. J Bone Joint Surg 1991; 73A:1251.

Brage ME, Hansen ST. Traumatic subluxation/dislocation of the peroneal tendons. Foot Ankle 1992; 13:423.

Cass JR, Morrey BF, Katoh Y, Chao EYS. Ankle instability: Comparison of primary repair and delayed reconstruction after longterm follow-up study. Clin Orthop 1985; 198:110.

Cheung Y, Rosenberg ZS, Magee T, Chiritz L. Normal anatomy and pathologic conditions of ankle tendons: Current imaging techniques. Radiographics 1992; 12:429.

Chrisman OD, Snook GA. Reconstruction of lateral ligament tears of the ankle. J Bone Joint Surg 1969; 51A:904.

Coker TM. Sports injuries to the foot and ankle. In: Jahss MH, ed. Disorders of the Foot and Ankle. Philadelphia: WB Saunders, 1991.

Drez D, Young JC, Waldman D, et al. Nonoperative treatment of double lateral ligament tears of the ankle. Am J Sports Med 1982; 10:197.

Dupont M, Bilibeau P, Theriault G. The efficacy of anti-inflammatory medication in the treatment of the acutely sprained ankle. Am J Sports Med 1987;15:41.

Evans GA, Hardcastle P, Frenyo AD. Acute ruptures of the lateral ligament of the ankle: To suture or not to suture. J Bone Joint Surg 1984; 66B:209.

Greene TA, Hillman SK. Comparison of support provided by a semirigid orthosis and adhesive ankle taping before, during and after exercise. Am J Sports Med 1990; 18:498.

Hocutt JE, Jaffe R, Rylander CR, Beebe JK. Cryotherapy in ankle sprains. Am J Sports Med 1982; 10:316.

Hopkinson WJ, St. Pierre P, Ryan JB, Wheeler JH. Syndesmosis sprains of the ankle. Foot Ankle 1990; 10:325.

Kannus P, Renstrom P. Treatment for acute tears of the lateral ligaments of the ankle: Current concepts review. J Bone Joint Surg 1991; 73A:305.

Marotta JJ, Micheli LJ. Os trigonum impingement in dancers. Am J Sports Med 1992, 20:533.

Rovere GD, Clarke TJ, Yates, CS, Burley K. Retrospective comparison of taping and ankle stabilizers in preventing ankle injuries. Am J Sports Med 1988; 16:228.

Ruben K, McCarthy S, Dietz MJ, Rudicel S. MRI appearance of painful conditions of the ankle. Radiographics 1991; 11:401.

St. Pierre R, Allman F, Bassett FH, et al. A review of lateral ankle ligamentous reconstruction. Foot Ankle 1982; 3:114.

St. Pierre, RK, Andrews L, Allman F, Fleming LL. The Cybex II evaluation of lateral ankle ligamentous reconstructions. Am J Sports Med 1984; 12:52.

Smith RW, Reischl SF. Treatment of ankle sprains in young athletes. Am J Sports Med 1986; 14:465.

Snook GA, Chrisman OD, Wilson TA. Longterm results of the Chrisman-Snook operation for reconstruction of the lateral ligaments of the ankle. J Bone Joint Surg 1985; 67A:1.

Snyder RB, Lipscomb AB, Johnston RK. The relationship of tarsal coalitions to ankle sprains in athletes. Am J Sports Med 1981; 9:313.

OVERUSE INJURIES OF THE ELBOW

A. The elbow serves as a link between the shoulder and the hand. As such, particularly in throwing sports, repetitive and often supraphysiologic loads are placed on various components of this joint. Pitchers and tennis players are the most likely groups to develop these problems, but they can be found in any throwing sports.

B. The elbow can be divided into four compartments—medial, lateral, anterior, and posterior. The predicted involvement of a given compartment depends on the nature of the repetitive activity undertaken. For instance, most high-level older pitchers will have overuse changes in their medial and posterior compartments. Joint effusions and a history of locking usually suggest intra-articular pathology. Localized soft tissue swelling and tenderness are found with muscular and ligamentous injuries. Differentiating neural entrapment is difficult because the findings are frequently the same as soft tissue injuries. However, the presence of Tinel's sign is helpful.

C. Intra-articular and bony overuse injuries include spurs, osteochondritis, loose bodies, and, in children, apophyseal injuries. Spurs are usually secondary to either traction or intra-articular degenerative changes. Osteochondritis, usually involving the lateral or radiocapitellar compartment, is thought to be caused by chronic forceful impingement of the radial head on the capitellum. This process may progress to the point where loose osteocartilaginous fragments are shed into the joint. Chronic strain in children often leads to undisplaced fractures in the apophysis of the elbow—the most commonly injured being the medial epicondyle. Recently, injuries to the olecranon apophysis in athletes have also been reported.

D. Recurrent mechanical locking of the elbow is usually secondary to either an intra-articular loose body or a spur impinging on adjacent structures. A reliable history of locking with objective evidence of a lesion mandates surgical treatment to allow return of function. Most loose bodies can be removed arthroscopically. If a spur is the definite cause, small lateral or medial incisions are recommended so as to not interfere with muscle function and to allow rapid return of motion.

E. Musculotendinous units such as the biceps or the common extensor origin and the collateral ligaments of the elbow joint are the most common sites of overuse injury in this area. Most present as chronic inflammation and respond well to nonoperative treatment. Overuse injuries are felt to be the result of repeated microtrauma. The tendon or ligament is momentarily elongated past its elastic limit and sustains a microscopic tear. Normally, with rest, these tears heal uneventfully. In these athletes, the healing process is only partially complete when another microscopic tear is sustained. These repeat injuries set up a chronic inflammatory process that requires anti-inflammatory medications and no further injury to allow healing. Although there are no known anatomic predisposing factors, a good number of these problems are secondary to improper technique or too vigorous a training schedule.

F. Repetitive overload, the most common cause of overuse, must cease during the healing phase. The rest prescribed is only for the involved elbow and only with regards to those motions that produce the overload. Maintaining fitness, especially cardiovascular, is crucial for the high-level athlete. Initial modalities of therapy should aim at reducing pain and inflammation and returning range of motion. These modalities include ultrasound, anti-inflammatory medications, and hydrotherapy. Once pain has subsided and motion returned, strengthening and flexibility can be addressed. Most of these injuries are secondary to improper technique and coaching assessment prior to returning to training should be encouraged. Only in a few types of injuries has bracing been shown to possibly be effective.

G. Instability, both acute and chronic, can occur at the elbow. Chronic instability usually occurs when the medial collateral ligament has undergone repetitive trauma. Surgical repair can be attempted, but has mixed results. Jobe requires that his patients have failed a 6- to 10-month rehab program, be high caliber athletes, and not be able to throw effectively before he will consider them for reconstruction. Acute collateral instability and acute tendon ruptures require early surgical repair followed by early motion.

H. Neural entrapment around the elbow mimics common overuse syndromes and as a result, the diagnosis is frequently missed. Entrapment of all three nerves at the elbow have been described. Classic neural compression within a confined space such as the cubital tunnel can occur; or the nerve may be compressed as it passes through muscle bellies. More frequently local inflammation, such as bursitis or tenosynovitis in adjacent structures, leads to neural compression. Differentiation of neural involvement is difficult, but the pattern of pain radiation and a positive Tinel's sign will help. A good portion of these will respond to nonoperative treatment.

I. Refractory neural entrapment should be documented by nerve conduction studies and have failed a reliable therapy regime prior to surgical exploration. Therapy should include methods of reducing local inflammation such as ultrasound, methods for reducing neural irritation such as transcutaneous nerve stimulation, and splinting to prevent further irritation. If surgical release is necessary, the approaches at the elbow are well outlined in Dawson et al (see References).

OVERUSE INJURY OF THE ELBOW

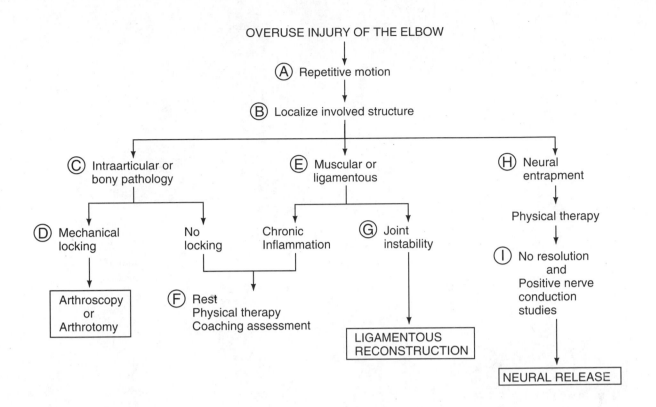

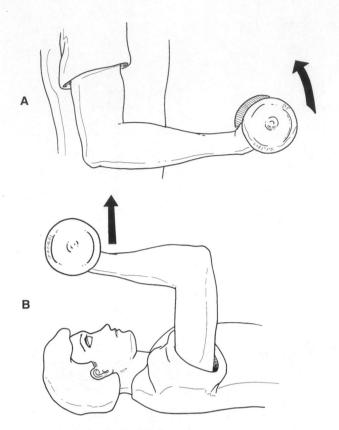

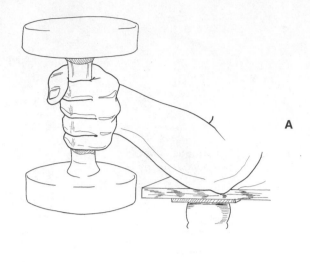

Figure 1 Elbow strengthening with weights. Weight should start small and slowly increase. Series should include at least two sets of fifteen repetitions. **A,** Elbow flexion done with elbow held at side. **B,** Elbow extension done supine with opposite hand stabilizing upper arm.

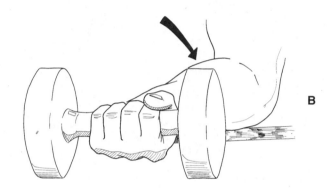

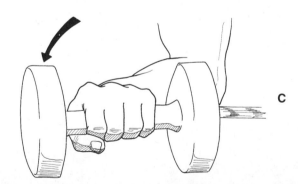

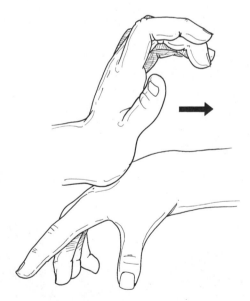

Figure 2 Forearm stretching.

Figure 3 Forearm strengthening done with proximal forearm on a flat surface, weight and hand free off the end of the surface. **A,** Forearm in neutral. **B,** Forearm to full supination. **C,** Forearm to full pronation.

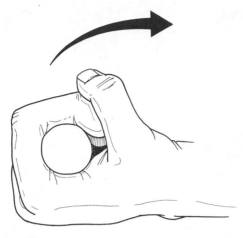

Figure 4 Wrist flexor and extensor strengthening. Flexion is demonstrated; extension is the opposite. The forearm should be stabilized.

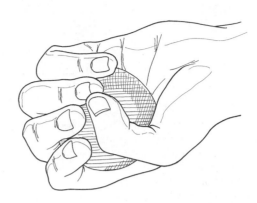

Figure 5 Grip strengthening works best with semirigid objects such as tennis balls or practice hockey pucks.

References

Dawson DM, Hallet M, Millender LH, eds. Entrapment Neuropathies. Boston: Little, Brown, 1990.

El-Hadidi S, Burke FD. Posterior interosseous nerve syndrome caused by a bursa in the vicinity of the elbow. J Hand Surg 1987; 128:33.

Gouldesbrough DR, Kinny SJ. Lipofibromatous hamartoma of the ulnar nerve at the elbow: a brief report. J Bone Joint Surg 1989; 718:331.

Groppel JL, Nirschl RP. A mechanical and electromyographical analysis of the effects of various joint counterforce braces on the tennis player. Am J Sports Med 1986; 14:195.

Gudmundsen TE, Ostensen H. Accessory ossicles in the elbow. Acta Orthop Scand 1987; 58:120.

Heller CJ, Wiltse LL. Avascular necrosis of the capitellum humeri. A report of a case. J Bone Joint Surg 1960; 42A:513.

Herrick RT, Herrick S. Ruptured triceps in a powerlifter presenting as cubital tunnel sydrome. Am J Sports Med 1987; 15:514.

Hirasawa Y, Sakakida K. Sports and peripheral nerve injury. Am J Sports Med 1983; 11:420.

Jobe FW, Stark H, Lombardo SJ. Reconstruction of the ulnar collateral ligament in athletes. J Bone Joint Surg 1986; 68A:1158.

Johnson RK, Spinner, Morton, Shrewsburg MM. Median nerve entrapment syndrome in the proximal forearm. J Hand Surg 1979; 4:48.

Jones JR, Evans DM, Kaushik A. Synovial chondromatosis presenting with peripheral nerve compression—a report of two cases. J Hand Surg 1987; 12B:25.

Karangia ND, Stiles PJ. Cubital bursitis. J Bone Joint Surg 1988; 70B:832.

Nielson K. Partial rupture of the distal biceps brachii tendon. Acta Orthop Scand 1987; 58:287.

Panner JJ. An affection of the capitellum humeri resembling Calvé-Perthes disease of the hip. Acta Radiol 1929; 10:234.

Roles NC, Maudsley RH. Radial tunnel syndrome. Resistant tennis elbow as a nerve entrapment. J Bone Joint Surg 1972; 54B:499.

Thompson WAL, Kopell HP. Peripheral entrapment neuropathies of the upper extremity. New Engl J Med 1959; 260:1261.

Torg JS, Pollock H, Sweterlitsch P. The effect of competitive pitching on the shoulders and elbows of preadolescent baseball players. Pediatrics 1972; 49:267.

Torg JS, Moyer RA. Nonunion of a stress fracture through the olecranon epiphyseal plate observed in an adolescent baseball pitcher: A case report. J Bone Joint Surg 1977; 59A:264.

Tullas HS, King JW. Lesions of the pitching arm in adolescents. JAMA 1972; 264.

Wilkerson RD, Johns JC. Nonunion of an olecranon stress fracture in an adolescent gymnast: A case report. Am J Sports Med 1990; 18:432.

Wilson FA, Andrews JR, Blackburn TA, McCluskey G. Valgus extension overload in the pitching elbow. Am J Sports Med 1983; 11:83.

Wojtys EM, Smith PA, Hankin FM. A cause of ulnar neuropathy in a baseball pitcher. A case report. Am J Sports Med 1986; 14:422.

SHOULDER PAIN IN THE THROWING ATHLETE

Forces on the shoulder girdle during athletic events, in particular throwing, often exceed the physiologic limits of the tissues involved and result in significant injury. Overuse and eccentric overload is a common etiology of rotator cuff dysfunction. Most commonly, the differential diagnosis deals with impingement or instability. Rotator cuff fiber fatigue results in partial or full-thickness tears. The rotator cuff can fail from tensile overload or from compressive forces of mechanical impingement from the subacromial arch. Lesions of the glenoid labrum can occur as isolated events or secondary to instability. Shoulder pain in the throwing athlete can be attributed to calcific tendinitis and compressive neuropathy such as suprascapular neuropathy. The use of tools such as motion analysis and synchronized EMG have significantly added to the knowledge base and understanding of the throwing motion. Throwers with painful shoulders can prolong their careers and improve their performance with changes in throwing mechanics, sports specific training and rehabilitation, and surgical intervention when necessary.

A. Because the extreme forces of the throwing mechanism cannot be recreated during a typical examination, the history is extremely important. Characteristics of the pain, such as the exact phase of the throwing motion in which it occurs (Fig. 1), are important clues to the pathology. The pattern of pain is also important. "Dead-arm" feeling at the deceleration phase of the throwing mechanism warrants a work-up for anterior subluxation. Resting night pain may be a clue for rotator cuff pathology. Apprehension in the abducted externally rotated position is characteristic of anterior instability. Throwers with quadrilateral space syndrome complain of dull aching exacerbated by abduction and external rotation.

B. Physical examination of the painful shoulder in a thrower should be organized and detailed. Great variability exists from athlete to athlete in range of motion (ROM), inherent joint laxity, and strength. Hyperelasticity of peripheral joints or abnormal widening or spreading of previous scars may represent a collagen abnormality as seen in athletes with multidirectional instability. Scapular winging or disruption of normal scapulothoracic rhythm during the examination is often seen in the painful thrower. Deltoid wasting and squaring of the acromial borders may represent axillary nerve injury. Infraspinatus wasting may be a clue to suprascapular nerve entrapment. During ROM examination, many throwers present with excessive external rotation on the throwing side, often at the expense of internal rotation. Posterior capsular tightness often presents as lack of internal rotation and should be noted. Glenohumeral stability assessment should be compared to the contralateral shoulder. Re-creation of the thrower's symptoms with provocative testing during the stability examination leads to a presumptive diagnosis of instability.

C. A typical shoulder series includes an anteroposterior view (AP) of the glenohumeral joint, axillary lateral, and trans-scapular lateral outlet views. The presence of a Type III hooked acromion, os acromiale, degenerative acromioclavicular (AC) joint or acromial spurs can create a compressive lesion of the rotator cuff. Calcium deposits in the rotator cuff mechanism are diagnosed by plain film radiograph. The Stryker notch view and the West Point view also give assessment for instability episodes noting the presence of Hill Sach's lesions or changes in the anterior inferior glenoid rim.

D. Calcifying tendinitis is a relatively uncommon source of a painful shoulder in the thrower. Calcifications are most commonly found in the supraspinatus tendon and may relate to direct pressure leading to tearing either by traction or compression or mechanical impingement to the blood supply of the cuff. A diagnosis is made by presentation of painful episodes similar to that of other rotator cuff dysfunctions along with radiographic calcifications within the tendon complex.

E. The great majority of pain in the athlete's shoulder relates to rotator cuff tendinitis secondary to impingement or instability. Assessment of the pain generator can often be aided with differential injections of the AC joint, subacromial space, and glenohumeral space with lidocaine. Assessment of instability with examination techniques assist in the differential but are not specific. Significant posterior shear forces also are present during the throwing motion and create posterior labral pathology. Superior labral avulsion is seen at the biceps insertion, the so-called slap-lesion (superior labral, anterior to posterior). During the workup of this complex pathology, throwers undergo a rehabilitation program, frequent examination and differential injections. If, for example, physical examination findings and radiographic findings are consistent with AC joint pathology and the differential injection of that joint alleviates 100% of the pain and, if those throwers fail at rehabilitative efforts, distal clavicle resection can result in complete relief of symptoms. If rehabilitation is successful, these throwers then continue with the maintenance program during their career.

SHOULDER PAIN IN THE THROWING ATHLETE

(A) History — (C) Shoulder series

(B) Physical exam

(D) Calcifying tendinitis

(E) Possible impingement vs. instability vs. rotator cuff tear

(F) Rehabilitation Injections

No improvement ← → Improved

(F) Rehabilitation:
Active Rest
NSAIDs
Lidocaine Injections
Rotator Cuff Scapular Stabilization
Posterior Capsular Stretching

Acromioclavicular DJD

Maintenance

(H) Ancillary Injections
MRI
Double Contrast
CT Arthrography

DISTAL CLAVICLE RESECTION

Improved   No improvement   Pure impingement   Instability   Rotator cuff tear   Labral pathology Loose bodies

(I) ARTHROSCOPIC DEBRIDEMENT
+/-ACROMIOPLASTY
+/- DISTAL CLAVICLE

(K) DEBRIDEMENT
ROTATOR CUFF REPAIR

(G) Maintenance Program:
Stretching
Rotator Cuff Strengthening

(J) STABILIZATION PROCEDURE

(L) ARTHROSCOPY REPAIR VS. DEBRIDEMENT

F. Throwers with painful shoulders commonly demonstrate scapular winging, scapular dyskinesia, subtle impingement signs, loss of internal rotation, and weakness in external rotation. These specific findings are the focus of the rehabilitation program. Short lever arms are used to strengthen the shoulder. Focus initially is on the eccentric control of the rotator cuff, in particular the subscapularis. Also included are exercises for a stable scapular platform. Stretching is also an important part of the program. Elimination of posterior capsular tightness and increasing internal rotation enhances performance. Included in the rehabilitation is a step-wise consistent exercise program that progresses toward return to the throwing mechanism. Sports specific exercises are gradually introduced in which throwing motion again becomes part of the program.

G. A maintenance program consists of neuromuscular control exercises for joint stability, continued proprioceptive training, strengthening of the rotator cuff musculature, scapular stabilization, and stretching exercises to maintain full ROM. Interim weight training, if done properly, also assists in those muscles about the shoulder girdle that act as decelerators and should be strengthened in an eccentric manner.

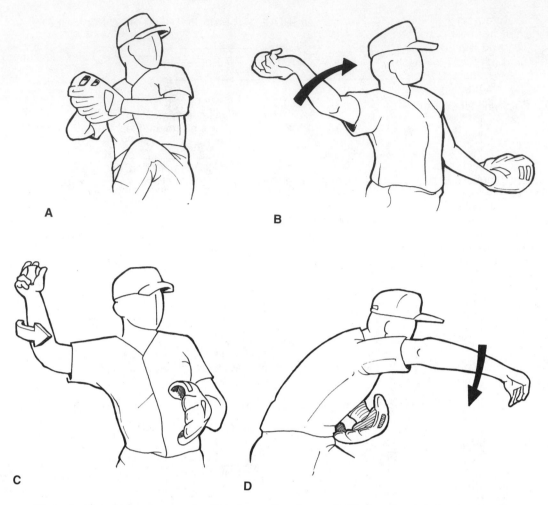

Figure 1 Throwing can be organized into four or five phases. **A,** Windup. **B** and **C,** Acceleration. **D,** Deceleration and follow-through.

H. Improved accuracy of shoulder magnetic resonance imaging (MRI) has been accomplished by the use of surface coils. MRI is a useful adjunct in the diagnosis of partial- and full-thickness rotator cuff tears and impingement. Assessment of the glenoid labrum, biceps tendon, and chondral surface of the joint also is helpful. Double-contrast computed tomography (CT) arthrography is beneficial for analysis of the labral structures and bony anatomy about the shoulder girdle.

I. In the case of subacromial pathology, either calcific tendinitis or, more commonly, impingement syndrome of the shoulder, arthroscopically assess the glenohumeral joint, followed by arthroscopic calcium excision in calcific tendinitis or arthroscopic acromioplasty with or without distal clavicle resection in cases of mechanical impingement. Arthroscopic acromioplasty should be successful in 80%–90% of patients with Stage II impingement.

J. Throwers with a diagnosis of refractory instability should undergo stabilization procedures in an attempt to recreate normal anatomy. Techniques have been developed to minimize soft tissue trauma by the surgical procedure such as capsulolabral reconstruction as described by Jobe. Arthroscopic techniques are presently being developed to further limit the morbidity of surgical dissection.

K. Rotator cuff tears in throwers that are symptomatic and resist conservative efforts are treated with arthroscopic evaluation, debridement or repair of the rotator cuff, analysis of the necessity of subacromial decompression, distal clavicle excision, and intra-articular debridement.

L. Glenoid labral injuries appear in various circumstances. Injury to the anterior inferior glenoid capsulolabral complex is seen with anterior instability. Bucket handle tears and detachments of the labrum can cause a mechanical-type instability as the labrum becomes interposed between the joint surfaces. Treatment is based on the type of lesion involved. Many lesions can be successfully treated with arthroscopic debridement such as a bucket handle tear. Slap lesions that involve the biceps insertion, and the Bankart type lesion should be repaired when technically possible.

References

Abrams JS. Special shoulder problems in the throwing athlete: Pathology, diagnosis, and non-operative management. Clin Sports Med 1991; 10(4):839.

Altchek DW, Warren RF, Wickiewicz TL, et al. Arthroscopic acromioplasty: technique and results. J Bone Joint Surg 1990; 72A:1198.

Andrews JR, Carson WG. The arthroscopic treatment of glenoid labral tears in the throwing athlete. Orthop Trans 1984; 8:44.

Andrews JR, Carson WG, McLeod WD. Glenoid labral tears related to the long-head of the biceps. Am J Sports Med 1985; 13:337.

Andrews JR, Gidamal RH. Shoulder arthroscopy in the throwing athlete: Prospectives and prognoses. Arthroscopy 1987; 6:565.

Baker CL, Liu SH, Blackburn TA. Neurovascular compression syndrome of the shoulder. In: Andrews JR, Wilk KE (eds). The Athlete's Shoulder. New York: Churchill Livingstone, 1994.

Burk DL Jr, Karasick D, Mitchell DG, Rifkin MD. MR imaging of the shoulder: A correlation with plain radiography. AJR 1990; 154:121.

Burkhart SS. Arthroscopic treatment of rotator cuff tears. Clin Orthop 1991; 267:45.

Callahan JD, Scully TB, Shapiro SA, et al. Suprascapular nerve entrapment. J Neurosurg 1991; 74:893.

Farley TE, Neumann CH, Steinbach LS, et al. Full-thickness tears of the rotator cuff of the shoulder: Diagnosis with MR imaging. AJR 1992; 158:347.

Fleisig GS, Dillman CJ, Andrews JR. Biomechanics of shoulder during throwing. In: Andrews JR, Wilk KE (eds). The Athlete's Shoulder. New York: Churchill Livingstone, 1994.

Fritz RC, Helms CA, Steinbach LS, et al. Suprascapular nerve entrapment: Evaluation with MR imaging. Radiology 1992; 182:437.

Gartsman GM: Arthroscopic acromioplasty for lesions of the rotator cuff. J Bone Joint Surg 1990; 72A:169.

Hawkins RJ, Schutte JP, Huckell GH, Abrams J. The assessment of glenohumeral translation using manual and fluoroscopic techniques. Orthop Trans 1988; 12:727.

Jobe FW, Giangarra CE, Kvitne RS. Anterior capsulolabral reconstruction of the shoulder in athletes in overhead sports. Am J Sports Med 1991; 19:428.

Jobe FW, Tibone JE, Jobe CM, et al. The shoulder in sports. In: Rockwood CA, Matsen FA (eds). The Shoulder. Philadelphia: WB Saunders, 1990.

Kibler BW, McQueen C, Uhl T. Fitness evaluations and fitness findings in competitive junior tennis players. Clin Sports Med 1988; 7:403.

Klicoyne RF, Reddy PK, Lyons F, Rockwood CA Jr. Optimal plain film imaging of the shoulder impingement syndrome. AJR 1985; 153:795.

Litchfield R, Hawkins RJ, Dillman CJ, et al. Rehabilitation of the overhead athlete. JOSPT 18:433.

Post M, Mayer J. Suprascapular nerve entrapment. Clin Orthop 1987; 223:126.

Redler MR, Ruland LJ, McCue SC. Quadrilateral space syndrome in the throwing athlete. Am J Sports Med 1986; 14:511.

Rowe CR: Recurrent transient anterior subluxation of the shoulder: The "dead-arm" syndrome. Clin Orthop 1987; 223:11.

Silliman JF, Hawkins RJ. Clinical examination of the shoulder complex. In: Andrews JR, Wilk KE (eds). The Athlete's Shoulder. New York: Churchill Livingstone, 1994.

Silliman JF, Hawkins RJ. Current concepts and recent advances in the athlete's shoulder. Clin Sports Med 1991; vol 10.

Snyder SJ. Slap lesions of the shoulder. Arthroscopy 1990; 6:274.

Snyder SJ, Karzel RP, Del Pizzo W, et al. Slap lesions of the shoulder. Arthroscopy 1990; 6:274.

Snyder SJ, Pachelli AF, Del Pizzo W, et al. Partial thickness rotator cuff tears: Results of arthroscopic treatment. Arthroscopy 1991; 7:1.

Uhthoff HK, Sarkar K, Maynard JA. Calcifying tendinitis: A new concept of pathogenesis. Clin Orthop 1976; 188:164.

Warner JJP, Warren RF. Arthroscopic Bankart repair using a cannulated, absorbable fixation device. Operative Tech Orthop 1991; 1:192.

INDEX

Avulsion—cont'd
  of interphalangeal joint, 352-354
  of posterior cruciate ligament, 494, 496
  of shoulder, 478
Avulsion fracture
  of calcaneal tendon, 86
  of tibial plateau, 70
Axis fracture, 420-423

B

Back pain; *see also* Spine
  acute, 434-436
  chronic, 438-441
  evaluation of, 430-433
  thoracic, 472-475
Band wire, for patellar fracture, 66, 68
Bankart lesion of shoulder, 478
Bar, physeal, 346
Barlow's sign, 304
Barton fracture, 398
Basilar invagination in spinal arthritis, 446, 448
Bead, antibiotic, in hip replacement, 146
Bed rest, for back pain, 434
Bennett's fracture
  fixation of, 382
  reverse, 366
  of thumb, 380
Bicondylar tibial fracture, 70
Biopsy
  for focal bone lesion, 192
  for soft tissue mass, 198
  spinal, 460
Bleeding disorder, arthropathy of knee from, 156-159
Blood pressure, compartment syndrome and, 78, 80
Blount's disease
  adolescent, 342-345
  infantile, 338-340
Bone; *see also specific bone*
  focal lesion of, 192-194
  metastasis to, 200-202
Bone graft, tibial shaft fracture and, 74
Bone scan, for thoracic pain, 472
Bone spur, heel pain from, 172
Boutonniere deformity, 410, 413
Bracing
  for back pain, 434
  for Blount's disease, 338
  for Legg-Calvé-Perthes disease and, 290, 292
  for pseudarthrosis of tibia, 274
  for Scheuermann's kyphosis, 330
  for scoliosis, 314, 318
Brooks fusion, axis fracture and, 420
Brown procedure for tibial hemimelia, 282, 284
Bryant's traction, 224
  for hip dysplasia, 306
Bunionectomy, 188-191
Bursitis, retrocalcaneal, 176
Burst fracture
  of atlas, 416
  of lower cervical spine, 424
  thoracolumbar, 428

C

Calcaneal fracture, 86-88
Calcaneo-fibular ligament, 166
Calcaneonavicular coalition, 168, 264, 508
Calcaneovalgus deformity, 242, 244
Calcifying tendinitis of shoulder, 516
Capital femoral epiphysis, slipped, 294-297
Capsule, shoulder; *see* Shoulder
Carpal injury, 376-379

Carpometacarpal injury, 364-366
  of thumb, 380-382
Cartilage, meniscal, 504-506
Cast
  for carpometacarpal joint injury, 364
  for hip dysplasia, 306
  for Legg-Calvé-Perthes disease, 290
  for patellar fracture, 66
  for scoliosis, 318
  of tibial plateau, 70
Catching, of knee, 500
Catheter, compartment syndrome and, 78
Cauda equina syndrome, 434
Cavovarus deformity of foot, 183
Cavovarus foot, 242
Cavus foot, 254-256
Cerebral palsy, scoliosis in, 322
Cervical spine
  atlas fracture of, 416-419
  axis fracture of, 420-423
  congenital fusion of, 230
  Klippel-Feil syndrome of, 238-240
  lower, injury to, 428-429
  myelopathy of, 450-453
  rheumatoid arthritis of, 446-449
  whiplash of, 464-470
Chance fracture, 428
Charcot joint, 103
Chauffer's fracture, 398
Cheilectomy, dorsal, 182
Chest injury, pelvic fracture with, 22
Chevron osteotomy, for hallux valgus, 190
Child
  angular deformity in, 334-337
  Blount's disease in
    adolescent, 342-344
    infantile, 338-340
  elbow fracture in, 218-221
  femoral fracture in
    distal, 226-228
    of shaft, 222-224
  foot deformity in, 242-245; *see also* Foot *entries*
  growth plate injury in, 206-208
  hip disorder in
    dysplasia as
      before 6 months of age, 302-305
      after 6 months of age, 306-309
    Legg-Calvé-Perthes disease and, 290-293
  humeral fracture in
    distal, 214-216
    proximal, 210-212
  leg disorder in; *see* Leg disorder
  limb length inequality in; *see* Limb length inequality
  neck deformity in
    Klippel-Feil syndrome and, 238-240
    torticollis and, 230-236
  spinal disorder in, 310-333; *see also* Spine, pediatric disorders involving
  torticollis in, 234
Chip fracture, calcaneal, 86
Chondrolysis, slipped capital femoral epiphysis and, 294
Chondromatosis, of knee, 500
Chronic pain syndrome, 439
Claudication, in spondylolisthesis, 454
Clavicle, 2-4
Closed intramedullary nailing of femur, 54-57
Closed reduction; *see* Reduction
Clubfoot deformity, 244, 246-248
Coalition
  calcaneonavicular, 168
  tarsal, 168, 262-264
    sports injury and, 508

Fixation—cont'd
  phalangeal fracture and, 368, 370, 371
  plate; *see* Plate fixation
  proximal humerus and, 14
  radial fracture and, 399
    distal, 396
  screw; *see* Screw fixation
  subtrochanteric fracture and, 49
  wire; *see* Wire fixation
Flake fracture, 90
Flap, for fingertip injury, 400-405
Flatfoot, peroneal spastic, 263
Flatfoot deformity, 258-261
Flexible flatfoot, 258-261
Flexion injury to spine, 428
  cervical, 424
Flexor tendon injury, of hand, 406-408
Focal bone lesion, 192-194
Foot
  Achilles tendinitis of, 176-179
  deformity of, 242-268
    algorithms for, 243
    cavovarus and, 183
    cavus foot as, 254-256
    flatfoot, 258-261
    Haglund's, 172
    metatarsus adductus and, 250-252
    tarsal coalition as, 262-264
    types of, 242-244
    vertical talus and, 266-268
  diabetic, 184-186
  femoral shaft fracture in child and, 222
  hallux valgus of, 188-191
  heel pain in, 172-175
  medial arch pain in, 168-171
  metatarsalgia and, 180-183
Foraminal herniation of cervical spine, 444
Forefoot deformity
  cavovarus, 242
  cavus, 254
Fracture
  acetabular, 30-32
  of ankle, 82-84
    pain after, 164
  bone metastasis and, 200
  burst
    of atlas, 416
    of lower cervical spine, 427
    thoracolumbar, 428
  calcaneal, 86-88
  of elbow, in child, 218-221
  femoral; *see* Femoral fracture
  glenohumeral joint dislocation and, 10
  growth plate injury and, 206-208
  of hand
    carpometacarpal joint, 364
    interphalangeal joint, 352
    metacarpal, 372-375
    phalangeal, 368-371
    proximal interphalangeal joint, 356-358
    radial, 396-399
    scaphoid, 384-387
  humeral; *see* Humeral fracture
  intertrochanteric, 42-44
  knee joint dislocation and, 62
  patellar, 66-68
  pelvic, 22-24
    hemorrhage from, 26-28
  Salter-Harris, 206, 208
    of proximal humerus, 210, 212
  spinal
    of atlas, 416-419

Fracture—cont'd
  spinal—cont'd
    of axis, 420-423
    lower cervical, 424-427
    spondylolisthesis and, 454
    thoracolumbar, 428-429
  spondylolisthesis and, 446
  stress
    heel pain from, 175
    of knee, 500
    in metatarsal, 180
  subtrochanteric, 46-49
  of talus, 90-92
  tibial
    of plateau, 70-72
    of shaft, 74-77
  trochanter, 124, 126
    dislocation after hip replacement and, 140
    total hip replacement and, 136
Fracture-dislocation
  of carpometacarpal joint
    of finger, 364-366
    of thumb, 380
  of metacarpophalangeal joint, of finger, 392
  of spine, 428
  tarsometatarsal, 94-96
Fragment, malleolar, 82
Freiberg's disease, 180
Fusion; *see also* Arthrodesis
  cervical myelopathy and, 456
  of knee
    for hemophilic arthropathy, 159
    for proximal femoral focal deficiency, 278, 280
  spinal
    for arthritis, 446, 447
    cervical, 230
    for Scheuermann's kyphosis, 330
    for scoliosis, 314, 315, 322
    for spondylolysis/spondylolisthesis, 326

G

Gallie fusion for axis fracture, 420
Gamma nail, 46
Garden classification of femoral neck fracture, 38, 40
Garment, antishock, 26
Gastrocnemius muscle, 179
Genu valgum, 334, 336, 337
Geriatric patient, hallux valgus in, 191
Giant cell tumor, of knee, 500, 501
Glenohumeral joint, 478
  dislocation of, 10-12
    in child, 210
Glenoid labral injury, 519
Graft
  flexor tendon injury of hand and, 406
  tibial shaft fracture and, 74
Granulomatous spinal infection, 458, 460
Great toe, hallux valgus of, 188-191
Greater tuberosity, humeral, 14
Grice subtalar arthrodesis
  for flatfoot, 258
  for vertical talus, 266
Groin pain, hip disorder causing, 124
Growth, physeal arrest and, 346
Growth plate
  Blount's disease and, 338-340
  injury to, 206-208

H

Haglund's deformity, 172
Hallux, pain in, 180
Hallux rigidus, 182